ANNUAL REVIEW OF
PHARMACOLOGY
AND TOXICOLOGY

ANNUAL REVIEW OF PHARMACOLOGY AND TOXICOLOGY

VOLUME 24, 1984

ROBERT GEORGE, *Co-editor*

University of California School of Medicine, Los Angeles

RONALD OKUN, *Co-editor*

University of California School of Medicine, Los Angeles

ARTHUR K. CHO, *Associate Editor*

University of California School of Medicine, Los Angeles

ANNUAL REVIEWS INC.   4139 EL CAMINO WAY   PALO ALTO, CALIFORNIA 94306 USA

Ŗ ANNUAL REVIEWS INC.
Palo Alto, California, USA

International Standard Serial Number: 0362–1642
International Standard Book Number: 0–8243–0424–1
Library of Congress Catalog Card Number: 61–5649

Annual Review and publication titles are registered trademarks of Annual Reviews Inc.

Annual Reviews Inc. and the Editors of its publications assume no responsibility for the statements expressed by the contributors to this *Review*.

Typesetting by Kachina Typesetting Inc., Tempe, Arizona; John Olson, President Typesetting coordinator, Jeannie Kaarle

PRINTED AND BOUND IN THE UNITED STATES OF AMERICA

Annual Review of Pharmacology and Toxicology
Volume 24 (1984)

CONTENTS

vi   CONTENTS   *(Continued)*

SOME RELATED ARTICLES IN OTHER *ANNUAL REVIEWS*

From the *Annual Review of Neuroscience,* Volume 6 (1983)

The Classification of Dopamine Receptors: Relationship to Radioligand Binding, Ian Creese, David R. Sibley, Mark W. Hamblin, and Stuart E. Leff

Clinical Implications of Receptor Sensitivity Modification, Arnold J. Friedhoff and Jeannette C. Miller

Experimental Approaches to Understanding the Role of Protein Phosphorylation in the Regulation of Neuronal Function, Mary B. Kennedy

From the *Annual Review of Neuroscience,* Volume 7 (1984)

Endogenous Opioids: Biology and Function, Huda Akil, Stanley J. Watson, Elizabeth Young, Michael E. Lewis, Henry Khachaturian, and J. Michael Walker

Endogenous Pain Control Systems: Brainstem Spinal Pathways and Endorphin Circuitry, Allan I. Basbaum and Howard L. Fields

Gonadal Steroid Induction of Structural Sex Differences in the Central Nervous System, Arthur P. Arnold and Roger A. Gorski

Multiple Mechanisms of Withdrawal from Opioid Drugs, D. E. Redmond, Jr. and J. H. Krystal

Intracerebral Neural Implants: Neuronal Replacement and Reconstruction of Damaged Circuitries, Anders Björklund and Ulf Stenevi

Proteolysis in Neuropeptide Processing and Other Neural Functions, Y. Peng Loh, Michael J. Brownstein, and Harold Gainer

From the *Annual Review of Immunology,* Volume 1 (1983)

Complement Ligand-Receptor Interactions that Mediate Biological Responses, Douglas T. Fearon and Winnie W. Wong

Mediators of Inflammation, Gary L. Larsen and Peter M. Henson

From the *Annual Review of Physiology,* Volume 46 (1984)

Interactions of Stress, Salt, and Blood Pressure, David E. Anderson

Behavioral Stress and Cardiac Arrhythmias, Richard L. Verrier and Bernard Lown

Patch Clamp Techniques for Studying Ionic Channels in Excitable Membranes, B. Sakmann and E. Neher

Gramicidin Channels, Olaf S. Andersen

The Brain Renin-Angiotensin System, William F. Ganong

Effects of Molybdate and Endongenous Inhibitors on Steroid-Receptor Inactivation, Transformation, and Translocation, Mary K. Dahmer, Paul R. Housley, and William B. Pratt

From the *Annual Review of Medicine*, Volume 35 (1984)

ERRATUM

Volume 23 (1983)

J. Bolard of the Département de Recherches Physiques, Université Pierre et Marie Curie, Paris, France, is co-author of the review, "Antifungal Agents Useful in Therapy of Systemic Fungal Infections," pages 303–30. His name was inadvertently omitted from the Table of Contents listing of his article, page v, and on the front cover. The editors apologize to Dr. Bolard for this oversight.

For the convenience of readers, a detachable order form/envelope is bound into the back of this volume.

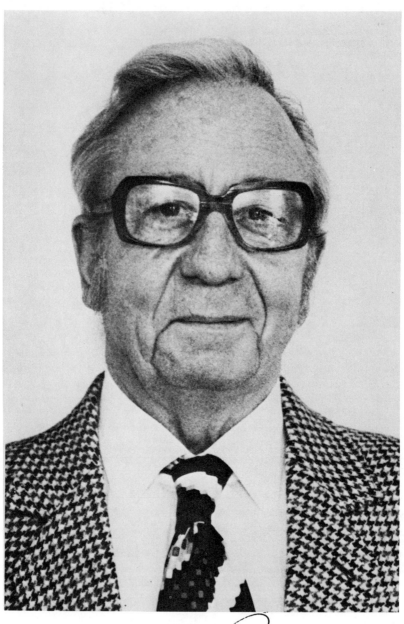

Ann. Rev. Pharmacol. Toxicol. 1984. 24:1–18
Copyright © 1984 by Annual Reviews Inc. All rights reserved

FROM PHYSIOLOGIST TO PHARMACOLOGIST— PROMOTION OR DEGRADATION? FIFTY YEARS IN RETROSPECT

Börje Uvnäs

Department of Pharmacology, Karolinska Institute, Stockholm, Sweden

When I studied medicine in the thirties at the University of Lund, an old provincial university in southern Sweden, pharmacology was a neglected discipline carrying on its activities on the outskirts of physiology. And to be sure, most pharmacologists of the time, with illustrious (notable) exceptions, expended their efforts on rather unimaginative, qualitative studies of the actions of drugs on animals and isolated organs, the classic targets of physiological research. Trained pharmacologists were nonexistent at Lund—they were rare birds in the whole of Scandinavia—and the pharmacology chair was held by a young physiologist with an interest in tissue respiration, which he studied with the Warburg and methylene blue techniques, in those days the highest fashion in metabolic research. To enter an academic institution a student had to serve as an unpaid assistant, an apprenticeship that could last for months or years. Such positions were very popular, with professors because they meant cheap teaching and research assistance and with students because they could mean the beginning of an academic career. Usually students who had done well on their examinations were offered these jobs. Since there were only about 20 students in our annual courses, the clever ones were chosen before they reached the pharmacology course, the last course of the three preclinical years. In my case, however, even after the pharmacology examination no professor offered me a position, so in desperation I took the rather unconventional step of asking for permission to begin in pharmacology.

My mind was not ready for a scientific career, however, and after one or two years of half-hearted contributions—I collaborated in some minor papers—I left science, temporarily as it turned out. Even though my scientific achieve-

1

ments during these early years in pharmacology were negligible, I made a contact that was of the utmost importance for my future. Into the little university town a young man arrived one day in answer to an invitation. His name was Georg Kahlson—generally called G. K.—and he was to become a very disturbing and at the same time stimulating member of the little medical faculty. G. K. was preceded by his reputation as an outstanding scientist, with ten years of scientific education in Jena and Göttingen. When he arrived in Lund with his very charming and beautiful wife, Louise, and their fox terrier, Grock, he was received with great expectation. Once he was installed in the department of pharmacology, I found him a stimulating teacher, a generous supporter, and a very good friend. He was to remain all these things to me until personal differences separated us several years later.

G. K. influenced my scientific career considerably. In 1938, when he was appointed professor of physiology in Lund, he invited me to join his staff and I accepted. I stayed in his department for almost 15 years and held a chair in physiology from 1949 to 1953 until I returned to pharmacology, this time in Stockholm, as will be described below.

It is interesting to note the absence of distinct boundary lines between physiology and pharmacology in the middle of the century. The three Swedish chairs in pharmacology were held by physiologists by training: Gunnar Ahlgren at Lund, myself in Stockholm, and Ernst Barany at Uppsala. Of the three Swedish professors in physiology two were trained pharmacologists: Ulf von Euler in Stockholm and Georg Kahlson in Lund. Today trained pharmacologists sit in all the pharmacology chairs in Sweden, at present more than a score of them.

During the thirties the German cultural influence was still very strong in Sweden, as it was in all the Scandinavian countries. Most medical text books were in German and the scientific journal, *Skandinavisches Archiv für Physiologie,* was published in German. Practically all visiting lecturers were from German-speaking countries; few professors and students could follow a lecture in English or French. In this way we were isolated from the English-speaking scientific world before the last world war. With the war things changed rapidly.

As was customary at that time, my work with Kahlson included a scientific problem whose investigation might become a dissertation. Neurophysiology was developing rapidly. Erlanger & Gasser had received the Nobel Prize in 1944 in physiology or medicine "for their discoveries relating to the highly differential functions of single nerve fibers." The relationship between the thickness of a nerve fiber and its excitability afforded the possibility of selectively exciting the fibers with electrical stimuli of selected characteristics. At that time little was known about nervous control of the acid- and pepsin-secreting glands of the gastric mucosa. I was to attack this problem by the selective activation of vagal fibers and was sent to Ragnar Granit at Karolinska

Institute in Stockholm for guidance. Granit was considered a coming man in neurophysiology: with Hartline & Wald he became Nobel Laureate in 1967 "for their discoveries concerning the primary physiological and chemical visual processes in the eye." I spent six months with Granit while one of his engineers worked on constructing a stimulator that would deliver all kinds of impulses— triangular, rectangular, circular, for example—of varying duration, frequency, steepness, etc. Time went by, the apparatus became more and more compli- cated, and its completion was repeatedly delayed. I became impatient and returned to Lund. There while waiting for the stimulator I began some basic experiments for practice. With an induction coil yielding an alternating current of about 40 periods per second and a metronome for the rhythmic alternating stimulation of the cat's vagus nerves with about one impulse volley per second, I was able to obtain a profuse gastric acid secretion that lasted for hours. In fact, my stimulation technique was a direct copy of the one described by Pavlov at the turn of the century.

What to do next to fulfill my professor's expectations? An accidental observation answered my question. Suddenly my experiments failed; vagal stimulation no longer aroused gastric secretion, and I realized that in order to improve the collection of gastric secretion I had ligated the pyloric area and probably interfered with the antrum vascular supply. Further analysis showed that interference with antrum function either by cocainization of the antral mucosa or extirpation of the antrum abolished or strongly reduced the secretory response to vagal stimulation. Pavlov had already observed that cocainization of the antrum of dogs blocked the gastric secretory response to feeding or sham feeding. He assumed the effect to be due to paralysis of antral secreting reflexes. In 1906, however, Edkins presented his "gastrin" theory according to which gastric secretion was under the control of the antral hormone gastrin, similar to the way pancreatic secretion was controlled by secretin, as postulated by Bayliss & Starling a few years earlier. Edkins's gastrin theory was never accepted by his contemporaries and more or less died. The American phys- iologist Ivy denied the existence of gastrin in numerous articles and considered histamine the sole humoral agent operating to control gastric secretion.

I postulated that my manipulations with the cat antrum area in some way had interfered with the gastrin mechanisms and I tried to prove it in cross- circulation experiments between two cats. The recipient cat had a cocainized antrum and no gastric secretory response to vagal stimulation; the antrum of the donor cat was intact. As I had observed earlier, vagal stimulation in the recipient cat did not evoke gastric secretion, but in the donor cat, to my delight, gastric acid flowed, indicating the presence of a blood-borne secretagogue.

Current American scientific literature was hard to come by at Lund, but about this time, I happened to come across a proceedings abstract by Komarov, a pupil of Pavlov who had emigrated to the U.S.A., in which he described the extraction of a secretory principle from the dog's antral mucosa. Komarov assumed this principle to be identical with Edkins's gastrin. I made similar extracts from the cat's antral mucosa and found that, even though such extracts did not evoke gastric secretion in cocainized cats, the accompanying infusion of such "gastrin" preparations and vagal stimulation induced profuse gastric secretion. These observations were presented in my thesis, "The Part Played by the Pyloric Region in the Cephalic Phase of Gastric Secretion" (1942), in which I postulated that gastrin was released by vagal impulses and that gastrin and vagal impulses in some way potentiated each other's effects. Unfortunately, radioimmunoassay (RIA) had not been invented at that time and the occurrence of gastrin could not be directly proven, but shown only indirectly as a gastric secretory response. It would take more than 30 years for my daughter Kerstin and I, using an RIA worked out by Berson & Yalow in New York, to directly demonstrate the vagal release of gastrin in cats.

My thesis, published as was customary as a monograph, met with strong criticism and was passed by the faculty only after several stormy meetings. The criticism with which the faculty at Lund received my thesis hurt me very much, it is true. But what almost broke me was the negative attitude I met abroad. When his gastrin theory was rejected, Edkins left science, married his laboratory assistant, and dedicated his life to university politics. I felt inclined to follow his example, but I resisted the temptation and fought on.

I have dwelled so long on the problems surrounding my dissertation because they illustrate a situation common to young scientists in those days. Young scientists were at the mercy of one or a handful of professors who were quick to criticize and loathe to praise. Most young scientists need positive criticism and encouragement, and my chief, G. K. gave me these. With his support I decided not to give up and become a practitioner, but to continue my research despite the criticism with which it had been received.

Although Sweden was not drawn into World War II, the war period meant almost total isolation from the outside world. Foreign scientific journals— especially English-written ones, of course—arrived only occasionally. At the end of the war, a number of Danish scientists of Jewish birth fled to Sweden and found refuge at Lund. Among them were well-known physiologists like August Krogh and Fritz Buchtal. Despite the unfortunate circumstances under which they came, they brought fresh air and a fighting spirit to the somewhat musty atmosphere of the little university town.

Once the war was over and the borders opened again, Swedish scientists hurried abroad. Now, however, their destinations were not Germany and Great Britain, both devastated and impoverished by the fighting, but to the undamaged and prosperous United States. Since I had been working on gastric secretion, it was natural that I choose to study with a specialist in gastric physiology. In those days, there were two alternatives: Ivy, whose laboratory was at Northwestern University in Chicago, and Babkin at McGill University in Montreal.

Ivy was a student of a famous Swedish physiologist, Anton Julius Karlsson, who was still alive at that time. Babkin was a Russian refugee, a student of Pavlov. I chose to work with Ivy, unfortunately, as it turned out, inasmuch as I got neither education nor ideas from him. Ivy was a hard worker. One found him at his desk practically day and night, Sundays as well as weekdays. He had many young scientists in his laboratories but rarely appeared there himself. These young guests were all working busily by themselves in some corner on problems Ivy had given them. He took their reports and wrote papers on their findings. My ticket of admission was to demonstrate my technique for the isolation of gastrin and its secretory activity. For that purpose, I was given a little dark closet, 2 × 2 m, without a window or equipment. Evidently, no one had worked with a cat in Ivy's laboratory before, and it took months to get the necessary equipment, in fact very simple things, not to mention getting cats. Since I had no technical assistance, my wife helped me, very bravely indeed since she had never set foot in a laboratory. When after a few months I had prepared my first gastrin extracts and could demonstrate their secretory effect on the cat's stomach, I called for Ivy. He had lost interest by that time, however, and flatly denied that the secretory effect could be due to gastrin. Instead he insinuated that it was due to contamination with histamine.

My main purpose in visiting Ivy's laboratory was to have an opportunity to work with conscious dogs. Ivy was especially famous for his studies on pouch dogs. In some preliminary experiments in Lund I had observed that the gastric secretory response to sham feeding of dogs was inhibited by antrectomy. I wanted to confirm these preliminary observations. However, the dogs at Ivy's laboratory—stray dogs caught by the Chicago police—were so filled with lice and the animal quarters were so filthy that I could not allow my wife to work there. Without assistance in the operative procedures I had to give up. After some months Ivy left his laboratory to assume a position in physiology at the University of Illinois. I felt forsaken and began looking for other scientific contacts at Northwestern.

One day I passed a laboratory in which a bald, kind-looking man was sitting bent over his desk. His name was Horace W. Magoun and he was well known for his experiments with stereotactic instruments, with which he could stimulate well-defined areas in the brain. I went in and asked if I could work in his laboratory. He was busy writing a book, he said, but I was welcome to practice with his instruments. I did so and, lacking any real idea of what to do, I put the electrode into the hypothalamus of a cat. To my surprise, the stimulation induced blood-pressure fall and bradycardia instead of what I expected, blood-pressure rise and tachycardia. My curiosity was stimulated and I continued for a few weeks just mastering the technique. The small observations I made were presented with the kind help of Magoun in the proceedings of the Society of Experimental Biology and Medicine.

In another corridor I found pharmacologist C. A. Dragstedt, who was well known for his studies on the role of histamine in anaphylactic reactions. He and Magoun were my first important contacts in the American scientific community. With their help I made many American acquaintances who would be of the greatest importance for my career, and a few months later, after a tour around the country, I left the States.

Back in Lund after the year abroad, we started enthusiastically to explore the possibilities of Magoun's stereotactic instruments. I was very lucky to have as my collaborator a very able young man, Björn Folkow, who later became professor of physiology in Gothenburg with an international reputation for his studies on circulation and hypertension. Our first experiment hit an area in the hypothalamus of the cat—later defined as the defense area—from which a specific reaction pattern, including rather selective vasodilator responses in the skeletal muscles, was induced. We had discovered what was later described as a cholinergic vasodilator outflow in the sympathetics. We worked happily for several years on the distribution and function of this cortico-spinal vasodilator outflow to the skeletal muscles of the cat and dog. We had (to us) exciting skirmishes with the Nestor of British pharmacology, J. H. Burn, who for many years had defended the existence of adrenergic vasodilator fibers. His main argument was the well-known vasodilator action of adrenaline on the skeletal muscle blood vessels. After reciprocal laboratory visits the dispute was settled and the existence of cholinergic vasodilator fibers recognized.

Our vasodilator research led successively to extensive studies on central and peripheral nervous vasomotor control. Both in Lund and later in Stockholm many dissertations were published in this field. I would like to mention two students, Percy Lindgren and Sune Rosell, who were my collaborators in Stockholm for many years. We found later that the vasodilator action of adrenaline occurring after intravenous injection is transformed into vasoconstriction upon stimulation of sympathetic nerves depleted of their noradrenaline by reserpinization and then reloaded with adrenaline. Apparently, the adrenaline released by sympathetic nerve stimulation hits vascular receptors different from the receptors stimulated by adrenaline given intravenously.

Concomitant with these scientific events, things were happening on the political front. G. K. was very active in the developments to come. In large part due to his forceful propaganda and his good relations with influential members of the sitting Social Democratic government, a Swedish Medical Research Council was formed patterned after the corresponding British organization. Increased resources were given to natural science and medical research and new chairs were instituted at the national universities. As a result of this new commitment to research, Sweden took the scientific lead in Scandinavia, and in some disciplines Swedish scientists have reached the international fore-front.

I was lucky enough to profit from these favorable developments and was appointed to the new chair in physiology at Lund University. Plans were also developed to build a new physiology department at Lund and, as G. K.'s favored assistant, I became deeply involved in preparatory negotiations with governmental authorities, architects, contractors, and others. Building began, but I was never to move into the new laboratories. The partnership with my old teacher and benefactor came to a sudden end. I was made uncomfortable by this development and looked for a way out. What I found changed my life. The chair in pharmacology at Karolinska Institute had been vacated with the retirement of Göran Liljestrand. I applied for the position and to my relief—and to the disappointment of others—I was invited to Stockholm in the summer of 1953.

Karolinska Institute was a new world to me. The faculty for generations had been composed of eminent and forceful scientists enthusiastically and success-fully engaged in developing the institute into a scientific medical center of international repute. To sit on this faculty was a tremendous opportunity for a young professor in pharmacology. My predecessor had been a very forceful and influential member of the faculty, but he was not to witness the great expansion in the science of pharmacology waiting around the corner. I was the lucky one who entered the scene at the right moment.

In the stimulating atmosphere of Karolinska Institute, with its recognized international position, I was able to recruit a group of enthusiastic young collaborators within a few years. The competition among disciplines for young talent was tough, and pharmacology was the last course in the preclinical curriculum—two months at the end of the third year. But I had a few tricks to help to attract some of the better students. One I had learned from G. K. in Lund. On his initiative there we bought a sailing boat for the use of staff members and their groups. It was a 40-foot sailing yacht especially built for sailing in the Swedish archipelago. Since histamine was one of the main interests in our department, the ship was named the *Histamina* and its dinghy the *Histaminase*. From the masthead flew our ensign, in honor of our favorite experimental animals two red cross-laid cats on a white ground. Many agree-able summer adventures at sea created a feeling of solidarity and a community of interests among us that were of great value during the everyday activities of the rest of the year.

When I took over the pharmacology department in Stockholm, I repeated the trick. With some friends I bought a sailing vessel, this time a rather large one that could accommodate quite a few people. It was a 30-ton revenue cutter that we rebuilt ourselves into a ketch, with three foresails on a long bowsprit. It was both fast and easy to maneuver. Many young pharmacologists got their training in seamanship on board this ship and our adventures were legion. I remember especially a trip to Åbo in Finland in 1966, where the 12th Scandinavian Congress for Physiology was to be held. We left Stockholm in fine weather with 12 Swedish scientists on board. We never reached Åbo, however. Instead we ran into a hurricane and almost went down, but we found a port of refuge and some leading members of Sweden's scientific community survived to continue their work.

The Department of Pharmacology in Stockholm was relatively new. It was built in 1948 when Karolinska Institute moved from its old site close to Stockholm's center to its new grounds at Norrbacka just north of Stockholm. Unfortunately, the original building plans had for economic reasons been reduced by 50% and as a result the animal quarters and the laboratory equipment, among other things, did not fulfill modern requirements, at least not in my opinion. My first step as chairman was to deliver an address to the faculty in which I presented the future of pharmacology as I saw it. I anticipated the development of various fields of pharmacology, such as biochemical pharmacology, neuropsychopharmacology, clinical pharmacology, and toxicology, and recommended the eventual establishment of chairs in these fields. I also asked for the immediate enlargement of the pharmacology department, especially its animal quarters, and for money to modernize the equipment. Many faculty members shook their heads at this presumptuous newcomer, but I must say to their credit that they were very cooperative; two decades later my demands were fulfilled in good measure, including chairs at the institute in all the subdisciplines I had mentioned.

In retrospect, the pharmacology department at the institute seems to have developed rather smoothly, but at the time some of our victories seemed hard won. Especially difficult was convincing the Ministries of Education and Finance to support our growth. I remember particularly the resistance that met our plans to enlarge the department. When the ministeries rejected even our request for a barrack to be used as temporary animal quarters and erected at our own expense, we were discouraged. But the stricture "that any animal quarters, even temporary ones, should be removable without any delay in case the grounds were requested by the building board for other purposes" gave us an idea. We bought circus wagons from the Stockholm amusement park—the original horse-drawn ones—equipped them with cages for rats, cats, and dogs, painted them bright red with white windowframes, and placed them in a semicircle outside the pharmacology department. This anachronistic sight aroused the public and angered the government authorities. They never forced us to remove the wagons, however, and after a few years of publicity in the leading newspapers we were allowed to build not only new animal quarters but new laboratories. The next problem was equipment. Fortunately, generous support from the National Institutes of Health saved us. In this context, I want to emphasize that financial help from the U.S. in the two decades after the war was of inestimable value in expanding the institute's scientific activities during these years. Unfortunately, Swedish political concerns forced a gradual decline in U.S. financial support. In fact, for a time such support practically disappeared.

Another important force in the development of Karolinska's scientific potential has been its participation in the Nobel Prize Awards in physiology or medicine. In the beginning the institute was reluctant to accept the responsibility, but over the years it has been very well managed and put to profitable use. Serving on the Nobel Committee, as I have done for decades, is an inestimable opportunity to watch international scientific developments. Moreover, studying the achievements of eminent colleagues has been both rewarding and stimulating to my own ambitions.

As I mentioned earlier, of primary interest at the Department of Physiology in Lund in the 1940s was histamine. This amine has intrigued physiologists since its synthesis by Windaus & Vogt in 1907, but its functional role was and still is obscure. Histamine was known to be distributed in tissues all over the body but its precise localization or mode of storage was still unknown, although it was believed to be stored in some way chemically linked to protein. The new extraction technique elaborated by Charles Code at the Mayo Clinic raised new expectations among histamine enthusiasts, but it had still to be assayed biologically on the guinea-pig ileum, which had been found to be especially sensitive to it. This biological assay was both time-consuming and tedious and I felt sorry for my young colleagues, who spent their time on these boring assays. I had resisted all invitations to join the histamine gang, but by the time I arrived in Stockholm things were changing. Chemical techniques had been developed for determining histamine, specific histamine releasers like compound 48/80—discovered by MacIntosh & Paton in 1949—had appeared, and histamine was found to be localized in mast cells by Riley & West in 1953.

Ever since my "gastrin period" in Lund, storage and release phenomena had spurred my interest. How could biologically active substances be stored in an inactive form and "reactivated" immediately on release? In our laboratory cat consumption was high but the rewards were considerable. To make better use of the animals, we decided to perfuse cat limbs in histamine-release studies. Cat skin turned out to be very rich in histamine, as well as a rich source of slow-reacting substance (SRS), so-called because it induces a slow contraction of guinea-pig ileum. SRS was known to accompany histamine release in anaphylactic reactions and was assumed to be at least partly responsible for anaphylactic symptoms. During the 1960s and 1970s we studied the chemical and biological characteristics of cat SRS, and quite a few young scholars defended their theses on SRS problems. We had an almost pure SRS preparation, its UV spectrum identified and ready for mass-spectrographic study, when Samuelsson and his group very elegantly solved the problem and developed the now well-known leucotriene hypothesis that won him the Nobel Prize in 1982. Samuelsson isolated leucotrienes from leucocytes, but in my mind there is no doubt that the cat SRS belongs to the leucotriene family.

Parallel with our research on SRS, our study of histamine developed nicely. Since histamine is located in mast cells, a rational approach to problems concerning its storage and release required access to isolated mast cells. Somewhat pure suspensions of rat mast cells had been obtained by gradient centrifugation of mixed cell populations from rat peritoneal washings on sugar. Unfortunately, such cells, although morphologically seemingly intact, were insensitive to compound 48/80 and other histamine-releasing agents. In our search for other density gradients we decided to try dextran, but by mistake the pharmacological company delivered ficoll. This new polymere turned out to be an excellent gradient material and we were able to obtain up to 95% pure mast cell suspensions. Bertil Diamant, now professor of pharmacology in Copenhagen, many other young collaborators, and I experimented with these mast cells.

In the beginning, our interest focused on the mechanism of mast-cell response to "degranulating" agents like compound 48/80 and antigens. The dependence of the response on oxidative and glucolytic energy production and the role of ATP in the release process were among the questions studied. We theorized that lecithinase A (later phospholipase A) played a role in an initial step of mast-cell reaction. Recently, phospholipase A activation has again been the focus of attention, this time as one of the initial processes in release mechanisms.

As years went on, our interests shifted from mast-cell response to the mechanism of histamine storage and release in mast-cell granules. We observed one day that granules isolated directly from mast cells lysed in deionized water still contained histamine but that they immediately lost their histamine when suspended in salt solutions like 0.9% NaCl or serum. This observation indicated to us that the histamine in the granules was stored in weak ionic linkage to the granule matrix and was then released by cation exchange once the granules were exposed to cation-containing media. For the next 20 years we were spellbound by the idea that the storage and release not only of histamine but also of other biogenic amines and other charged substances, for example neuropeptides, might be effected according to the cation-exchange principle.

The idea that histamine is stored in ionic linkage to anions in mast-cell granules was not original. The presence of heparin in the granules led early to the assumption that histamine is stored in ionic linkage with this strongly acid polysaccharide. We soon found that this was a premature conclusion, however. An analysis of the binding properties of isolated granules showed stoichiometric relationships and pH-dependence, for example, indicating histamine's ionic binding not to the sulphated groups in heparin but to the carboxyl groups. Chemical analysis of the granule matrix, as well as quantitative studies of the storage capacity of isolated granules and of "artificial granules" (a heparin-protein complex) supported our idea that histamine is stored in ionic linkage to carboxyls in a protein-heparin complex in which the sulphated groups of heparin are masked by strong ionic binding to the amino groups of the protein. The fact that histamine is bound in weak ionic linkage to protein carboxyls and not to the strong acidic groups of heparin was an essential observation of importance for our later speculations about the cation-exchange process as a general principle in storage and release mechanisms.

Quantitative studies of the storage capacity of mast-cell granules for histamine and sodium, the stoichiometric relationships between sodium uptake and histamine release and other questions led to the conclusion that in vitro mast-cell granules behave as weak cationic exchangers with carboxyls as the ionic binding sites. Electron microscopic studies strengthened our belief that the release of histamine from the "degranulating" cell also occurs as a cation exchange sodium $\rightleftharpoons$ histamine. Later, a closer inspection of our electron microscopic pictures—the result of a collaboration with the eminent Hungarian specialist Pal Röhlich—cast some doubt on the current idea that degranulation of the mast cell is a primary and histamine release from the expelled granules a secondary step in the release response. Through electron microscopic auto-radiography we observed that granules in the periphery of the cell may swell and loosen their histamine in spite of the fact that they have not yet lost their membranes. In other words, the electron microscopic pictures indicated that histamine release—probably by cation exchange across membranes with increased permeability or through newly formed pores—might occur as the primary step, with the expulsion of granules a secondary phenomenon. I mention this observation because I later defended the idea that the release of neurotransmitters might occur not as an exocytosis but as a fractional release of the transmitter by cation exchange initiated by the nerve impulse. I will come back to these recent studies below.

The observation that led to the idea of cation exchange being a general principle of amine storage and release was the observation that mast-cell granules in vitro take up not only sodium and histamine in a competitive way, but also other amines, biogenic as well as synthetic, as long as they contain a charged amino group. All these amines, among them the transmitter amines noradrenaline, adrenaline, dopamine, serotonin, and acetylcholine, seemingly compete for the same ionic sites in the mast-cell granules and are released by sodium and other inorganic cations. Therefore might the matrix of other amine-storing granules also have properties similar to cation-exchanger materials?

So far we have studied chromaffin granules and adrenergic nerve granules from this point of view. We discovered that the matrices of these two types of granules show properties reminiscent of cation-exchanger materials, with carboxyls as the ionic binding sites. Of special interest to us were experiments that demonstrated great similarities in the cation-exchange properties of the synthetic carboxyl resins, e.g. the Amberlite IRC-50 and Sephadex C-50, and the matrices from these granules. When the synthetic resins and isolated granules from chromaffin cells and nerves were exposed to isotonic NaCl by superfusion, the release of catecholamines and noradrenaline showed the same kinetics. Recently, the in vivo release of catecholamines from cat and pig adrenals induced by supramaximal splanchnic nerve stimulation shows the same kinetics observed in vitro. At present, we are looking for further evidence that the storage and release of transmitter amines follow the principles of cation exchange and that the transmitter release and perhaps the release of other amines and neuropeptides occur not by exocytotic emptying of a few granules but by cation exchange as a fractional release from multiple granules.

The modern and roomy animals quarters approved by the authorities in the face of our circus wagons provided the facilities for gastrointestinal research on conscious animals. Gastrin research began to see movement again with the important contributions of C. A. Dragstedt, previously professor of surgery in Chicago, who was very active after his retirement in experimental gastrointestinal surgery in Gainesville, Florida. He manipulated the dog antrum surgically and found that excluding the antrum either as a separated pouch or as a transplant in the colon led to a hypersecretion of HCl in the remaining stomach, frequently followed by penetrating peptic ulcers. This hypersecretion disappeared when antrum mucosa was acidified or extirpated. Dragstedt considered that the changes in HCl secretion he observed reflected disturbances in the gastrin mechanism, since gastrin release from the antrum is inhibited by acid pH.

These findings revived my old interest in gastrin and we decided to confirm and if possible extend the observations I had made in Lund that the acid secretory response to sham feeding disappears after antrectomy. My young collaborator, Lars Olbe, did an excellent job in conducting the experiments. He invented an esophagal cannula of plastic that allowed the dogs to feed themselves and survive in good health for years. Olbe found not only that antrectomy practically terminates the acid secretory response to sham feeding but also that intravenous infusion of subthreshold doses of gastrin *during* sham feeding induces a dose-dependent acid secretory response. In other words, my previous observations on the interaction between gastrin and vagal impulses in anesthetized cats were fully confirmed in conscious dogs.

There still was no technique for determining gastrin in the blood, but it would come soon. Solomon Berson & Rosalyn Yalow reported in 1955 that they had developed antibodies against insulin and had used them to develop a radioimmunoassay. Their report caused a sensation, since it was considered impossible to induce antibody production against such small protein molecules. In fact, a respected scientific journal refused to publish Berson & Yalow's first paper unless they changed the term *antibody* to a more neutral term. Today everyone knows that Berson & Yalow were correct; their radiommunoassay for insulin revolutionized the whole polypeptide area. Unfortunately, Berson died unexpectedly of a heart attack—he worked himself to death—but Yalow was awarded the Nobel Prize "for the development of radioimmunoassays of peptide hormones" in 1977, a prize meant for both of them.

I met Berson before his death, when he gave the Ihre lecture at a Nobel symposium in Stockholm in 1970. At a dinner at Bengt Ihre's home I asked him to work out a radioimmunoassay for gastrin. He promised to try and a few months later he called me from New York to say that he had a gastrin RIA ready for me, would I come to New York to see it? Although I did not consider it possible to go myself, I sent one of my young pupils, Göran Nilsson. A few months later in Berson's laboratory, Nilsson and Berson were able to show that sham feeding induces a rise in plasma gastrin level. When the gastrin RIA was brought home to Stockholm, my daughter Kerstin, as already mentioned, demonstrated that vagal stimulation in the cat causes a considerable output of gastrin-17 not only into the blood but also into the stomach. Since then, in our laboratory as well as in others, researchers have shown that the vagus nerve contains several polypeptides—cholecystokinin, vasointestinal peptide, substance P, insulin, somatostatin, gastrin, and many others—that appear in the blood and gastrointestinal canal when the vagus nerve is activated. In fact, in addition to sham feeding, suckling leads to a hormonal release pattern with a concomitant occurrence of gastrointestinal and hypophyseal hormones, indicating an intimate central coordination between these hormonal delivery sources.

Our gastrin studies stimulated our interest in the role of the antrum-duodenum area in controlling gastric acid secretion. The Pavlov school considered this area a reflex center for the excitatory and inhibitory control of gastric secretion.

We were able to confirm previous observations that acidification of duodenal content leads to a pronounced inhibition of acid secretion in Pavlov and Heidenhain pouches. However, this inhibition does not occur until the pH is suppressed 2–3. Since such a low duodenal pH is never observed under normal conditions, the functional role of the duodenal inhibitory mechanism has been seriously doubted. However, between meals the stomach empties its acid content into the duodenum, and as a result there might be an acidity gradient with low pH close to the pylorus, the pH rising with increasing neutralization during the distal passage of duodenal content. Could the inhibitory mechanism be located in the bulb and, if so, does bulbar pH reach the required low values? We found in fact that acidification of the duodenal bulb to pH 3–2 or lower does activate the inhibitory mechanism. Moreover, with a series of technically advanced surgical procedures it could be shown that the bulbar inhibitory mechanism is humoral. We baptized the unknown inhibitory principle *bulbogastrone*, but our attempts to identify it chemically in duodenal extracts failed.

In the meantime another of our colleagues, Sven Andersson, was sent to Los Angeles, where Morton Grossman of UCLA had perfected a technique with which it was possible to register the pH-gradient in the duodenum. They found that in both man and dog postprandial pH in the duodenal bulb decreases to 2–3. In other words, the bulbogastrone mechanism might play a physiological role in the inhibitory gastric acid secretion. Later my daughter Kerstin observed that acidification of the duodenal bulb leads to increased somatostatin levels in the peripheral blood. These levels are high enough to exert inhibitory actions. Whether bulbogastrone is identical with somatostatin remains to be established.

As is evident from this somewhat rhapsodic narrative, my scientific activities and those of my collaborators were physiological in nature. One is justified to ask what my department has done for the field of pharmacology. In fact, rather much.

The scientific staff in the Department of Pharmacology at Karolinska Institute has reached considerable size. Last year the list included four professors, four senior lecturers, four assistant professors, two adjunct professors (part-time scientists from the pharmaceutical industry), seven research fellows, and twenty-five postgraduate students. More than 150 scientific papers were published. Out of 80 postgraduate students who have defended their theses at the department in the last 30 years, 25 are professors of pharmacology or of related theoretical and clinical disciplines. Our research activities cover such diverse fields as biochemical pharmacology, cancer chemotherapeutics, prostaglandins, the physiology and pharmacology of adrenergic transmitter mechanisms and of purines, neurohumoral peptide physiology, the pharmacology of gastric secretion, dental pharmacology, and neuropsychopharmacology. If the two chairs in clinical pharmacology and one in toxicology are included—they have branched off to form their own departments—the scientific output is very high indeed.

I suppose such a large and diverse department reflects favorable developments in the pharmacological field, but at the same time the growth of huge departments with many independent research groups has its risks. The diversification of scientific interests can lead to in-fighting among special interests. Harmony and communication among individuals can be jeopardized. Without common goals, the strength and in the long run the future of the department are endangered. I have no solution to the problem, but I can recommend one rather effective measure to prevent or at least retard such an undesirable development. This is the organization of what we have called a manuscript committee, whose members are the "grown up" scientists in the department. This committee reads and edits all manuscripts emanating from the department before they are published. Such a procedure is a great help to young researchers and effectively serves to uphold high scientific standards for the publications, since nobody— especially not the older professors—wants to present bad papers. What is more important, however, is that everyone gets to know what work is being done throughout the department, an effective measure against the isolationism and self-sufficiency that often occur in large organizations.

Teaching pharmacology to medical students, one was confronted with how little doctors, clinicians as well as practioners, knew about drugs. Refresher courses in pharmacology for doctors were instituted to rectify this situation, and such courses led directly to the development of clinical pharmacology, today a strong discipline in Sweden, with chairs and head positions at every teaching hospital in the country. In the beginning, clinical pharmacology met with scepticism, especially from internists, but resistance disappeared when clinical pharmacologists were relieved of their hospital duties to serve as teachers and advisers in drug therapy and drug research. It is still that way in Sweden, and the collaboration between clinicians and clinical pharmacologists is intimate and profitable.

The growth of the medicinal industry and the introduction of chemical and biochemical techniques after World War II opened up new ways to study the pharmacodynamic properties of drugs. Increased insight in the quantitative aspects of drug action on animals and man paved the way for quantitative drug therapy and the development of clinical pharmacology.

These new dimensions within pharmacology weakened the traditional ties between pharmacologists and physiologists. In fact, the new generation of biochemical pharmacologists and other scientists felt no loyalty to physiology at all. Physiologists and the older generation of pharmacologists, who had received their scientific training in physiology, did not seem to realize the explosive power of these new trends.

Except in the leading scientific communities in France, Germany, Great Britain, and the U.S., national pharmacological societies were formed slowly. Nationally and internationally, pharmacologists were represented by physiological societies and there was growing dissatisfaction among pharmacologists with their inability to influence the scientific program at physiology congresses.

In the 1950s, beginning at the 18th congress of the International Union of Physiological Sciences (IUPS) in Copenhagen in 1950, a special pharmacology day was arranged at the end of the meetings. At these gatherings, the question of an independent international organization of pharmacologists was repeatedly put on the agenda. An international committee was set up with Corneille Heymans of Ghent as chairman and Carl F. Schmidt of Philadelphia as secretary. After nearly ten years of discussions and negotiations, IUPS in 1959 agreed to the formation of an independent division for pharmacologists within the organization, the Section on Experimental Pharmacology (SEPHAR). The agreement was a typical compromise. The constitution of IUPS was revised to authorize SEPHAR to "organize international conferences, symposia and congresses and to carry on other activities provided that they do not conflict with the aims and principles of IUPS." This objection led to an agreement that SEPHAR "would do its best not to compete with or otherwise weaken the triennial congresses of IUPS whenever it arranges separate international pharmacological programs." Carl Schmidt was elected the first president of SEPHAR, with Daniel Bovet as secretary. The SEPHAR council had its first meeting in Stockholm in 1961. Council loyalty to IUPS was demonstrated by its appointment of a liaison officer, E. J. Ariëns, as a member of the local organizing committee for the next physiology congress in Leyden in 1962. The council also decided to continue pharmacology day at future physiology congresses.

As years passed and increasing contacts with foreign colleagues widened my horizons, I could not avoid recognizing the increasing tension between physiologists and pharmacologists, as the repeated proposals for an idependent international pharmacological organization showed. The notion of holding an international meeting of pharmacologists in Stockholm was born over a drink in my home one fall evening in 1958. My friend Tom Maren, professor of pharmacology in Gainesville, Florida, and I were discussing the unsatisfactory international position of pharmacology. True, negotiations had by then begun to form a pharmacology division within IUPS. Even so, dissatisfaction was widespread, especially among biochemically oriented pharmacologists, who felt no community with physiologists and who wanted to break loose completely to organize their own scientific programs.

Tom Maren belonged to the group of young non-traditional biochemical pharmacologists who pleaded for the independence of pharmacology. Tom and I decided to make inquiries on the question among prominent friends and colleagues. The correspondence in my files reveals little enthusiasm and encouragement for the formation of an independent pharmacological association. Most responses were ambiguous or passive. Some were directly negative. Most felt that to break with the physiologists was a mistake; many predicted difficulty in raising the necessary funds.

In the meantime SEPHAR was officially established—not without opposition within the parent organization—at the IUPS congress in Buenos Aires in 1959. As mentioned above, according to the revised IUPS statutes, the new division was authorized to organize its own international meetings.

The formation of SEPHAR paved the way for international pharmacological activities. But when we in Stockholm undertook to arrange the first international pharmacological meeting, we were well aware of the divergences of opinion, not only about what form such a meeting should assume but even about whether it should be held at all. Some pharmacologists were enthusiastic advocates of an international pharmacological congress of the conventional kind. Others favored the organization of symposia. Lastly, there were those who rejected the whole idea. In particular I understood the apprehensions of those who felt that an international congress of pharmacologists would weaken the valuable communication between physiologists and pharmacologists long fostered by the international physiological conventions. As a physiologist by training I could well appreciate that point of view. However, like many others, I felt that the danger of a schism among the pharmacologists themselves was so great that some form of an international gathering should be arranged. A feasible compromise solution—at least for the time being—was to organize pharmacological meetings that would provide satisfactory interchange between older and younger generations and offer opportunities for contact not only with physiologists but with biochemists and representatives of other allied disciplines.

At a preliminary informal meeting in Washington early in the winter of 1959, I declared my willingness to arrange a pharmacological program in Stockholm. SEPHAR's agreement not to compete with the 1962 IUPS congress precluded emphasis on physiological presentations. The recent outstanding developments in biochemical pharmacology spoke in favor of a biochemical approach. We therefore decided to put together a series of symposia on the topic, "Modes of Actions of Drugs." One of the most active spokesmen for this program was Bernard B. Brodie, at that time head of the Department of Chemical Pharmacology at the National Institutes of Health in Bethesda, who gave us his enthusiastic and invaluable support from the beginning. K. K. Chen from the Lilly Company in Indianapolis was another indefatigable and influential supporter. C. Heymans of Ghent and C. Schmidt of Philadelphia, who joined when we were well embarked on the adventure, also gave full and unflinching assistance. Even IUPS contributed 2,500 U.S. dollars for preliminary expenses.

In spite of the efforts of the organizing committee to give the program an international character, scientifically as well as geographically, Americans clearly dominated the meetings. Five out of eight organizers and 478 out of 1483 attendees were Americans. In angry letters the Russians, French, Belgians, and others accused us of favoring or giving in to the Americans. The fact is, however, that the program committee's decision to emphasize biochemical pharmacology was more or less forced upon us by our agreement with the IUPS not to focus on physiology and the Americans, and to a certain extent the Germans, were the leaders in biochemical pharmacology at that time. This new branch of pharmacology was still rather undeveloped in most European countries, especially in those where the complainers came from.

The Stockholm meeting was to become not only the first in a series of successful international pharmacological congresses and a strong impetus to the development of the field. It also led to the formation of the International Union of Pharmacologists (IUPHAR). IUPHAR was officially inaugurated by the General Assembly of the IUPS in Tokyo on September 2, 1965. The first ordinary meeting of the IUPHAR council was held in Sao Paulo on July 28, 1966. Since then seven IUPHAR congresses have been held, in Stockholm in 1961, headed by myself; in Prague in 1963, headed by H.·Rašková; in Sao Paulo in 1966, headed by M. Rocha e Silva; in Basel in 1969, headed by K. Bucher; in San Francisco in 1972, headed by R. Featherstone; in Helsinki in 1975, headed by K. Paasonen; in Paris in 1978, headed by P. Lechat; and in Tokyo in 1981, headed by S. Ebashi.

Within IUPHAR, the divisions of clinical pharmacology and of toxicology demonstrate not only the growth of pharmacology as a field, but also IUPHAR's commitment to represent all aspects of the discipline, allowing new branches independence within the framework of the parent organization. With its membership in ICSU, WHO, CIOMS, and various other international scientific organizations, IUPHAR belongs to a global network of government, academic, industrial, and other organizations through which it exerts worldwide influence on all aspects of pharmacological research and teaching as well as on drug development and pharmacotherapy.

My years as secretary of SEPHAR and then as president of IUPHAR were a very challenging and profitable time, both scientifically and personally. My understanding has widened; my circle of friends includes people from all over the world. The steady growth of IUPHAR and the success of its congresses, begun so modestly in Stockholm over 20 years ago, has given me great personal satisfaction.

To be a retired professor in Sweden has its advantages. The law provides an emeritus professor a laboratory and office space for research and teaching activities, that is, if the available resources allow. I am a very lucky man to have retired from a department with such resources, so I spend my time more or less as before, in my office and in my labs, aided by kind, loyal, and experienced assistants and coworkers. My three hunting dogs accompany me to my office and home as well as hunting, and I can work undisturbed by committee meetings and the other official duties that previously were a heavy burden. I consider myself lucky to have entered pharmacology at the beginning of its rise to an independent discipline and to have witnessed its enormous national and international growth from a branch of physiology to an important discipline in the forefront of medical research. I have never regretted my desertion of physiology for pharmacology.

Ann. Rev. Pharmacol. Toxicol. 1984. 24:19–42

THE METABOLISM OF INSECTICIDES: THE ROLE OF MONOOXYGENASE ENZYMES

A. P. Kulkarni

Toxicology Program, Department of Environmental and Industrial Health, University of Michigan, Ann Arbor, Michigan 48109

E. Hodgson

Interdepartmental Toxicology Program, North Carolina State University, Raleigh, North Carolina 27650

INTRODUCTION

Although cytochrome P-450-dependent xenobiotic-metabolizing monooxygenase systems have been investigated extensively and reviewed frequently, this is not true of their role in insecticide metabolism. In the majority of the investigations reported, the substrates of choice are drugs, carcinogens, or compounds related to them. The last comprehensive review of the oxidative metabolism of insecticides was published in 1980, with the review of the literature extending only through 1978 (1). Since that time it has become apparent that the FAD-containing monooxygenase is of considerable importance (2) in insecticide metabolism and that its role relative to that of cytochrome P-450 needs to be redefined. Co-oxidation during prostaglandin synthesis (3) has also emerged as a new metabolic route and our knowledge of some other aspects of insecticide oxidation has been extended.

Even though insecticides are subject to the whole array of phase I and phase II xenobiotic-metabolizing enzymes, the role of monooxygenases is of primary and critical importance. In addition to their role in detoxication, their production of highly reactive intermediates plays an important part in activation reactions and hence in both acute and chronic toxicity. Since the monooxygenases are a common locus for the metabolism of many types of xenobiotics,

19

most of which can act as inducers or inhibitors as well as substrates, they are the most important locus for interactions between different compounds (4). Their role as activating systems in genotoxicity testing has also been extended to include insecticides (5). In insects, the target organisms, they play a role in resistance, hormone metabolism, and polyphagy (6) in addition to their role in the detoxication and activation of xenobiotics.

This review consists of aspects of the topic on which our information has been extended since the last comprehensive review (1). Due to space limitations, citation of the literature is selective rather than comprehensive.

MONOOXYGENASE SYSTEMS

Despite considerable effort by many investigators, the mechanism of action of cytochrome P-450 has not been completely elucidated. However, the current status of our knowledge is summarized in Figure 1. It is apparent that insecticides, while acting as substrates or inhibitors, may also play a role in lipid peroxidation and in the generation of active oxygen species. We now know that cytochrome P-450 exists as a number of isozymes (7) that vary in their distribution between species, strains, and organs as well as in their substrate specificities, physical properties, and inducibility, although the importance of this multiplicity in insecticide metabolism is not yet clear. Many of the studies to date have been carried out on induced isozymes, but recently we have purified several constitutive forms from the livers of untreated mice (8) and are currently investigating their specificity vis-a-vis insecticide substrates (9). Multiplicity is also known in insects (10), although in this case the isozymes have been less well defined. It is apparent, however, that neither aryl hydrocarbon hydroxylase activity (11), nor cytochromes found in insect microsomes with λ_{max} lower than 450 nm (12), should be equated with the cytochrome P-448 induced in mammalian liver by polycyclic aromatic hydrocarbons.

The basic distribution of cytochrome P-450 between cell types, organs, strains, and species has been known for some time, but less is known about these aspects as they relate to insecticide metabolism. Most previous studies have been carried out on rodent liver or insects (1), but recently some emphasis has been placed on fish and birds. In the former case, this includes the demonstration of aldrin epoxidation in carp *(Cyprinus carpio)*, grass carp *(Ctenopharyngodon idella)*, tilapia *(Tilapia aurea)*, and trout *(Salmo trutta)*, as well as parathion desulfuration in the carp (13) and the oxidation of diazinon by five species of marine and saltwater fish: carp, rainbow trout *(Salmo gairdneri)*, channel catfish *(Ictalurus punctatus)*, dace *(Tribolodon hakonensis)*, and yellow tail *(Seriola quinqueradiata)* (14).

An extensive study of wild sea birds and one land bird (15, 16) showed the oxidation of the cyclodienes, aldrin, and HCE by liver microsomes from the

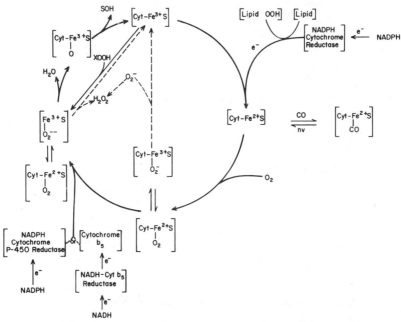

Figure 1   Reaction sequence of the cytochrome P-450-dependent monooxygenase system.

puffin *(Fratercula arctica)*, the razorbill *(Alca torda)*, the guillemot *(Uria aalge)*, the shag *(Phalacrocorax aristotelis)*, the cormorant *(Phalocrocorax carbo)*, the Manx shearwater *(Puffinus puffinus)*, the black-headed gull *(Larus ridibundus)*, and the rook *(Corvus frugilegus)*. Aldrin epoxidation has also been demonstrated in several organs of Japanese quail (17), and naphthalene has been shown to be oxidized to 1-naphthol and the 1,2-diol by liver microsomes of the pigeon (18). Both oxidative dearylation and oxidative desulfuration cf parathion was demonstrated in liver microsomes of four species of wild birds: the barn-owl *(Tyto alba)*, the blackbird *(Turdus merula)*, the African bulbul *(Pycnonotus capensis)*, and the house sparrow *(Passer domesticus)* (19).

The status of cytochrome P-450-dependent monooxygenase systems in insects has recently been reviewed (6, 10, 12).

The other microsomal monooxygenase of importance is the FAD-containing monooxygenase. This enzyme, first described as an amine oxidase and later shown to oxidize a variety of sulfur compounds, is widely distributed in vertebrate species and occurs in several tissues (20). It has not to date been identified in invertebrates. The mechanism of action is illustrated in Figure 2. It can be seen that the oxidizable xenobiotic is the third substrate to combine with the enzyme (NADPH, then oxygen, and then the oxidizable substrate). According to the proposed mechanism, it appears that V_{max} should be similar for all

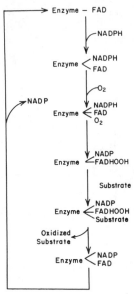

Figure 2   Reaction sequence of the FAD-containing monooxygenase.

substrates, with K_m being variable (20). In the case of insecticides, the low solubility in water frequently makes determination of kinetic constants difficult.

CYTOCHROME P-450 REACTIONS

Desulfuration and Ester Cleavage

The enzymatic substitution of a sulfur atom by an oxygen atom typifies bioactivation of all phosphorothioate and phosphorodithioate insecticides. Initial studies (21) on the characterization of parathion desulfuration by mammalian liver implicated cytochrome P-450, as they indicated that the activity resides in microsomes, requires NAD(P)H and molecular oxygen, and is inhibited by CO, SKF 525-A, methylenedioxyphenyl compounds, and substituted imidazoles.

Conclusive evidence for the monooxygenase nature of the parathion activation was provided by the use of reconstituted systems consisting of homogeneous hepatic microsomal cytochrome P-450 from rat or rabbit liver, NADPH cytochrome P-450 reductase, NADPH, and phospholipid (21). The reaction mechanism proposed for the formation of paraoxon from parathion includes initial donation of a singlet oxygen atom to the sulfur atom of parathion to yield a compound analogous to S-oxide. One of the four resonance forms of the proposed intermediate rearranges internally to form a cyclic P-S-O intermediate. This resultant phosphooxathiiran then undergoes a cyclic electron shift with the loss of elemental sulfur, forming paraoxon.

Parathion is metabolized in vitro by the microsomal monooxygenase system to paraoxon, diethyl phosphorothioic acid, diethyl phosphoric acid, and *p*-nitrophenol. Similar metabolic patterns consisting of both activation by desulfuration and detoxication by oxidative ester cleavage have now been demonstrated by in vitro studies on several organophosphorus (OP) insecticides (1). These observations led to the question of whether these two reactions are catalyzed by the same enzyme or each is catalyzed by a separate system involving different cytochrome P-450 species. Neal and co-workers (21) have proposed that all of these products originate non-enzymatically from the enzymatically produced phosphooxathiiran intermediate. Both molecular oxygen and oxygen from water participate in metabolite production, and the accessibility of water to the active site of cytochrome P-450 and the *cis* or *trans* position of the sulfine with respect to the *p*-nitrophenyl group seem to determine their relative proportions. Whether this hypothesis is applicable to the metabolism of other OP insecticides under different experimental conditions (1) is not yet clear.

In addition to the monooxygenase-catalyzed dearylation of phosphorothionate insecticides, oxidative disruption of the acid-anhydride bond of phosphates has been observed in a few cases (1), although in general oxons are considered poor substrates for the microsomal monooxygenase system. Recently, an unusual substrate specificity in the oxidative dearylation of paraoxon analogs was described (22). The dearylation process in question is a typical monooxygenase reaction, since it requires NADPH and oxygen and is inhibited by CO, SKF 525-A, and piperonyl butoxide. Although methyl-, ethyl-, n-butyl-, and n-amyl-paraoxon were not readily metabolized, considerable dearylation of n-propyl paraoxon was observed. When the two alkyl substituents were not identical, only the compounds with an n-propyl group were metabolized. Dearylation was also observed with analogs containing certain branched chains or modified ethyl groups. This unusual substrate specificity is associated with the presence of a 3-carbon chain or its steric equivalent. The reaction mechanism is probably different from that for the monooxygenase-catalyzed dearylation of phosphorothioates, since *p*-nitrophenol production from the paraoxon analogs is not accompanied by release of the corresponding dialkyl phosphate.

A number of reports are available indicating the role of species, strain, tissues, sex, and other factors on desulfuration and ester cleavage of OP insecticides (1, 13, 14, 23–35).

Epoxidation and Aromatic Hydroxylation

As early as 1951, the accumulation of a metabolite was observed in different tissues of rats treated with chlordane. The isolation and identification of the metabolite as an epoxide was reported later. Since then, as indicated in our earlier review (1), at least 75 animal species capable of epoxidation of organochlorine insecticides have been reported in the literature. Now the list is further extended by 26 animal species (13, 15, 16, 36–42).

The epoxidation of aldrin can be quantified with high sensitivity and reproducibility by gas chromatography, requires minimal amounts of liver microsomes or liver tissue, and the product, dieldrin, is stable and rather refractive to further metabolism. As a result, this reaction may prove a useful index for the routine clinical evaluation of the status of the human liver endoplasmic reticulum. Two reports on aldrin epoxidase activity using needle biopsy samples of liver from monkey (43) and human (44) have already appeared. The obvious utility of this monooxygenase reaction is now being exploited in studies using isolated hepatocytes from rodents and humans (45, 46).

Reports indicating that epoxidation can be observed in vitro when liver microsomes and cyclodiene insecticides are incubated in the presence of NADPH and air first appeared in 1965. The monooxygenase nature of the epoxidation reaction was later confirmed by the demonstration of obligatory requirements for reduced pyridine nucleotides, NADPH-cytochrome P-450 reductase, and molecular oxygen. Further supportive evidence for the involvement of cytochrome P-450 comes from the fact that epoxidation proceeds most actively with microsomes compared to other subcellular fractions and is significantly inhibited by several classical specific inhibitors of the monooxygenase system: CO, methylenedioxyphenyl compounds, substituted imidazoles, SKF-525A, and metyrapone (1).

The most conclusive evidence for the monooxygenase nature of the epoxidation reaction comes from reconstitution studies utilizing purified cytochrome P-450. Yu & Terriere (47) isolated six chromatographically distinct forms of microsomal cytochrome P-450 (A_1, A_2, B_1, B_2, C_1, and C_2) from NAIDM and Rutger's strains of housefly. In reconstitution experiments they used these fractions, rat liver NADPH-cytochrome P-450 reductase, and a synthetic phospholipid. The highest activity reported was for the B_1 and C_1 fractions of Rutger's and NAIDM houseflies respectively. Levi & Hodgson (9) investigated aldrin epoxidation in cytochrome P-450 systems reconstituted from uninduced mouse liver. Of five cytochrome P-450 fractions designated A_1, A_2, B_1, B_2, and B_3, according to the order of elution from DEAE cellulose columns, the A_1 fraction showed the highest activity in epoxidation of aldrin to dieldrin. A_2 and B_3 fractions also showed some activity, while B_1 and B_2 were inactive. A report on the evaluation of aldrin epoxidation in monooxygenase systems reconstituted from purified rat liver microsomal cytochrome P-450 or P-448 is also available (48). Either phenobarbital or 3-methylcholanthrene-pretreated rats were used. Considering the turnover numbers, the cytochrome P-448-dependent rate of aldrin epoxidation was less than 3% of the cytochrome P-450-dependent activity when the highest value determined for cytochrome P-448 was compared to the lowest value obtained in the cytochrome P-450 system. The apparent Km for aldrin in the complete P-450 system was 7 μM and the maximum value reported for turnover number was 2.2 mol. dieldrin/min/mol. cytochrome P-450. A marked stimulation by ethanol, significant inhibition by SKF 525-A, and no effect of 7,8-benzoflavone on cytochrome P-450-dependent epoxidase activity was noted, while ethanol and 7,8-benzoflavone caused significant inhibition in the P-448 system. These results clearly indicate that aldrin is a selective substrate for phenobarbital-induced cytochrome P-450 as compared to the P-448 species induced by 3-methylcholanthrene.

In rat liver microsomes (49), the singlet oxygen quencher 1,4-diazabicyclo (2, 2, 2) octane inhibited epoxidation, while guanosine had no effect. While tiron and superoxide dismutase are known to inhibit reactions mediated by superoxide anion, the former stimulated aldrin epoxidation and the latter had no effect. The participation of neither H_2O_2 nor OH· was examined and the oxygen species responsible for aldrin epoxidation remains far from being clearly established.

Besides aldrin, heptachlor, isodrin, and photoaldrin can also serve as substrates for microsomal epoxidase activity. Except for chlordene, epoxidation occurs by oxygen attack at the C_6 and C_7 position in the substrate molecule. Methylated analogs of aldrin, however, do not undergo epoxidation. With chlordene, formation of 2,3-epoxide was noted with fish and mouse liver microsomes. Apart from this, an additional route leading to the formation of hydroxyepoxide via a hydroxychlordene intermediate has also been observed with pig liver and housefly microsomes. Although these observations tend to suggest that epoxidation occurs only if a reactive double bond is present in the substrate molecule, this becomes questionable when the results of studies with chlordane, a member of the cyclodiene family with a saturated ring, are considered. Both α- and β-chlordane isomers undergo initial desaturation to an intermediate 1-exo-2-dichlorochlordene that is subsequently epoxidized to oxychlordane. Subsequently, another pathway was proposed (50) in which chlordane undergoes reductive dehalogenation to give dihydroheptachlor or dihydrochlordene, which are oxidized to their respective epoxides after desaturation.

Lindane and other isomers of hexachlorocyclohexane produce 2,4,6-trichlorophenol as the major oxidation product when metabolized by either housefly or rat liver microsomes in the presence of oxygen and NADPH (51). The reaction was inhibited by CO; the order of reactivity was $\delta > \epsilon > \alpha > \lambda > \beta$. A direct insertion of oxygen into the cyclohexane ring to yield pentachlorocyclohexanone-gem-chlorohydrins was proposed as the reaction mechanism. The labile chlorohydrins are subsequently converted to corresponding cyclohexanones, which undergo two-step dehydrochlorinations via their enol forms to yield 2,4,6-trichloro-phenol. Mouse hepatic microsomal enzymes were shown to convert 1,1-bis(p-chlorophenyl) ethylene, an mammalian metabolite of DDT, into 1,1-bis(p-chlorophenyl)-1,2-ethanediol (52). The putative epoxide intermediate, however, was not isolated.

The susceptibility of aromatic rings to oxidative attack by microsomal monooxygenase systems is well known, but there are relatively few examples involving insecticides, although naphthalene was a early example of arene oxide formation. This reaction has recently been studied in birds (18). The relative scarcity of examples of arene oxide formation is probably because various ring substituents offer more favorable sites for hydroxylation. Carbaryl metabolism does, however, proceed via this pathway. Aerobic incubation of carbaryl with NADPH fortified liver microsomes yields 4,5-hydroxy-1-naphthyl methylcarbamate and 5,6-dihydro-5,6-dihydroxy-1-napthyl methylcarbamate. The production of these metabolites of carbaryl was envisioned to proceed via an epoxide intermediate. Apart from carbaryl, ring hydroxylation is also known to occur in some other carbamate insecticides such as Landrin®, propoxur, Tsumacide®, and Pyramat®. In none of these cases has the postulated epoxy intermediate been isolated. Ring hydroxylation is rarely observed with OP insecticides and usually represents a minor pathway. Available reports include ring hydroxylation of phosmet, the thiophenol moiety of fonofos and its chloro analog (1).

Several synthetic pyrethroids undergo ring hydroxylation of the alcohol moiety before or after ester cleavage, yielding a variety of metabolites. The hydroxylation rates are usually higher with *cis* than with *trans* isomers and the preferred sites of hydroxylation vary in different animal species (53–55). For example, both *cis*- and *trans*-permethrin give rise to 4'-hydroxy metabolites with microsomal preparations from carp or trout and to 6-hydroxy derivatives with mouse or housefly preparations. Hydroxylation at the 2' position is observed only with the *cis* isomer and only with mouse liver microsomes. Both 4' and 5-hydroxy derivatives are produced from cypermethrin by mouse liver microsomes. Kadethrin and decamethrin were shown to be hydroxylated at the 4' position by microsomal oxidases.

Aliphatic Hydroxylation

Aliphatic C-H bonds not adjacent to hetero atoms are susceptible to initial oxidative attack, yielding stable alcohols that may in certain cases be the subject of further oxidation or conjugation. Several studies have firmly established that aliphatic hydroxylation of alkyl side chains represents the predominant route for oxidative biotransformation of carbamate insecticides. The chemical nature of the metabolites produced depends upon the kind and number of substituents. Thus, oxidation of the methyl group may stop at the alcohol step, as in case of Tsumacide®, or may proceed to the carboxy analog with compounds such as Banol. In carbamates such as in Landrin®, Bux®, UC-

10854, RE-11775, RE-5365, carbofuran, and N-(2-toluenesulfenyl) carbofuran, there may be simple hydroxy analog formation (1).

Aliphatic hydroxylation of alkyl ring substituents of some OP insecticides, such as O, O, O-tri-o-tolyphosphate (TOCP) and O, O, O-tri-(p-ethylphenyl)-phosphate (TPEP), results in activation, while oxidation of the 3-methyl group of fenitrothion to a carboxyl group leads to detoxication. The side chain on the heteroaromatic ring of diazinon and diazoxon also undergoes hydroxylation to produce hydroxydiazinon and isohydroxydiazinon, metabolites B and C. The involvement of cytochrome P-450 is suggested from the observed inhibition by CO, piperonyl butoxide, and substituted imidazoles. All oxidation products with intact ester linkages exhibit anticholinesterase activity.

For some time, epoxides were thought to be the terminal residues of cyclodiene insecticides such as aldrin. However, several studies have indicated the production of small amounts of 2-hydroxy, 4-hydroxy derivatives or Klein's metabolite from dieldrin following attack by microsomal monooxygenases. Similar to dieldrin, the rat hepatic microsomal system has also been found to catalyze conversion of endrin to four monohydroxylated products. Related cyclic compounds vulnerable to hydroxylation by the microsomal monooxygenase systems include dihydroaldrin, dihydroisodrin, HCE, photoisodrin, chlordene, dehydrochlordene, photoheptachlor, toxaphene, and methylated analogs of aldrin and dieldrin (1, 56, 57).

Extensive investigations on the in vitro metabolism of pyrethroids were carried out by Casida, Elliott, Miyamoto, and co-workers [cited in (1)]. On the basis of recovered radiocarbon in various metabolites, hydroxylation of the *trans* methyl group of the isobutyl side chain in the acid moiety represents the major pathway of metabolism with compounds like allethrin, while that of *cis* methyl group appears to be a minor site. This oxidation results in the sequential formation of the corresponding hydroxymethyl, aldehyde, and carboxylic acid. These or similar pathways have been found to be operative in the case of natural pyrethroids as well as in that of synthetic compounds.

Heterocyclic Ring Hydroxylation

Heterocyclic ring hydroxylation represents a rare reaction in insecticide metabolism and is best studied in the case of nicotine. Earlier reports indicated that rabbit liver microsomes can catalyze hydroxylation at the α-carbon of the pyrrolidine ring in the nicotine molecule. This biotransformation required NADPH and oxygen, and the hydroxynicotine produced was further oxidized by aldehyde oxidase to cotinine. Cotinine formation, but not the disappearance of nicotine, was inhibited by SKF 525-A and KCN. Reconstitution studies (58) have provided further evidence for the participation of cytochrome P-450 in nicotine oxidation. The reaction depends on cytochrome P-450, NADPH cytochrome P-450 reductase, and NADPH. Despite the several known metabolites of nicotine (1, 59), the authors monitored the disappearance of substrate to quantitate activity. Heterocyclic ring hydroxylation has also been shown as an intermediate metabolic step in the metabolism of anabasine analogs and an experimental insecticide, R-16661 (1).

Dealkylation

The oxidative cleavage of alkyl groups attached to electronegative heteroatoms such as nitrogen and oxygen is a metabolic reaction frequently encountered with insecticides. Since all the commercial carbamate insecticides contain N-alkyl groups in their molecules, the N-dealkylation reaction first reported by Hodgson & Casida (60, 61) assumes major significance in their metabolism. Using rat liver microsomes, the enzymatic splitting of the C-N bond in 4-nitrophenyl-N,N-dimethylcarbamate was found to require NADPH and molecular oxygen. The reaction was inhibited by classical inhibitors of the monooxygenase system such as piperonyl butoxide and SKF 525-A.

From the mechanistic point of view, the initial attack may occur either at the carbon attached to the nitrogen or at the nitrogen itself. Thus, initial α-carbon oxidation directly yields a carbinolamine that ultimately rearranges to liberate a carbonyl compound and the dealkylated amine, while prior N-oxidation leading to carbinolamine formation represents another route. The experimental evidence, however, is strongly in favor of C-oxidation leading to N-hydroxyalkyl metabolites. Although dimethyl as well as monomethyl carbamates serve as substrates for the monooxygenase-catalyzed N-dealkylation reaction, only one methyl group of dimethylcarbamates participates in hydroxylation, yielding an N-methylcarbamate, and there is no evidence for the further oxidation of the remaining N-methyl group to yield the primary carbamate. In some cases, the N-hydroxymethyl derivatives are sufficiently stable to be isolated following either in vivo or in vitro oxidation (1).

In contrast to carbamates, in which N-dealkylation usually results in detoxication, oxidation of certain OP insecticides such as scradan and dimefox via postulated N-oxide intermediates leads to the formation of highly potent anticholinesterase agents, while detoxication involving carbinolamine intermediates occurs with others. Some data on the N-dealkylation of cotinine and nicotine are also available (1, 32, 62, 63).

The O-dealkylation of OP triesters to the corresponding diester is a major mechanism of detoxication and is seen in both insects and mammals. It differs from other O-dealkylations in that the oxygen attack is on an ester linkage rather than on an ether. The reaction mechanism is analogous to N-dealkylation except that the hydroxy or diol intermediates of an O-dealkylation reaction are extremely unstable and undergo spontaneous rearrangement to liberate the dealkylated substrate. Paraoxon serves as a substrate for microsomal monooxygenase-catalyzed O-deethylation and leads to the production of either ethanol, acetaldehyde, or acetate in different animal species. Although this reaction has been extensively studied with a number of OP triesters, the obligatory requirement for cytochrome P-450 remains uncertain, at least in the case of chlorfenvinphos (1).

Although O-dealkylation is a rather common reaction in the case of OP triesters (1,64), its occurrence in the metabolism of other classes of insecticides appears rare. Several reports (1, 65, 66) indicate that one or both *para* substituted methoxy groups of methoxychlor are readily cleaved off by liver microsomes in the presence of NADPH and air. The same degradative pathway was implicated in the metabolism of ethoxychlor, in the formation of 2-hydroxyphenyl N-methylcarbamate from propoxur, and in the oxidation of 3-methyoxy group of rotenone (1).

Dehydrogenation

Desaturation, a novel reaction mechanism first discovered during in vitro enzymatic conversion of α- and β-chlordane to 1,2-dichlordene, is now firmly established as a typical monooxygenase reaction catalyzed by microsomal cytochrome P-450. The necessary evidence for the oxidative dehydrogenation was presented in the case of lindane. The reaction required NADPH and molecular oxygen and was inhibited by CO and SKF 525-A (67). Lack of inhibition by KCN further differentiates this dehydrogenase system from the cytochrome b_5-dependent fatty acid desaturase system. In the proposed mechanism, the oxenoid, generated from oxygen and the enzyme(s), abstracts two hydrogen atoms from the substrate to yield water and the alkene directly. It now appears that chlordane isomers and hexachlorocyclohexene also serve as substrates for microsomal enzymes isolated from the housefly (49, 51, 68) and the rat (49–51, 69). Recently dehydrogenation, dehydrochlorination, and hydroxylation were found to be involved in the metabolism of lindane by human liver microsomes. The rates were found to be comparable to those reported for rats and insects despite considerable quantitative variation between individuals (70).

INSECTICIDE METABOLISM DURING PROSTAGLANDIN BIOSYNTHESIS

In addition to the cytochrome P-450-dependent monooxygenase system, coupling of the N-dealkylation of an insecticide to prostaglandin biosynthesis has recently been described (3). The reconstituted prostaglandin endoperoxide synthetase involves two enzyme activities, fatty acid cyclooxygenase that catalyzes bis-dioxygenation to produce the hydroperoxy endoperoxide PGG_2, and hydroperoxidase, the reduction of PGG_2 to PGH_2. A variety of xenobiotics that can provide the requisite pair of electrons for the last step of the reaction are themselves co-oxidized. Ram seminal vesicle microsomes, when incubated in the presence of air and arachidonic acid, effected the N-dealkylation of amino-carb as measured by formaldehyde production. Besides aminocarb, several mono- and di-methyl substituted model compounds were found to be sub-strates. However, S- or O-dealkylation was not observed with the compounds tested. The N-demethylation rate was comparable to that observed with NADPH-dependent hepatic microsomal cytochrome P-450-mediated monoox-ygenase reactions and detectable amounts of neither cytochrome P-450 nor NADPH-dependent dealkylation were present. Although the reaction mecha-nism is not yet precisely understood, the proposed dehydrogenase mechanism of N-dealkylation for the prostaglandin synthetase coupled system is expected to be very different from that suggested for the cytochrome P-450 system. Since prostaglandin biosynthesis occurs in many cell types in various tissues such as lung, kidney, and skin, xenobiotic metabolism via this alternate pathway could conceivably play a significant role in determining the suscepti-bility of target organs lacking monooxygenase activity.

FAD-CONTAINING MONOOXYGENASE REACTIONS

Sulfoxidation

In the presence of NADPH and oxygen, thioether-containing OP insecticides are oxidized by the FAD-containing monooxygenase purified from pig liver microsomes. The stoichiometry between NADPH and substrate consumed is 1:1 and the product, in the case of phorate and disulfoton, is the sulfoxide (71, 72). The sulfoxides are optically active and further oxidation to the sulfone is not apparent. n-Octylamine, which inhibits cytochrome P-450 and activates the FAD-containing monooxygenase, increases the rate of sulfoxidation. Structur-al changes around the thioether sulfur that affect nucleophilicity or cause steric hindrance tend to decrease the rate of sulfoxidation. Although neither thiono nor thiolo sulfur atoms of phosphorodithioates are attacked, substitution of either by oxygen decreases thioether oxidation. O,O-dimethyl compounds that contain thioether sulfur are not oxidized as readily as their O,O-diethyl ana-logs.

The (−) isomer of profenofos is activated to a more potent cholinesterase inhibitor by an oxidative attack on the thiolo sulfur that, in the case of the less toxic (+) isomer, results in detoxication (73). We have recently shown (Levi & Hodgson, unpublished information) that this reaction is catalyzed primarily by cytochrome P-450, with only a small contribution due to the FAD-containing monooxygenase. Furthermore, one of the cytochrome P-450 isozymes purified from the hepatic microsomes of uninduced mice (8) is more active in this regard than the others.

Sulfur-containing carbamates are not as effectively metabolized by the

FAD-containing monooxygenase as OP insecticides but some, including thiofanox, aldicarb, methiocarb, and croneton, are oxidized at appreciable rates (71, 72).

Methiochlor and its analog containing one $-SCH_3$ and one $-OCH_3$ group are both readily oxidized by the pig liver FAD-containing monooxygenase (2), the product presumably being the monosulfoxide, since one mole of NADPH is consumed per mole of substrate oxidized. This leaves unanswered the question of the origin of the sulfones known to be formed in vivo.

Many microsomal sulfur oxidations have been attributed to cytochrome P-450 (1) and, by comparison with non-insecticidal substrates, it appears probable that this may often be the case. The relative importance of these two metabolic routes for common substrates is presently unknown. We have addressed this problem in the case of the hepatotoxicant thiobenzamide, and we find that the relative contributions vary from species to species and organ to organ (74). In the mouse their contributions are approximately equal in the liver, while in the lung 85% of thiobenzamide oxidation proceeds via the FAD-containing enzyme.

In view of the well-known formation in vivo of sulfones (1) and the apparent inability of the FAD-containing monooxygenase to carry insecticide oxidations beyond the sulfoxide, it can be speculated that the second step is catalyzed by cytochrome P-450.

In this regard it is interesting that, although methidathion is not a substrate for the FAD-containing monooxygenase, the S-methyl derivative of its hydrolysis product is. This compound, which is formed in vivo, is metabolized to the sulfoxide by the FAD-enzyme, but further oxidation to the sulfone is apparently mediated by the cytochrome P-450-dependent system (27).

Desulfuration

The FAD-containing monooxygenase catalyzes the oxidation of fonofos and phenyl fonofos. Reaction stoichiometry, product identification, and the formation of a potent cholinesterase inhibitor all indicate that the reaction is an oxidative desulfuration producing the oxon as the principal product (75). Previous studies on fonofos activation (76–79) all implicate the cytochrome P-450-dependent monooxygenase system and propose a mechanism involving a cyclic phosphooxathiran intermediate similar to that proposed for parathion (21). Since previous studies on fonofos were carried out with microsomal preparations and, since both the FAD-dependent monooxygenase and the cytochrome P-450-dependent monooxygenase system are NADPH and O_2 dependent, the relative roles of the two systems were not defined. It is clear, however, that cytochrome P-450 is responsible for the oxidative desulfuration of phosphorothioates, such as parathion, since this reaction has been carried out with purified, reconstituted cytochrome P-450 (21). It is possible that phosphonates, such as fonofos and its phenyl analogs, are metabolized by both systems. Lee et al (78) showed that retention of configuration, considered to be consistent with the above mechanism for cytochrome P-450, was the principal stereochemical course for the activation of fonofos isomers by rat liver microsomes. They speculated that the 21–28% inversion observed was due to a second mechanism involving an initial attack on the phosphorus atom.

The phosphorodithioate analog of fonofos is neither a substrate nor an inhibitor for the FAD-containing monooxygenase. It is not understood why, with this enzyme, oxidative desulfuration occurs with phosphonates but not with phosphorothioates. Although the former lack p^π-d^π bonding due to the absence of free electrons in the carbon atom covalently bound to the phosphorus, in contrast to the oxygen atom in the latter, the significance of this in the reaction mechanism is as yet unknown.

Indirect support for an attack on phosphorus is provided by the observation that this enzyme also catalyzes the oxidation of the phosphines, diphenyl-methylphosphine and the CNS depressant 3-dimethylamino-propyl-diphenylphosphine, the products being diphenylmethylphosphine oxide in the former and both the P-oxide and the N,P-dioxide in the latter (2). Since diphenylmethylphosphine does not contain either sulfur or nitrogen, the attack is presumably on the phosphorus atom. Moreover, the pentavalent sulfide of diphenyl methylphosphine is metabolized by this enzyme to its oxygen analog, the phosphine oxide. These two observations, taken together, increase the probability that the activation of fonofos and other phosphonates is via an attack on the phosphorus atom.

Amine Oxidation

Tetram and its analogs are also substrates for the FAD-containing monooxygenase and the product appears to be the corresponding N-oxide (71, 72).

MONOOXYGENASES AND NEWER INSECTICIDES

The following are some brief remarks concerning monooxygenation of some of the newer insecticides or compounds of potential importance in insecticide development. They include synthetic pyrethroids, juvenile hormones and hormone analogs, anti-juvenoids, and an insect growth regulator, diflubenzuron.

Pyrethroids

Although oxidation of pyrethroids is well known and many of the reactions, and the structural basis for them, have been reviewed either in reference (1) or in the section on cytochrome P-450 reactions above, it is now clear that hydrolysis is the most important route for the metabolism of the majority of the synthetic pyrethroids (53, 80–82). Inhibition of the esterases involved, by other insecticides or related compounds, raises the possibility of synergistic interactions (82).

The rapid and complete debromination of tralomethrin and thalocythrin to yield deltamethrin and cypermethrin is apparently non-enzymatic, but the two products and their subsequent enzymatic hydrolysis products are subject to oxidative metabolism (83, 84).

Hormones and Hormone Analogs

The final step in the biosynthesis of juvenile hormones is epoxidation, and monooxygenases are involved in this and in their deactivation in insects. It is apparent, however, that epoxide hydrolase and esterase action are more important in their metabolic deactivation in insects. The low toxicity of juvenile hormones and hormone analogs to mammals, however, may be due to the rapidity with which they are oxidized in mammalian preparations. These and other aspects have recently been reviewed (10).

Anti-juvenoids, the precocenes, appear to function as suicide substrates for the monooxygenases of the corpus allatum, blocking hormone production and causing necrosis of the gland. Although the postulated epoxide has not been isolated, the resultant diol has. The early studies leading to these conclusions have recently been reviewed (10). Because of the potential for applied use this area has been one of intense interest. Recently (85), synthetic analogs of precocenes, such as substituted isopentenylphenols, have been synthesized whose mode of action is indistinguishable from the natural precocenes. However, precocenes are known to be hepatotoxic (86) and nephrotoxic (87) in rats, although at high dose levels, effects possibly mediated through oxidative formation of reaction intermediates similar to those formed in the corpus allatum. If this is the case, the selective difference in sensitivity between the insect gland and the mammalian tissue is remarkable.

Insect Growth Regulators

Diflubenzuron [1-(2,6-difluorobenzoyl)-3-3(4-chlorophenyl)urea], a compound that affects chitin formation in insects, is one of the growth regulators currently of much interest as an insecticide. On the basis of in vivo studies in houseflies (88, 89) it is known to produce a number of metabolites characteristic of monooxygenase activity, including 2,6-difluorobenzamide, 2,6-difluorobenzoic acid, 4-chlorophenyl urea, and several ring hydroxylated species. The monooxygenase nature of this metabolism is supported by sesamex inhibition (89).

Similar pathways are known in domestic animals, but frequently the bulk of the administered dose is excreted in the feces unchanged (90). In chickens diflubenzuron is particularly refractory to metabolism, the small amount broken down by microsomal metabolism being apparently the result of non-oxidative pathways (91).

INDUCTION

Effect of Induction

Induction or inhibition of the cytochrome P-450-dependent monooxygenase system following chemical pretreatment of animals might be expected to be reflected in an increased or decreased monooxygenase activity in vitro. This does appear to be the case in several animal species (1). In addition, phenobarbital induces cyclodiene epoxidase activity in three species of blow fly (39), rat (92), and mouse hepatocytes in culture (45) as well as induces cytochrome P-450 in susceptible houseflies (93). Liver microsomal aldrin epoxidase is significantly increased in nestling and adult barn owls by Aroclor-1254 (94) and in rats by either toxaphene or (non)polar extracts of toxaphene (95). On the other hand, 3-methylcholanthrene (92) or α- or β-endosulfan (96) exposure lowers hepatic aldrin epoxidase activity. In blow flies, β-naphthoflavone induction of aldrin epoxidase was found to be relatively minor (39), while this inducer had no effect on mouse hepatocytes in culture (45). There is evidence, in addition to that previously summarized (10), that aldrin epoxidase in insects can also be induced by the allelochemicals present in plants (38, 40, 41).

A significant induction of in vitro liver microsomal metabolism of OP compounds via O-dealkylation and dearylation pathways has been reported when rats or mice were pretreated with either phenobarbital (30), halobenzenes (97), DDE (98), or different pesticides (31, 99).

Induction studies also suggest that constitutive and phenobarbital-induced forms of hepatic microsomal enzymes, which can be inhibited by α-naphthoflavone, participate in nicotine oxidation (100). After either 3-methylcholanthrene or β-naphthoflavone treatment nicotine oxidase activity per cytochrome P-448 molecule was actually decreased but the specific activity of the enzyme remained unchanged. Female rats, fed on a diet containing either Aroclor-1254, phenobarbital, or β-naphthoflavone for one week, followed by oral lindane administration, showed induction of liver microsomal lindane dehydrogenase activity by Aroclor-1254 and phenobarbital, while β-naphthoflavone pretreatment impaired the enhancement of dehydrogenase activity (69).

Insecticides as Inducers

Subsequent to previous reviews (1, 31, 99) a number of reports have appeared on induction by insecticides. Generally they fall into three areas: effects on the LD_{50} of other insecticides; effects of kepone, mirex, and related compounds on liver function; general induction of xenobiotic-metabolizing enzymes and its possible consequences. Space limitations preclude a complete review but a brief summary with selected references follows.

Dieldrin was shown to protect against the acute toxicity of chlorfenvinphos, the effect due to increased metabolism (101), while large doses of carbaryl provided only marginal protection against the acute effects of parathion and propoxur (102).

Kepone (chlordecone) is a potent inducer of microsomal cytochrome P-450 and monooxygenase activity (99, 103). In addition, it causes a dramatic enhancement of the hepatotoxicity of haloalkanes such as carbon tetrachloride (104). However, it is not immediately obvious that the latter activity is related to enzyme induction (104, 105). The related compound, mirex, is a more potent inducer than kepone, although it does not cause the enhancement of haloalkane toxicity. It is, in fact, the most potent inducer of cytochrome P-450 among pesticides (99). The inducing effect of mirex and related compounds on various aspects of xenobiotic metabolism have frequently been demonstrated (99, 106–108).

Many insecticides have been shown to induce cytochrome P-450 and associated monooxygenase activities (99). These investigations continue to be extended and recent studies include the following: the effect of lindane on CF1 mice (109); induction of cytochrome P-450 by methylenedioxyphenyl synergists such as piperonyl butoxide and the possible role of the methylene carbon (110, 111); the possible role of induction by dieldrin (112), toxaphene, and carbaryl (113) on the expression of carcinogenicity caused by other compounds; an attempt to classify pesticide inducers according to the pattern of activities induced (114, 115).

INHIBITION

Inhibition of Insecticide Metabolism

Although much of the current literature on monooxygenase inhibition concerns compounds related to insecticides, this topic is beyond the scope of this review. Either the compounds are not themselves synergists or the inhibited reactions do not involve insecticides. For example, much of the work on methylenedioxyphenyl compounds concerns safrole and isosafrole. A comprehensive review of these aspects, which are of great importance in consideration of the mode of action of synergists, is in press (116).

Some findings directly related to insecticide action are summarized below. Pretreatment with piperonyl butoxide was found to result in different levels of inhibition of desulfuration and hydroxylation of azinphosmethyl and azinphosethyl by mouse hepatic microsomes (24). Piperonyl butoxide was also shown to block the metabolism in vivo of the hormone analog methoprene in the imported fire ant, *Solenopsis invicta* (117). In the housefly, juvenile hormone I was shown to be a competitive inhibitor for the formation of the metabolite-inhibitory complex formed by piperonyl butoxide (118), a finding that tends to confirm that monooxygenases are involved in juvenile hormone inactivation and that the sometimes reported hormone-like activity of methylenedioxyphenyl compounds may be due to their ability to block hormone degradation. Several naturally occurring methylenedioxyphenyl compounds have been shown to affect insecticide metabolism. This includes the effect of myristicin on parathion and paraoxon metabolism (119) and the effect of dillapiole (2,3-dimethoxy-4,5-methyldioxyallylbenzene) and several of its synthetic analogs on pyrethrin toxicity (120).

5,6-Dichloro-1,2,3-benzothiadiazole has been shown to form a metabolite-inhibitory complex with cytochrome P-450 (121), a finding that presumably explains its activity as an insecticide synergist.

Insecticides as Inhibitors

In vitro, insecticides are frequently competitive inhibitors of the metabolism of related compounds, but these interactions are usually marginal in vivo. They will not be discussed further. Of greater interest is the ability of some insecticides to inactivate cytochrome P-450 during the course of their metabolism and as a result affect the metabolism and toxicity of other compounds.

Parathion inactivates the microsomal cytochrome P-450-dependent monooxygenase system when administered in vivo or when incubated in vitro with microsomes NADPH and O_2 (21, 122). This metabolism-dependent inactivation is brought about by the interaction of an active metabolite (probably singlet sulfur) with the heme iron, which results in a loss of heme. Other interactions include the formation of hydrodisulfide (R-S-SH) linkages with cysteine residues in the protein moiety of cytochrome P-450. These latter reactions are apparently of less importance in the inactivation mechanism (21, 122).

This inactivation mechanism probably also explains the results of in vitro studies that have shown that aldrin epoxidation, parathion oxidation (25, 26), and chlorpyrifos desulfuration (123) are inhibited by parathion, as well as the effect of fenitrothion on monooxygenases in weanling rats (124).

Phenolphthalein, halogenated fluoresceins, and di- and triphenylmethane derivatives have also been shown to be inhibitors of aldrin epoxidase (125).

SUMMARY AND CONCLUSIONS

In summary, it can be said that advances have been made in understanding the range and significance of monooxygenase reactions involving insecticides in both target and non-target species and that some specific aspects emerge that should command the attention of insecticide toxicologists and others in the immediate future.

The role of co-oxidation of insecticides during prostaglandin synthesis has just emerged as an issue but, if we can extrapolate from other xenobiotics

(126), we can predict with some confidence that it will assume major proportions.

It is also apparent that both activation and detoxication reactions are catalyzed by the FAD-containing monooxygenase and that many of these reactions were formerly attributed to the cytochrome P-450-dependent monooxygenase system. Since any particular substrate may be oxidized by either or both of these two routes, it is essential that studies be conducted to define their relative contributions to xenobiotic oxidation in microsomal preparations and ultimately in vivo.

The area of interactions and the mechanisms behind them is also of importance, from the public health point of view in the case of multiple exposures, and from the practical viewpoint in the case of insecticide synergists.

While the above aspects are not the only ones of future importance, they should contribute to the ultimate goal of insecticide toxicology: practical, safe use of chemicals for the control of insect pests.

Literature Cited

1. Kulkarni, A. P., Hodgson, E. 1980. Metabolism of insecticides by mixed function oxidase systems. *Pharmacol. Ther.* 8:379–475

2. Hodgson, E. 1982–83. Production of pesticide metabolites by oxidative reactions. *J. Toxicol. Clin. Toxicol.* 19:609–21

3. Sivarajah, K., Lasker, J. M., Eling, T. E., Abou-Donia, M. B. 1982. Metabolism of N-alkyl compounds during the biosynthesis of prostaglandins. N-dealkylation during prostaglandin biosynthesis. *Mol. Pharmacol.* 21:133–41

4. Hodgson, E. 1980. Chemical and environmental factors affecting metabolism of xenobiotics. In *Introduction to Biochemical Toxicology*, ed. E. Hodgson, F. E. Guthrie, pp. 143–61. New York: Elsevier Biomedical. 437 pp.

5. Gentile, J. M., Gentile, G. J., Bultman, J., Sechriest R., Wagner, E. D., Plewa, M. J. 1982. An evaluation of the genotoxic properties of insecticides following plant and animal activation. *Mutat. Res.* 101:19–29

6. Hodgson, E. 1983. The significance of cytochrome P-450 in insects. *Insect Biochem.* 13:237–46

7. Lu, A. Y. H. 1979. Multiplicity of liver drug metabolizing enzymes. *Drug Metabol. Rev.* 10:187–208

8. Levi, P. E., Hodgson, E. 1983. Purification and reconstitution of the cytochrome P-450 monooxygenase system from un-induced mouse liver. *Int. J. Biochem.* 15:349–53

9. Levi, P. E., Hodgson, E. 1983. Metabolism of pesticides by purified reconstituted cytochrome P-450 dependent monooxygenase systems. *Toxicologist* 3:78(Abstr. 309)

10. Hodgson, E. 1984. Microsomal monooxygenases. In *Comprehensive Insect Physiology, Biochemistry and Pharmacology*, ed. G. A. Kerkut, L. I. Gilbert. Oxford: Pergamon press. In press

11. Chang, K-M., Wilkinson, C. F., Hetnarski, K., Murray, M. 1983. Aryl hydrocarbon hydroxylase in larvae of the southern armyworm *(Spodoptera eridania)*. *Insect Biochem.* 13:87–94

12. Hodgson, E. Kulkarni, A. P. 1983. Characterization of cytochrome P-450 in studies of insecticide resistance. In *Pest Resistance to Pesticides*, ed. G. P. Georghiou, T. Saito, pp. 207–28. New York: Plenum. 809 pp.

13. Yahalomi, Z., Perry, A. S. 1981. Microsomal mixed-function oxidases in fish in relation to environmental contamination by organochlorine insecticides. *Comp. Biochem. Physiol.* c70:97–102

14. Fujii, Y., Asaka, S. 1982. Metabolism of diazinon and diazoxon in fish liver preparations. *Bull. Environ. Contam. Toxicol.* 29:455–60

15. Knight, G. C., Walker, C. H., Cabot, D. C., Harris, M. P. 1981. The activity of two hepatic microsomal enzymes in sea

birds. *Comp. Biochem. Physiol.* c68: 127–32
16. Knight, G. C., Walker, C. H. 1982. A study of the hepatic microsomal monooxygenase of sea birds and its relationship to organochlorine pollutants. *Comp. Biochem. Physiol.* c73:211–21
17. Riviere, J. L., Bach, J. 1979. Aldrin epoxidase in liver and small intestine of rat and Japanese quail. *Bull. Environ. Contam. Toxicol.* 21:498–501
18. Grossman, J. C., Khan, M. A. Q. 1979. Metabolism of naphthalene by pigeon liver microsomes. *Comp. Biochem. Physiol.* c63:251–60
19. Yawetz, A., Agosin, M., Perry, A. S. 1979. Metabolism of parathion and brain cholinesterase inhibition in four species of wild birds. *Pestic. Biochem. Physiol.* 11:294–300
20. Ziegler, D. M. 1980. Microsomal flavin-containing monooxygenase: Oxygenation of nucleophilic nitrogen and sulfur compounds. In *Enzymatic Basis of Detoxication,* ed. W. B. Jakoby, 1:201–27. New York: Academic. 415 pp.
21. Neal, R. A., Halpert, J. 1982. Toxicity of thiono-sulfur compounds. *Ann. Rev. Pharmacol. Toxicol.* 22:321–39
22. Cammer, P. A., Hollingworth, R. M. 1976. Unusual substrate specificity in the oxidative dearylation of paraoxon analogs by mouse hepatic microsomal enzymes. *Biochem. Pharmacol.* 25:1799–807
23. Lin, S. N., Chen, C. Y., Murphy, S. D., Caprioli, R. M. 1980. Quantitative high performance liquid chromatography and mass spectroscopy for the analysis of the *in vitro* metabolism of the insecticide azinphos-methyl (Guthion) by rat liver homogenates. *J. Agric. Food Chem.* 28:85–88
24. Lin, S., Murphy, S. D. 1983. Correlation of inhibitory enzyme kinetics with altered toxicities of azinphosmethyl (AM), azinphosethyl (AE) and their oxygen analogues (AMO and AEO) induced by piperonyl butoxide. *Toxicologist* 3:77 (Abstr. 306)
25. Morelli, M. A., Nakatsugawa, T. 1978. Inactivation *in vitro* of microsomal oxidases during parathion metabolism. *Biochem. Pharmacol.* 27:293–99
26. Morelli, M. A., Nakatsugawa, T. 1979. Sulfur oxyacid production as a consequence of parathion desulfuration. *Pestic. Biochem. Physiol.* 10:243–50
27. Chopade, H. M., Dauterman, W. C. 1981. Studies on the *in vitro* metabolism of methidathion by rat and mouse liver. *Pestic. Biochem. Physiol.* 15:105–19

28. El-Oshar, M. A., Dauterman, W. C. 1979. *In vitro* metabolism of O,O-diethyl-S-(N-methylcarbamoylmethyl) phosphorodithioate by mouse liver. *Pestic. Sci.* 10:14–18
29. Nomeir, A. A., Dauterman, W. C. 1979. *In vitro* metabolism of EPN and EPNO by mouse liver. *Pestic. Biochem. Physiol.* 10:190–96
30. Venera, G. D., Morisoli, L. S., Rodriguez, G. E. A. 1978. Degradation of parathion to paranitrophenol by livers of rats treated with phenobarbital. *Farmaco* 33:549
31. Robacker, K. M., Kulkarni, A. P., Hodgson, E. 1981. Pesticide induced changes in the mouse hepatic microsomal cytochrome P-450-dependent monooxygenase system and other enzymes. *J. Environ. Sci. Health B* 16:529–45
32. Kulkarni, A. P., Hodgson, E. 1982. Mouse liver microsomal hexose-6-phosphate dehydrogenase: NADPH generation and its utilization in monooxygenation reactions. *Biochem. Pharmacol.* 31:1131–37
33. Halpert, J., Hammond, D., Neal, R. A. 1980. Inactivation of purified rat liver cytochrome P-450 during the metabolism of parathion (diethyl p-nitrophenyl phosphorothionate). *J. Biol. Chem.* 255:1080–89
34. Lasker, J. M., Graham, D. G., Abou-Donia, M. B. 1982. Differential metabolism of O-ethyl-O-4-nitrophenyl-phenylphosphonothioate by rat and chicken hepatic microsomes. *Biochem. Pharmacol.* 31:1961–67
35. Hughes, P. B., Devonshire, A. L. 1982. The biochemical basis of resistance to organophosphorus insecticides in the sheep blow fly, *Lucillia cuprina. Pestic. Biochem. Physiol.* 18:289–97
36. Yawetz, A., Agosin, M., Perry, A. S. 1978. Components of electron transport system in the microsomal mixed function oxidase system in wild birds. *Pestic. Biochem. Physiol.* 8:44–52
37. Mullin, C. A., Croft, B. A., Strickler, K., Matsumura, F., Miller, J. R. 1982. Detoxication enzyme differences between a herbivorous and predatory mite. *Science* 217:1270–72
38. Yu, S. J., Berry, R. E., Terriere, L. C. 1979. Host plant stimulation of detoxifying enzymes in a phytophagus insect. *Pestic. Biochem. Physiol.* 12:280–84
39. Rose, H. A., Terriere, L. C. 1980. Microsomal oxidase activity of three blow fly species and its induction by phenobarbital and β-naphthoflavone. *Pestic. Biochem. Physiol.* 14:275–281

40. Farnsworth, D. E., Berry, R. E., Yu, S. J., Terriere, L. C. 1981. Aldrin epoxidase activity and cytochrome P-450 content of microsomes prepared from alfalfa and cabbage looper larvae fed various plant diets. *Pestic. Biochem. Physiol.* 15:158–165

41. Yu, S. J. 1982. Induction of microsomal oxidases by host plants in the fall armyworm, *Spodoptera frugiperda* (J. E. Smith). *Pestic. Biochem. Physiol.* 17: 59–67

42. Yu, S. J. 1982. Microsomal oxidases in the mole crickets, *Scapteriscus acletus*. Rehn and Hebard and *Scapteriscus vicinus* Scudder. *Pestic. Biochem. Physiol.* 17:170–76

43. Krieger, R. I., Gee, S. J., Miller, J. L., Thongsinthusak, T. 1976. Monooxygenase-catalyzed aldrin epoxidation and dihydroisodrin hydroxylation in monkey liver needle-biopsy specimens. Assay and properties. *Drug Metab. Dispos.* 4:28–34

44. Williams, F. M., Woodhouse, K. W., Middleton, D., Wright, P., James, O., Rawlins, M. D. 1982. Aldrin epoxidation kinetics in small samples of human liver. *Biochem. Pharmacol.* 31:3701–03

45. Parker, G. L., Bridges, J. W., Elcombe, C. R. 1983. Stimulation of cytochrome P-450-mediated monooxygenase activity in primary mouse hepatocyte cultures. *Toxicologist* 3:94 (Abstr. 373)

46. Elcombe, C. R., Canning, P. M., Parker, G. L. 1983. Xenobiotic metabolism in isolated human hepatocytes and microsomes. *Toxicologist* 3:161 (Abstr. 643)

47. Yu, S. J., Terriere, L. C. 1979. Cytocrome P-450 in insects. 1. Differences in the forms present in insecticide resistant and susceptible houseflies. *Pestic. Biochem. Physiol.* 12:239–48

48. Wolff, T., Greim, H., Huang, M. T., Miwa, G. T., Lu, A. Y. H. 1980. Aldrin epoxidation catalyzed by purified rat liver cytochromes P-450 and P-448. High selectivity for cytochrome P-450. *Eur. J. Biochem.* 111:545–51

49. Tanaka, K., Kurihara, N., Nakajima, M. 1979. Oxidative metabolism of tetrachlorocyclohexenes, pentachlorocyclohexenes, and hexochlorocyclohexenes by microsomes from rat liver and housefly abdomen. *Pestic. Biochem. Physiol.* 10:79–95

50. Brimfield, A. A., Street, J. C. 1979. Mammalian biotransformation of chlordane: *In vivo* and primary hepatic comparisons. *Ann. NY Acad. Sci.* 320:247–56

51. Tanaka, K., Kurihara, N., Nakajima, M. 1979. Oxidative metabolism of lindane and its isomers with microsomes from rat liver and housefly abdomen. *Pestic. Biochem. Physiol.* 10:96–103

52. Planche, G., Croisy, A., Malaveille, C., Tomatis, L., Bartsch, H. 1979. Metabolic and mutagenic studies on DDT and 15 derivatives. Detection of 1,1-bis(p-chlorophenyl)-2,2-dichloro-ethane and 1,1-bis(p-chlorophenyl)-2,2,2-trichloroethylacetate (Kelthane acetate) as mutagens in *Salmonella typhimurium* and of 1,1-bis(p-chlorophenyl) ethylene oxide, a likely metabolite, as an alkylation agent. *Chem. Biol. Inter.* 25:157–75

53. Glickman, A. H., Weitman, S. D., Lech, J. J. 1982. Differential toxicity of trans-permethrin in rainbow trout and mice. 1. Role of biotransformation. *Toxicol. Appl. Pharmacol.* 66:153–61

54. Shono, T., Ohsawa, K., Casida, J. E. 1979. Metabolism of trans and cis-permethrin, trans and cis-cypermethrin, and decamethrin by microsomal enzymes. *J. Agric. Food Chem.* 27:316–25

55. Ohsawa, K., Casida, J.E. 1980. Metabolism in rats of the potent knockdown pyrethroid kadethrin. *J. Agric. Food Chem.* 28:250–55

56. Chandurkar, P. S., Matsumura, F. 1979. Metabolism of toxaphene components in rats. *Arch. Environ. Contam. Toxicol.* 8:1–24

57. Chipman, J. K., Walker, C. H. 1981. Metabolism and route of excretion of the chloro-cyclodiene HCE in the pigeon. *Arch. Environ. Contam. Toxicol.* 10:755–64

58. Nakayama, H., Nakashima, T., Kurogochi, Y. 1982. Participation of cytochrome P-450 in nicotine oxidation. *Biochem. Biophys. Res. Commun.* 108: 200–05

59. Schievelbein, H. 1982. Nicotine, resorption and fate. *Pharmacol. Ther.* 18:233–48

60. Hodgson, E., Casida, J. E. 1960. Biological oxidation of N, N-dialkyl carbamates. *Biochim. Biophys. Acta* 42:184–86

61. Hodgson, E., Casida, J. E. 1961. Metabolism of N, N-dialkyl carbamates and related compounds by rat liver. *Biochem. Pharamcol.* 8:179–91

62. Dahl, A. R., Hadley, W. M. 1983. Formaldehyde production promoted by rat nasal cytochrome P-450-dependent monooxygenases with nasal decongestants essences, solvents, air pollutants, nicotine and cocaine as substrates. *Toxicol. Appl. Pharmacol.* 67:200–05

63. Nguyen, T-L., Gruenke, L. D., Castag-

noli, N. 1979. Metabolic oxidation of nicotine to chemically reactive intermediates. *J. Med. Chem.* 22:259–63

64. Braun, R., Schoneich, J., Weissflog, L., Dedek, W. 1983. Activity of organophosphorus insecticides in bacterial tests for mutagenicity and DNA repair—Direct alkylation versus metabolic activation and breakdown. II. O,O-demethyl -O- (1, 2-dibromo-2, 2- dichloroethyl)-phosphate and two O-ether derivatives of trichlorfon. *Chem.-Biol. Inter.* 43:361–70

65. Bulger, W. H., Muccitelli, R. M., Kupfer, D. 1978. Studies on the *in vivo* and *in vitro* estrogenic activities of methoxychlor and its metabolites. Role of hepatic monooxygenase in methoxychlor activation. *Biochem. Pharmacol.* 27:2417–23

66. Bulger, W. H., Temple, J. E., Kupfer, D. 1983. Covalent binding of [14C] methoxychlor metabolite(s) to rat liver microsomal components. *Toxicol. Appl. Pharmacol.* 68:367–74

67. Chadwick, R. W., Chadwick, C. J., Freal, J. J., Bryden, C. C. 1977. Comparative enzyme induction and lindane metabolism in rats pretreated with various organochlorine pesticides. *Xenobiotica* 7:235–46

68. Tanaka, K., Nakajima, M., Kurihara, N. 1981. The mechanisms of resistance to lindane and hexadeuterated lindane in the third Yumenoshima strain of housefly. *Pestic. Biochem. Physiol.* 16:149–57

69. Chadwick, R. W., Copeland, M. F., Mole, M. L., Nesnow, S., Cooke, N. 1981. Comparative effect of pretreatment with phenobarbital, Aroclor-1254, and β-naphthoflavone on the metabolism of lindane. *Pestic. Biochem. Physiol.* 15: 120–36

70. Fitzloff, J. F., Protig, J., Stein, K. 1982. Lindane metabolism by human and rat liver microsomes. *Xenobiotica* 12:197–202

71. Hajjar, N. P., Hodgson, E. 1980. Flavin adenine dinucleotide-dependent monooxygenase: Its role in the sulfoxidation of pesticides in mammals. *Science* 209: 1134–36

72. Hajjar, N. P. Hodgson, E. 1982. Sulfoxidation of thioether-containing pesticides by the flavin adenine dinucleotide-dependent monooxygenase of pig liver microsomes. *Biochem. Pharmacol.* 31: 745–52

73. Wing, K. D., Glickman, A. H., Casida, J. E. 1983. Oxidative bioactivation of S-alkyl phosphorothiolate pesticides: Stereospecificity of profenofos insecticide activation. *Science* 219:63–65

74. Tynes, R. E., Hodgson, E. 1983. The S-oxidation of thiobenzamide by the FAD-containing and cytochrome P-450-dependent monooxygenases of liver and lung microsomes. *Biochem. Pharmacol.* In press

75. Hajjar, N. P., Hodgson, E. 1982. The microsomal FAD-dependent monooxygenase as an activating enzyme: fonofos metabolism. In *Biological Reactive Intermediates II, Part B,* ed. R. Snyder, D. V. Parke, J. J. Kocsis, D. J. Jollow, C. G. Gibson, C. M. Witmer, p. 1245–53. New York: Plenum. 1476 pp.

76. McBain, J. B., Yamamoto, I., Casida, J. E. 1971. Mechanism of activation and deactivation of dyfonate (O-ethyl S-phenyl ethylphosphonodithioate) by rat liver microsomes. *Life Sci.* 10(2):947–57

77. McBain, J. B., Hoffman, L. J., Menn, J. J., Casida, J. E. 1971. Dyfonate metabolism studies 2. Metabolic pathway of O-ethyl S-phenyl ethylphosphonodithioate in rats. *Pestic. Biochem. Physiol.* 1:356–67

78. Lee, P. W., Allahyari, R., Fukuto, T. R. 1978. Studies on the chiral isomers of fonofos and fonofos oxon: *In vitro* metabolism. *Pestic. Biochem. Physiol.* 8: 158–69

79. Lee, P. W., Allahyari, R., Fukuto, T. R. 1978. Studies on the chiral isomers of fonofos and fonofos oxon: 3. *In vivo* metabolism. *Pestic. Biochem. Physiol.* 9:23–34

80. Ishaaya, I., Casida, J. E. 1980. Properties and toxicological significance of esterases hydrolyzing permethrin and cypermethrin in *Trichoplusia ni* larval gut and integument. *Pestic. Biochem. Physiol.* 14:178–84

81. Chang, C. K., Jordan, T. W. 1983. Inhibition of permethrin hydrolyzing esterases from *Wiseana cervinata* larvae. *Pestic. Biochem. Physiol.* 19:190–95

82. Soderlund, D. M., Abdel-Aal, Y. A. I., Helmuth, D. W. 1982. Selective inhibition of separate esterases in rat and mouse liver microsomes hydrolyzing malathion, trans-permethrin and cis-permethrin. *Pestic. Biochem. Physiol.* 17:162–69

83. Ruzo, L. O., Gaughan, L. C., Casida, J. E. 1981. Metabolism and degradation of the pyrethroids tralomethrin and tralocythrin in insects. *Pestic. Biochem. Physiol.* 15:137–42

84. Cole, L. M., Ruzo, L. O., Wood, E. J., Casida, J. E. 1982. Pyrethroid metabolism: Comparative fate in rats of tralomethrin, tralocythrin, deltamethrin and (1R, S)-cis-cypermethrin. *J. Agric. Food Chem.* 30:631–36

85. Bowers, W. S., Evans, P. H., Marsella, P. A., Soderlund, D. M., Bettarini, F. 1982. Natural and synthetic allotoxins: Suicide substrates for juvenile hormone biosynthesis. *Science* 217:647–48

86. Hsia, M. T. S., Grossman, S., Schrankel, K. R. 1981. Hepatotoxicity of the anti-juvenile hormone precocene II and the generation of dihydrodiol metabolites. *Chem.-Biol. Inter.* 37:265–77

87. Schrankel, K. R., Grossman, S. J., Hsia, M. T. S. 1982. Precocene II nephrotoxicity in the rat. *Toxicol. Lett.* 12:95–100

88. Pimprikar, G. D., Georghiou, G. P. 1979. Mechanisms of resistance to diflubenzuron in the housefly, *Musca domestica* (L.). *Pestic. Biochem. Physiol.* 12:10–22

89. Pimprikar, G. D., Georghiou, G. P. 1982. Effect of sesamex on the *in vivo* metabolism of diflubenzuron in larvae of susceptible and resistant strains of the housefly, *Musca domestica* (L.). *J. Agric. Food Chem.* 30:615–18

90. Opdycke, J. C., Miller, R. W., Menzer, R. E. 1982. Metabolism and fate of diflubenzuron in swine. *J. Agric. Food Chem.* 30:1223–27

91. Opdycke, J. C., Miller, R. W., Menzer, R. E. 1982. *In vivo* and liver microsomal metabolism of diflubenzuron by two breeds of chickens. *J. Agric. Food Chem.* 30:1227–33

92. Wolff, T., Demf, E., Wanders, H. 1979. Aldrin epoxidation, a highly sensitive indicator specific for cytochrome P-450-dependent monooxygenase activities. *Drug Metab. Dispos.* 7:301–05

93. Moldenke, A. F., Terriere, L. C. 1981. Cytochrome P-450 in insects 3. Increase in substrate binding by microsomes from phenobarbital-induced house flies. *Pestic. Biochem. Physiol.* 16:222–30

94. Rinsky, A., Perry, A. S. 1981. Induction of mixed function oxidase system in the liver of the barn owl *Tyto alba* by PCBs. *Pestic. Biochem. Physiol.* 16:72–78

95. Pollock, G. A., Krasnec, J. P., Niemann, B. R. 1983. Rat hepatic microsomal enzyme induction by pretreatment with toxaphene and toxaphene fractions. *J. Toxicol. Envir. Health* 11:355–65

96. Dorough, H. W., Huhtanen, K. Marshall, T. C., Bryant, H. E. 1978. Fate of endosulfan in rats and toxicological considerations of apolar metabolites. *Pestic. Biochem. Physiol.* 8:241–49

97. Townsend, B. A., Carlson, G. P. 1981. Effect of halogenated benzene on the toxicity and metabolism of malathion, malaoxon, parathion, and paraoxon in mice. *Toxicol. Appl. Pharmacol.* 60:52–61

98. Bradford, W. L., Nakatsugawa, T. 1982. Perfusion analysis of periportal and centrilobular metabolism of paraoxon in the rat liver. *Pestic. Biochem. Physiol.* 18:298–303

99. Hodgson, E., Kulkarni, A. P., Fabacher, D. L., Robacker, K. M. 1980. Induction of hepatic drug metabolizing enzymes in mammals by pesticides: A review. *J. Envir. Health* B15:723–54

100. Nakayama, H., Nakashima, T., Kurogochi, Y. 1982. Heterogeneity of hepatic nicotine oxidase. *Biochim. Biophys. Acta* 715:254–57

101. Hutson, D. H., Wright, A. S. 1980. The effect of hepatic microsomal monooxygenase induction on the metabolism and toxicity of the organophosphorus insecticide chlorfenvinphos. *Chem.-Biol. Inter.* 31:93–101

102. Neskovic, N. K. 1979. Effects of subacute feeding of carbaryl on mixed function oxidase and on acute toxicity of parathion and propoxur in rats. *Environ. Res.* 20:148–53

103. Ebel, R. E. 1982. Alterations in microsomal cytochrome P-450-catalyzed reactions as a function of chlordecone (kepone) induction. *Pestic. Biochem. Physiol.* 18:113–21

104. Mehendale, H. M. 1981. Chlordecone-induced hepatic dysfunction. *J. Toxicol. Environ. Health.* 8:743–55

105. Cianflone, D. J., Hewitt, W. R., Villenneuve, D. C., Plaa, G. L. 1980. Role of biotransformation in the alterations of chloroform hepatotoxicity produced by kepone and mirex. *Toxicol. Appl. Pharmacol.* 53:140–49

106. Mehendale, H. M., Onoda, K., Curtis, L. R., Ho, I. K. 1979. Induction of hepatic mixed function oxidases by photomirex. *J. Agric. Food. Chem.* 27:1416–18

107. Chambers, J. E., Trevathan, C. A. 1983. Effect of mirex, dechlorinated mirex derivatives and chlordecone on microsomal mixed-function oxidase activity and other hepatic parameters. *Toxicol. Lett.* 16:109–15

108. Havkin-Frenkel, D., Rosen, J. D., Gallo, M. A. 1983. Enhancement of hydroxyl radical formation in rat liver microsomes by mirex. *Toxicol. Lett.* 15:219–23

109. Oesch, F., Friedberg, T., Herbst, M., Paul, W., Wilhelm, N., Bentley, P. 1982. Effects of lindane treatment on drug metabolizing enzymes and liver weight of CF1 mice in which it evoked

hepatomas and in non-susceptible rodents. *Chem.-Biol. Inter.* 40:1–14

110. Fennell, T. R., Sweatman, B. C., Bridges, J. W. 1980. The induction of hepatic cytochrome P-450 in C57 B1/10 and DBA/2 mice by isosafrole and piperonyl butoxide. A comparative study with other inducing agents. *Chem.-Biol. Inter.* 31:189–201

111. Cook, J. C., Hodgson, E. 1983. Induction of cytochrome P-450 by methylenedioxyphenyl compounds: Importance of the methylene carbon. *Toxicol. Appl. Pharmacol.* 68:131–39

112. Tennekes, H. A., Wright, A. S., Dix, K. M., Koeman, J. H. 1981. Effects of dieldrin, diet and bedding on enzyme function and tumor incidence in livers of male CF-1 mice. *Cancer Res.* 41:3615–20

113. Triolo, A. J., Lang, W. R., Coon, J. M., Lindstrom, D., Herr, D. L. 1982. Effect of the insecticides toxaphene and carbaryl on induction of lung tumors by benzo[a]pyrene in the mouse. *J. Toxicol. Environ. Health* 9:637–49

114. Madhukar, B. V., Matsumura, F. 1979. Comparison of induction patterns of rat hepatic microsomal mixed-function oxidases by pesticides and related chemicals. *Pestic. Biochem. Physiol.* 11:301–08

115. Madhukar, B. V., Matsumura, F. 1981. Differences in the nature of induction of mixed-function oxidase systems of the rat liver among phenobarbital, DDT, 3-methylcholanthrene and TCDD. *Toxicol. Appl. Pharmacol.* 61:109–18

116. Wilkinson, C. F., Murray, M., Marcus, C. B. 1984. Interaction of methylenedioxyphenyl compounds with cytochrome P-450 and microsomal oxidation. *Rev. Biochem. Toxicol.* 6: In press

117. Bigley, W. S., Vinson, S. B. 1979. Effects of piperonyl butoxide and DEF on the metabolism of methoprene by the imported fire ant, *Solenopsis invicta* Buren. *Pestic. Biochem. Physiol.* 10:14–22

118. Fisher, C. W., Mayer, R. T. 1982. Characterization of housefly microsomal mixed function oxidases: inhibition by juvenile hormone I and piperonyl butoxide. *Toxicology* 24:15–31

119. Fuhremann, T. W., Lichtenstein, E. P. 1979. Insecticide toxicity and degradation in houseflies as affected by naturally occurring food plant components. *J. Agric. Food Chem.* 27:87–91

120. Mukerjee, S. K., Saxena, V. S., Tomar, S. S. 1979. New methylenedioxyphenyl synergists for pyrethrins. *J. Agric. Food Chem.* 27:1209–11

121. Ortiz de Montellano, P. R., Mathews, J. M. 1981. Inactivation of hepatic cytochrome P-450 by a 1,2,3-benzothiadiazole insecticide synergist. *Biochem. Pharmacol.* 31:1138–41

122. Halpert, J., Neal, R. A. 1981. Inactivation of rat liver cytochrome P-450 by the suicide substrates parathion and chloramphenicol. *Drug Metab. Rev.* 12:239–59

123. Sultatos, L. G., Murphy, S. D. 1983. Kinetic analyses of the microsomal biotransformation of the phosphorothioate insecticides chlorpyrifos and parathion. *Fund. Appl. Toxicol.* 3:16–21

124. Ecobichon, D. J., Zelt, D. 1979. The acute toxicity of fenitrothion in weanling rats and effects on tissue esterases and mono-oxygenases. *Toxicology* 13:287–96

125. Jordan, T. W., Smith, J. N. 1981. Inhibition of housefly oxidative detoxication by phthaleins, fluoresceins and related compounds. *Xenobiotica* 11:1–7

126. Marnett, L. J., Eling, T. E. 1983. Cooxidation during prostaglandin biosynthesis: A pathway for the metabolic activation of xenobiotics. In *Reviews in Biochemical Toxicology*, ed. E. Hodgson, J. R. Bend, R. M. Philpot, p. 135–72. New York: Elsevier Biomedical

Ann. Rev. Pharmacol. Toxicol. 1984. 24:43–64

THE EFFECTS OF DRUGS ON MEMBRANE FLUIDITY

Dora B. Goldstein

Department of Pharmacology, Stanford University School of Medicine, Stanford, California 94305

INTRODUCTION

Drugs will find their way into membranes. Any foreign molecules will distribute into the hydrophobic regions of cells according to their lipid solubilities, and it is reasonable to predict that their presence in adequate concentrations will disrupt the structure of the bilayer. Some drugs never reach effective concentrations in membranes because they are intercepted by chemical binding to sites in the aqueous phase. Such drugs may have dramatic pharmacological effects at doses much too low to affect membranes, so their membrane effects can only be observed in vitro. Drugs that are simple chemical molecules are likely to disrupt membranes because they have little effect in the aqueous phase and will do no harm until they partition into membranes in sufficient amounts. Some of these drugs are highly lipid soluble, but great lipid solubility is not a prerequisite for membrane action. All that is required is that the membrane effect not be preempted by stronger effects at lower doses.

This review will deal primarily with anesthetics and similar drugs, such as alcohols, for which we have long-standing evidence of action in some lipid phase as well as new information about the nature of the interaction. Anesthetics are the best known members of this class of drugs but they are not the only such agents.

It may be premature to take sides in the controversy about whether membrane lipids or membrane proteins are the site of drug action. The change that concerns us is physical and can occur in any hydrophobic phase. Drugs with high lipid solubility will enter hydrophobic regions of both proteins and lipids in the core of the membrane. Although it is too early to explain exactly how the hydrophobic interaction affects function, it is reasonable to predict that disrup-

43

tion of protein function will result from disorder in any of the hydrophobic regions. Some proteins presumably will be more affected than others.

Drugs that have receptors may have hydrophobic actions as well. Benzodiazepines and neuroleptics, for example, have high lipid solubilities that must affect their availability at the site of action. It is not yet known whether the actual binding sites are in the aqueous phase or in the membrane, although the natural ligands, such as GABA or dopamine, must bind in the aqueous phase since they are highly hydrophilic. The intramembrane concentrations of the lipophilic drugs are often hundreds of times higher than the aqueous concentration, a fact that is not always considered in binding experiments. Some of the equations for dealing with these drugs have been worked out (1), but the field is largely undeveloped.

Meaning of Membrane Fluidity

The concept of membrane fluidity lacks a precise definition but it can nevertheless be useful. In general, the term means a combination of different types of mobility of membrane components. These include the following: flexibility of acyl chains, lateral diffusion of molecules in the plane of the membrane, transverse diffusion of molecules from one monolayer to the other, and phase transitions leading to lateral phase separations. These are all anisotropic motions and cannot be considered measures of viscosity, which is a characteristic of isotropic resistance to flow. Any of these measures of fluidity may be affected by drugs.

The motion of phospholipid acyl chains in membranes can be observed with several commonly used techniques, such as nuclear magnetic resonance (NMR) and electron spin resonance (ESR). This motion is the basis for most pharmacological work on membrane fluidity. The acyl chains can be selectively deuterated at different positions, allowing the use of deuterium NMR to observe their motion. Spin labels, with nitroxide groups attached at different positions along a fatty acid chain, are used for the same purpose. Results of tests using both techniques agree that there exists a gradient of flexibility in the chains from the surface toward the core of the bilayer, with increasing freedom of motion near the center. However, the shape of the gradient appears different with each technique (2, 3). Order parameters used in NMR and ESR techniques are related to the angle of a particular chain segment to the membrane surface. The cumulative motion of segments produces the flexibility gradient. Transgauche isomerization about carbon-carbon bonds causes evanescent "kinks" in the chain (4) and cis double bonds produce permanent kinks. In this way, spaces are created and parts of adjacent chains can move in and out. Drugs can affect the probability of trans-gauche isomerizations (as cholesterol does, for example) and thus affect the fluidity gradient.

Lateral diffusion of phospholipids along the surfaces of the bilayer occurs rapidly, with diffusion constants on the order of 10^{-8} cm^2 sec^{-1} for phospholipids (5). Proteins also diffuse laterally; their rates are slower and more variable than those of lipids and some proteins are anchored in place by the cytoskeleton (6). Lateral diffusion of proteins is important for coupling receptors to enzyme catalytic units and in the ability of bivalent ligands (such as calcium or antibodies) to attach to the membrane surface. We have few experimental data on the effects of drugs on lateral diffusion in membranes, but it is reasonable to expect that drugs will alter diffusion rates and that membrane function will be affected.

Transverse diffusion from one surface of the bilayer to the other is extremely slow in model membranes (7) but may be faster in biomembranes (8). Since the different phospholipid head groups are of different size and charge, flipflop might serve to change the membrane properties substantially. A limited amount of flipflop is mediated by the phospholipid methyltransferases described by Hirata & Axelrod (9) that convert phosphatidylethanolamine to phosphatidylcholine and move it from the inner to the outer monolayer. The change in membrane fluidity reported to accompany this activity is discussed below.

Lateral phase separations must be critical to events occurring within membrane structures, but precise evidence on this topic is limited to model membranes of known composition. Shimshick & McConnell (10) demonstrated the coexistence of solid and fluid phases in binary mixtures of pure phospholipids at suitable temperatures, and there is evidence from freeze fracture studies (5) and fluorescence lifetimes (11) for patches of gel in otherwise fluid biomembranes. Exogenous compounds can increase the proportion of fluid lipid without changing the rate of lateral diffusion in the fluid phase (11). Since proteins are probably excluded from the gel domains, any increase in the amount of fluid lipid will decrease the effective concentration of proteins, which must affect cooperative interactions and coupling.

Thus the evidence to be discussed below that drugs "fluidize" or "disorder" membranes can be interpreted to mean that the drugs decrease the packing density of phospholipids, allowing all components of the membrane to jostle each other more often but less strongly than in the drug-free state. A quite different interpretation is that the frequency and vigor of such collisions is unaffected in the fluid domains but more of the membrane is free to engage in them. Either effect would have important implications for the function of membrane-bound proteins.

ENTRY OF DRUGS INTO MEMBRANES

Bulk Solvents

The lipid solubility of drugs is measured as their partition at equilibrium between aqueous and organic phases. A nonpolar or amphiphilic solute disrupts the network of hydrogen bonds in water and as a result is driven into a more favorable energy state in the organic solvent (12). In an initial approach to an investigation of drug concentrations in membranes, octanol is a useful model solvent; it accommodates both hydrogen-bonding and nonpolar solutes (13). The solubilities of hundreds of compounds in various solvents have been converted to octanol:water partition coefficients by Leo et al (14) using generally applicable equations. Lindenberg provides an unusually complete set of oil:water partition coefficients for alkanols (15). Solubility data can be predicted to some extent, because each moiety of a solute molecule contributes an incremental factor to the partition coefficient (16). A factor of two or three is usually observed for each additional methylene group (17), but the effect of additional hydroxyl groups varies widely in different solvents.

Model Membranes

The solvent properties of phospholipid bilayers resemble those of octanol, although lecithin is more like the lower alcohols than like octanol, at least for a series of hydrogen-bonding solutes (17). The measured solubility of any compound in a bilayer must be an average of its concentrations at different distances from the surface. Furthermore, the structured bilayer (unlike octanol) differentiates among solutes of different molecular shapes. For example, lecithin discriminates against branched solutes more than a bulk solvent does (17).

Biomembranes

Measurement of the solubility of drugs in biomembranes is more complex. Roth & Seeman (18) measured membrane:buffer partition coefficients for several alcohols and phenols in red cell ghosts and in some nerve and muscle membranes and found them to be about 20% of the corresponding octanol:water partition coefficients. Two negatively charged drugs, valerate and pentobarbital, were about ten times less soluble in membranes than in octanol. According to Diamond & Katz (17), the erythrocyte membrane is similar to dimyristoylphosphatidylcholine as a solvent for drugs, although the biomembrane is slightly more hydrophobic than lecithin and its additional surface charge (sialic acid and protein) must be taken into account. The partition coefficient of benzyl alcohol in erythrocytes increases at high drug concentrations (contrary to the definition of the partition coefficient) and also increases slightly with temperature (19), suggesting that a more fluid membrane may accommodate more drug.

The octanol:water partition coefficient of charged compounds is usually measured for the undissociated drug at least 4 pH units away from pK (14), and the overall partition at physiological pH can be calculated on the assumption that only the uncharged form of the drug enters the membrane. However, Miller & Yu (20) found that the charged form of pentobarbital has an appreciable solubility in egg phosphatidylcholine vesicles.

Amphiphilic drug molecules that have both polar and nonpolar moieties may accumulate at the surface of the bilayer, where they may act in both the aqueous and the membrane phase. The studies of Bienvenüe et al (21) illustrate the factors that affect the activity of such drugs. The potency of spin-labeled long-chain acylcholines in displacing acetylcholine from its membrane-bound receptor depends on the availability of bulk lipid to take up the drug as well as on its binding affinity to the receptor. Seeman's studies of the dopamine receptors (22) illustrate the same point.

Conrad & Singer (23) were unable to detect any entry of amphiphilic drugs into biomembranes under conditions where partition into liposomes was easily measurable. They used a gentle filtration technique rather than centrifugation. They concluded that a large internal pressure in biomembranes prevents uptake of drugs. However, there has been no confirmation of this surprising finding, and other laboratories have since reported contradictory results (24, 25). The known uptake of amphiphilic spin labels and fluorescent dyes, which can be measured in biomembranes without separating the phases, argues against the internal pressure concept.

Rottenberg et al (26) reported much higher partition coefficients of ethanol in mitochondrial and synaptosomal membranes than predicted from Seeman's conversion factor or from the known partition of longer-chain alkanols.

From the Meyer-Overton relation of 40 mmoles of anesthetic per kg of membrane to produce local anesthesia (27), one can calculate a mole fraction of 0.05 for the drug in membrane lipid (assuming a membrane that is half protein and half lipid by weight and a cholesterol/phospholipid molar ratio of 0.5) General anesthesia occurs at 10- to 20-fold lower membrane concentrations (27), about one drug molecule per 200 lipid molecules. Many studies of drug effects in membranes have been done at drug concentrations that are orders of magnitude higher than this.

The Meyer-Overton concept that anesthetic potency varies with lipid solubility has been repeatedly confirmed (27). Recently, McCreery & Hunt (28) and Lyon et al (29) used the Hansch equations and Seeman's factor to calculate membrane:buffer partition coefficients for many drugs and reported good correlations of central nervous system (CNS)-depressant activity with solubility in biomembranes.

DRUG EFFECTS MEASURED IN VITRO

Many different physicochemical techniques have been used to provide evidence that anesthetic agents and similar drugs have a biophysical action on cell membranes that can often be described as a disordering or fluidizing effect.

Nuclear Magnetic Resonance

Nuclear magnetic resonance (NMR) is a versatile but insensitive technique that has not yet made its main contributions to pharmacology. The first experiments on membrane disorder were done with proton NMR to study the effect of benzyl alcohol on red cell membranes (19). No probe was needed; the signal was derived from the drug itself. Rapid isotropic motion of the benzyl alcohol in solution produced a narrow signal line. On addition of erythrocytes the line broadened, indicating that the motion of the drug was constrained in the red cell membrane. However, when progressively higher concentrations of the drug were added, the line narrowed again, showing that the alcohol had increased the fluidity of its environment in the membrane. The membrane proteins did not contribute to this effect, as it occurred equally well in extracts of the membrane lipids. At very high drug concentrations, however, the membranes became stiffer, apparently because of irreversible changes in the proteins. Metcalfe et al (19) were the first to recognize that membrane disorder is the result of the addition of anesthetic agents.

In lecithin liposomes with selectively deuterated acyl chains, deuterium NMR can be used to locate a drug effect. The disordering effect of benzyl alcohol is maximal at midchain, even though benzyl alcohol is a fairly water-soluble compound and might be expected to remain near the membrane surface (30). The ordering effect of cholesterol is also maximal at midchain. The NMR data allow calculation of the orientation of each C-C segment of the acyl chain, from which it can be seen that benzyl alcohol decreases the thickness of the bilayer and cholesterol increases it. Drug concentrations above 0.5 mole of drug per mole of lipid were used in this study; no effects could be seen at anesthetic concentrations.

Vanderkooi et al (31) used proton NMR to show that anesthetic drugs increase the proportion of fluid lipid in phosphatidylcholine bilayers and in sarcoplasmic reticulum. Addition of halothane or chloroform increased the resolution of peaks attributed to the fatty acid chains of melted phospholipids, indicating increased mobility of the chains.

^{31}P NMR is a suitable technique for observing the presence of nonbilayer forms of phospholipids. Cullis and co-workers (32) have described the formation of hexagonal H_{II} forms of phosphatidylethanolamine and cardiolipin. It is not known whether these forms exist in vivo, but if they do they may promote membrane fusion. Calcium facilitates the formation of H_{II} and dibucaine (used here at a 1:1 molar ratio with phospholipid) antagonizes the calcium effect, stabilizing the bilayer form.

Electron Spin Resonance

Because of its sensitivity and its versatility, electron spin resonance (ESR) has been the most useful technique for studying drug effects on the physical properties of membranes. For excellent discussions of ESR principles and techniques in biological work, see McConnell (5), Griffith & Jost (33), and Smith & Butler (34). Suitable spin labels are derivatives of natural membrane components, such as fatty acids, phospholipids, or sterols, to which a nitroxide group is attached. Hydrophilic probes and those that bind to proteins have been less often used in pharmacological studies. The orientation and mobility of the probe are measured from the spectra by the amplitude of the peaks or the distances (splittings) between them. A commonly used measure is the order parameter of Hubbell & McConnell (35), which is related to the time-averaged angle that the probe nitroxide axis makes with the bilayer surface and is thus a measure of the flexibility of the probe. By definition, order parameters vary from 0 (completely free to move) to 1 (total rigidity).

GENERAL ANESTHETICS   Gaseous anesthetics reduce the order of pure lipid bilayers and biomembranes. Halothane and methoxyflurane have equal potencies at equivalent intramembrane concentrations (36) and are equally effective at different depths in phospholipid bilayer, as measured by phospholipids spin-labled at the 6 and 10 position of the acyl chain. The disordering can be measured at surgical concentrations (37), is not stereospecific (38), and can be partially reversed (as can anesthesia itself) by high hydrostatic pressure (39). In synaptic membranes, a greater disordering effect of halothane was seen deep in the bilayer (16-doxylstearic acid probe) than near the surface (5-doxyl) (40). These biomembranes were more sensitive to disordering by halothane than were lipids extracted from them. Concentration-related disordering of phosphatidylcholine bilayers and synaptic membranes is caused by other anesthetic agents, including trichloroethanol, α- (but not β-) chloralose, urethane, and ketamine (40, 41).

Rosenberg and coworkers reported an unusual ordering effect of halothane at low concentrations in lecithin vesicles or synaptic membranes (42, 43), reversing to disordering at higher (clinically irrelevant) concentrations. The ordering was detected by increased order parameters of 5-doxylstearic acid and by a decreased rate of lateral diffusion of the probe, measured by spin exchange. Boggs et al (44), using relatively insensitive methods, were unable to detect an effect of halothane, chloroform, or diethyl ether on order parameters of 5- , 8- , or 12-doxyl fatty acid spin labels.

LOCAL ANESTHETICS   The membrane order of oriented lipid films that contain very little cholesterol increases dramatically on addition of low concentrations of local anesthetics (45, 46). Calcium potentiates the ordering. The extent of ordering by tetracaine is greater at low than at high pH, suggesting that the ionized form of the drug orders the lipid. By contrast, at high drug concentrations and high pH, the undissociated drugs disorder the membranes (45). Hubbell et al (47) found that tetracaine and xylocaine had a mild disordering effect in red cell membranes, and Rosenberg et al (43) did not observe an effect of lidocaine on synaptic plasma membranes or liposomes. Ionizable local anesthetics probably will not show the same relation of membrane disorder to anesthetic potency as do neutral drugs—some specificity of binding is to be expected since these drugs interact with anionic sites on the cytoplasmic surface of the membrane (48).

Chlorpromazine has a local anesthetic action at concentrations far above those required for binding to dopamine receptors. At 0.1 mM it disorders erythrocyte membranes (49) but orders low-cholesterol brain lipids as other local anesthetics do (46). Much higher concentrations disorder the lipids. These findings agree with the observations of Pang & Miller (50), who reported that the ordering effect of chlorpromazine in low-cholesterol liposomes reversed to a disordering effect at higher cholesterol concentrations.

Propranolol is a cationic drug with a local anesthetic action independent of its adrenergic blocking effect. It dissolves in (or binds to) acidic phospholipids extremely strongly and has an ordering effect in liposomes of phosphatidylserine or phosphatidic acid, but it is much less soluble in neutral phospholipids and does not perturb them (51). Red cell membranes are slightly disordered by propranolol and some weakly immobilized protein sites are converted to strongly immobilized sites by the drug. The ordering effect is apparently not seen in red cells because of their high cholesterol content and low amounts of acidic phospholipids (52).

STEROID ANESTHETICS   These compounds show dramatic stereospecificity in their anesthetic potencies and corresponding differences in their effects on order parameters in high-cholesterol lecithin liposomes (53). The orientation of the 3-OH is critical; 3α-hydroxy-5α-pregnane-11,20-dione is a potent anesthetic and has a strong disordering effect, but the corresponding 3β isomer is inactive in both systems. (Other pairs of steroid isomers show less striking differences.) A convulsant steroid lacks disordering activity. These findings add weight to the hypothesis that hydrogen bonding is an important component of membrane perturbing action of some drugs (54) and that the disordering potency may depend partly on the orientation of a hydrogen bond.

CANNABINOIDS   The psychoactive cannabinoids disorder high-cholesterol phosphatidylcholine bilayers (55), but the inactive cannabinol is reported to order (55) or disorder (50) them.

BARBITURATES   It is not yet established whether barbiturates have relevant membrane-disordering actions. An ordering effect of pentobarbital in low-cholesterol phospholipids (46, 50, 56) or thiopental in synaptic membranes (43) has been reported. Unlike the effect of local anesthetics, this was not potentiated by calcium (46). However, the lipid composition of the bilayer strongly affects its response to barbiturates, and the ordering effect of barbiturates, like that of chlorpromazine and cannabinol, reverses to disordering when a high-cholesterol membrane is used (50, 56). Increasing the phosphatidic acid content of the vesicles from 4% to 10% changed the action of barbiturates from disorder to order. Three barbiturates were among the drugs that Pang et al (41) found to disorder spin-labeled lipid vesicles that contained 33 mol% cholesterol. In that study thiopental and pentobarbital seemed to be more potent as anesthetics in vivo than could be accounted for by their disordering potency in vitro, as would be expected if the drugs act via a specific receptor.

BENZYL ALCOHOL   Benzyl alcohol is often chosen as a prototype disordering drug for studies of membrane function. It consistently disorders membranes, but function may not change in parallel. Low concentrations of benzyl alcohol reduce order parameters and stimulate adenylate cyclase and sodium-potassium ATPase activities in liver plasma membranes (57). Higher concentrations inhibit the enzymes, whereas the disordering is stronger than ever. A problem arises when enzymes are inhibited by a disordering drug. For example, benzyl alcohol decreases order and inhibits glucose uptake in adipocyte membranes (58). It is unlikely that disorder causes the inhibition of glucose transport because an increase in temperature has the opposite effect. Drug-induced disorder can explain enzyme malfunction only if the enzyme is stimulated by the drug. Enzymes that are inhibited by disordering drugs are almost always stimulated by warming. For such enzymes the disorder hypothesis fails.

ALIPHATIC ALCOHOLS   The normal alcohols of length 3 to 8 carbon atoms increase the mobility of a spin label in phosphatidylserine vesicles (59), in lipids extracted from erythrocytes or from brain white matter (60), and in mitochondrial (61) or synaptic (29, 40) membranes. The log of the potency of the alcohols, like the log of their partition coefficient, is directly proportional to the chain length. Butanol is more potent in whole membranes (whether synaptic or mitochondrial) than in extracted phospholipids (40, 61).

Normal, branched, and secondary alcohols up to 8 carbons in length all disorder biomembranes, with potencies determined by their lipid solubilities (29). The magnitude of the effect is linearly related to the drug concentration, as would be expected for drugs that act by partitioning into their site of action. This is in contrast to the logarithmic dose response curve of drugs that act by binding to a specific receptor. For alkanols up to hexanol, the disordering potencies correlate well with hypnotic doses in mice. Heptanol and octanol are less potent; they may be too water-insoluble to be delivered to the brain in effective concentrations by intraperitoneal injections.

The alkanols up to decanol uniformly disorder membranes and are anesthetics (62, 63). Longer chains, however, are weak fluidizers (59, 63) or increase the order of membranes (62). They are not anesthetics in tadpoles (63). They do block nerve conduction in the system used by Richards et al (62) but with latencies of several hours. Pringle et al (63) and Lyon et al (29) explain the cutoff in anesthetic potency simply as an inability to achieve adequate membrane concentrations in vivo because of the very low water solubility of these drugs. Alternatively, Richards et al (62) conclude that anesthetic molecules (which are of many different chemical types) occupy multiple receptor sites in the hydrophobic regions of proteins. No data are presented to demonstrate a direct interaction with proteins.

Long-chain alkenols are more potent anesthetics than their saturated counterparts, perhaps because they perturb the bilayer more strongly. Alkenols with different orientation of the double bond differ in disordering potency in liposomes made of egg lecithin with 33 mol% cholesterol but they have the same anesthetic potency in tadpoles (63). This discrepancy may be explained by the observation that the isomers are equipotent in disordering liposomes with 50 mol% cholesterol.

ETHANOL   Because of its medical importance, ethanol has received extra attention in studies of membranes. Chin & Goldstein (64) showed that sublethal concentrations of ethanol reduce the order parameter of spin-labeled membranes. The effect is significant with mouse erythrocyte membranes and synaptosomal plasma membranes (but not with myelin) and is also seen in egg lecithin bilayers (65). The effect is stronger in the core of the bilayer than near the surface, as shown by comparing the motion of the 5- and 12-doxylstearic acid probes in model membranes (65) and in synaptosomal membranes (66), as previously reported for butanol (40). However, this does not tell us where the drug molecules actually reside, since we can only see where their effects are strongest. Ethanol is probably held near the membrane surface by hydrogen bonding. Its relatively slight disordering effect at that site may be magnified along the flexible acyl chains. Cholesterol, known to be located near the membrane surface (67), also has a greater effect on order parameters with 12-doxyl than with 5-doxylstearic acid (65).

In general, the more fluid regions in the membrane core are more easily perturbed by any agent than are the stiffer surface regions (65). This holds for the disordering effect of increased temperature and of ethanol and for the ordering effect of cholesterol (65). Furthermore, cholesterol, an ordering agent, blocks the ability of ethanol to disorder a lecithin bilayer (65). These observations suggest that ethanol has its greatest effect in regions of the membrane that are already relatively fluid, and also that the lipid composition of local regions of membranes may determine their vulnerability to ethanol.

Correlations between disorder and intoxication suggest a causal relation. Genetic correlations carry the idea further. Inherited traits greatly affect the sensitivity of mice to acute effects of ethanol, and the differential sensitivity is expressed in their membranes. For example, the most ethanol-sensitive individual mice in a genetically heterogeneous population have brain membranes that are disordered to a greater extent by ethanol in vitro than are membranes from ethanol-resistant mice (68). Furthermore, two lines of mice that have been selectively bred for differential sensitivity to the hypnotic effects of ethanol also show differential sensitivity of their membranes to ethanol in vitro (68). The correlation between disorder and intoxication also holds up when it is shown (see below) that ethanol-tolerant mice have brain membranes that are resistant to the disordering effects of ethanol in vitro.

Fluorescence Polarization

The polarization of fluorescence emitted by a membrane-bound dye reflects the mobility of the probe in its hydrophobic environment. Dye molecules immobilized in a rigid matrix and excited by polarized light emit fluorescence that is polarized parallel to the exciting light. To the extent that they move during the few nanoseconds' lifetime of the excited state the polarization of the emission is reduced (69). Thus, a decrease in fluorescence polarization (sometimes expressed as fluorescence anisotropy) is a measure of disordering. This technique is comparable to ESR in sensitivity to the membrane-disordering effects of drugs. It has been less used, perhaps because the available probes cannot be as accurately directed to exact locations in the bilayer. The most commonly used probe is 1,6-diphenyl-1,3,5-hexatriene (DPH), a rod-shaped molecule. Whether it remains oriented parallel to acyl chains or can "lie down" in the core of the membrane is unknown, and it is not yet certain whether DPH is distributed evenly throughout the bilayer. Stubbs et al (70) have shown that DPH partitions equally between liposomes and rod outer segment disk membranes, where essentially all of the lipid is associated with proteins, suggesting that this probe monitors different hydrophobic regions equally well. Klausner et al (71), in studies of the heterogeneity of fluorescence lifetimes of DPH, suggested that 10 or 20% of the signal comes from the edges of gel domains in biomembranes.

Jacobson & Wobschall (72) provide a thoughtful analysis of fluorescence polarization in lipid bilayers, including the reasons that it is inappropriate to convert the polarization or anisotropy data into units of microviscosity (poise). Shinitzky and co-workers (73) used the Perrin equation to convert polarization to viscosity, using a standard oil for calibration. However, this concept is only applicable to isotropic motion where the volume of rotation of the probe is the same as in the oil, and not in a bilayer where motion of the probe is anisotropic.

It is important to know whether the drug changes the lifetime of the excited state. The lifetime is the period during which motion of the dye can be detected; if the lifetime is shortened (for example, by energy transfer from the dye to the drug), the motion will appear to be slower and any disorder caused by the drug will be underestimated.

ANESTHETICS   Several inhalation anesthetics can disorder phospholipid vesicles (31). With the exception of halothane, which contains a fluorescence-quenching bromine atom, they do not affect the fluorescence lifetime of the dye pyrene. Dibucaine disorders acidic phospholipids (74); it partitions into acidic phospholipids much more strongly than to neutral phospholipids. Calcium orders the membranes and antagonizes the drug-induced disorder. Dibucaine, itself a fluorophore, quenches fluorescence and shortens the lifetime of DPH. Thus, an increased rate of probe rotation can be demonstrated after correcting for the altered lifetime, whereas the polarization actually increases in the presence of the drug.

BARBITURATES   Barbiturates reduce the polarization of DPH fluorescence in mouse synaptosomal membranes, with potencies proportional to their lipid solubilities (75). Both anesthetic and convulsant barbiturates disorder the membranes, and (unlike anesthesia) there is no stereospecificity. Intact synaptosomal plasma membranes are more easily disordered than lipids extracted from them, and a lipid extract containing only phospholipids (no cholesterol) is ordered by the drug, in agreement with Pang & Miller's ESR data on pure phospholipid vesicles (50).

BENZYL ALCOHOL   Cherenkevich et al (76) used DPH polarization data to calculate an order parameter in macrophage membranes. The order was reduced by benzyl alcohol in parallel with a change in oxidase activity.

ALIPHATIC ALCOHOLS   Kutchai and coworkers have studied a series of normal alkanols in red cells, using DPH polarization to measure disordering and relate it to changes in membrane function such as water permeability (77) or sugar transport (78). As expected, the intrinsic order of the membrane was increased by extra cholesterol, and the disordering potency of alkanols (pentanol through heptanol) increased with chain length. Despite their opposite effects on fluidity, cholesterol and alkanols sometimes had the same effect on function, so it was not possible to explain the relation between fluidity and the particular transport system under study. The alkanols from 4 to 8 carbons reduce the fluorescence anisotropy of DPH in chick embryo heart microsomes, an effect that is proportional to the lipid solubility of the drugs (79).

ETHANOL   Using fluorescence anisotropy of DPH, Harris & Schroeder (80) have shown that ethanol disorders biomembranes. In synaptosomal plasma membranes, the effects of 20 mM ethanol are significant, but lipids extracted from membranes are much less sensitive. Myelin is less affected than the plasma membranes. A probe of the membrane surface, 1-aminopyrene, is not much affected by ethanol, confirming ESR data about the relative sensitivity at different depths in the membrane.

A high concentration of ethanol, 1.8 M, can reduce the fluorescence lifetime of pyrene in phosphatidylcholine vesicles (31), but 0.32 M ethanol does not affect the fluorescence lifetime of DPH in synaptosomal plasma membranes (75).

PHOSPHOLIPID METHYLTRANSFERASES   Hirata & Axelrod have described a phospholipid methyltransferase system that converts phosphatidyl-ethanolamine to phosphatidylcholine and transfers the lipid from the cytoplasmic surface of the membrane to the outer surface. This reaction occurs in a great variety of cells in response to many pharmacological stimuli (9). In red cells it is reported to be accompanied by a large change in microviscosity, measured by polarization of DPH fluorescence (81). The increased fluidity is thought to be the mechanism for a number of events triggered by β-adrenergic receptors, mitogens, and chemotactic compounds. The change in membrane order accompanying the enzyme activity has not been found in kidney or brain membranes, however (82, 83). The methyltransferases are inhibited by ethanol in vitro (84).

Phase Transitions

Thermotropic phase transitions between the gel and liquid crystal forms of lipids are easily seen in pure lipid bilayers by a variety of methods such as differential scanning calorimetry, turbidimetry, and the spectra of spin labels that partition only into the fluid portion of a lipid.

GENERAL ANESTHETICS   Anesthetic drugs generally lower the temperature at which the phase transition takes place, an effect that increases the overall fluidity of the membrane at temperatures slightly below the original transition temperature. Inhalation anesthetics reduce the transition temperature of phosphatidylcholine vesicles (31, 85, 86); they are equally effective in phosphatidylcholines with chain lengths of 14, 16, or 18 carbons (87). These drugs also increase the width of the transition, which indicates that they reduce the size of the cooperative unit of lipids that participate in the melting. Mountcastle et al (88) suggest that the lipids exist in clusters the size of which influences the interactions between proteins. Both the decrease in transition temperature and the broadening of the transition are reversed by hydrostatic pressure (88–90), and pressure alone raises the transition temperature. Methoxyflurane lowers the transition temperature much further in phosphatidic acid membranes than in phosphatidylcholine (91), and pressure may be able to force the anesthetic out of phosphatidic acid but not out of phosphatidylcholine membranes.

LOCAL ANESTHETICS   Barbiturates depress phase transition temperatures of liposomes made of phosphatidylcholine or phosphatidylethanolamine but not phosphatidylserine (92). The uncharged form of the drug seems to be the active form. Lee (92) suggests that barbiturates and other local anesthetics block sodium conductance by melting the boundary lipids that surround the channel protein. In rat liver plasma membranes, phenobarbital depresses the temperature of the transition that has been assigned to the outer monolayer (93). Analysis of Arrhenius plots of enzymes that have known locations in this membrane led to the concept that outer-monolayer enzymes have a phase transition at about 28°. The transition is revealed by a change in slope of the Arrhenius plots and the break is shifted to a lower temperature by phenobarbital. Dibucaine reduces the transition temperature of acidic lipids (phosphatidylserine or phosphatidylglycerol) in which the drug is highly soluble, but does not affect that of phosphatidylcholine (74).

ALIPHATIC ALCOHOLS   Short-chain alkanols depress phase transitions of pure phospholipid vesicles (94). Hill (86, 95) and Rowe (96–97) followed phase transitions in liposomes by a simple optical method, and calculated the partition coefficients of alcohols by their ability to lower the phase transition temperature, assuming that the drugs are confined to the fluid phase. Compounds that reduce the transition temperature generally abolish the phosphatidylcholine pretransition.

In addition to reducing the transition temperature, some alcohols affect the width of the phase transition. Short chain alcohols, up to 5 carbons, do not affect the width of the phase transition in phosphatidylcholines (90, 97, 98). Alcohols or fatty acids of 5–10 carbons broaden the transition in phosphatidylcholine vesicles (94, 98) but not in phosphatidylethanolamine (94).

By contrast, long chain alcohols (or fatty acids) with more than 10 carbon atoms raise the transition temperature (94, 99). Alkanols affect long-chain phosphatidylcholines more than short chain phosphatidylcholines (87).

Jain & Wu (98) have classified a variety of drugs according to their ability to shift the midpoint of the transition and/or increase its width in an attempt to localize the drug action within the bilayer.

As a next step from pure lipids toward biomembranes, Lee has studied effects of alkanols on phase diagrams of binary mixtures of phospholipids (94). The drugs shifted downward the temperature range at which gel and fluid lipid coexist. Lee's data provide an illustration of the potential importance of phase transitions in terms of the overall fluidity of a biomembrane. About 40% of the lipid in a particular binary mixture was fluid at 30° C in the absence of drugs, but 63% was fluid in the presence of 0.8 mM octanol.

CHRONIC ADMINISTRATION OF MEMBRANE-DISORDERING DRUGS

Many of the drugs that act on cell membranes are capable of producing tolerance and physical dependence. These phenomena may be adaptive in nature, i.e. homeostatic mechanisms may allow the body to function fairly normally despite the continuous presence of initially toxic drug concentrations. On withdrawal of the drug a dangerous syndrome may ensue. Because these drugs have their primary action on the hydrophobic regions of cell membranes the same regions may be the locale of the adaptation, as was suggested in 1975 by Hill & Bangham (100).

Adaptation to a disordering drug may be analogous to temperature adaptation. Microorganisms and poikilothermic vertebrates compensate for changes in ambient temperature by altering the chemical composition of their membrane phospholipids, a process that Sinensky (101) has called *homeoviscous adaptation*. Bacteria accomplish this by increasing the degree of unsaturation of membrane acyl chains as the temperature falls. The lipids remain at roughly the same fluidity whatever the growth temperature. Homeoviscous adaptation has been observed in many species; even in mammals the degree of unsaturation of depot fats (triglycerides) can change to suit the temperature (102). Thus, it is reasonable to seek evidence that mammalian membrane lipids may adapt to the continuous presence of drugs that mimic warming. At present we have good evidence that chronic exposure to drugs alters the physical properties of membranes but the nature of the underlying chemical change is still in doubt. There may be many ways of accomplishing the same homeoviscous adaptation and they may occur simultaneously or in sequence.

Chronic administration of ethanol alters mammalian membranes both chemically and physically. The chemical composition may be adjusted in several respects simultaneously and the resultant change in membrane order (if any) is difficult to predict. Littleton & John (103) observed an increase in the degree of saturation in the fatty acids of brain phospholipids in mice treated chronically with ethanol. The ratio of linoleic to arachidonic acid increases in many tissues after chronic ethanol treatment of the animals. Similarly, the proportion of linolenic falls while more saturated acids accumulate in mitochondrial cardiolipin from alcohol-treated rats (104). Chin & Goldstein (105) have recently reviewed these changes in more detail than can be included here.

In mammals cholesterol is a major chemical determinant of membrane order. An increase in the membrane content of cholesterol, which is an appropriate response to the disordering effect of an anesthetic drug, sometimes occurs after chronic administration of ethanol. Treatment of mice or rats with ethanol in a liquid diet increases the cholesterol content of their synaptosomal (106–108), erythrocyte (106), and hepatic (109) membranes. However, when ethanol was administered by inhalation or injection, even when the regimen sufficed to produce changes in fatty acid content of membranes or to produce tolerance and physical dependence, the cholesterol:phospholipid ratio of synaptosomal plasma membranes was unchanged (110, 111).

Ethanol (like an increase in temperature) accelerates the transfer of cholesterol between membranes in vitro without affecting its equilibrium distribution (112). The end result in vivo might be a shift in the steady state distribution of cholesterol among different carriers and membranes. An increased content of cholesterol might account for tolerance, since cholesterol counteracts the disordering effect of ethanol in phosphatidylcholine vesicles (65) and reduces the partition of pentobarbital (and probably other drugs) into lipid vesicles (20). However, these effects are most evident at low concentrations of cholesterol, analogous to intracellular membranes. Liposomes with more than 30 mol% cholesterol, comparable to plasma membranes, are relatively insensitive to further increases.

Membranes isolated from ethanol-treated animals are often found to be resistant to the disordering effects of the drug in vitro. This represents tolerance of the membranes occurring in parallel with behavioral tolerance in the animals. This condition can be elicited in mice either by administration of ethanol in a liquid diet for 8–9 days (113), by a 3–day period of ethanol inhalation (111), or by a series of injections (107). In rats a month of liquid diet treatment accomplishes the same result (104). Membranes of brain, liver, and red cells show similar changes in sensitivity, and phospholipid extracts also show a decreased response to ethanol, indicating that the changes are not restricted to the proteins. Cross-tolerance to ethanol is seen in membranes of mice treated with pentobarbital but not in those treated with morphine (114), and membranes of ethanol-treated mice are cross-tolerant to t-butanol (111) and halothane (26).

Less consistently, the membranes from such animals have an increased intrinsic order, an abnormal rigidity that might perhaps mediate the hyperexcitability of the withdrawal reaction, since it is the opposite of the primary (sedative and disordering) effect of the drug. In mice after 3 days of ethanol inhalation we found an increase in intrinsic order in the region monitored by 12-doxylstearic acid but not in the regions monitored by 5- or 16-doxyl probes (111). Fluorescence polarization of DPH also showed increased intrinsic order in these synaptosomal plasma membranes (115), but not in lipid extracts of membranes from alcohol-treated mice or rats (116).

Rottenberg et al (26) reported that the partition coefficient of ethanol (and also that of halothane) was considerably lower in membranes from rats that had been chronically treated with ethanol than in controls. Such a change might explain the decreased slope of the ethanol concentration response curve but could not account for the changed intrinsic order.

SUMMARY

Anesthetics almost always disorder or "fluidize" membranes, i.e. the drugs increase the mobility of spin labels and reduce order parameters. This effect is universal at high concentrations above the clinical range, but in some kinds of membranes low concentrations of drugs have an ordering effect. Drugs that carry charges, including many local anesthetics, often stiffen membranes, as do long-chain alcohols or fatty acids that mimic natural membrane components. The potencies of short-chain alcohols correlate well with lipid solubility, but a cutoff is reached at 10–12 carbons, where pharmacological actions become weak or absent despite a progressive increase in lipid solubility. The cutoff is partly explained by the ordering action of the long chains and partly by the difficulty of administering such water-insoluble drugs in vivo.

The idea of membrane disorder does not exclude some specificity. Closely related drugs may have different molecular shapes and may be capable of forming hydrogen bonds with different orientations, affecting their ability to make membrane more fluid. Perhaps for this reason, there is a remarkable stereospecificity in the disordering effect of anesthetic steroids, chloralose, and long-chain alkenols.

Some specificity is mediated by different membrane environments. The drug action may actually reverse from order to disorder on addition of cholesterol, but in other experimental systems cholesterol blocks a disordering effect, and we cannot yet explain the action of drugs in different biomembranes. Further, drugs may have differential solubilities in membranes of different composition. This cannot always be predicted from octanol:water partition coefficients because branched molecules are differentially excluded from structured bilayers. Charged drugs react quite differently with charged and neutral phospholipids and may have differential actions on the two sides of the bilayer because of the asymmetry of the phospholipid distribution. The deeper reaches of the membrane seem particularly sensitive to disordering, even by drugs that presumably reside near the surface. Thus, proteins whose midregions are sensitive to disordering may be especially disrupted by drugs.

This is a new field of pharmacology, currently applied only to a small group of drugs. But an understanding of the physicochemical actions of drugs in hydrophobic regions of cells will clearly be needed for full understanding of membrane-bound drug receptors, enzymes, and transport systems. This is just a beginning.

ACKNOWLEDGEMENT

Our work has been supported in part by grants from USPHS, DA 02584, AA 01066, and a Research Scientist Award AA 00075.

Literature Cited

1. Parry, G., Palmer, D. N., Williams, D. J. 1976. Ligand partitioning into membranes: Its significance in determining K_m and K_s values for cytochrome P-450 and other membrane bound receptors and enzymes. *FEBS Lett.* 67:123–29

2. Hubbell, W. L., McConnell, H. M. 1969. Orientation and motion of amphiphilic spin labels in membranes. *Proc. Natl. Acad. Sci. USA* 64:20–27

3. Seelig, A., Seelig, J. 1974. The dynamic structure of fatty acyl chains in a phospholipid bilayer measured by deuterium magnetic resonance. *Biochemistry* 13:4839–45

4. Traüble, H., Haynes, D. H. 1971. The volume change in lipid bilayer lamellae at the crystalline-liquid crystalline phase transition. *Chem. Phys. Lipids* 7:324–35

5. McConnell, H. M. 1976. Molecular motion in biological membranes. In *Spin Labeling Theory and Applications*, ed. L. J. Berliner, pp. 525–60. New York/San Francisco/London: Academic. 592 pp.

6. Nicolson, G. L. 1975. Restrictions on the lateral mobility of cell membrane components. In *Functional Linkage in Biomolecular Systems*, ed. F. O. Schmitt, D. M. Schneider, D. M. Crothers, pp. 137–47. New York: Raven. 350 pp.

7. Kornberg, R. D., McConnell, H. M. 1971. Inside-outside transitions of phospholipids in vesicle membranes. *Biochemistry* 10:1111–20

8. McNamee, M. G., McConnell, H. M. 1973. Transmembrane potentials and phospholipid flip-flop in excitable membrane vesicles. *Biochemistry* 12:2951–58

9. Hirata, F., Axelrod, J. 1980. Phospholipid methylation and biological signal transmission. *Science* 209:1082–90

10. Shimshick, E. J., McConnell, H. M. 1973. Lateral phase separation in phospholipid membranes. *Biochemistry* 12:2351–60

11. Karnovsky, M. J., Kleinfeld, A. M., Hoover, R. L., Klausner, R. D. 1982. The concept of lipid domains in membranes. *J. Cell Biol.* 94:1–6

12. Tanford, C. 1980. *The Hydrophobic Effect. Formation of Micelles and Biological Membranes.* New York: Wiley, 233 pp. 2nd ed.

13. Hansch, C., Dunn, W. J. III. 1972. Linear relationships between lipophilic character and biological activity of drugs. *J. Pharm. Sci.* 61:1–19

14. Leo, A., Hansch, C., Elkins, D. 1971. Partition coefficients and their uses. *Chem. Rev.* 71:525–616

15. Lindenberg, B. A. 1951. Sur la solubilité des substances organiques amphipatiques dans les glycérides neutres et hydroxyles. *J. Chim. Phys.* 48:350–55

16. Cratin, P. D. 1968. Partitioning at the liquid-liquid interface. *Ind. Enq. Chem.* 60(9):14–19

17. Diamond, J. M., Katz, Y. 1974. Interpretation of nonelectrolyte partition coefficients between dimyristoyl lecithin and water. *J. Membr. Biol.* 17:121–54

18. Roth, S., Seeman, P. 1972. The membrane concentrations of neutral and positive anesthetics (alcohols, chlorpromazine, morphine) fit the Meyer-Overton rule of anesthesia: Negative narcotics do not. *Biochim. Biophys. Acta* 255:207–19

19. Metcalfe, J. C., Seeman, P., Burgen, A. S. V. 1968. The proton relaxation of benzyl alcohol in erythrocyte membranes. *Mol. Pharmacol.* 4:87–95

20. Miller, K. W., Yu, S.-C. T. 1977. The dependence of the lipid bilayer membrane:buffer partition coefficient of pentobarbitone on pH and lipid composition. *Br. J. Pharmacol.* 61:57–63

21. Bienvenüe, A., Rousselet, A., Kato, G., Devaux, P. F. 1977. Fluidity of the lipids next to the acetylcholine receptor protein of *Torpedo* membrane fragments. Use of amphiphilic reversible spin-labels. *Biochemistry* 16:841–48

22. Seeman, P. 1977. Anti-schizophrenic drugs—Membrane receptor sites of action. *Biochem. Pharmacol.* 26:1741–48

23. Conrad, M. J., Singer, S. J. 1979. Evidence for a large internal pressure in biological membranes. *Proc. Natl. Acad. Sci. USA* 76:5202–06

24. Bondy, B., Remien, J. 1981. Differential binding of chlorpromazine to human blood cells: Application of the hygroscopic desorption method. *Life Sci.* 28:441–49

25. Gaffney, B. J., Willingham, G. L., Schepp, R. S. 1983. Synthesis and membrane interactions of spin-label bifunctional reagents. *Biochemistry* 22:881–92

26. Rottenberg, H., Waring, A., Rubin, E. 1981. Tolerance and cross-tolerance in chronic alcoholics: Reduced membrane binding of ethanol and other drugs. *Science* 213:583–85

27. Seeman, P. 1972. The membrane actions

of anesthetics and tranquilizers. *Pharmacol. Rev.* 24:583–655

28. McCreery, M. J., Hunt, W. A. 1978. Physico-chemical correlates of alcohol intoxication. *Neuropharmacology* 17: 451–61

29. Lyon, R. C., McComb, J. A., Schreurs, J., Goldstein, D. B. 1981. A relationship between alcohol intoxication and the disordering of brain membranes by a series of short-chain alcohols. *J. Pharmacol. Exp. Ther.* 218:669–75

30. Turner, G. L., Oldfield, E. 1979. Effect of a local anaesthetic on hydrocarbon chain order in membranes. *Nature* 277:669–70

31. Vanderkooi, J. M., Landesberg, R., Selick, H. II, McDonald, G. G. 1977. Interaction of general anesthetics with phospholipid vesicles and biological membranes. *Biochim. Biophys. Acta* 464:1–6

32. Cullis, P. R., De Kruijff, B. 1979. Lipid polymorphism and the functional roles of lipids in biological membranes. *Biochim. Biophys. Acta* 559:399–420

33. Griffith, O. H., Jost, P. C. 1976. Lipid spin labels in biological membranes. See Ref. 5, pp. 453–523

34. Smith, I. C. P., Butler, K. W. 1976. Oriented lipid systems as model membranes. See Ref. 5, pp. 411–51

35. Hubbell, W. L., McConnell, H. M. 1971. Molecular motion in spin-labeled phospholipids and membranes. *J. Am. Chem. Soc.* 93:314–26

36. Trudell, J. R., Hubbell, W. L., Cohen, E. N. 1973. The effect of two inhalation anesthetics on the order of spin-labeled phospholipid vesicles. *Biochim. Biophys. Acta* 291:321–27

37. Mastrangelo, C. J., Trudell, J. R., Edmunds, H. N., Cohen, E. N. 1978. Effect of clinical concentrations of halothane on phospholipid-cholesterol membrane fluidity. *Mol. Pharmacol.* 14:463–67

38. Kendig, J. J., Trudell, J. R., Cohen, E. N. 1973. Halothane stereoisomers: Lack of stereospecificity in two model systems. *Anesthesiology* 39:518–24

39. Trudell, J. R., Hubbell, W. L., Cohen, E. N. 1973. Pressure reversal of inhalation anesthetic-induced disorder in spin-labeled phospholipid vesicles. *Biochim. Biophys. Acta* 291:328–34

40. Lenaz, G., Curatola, G., Mazzanti, L., Bertoli, E., Pastuszko, A., 1979. Spin label studies on the effect of anesthetics in synaptic membranes. *J. Neurochem.* 32:1689–95

41. Pang, K.-Y. Y., Braswell, L. M., Chang,

L., Sommer, T. J., Miller, K. W. 1980. The perturbation of lipid bilayers by general anesthetics: A quantitative test of the disordered lipid hypothesis. *Mol. Pharmacol.* 18:84–90

42. Rosenberg, P. H., Eibl, H., Stier, A. 1975. Biphasic effects of halothane on phospholipid and synaptic plasma membranes: A spin label study. *Mol. Pharmacol.* 11:879–82

43. Rosenberg, P. H., Jansson, J.-E., Gripenberg, J. 1977. Effects of halothane, thiopental, and lidocaine on fluidity of synaptic plasma membranes and artificial phospholipid membranes. *Anesthesiology* 46:322–26

44. Boggs, J. M., Yoong, T., Hsia, J. C. 1976. Sites and mechanism of anesthetic action. 1. Effect of anesthetics and pressure on fluidity of spin-labeled lipid vesicles. *Mol. Pharmacol.* 12:127–35

45. Butler, K. W., Schneider, H., Smith, I. C. P. 1973. The effects of local anesthetics on lipid multilayers. A spin probe study. *Arch. Biochem. Biophys.* 154: 548–54

46. Neal, M. J., Butler, K. W., Polnaszek, C. F., Smith, I. C. P. 1976. The influence of anesthetics and cholesterol on the degree of molecular organization and mobility of ox brain white matter. *Mol. Pharmacol.* 12:144–55

47. Hubbell, W. L., Metcalfe, J. C., Metcalfe, S. M., McConnell, H. M. 1970. The interaction of small molecules with spin-labelled erythrocyte membranes. *Biochim. Biophys. Acta* 219:415–27

48. Narahashi, T., Frazier, D. T., Yamada, M. 1970. The site of action and active form of local anesthetics. I. Theory and pH experiments with tertiary compounds. *J. Pharmacol. Exp. Ther.* 171:32–44

49. Giraud, F., Claret, M., Bruckdorfer, K. R., Chailley, B. 1981. The effects of membrane lipid order and cholesterol on the internal and external cationic sites of the Na^+-K^+ pump in erythrocytes. *Biochim. Biophys. Acta* 647:249–58

50. Pang, K.-Y. Y., Miller, K. W. 1978. Cholesterol modulates the effects of membrane perturbers in phospholipid vesicles and biomembranes. *Biochim. Biophys. Acta* 511:1–9

51. Surewicz, W. K., Leyko, W. 1981. Interaction of propranolol with model phospholipid membranes. Monolayer, spin label and fluorescence spectroscopy studies. *Biochim. Biophys. Acta* 643:387–97

52. Surewicz, W. K. 1982. Propranolol-induced structural changes in human

erythrocyte ghost membranes. A spin label study. *Biochem. Pharmacol.* 31:691–94

53. Lawrence, D. K., Gill, E. W. 1975. Structurally specific effects of some steroid anesthetics on spin-labeled liposomes. *Mol. Pharmacol.* 11:280–86

54. Brockerhoff, H. 1982. Anesthetics may restructure the hydrogen belts of membranes. *Lipids* 17:1001–3

55. Lawrence, D. K., Gill, E. W. 1975. The effects of Δ^1-tetrahydrocannabinol and other cannabinoids on spin-labeled liposomes and their relationship to mechanisms of general anesthesia. *Mol. Pharmacol.* 11:595–602

56. Miller, K. W., Pang, K.-Y. Y. 1976. General anaesthetics can selectively perturb lipid bilayer membranes. *Nature* 263:253–55

57. Gordon, L. M., Sauerheber, R. D., Esgate, J. A., Dipple, I., Marchmont, R. J., et al. 1980. The increase in bilayer fluidity of rat liver plasma membranes achieved by the local anesthetic benzyl alcohol affects the activity of intrinsic membrane enzymes. *J. Biol. Chem.* 255:4519–27

58. Sauerheber, R. D., Esgate, J. A., Kuhn, C. E. 1982. Alcohols inhibit adipocyte basal and insulin-stimulated glucose uptake and increase the membrane lipid fluidity. *Biochim. Biophys. Acta* 691:115–24

59. Pushkin, J. S., Martin, T. 1978. Effects of anesthetics on divalent cation binding and fluidity of phosphatidylserine vesicles. *Mol. Pharmacol.* 14:454–62

60. Paterson, S. J., Butler, K. W., Huang, P., Labelle, J., Smith, I. C. P., et al. 1972. The effects of alcohols on lipid bilayers: A spin label study. *Biochim. Biophys. Acta* 266:597–602

61. Lenaz, G., Bertoli, E., Curatola, G., Mazzanti, L., Bigi, A. 1976. Lipid protein interactions in mitochondria. Spin and fluorescent probe studies on the effect of n-alkanols on phospholipid vesicles and mitochondrial membranes. *Arch. Biochem. Biophys.* 172:278–88

62. Richards, C. D., Martin, K., Gregory, S., Keightley, C. A., Hesketh, T. R., et al. 1978. Degenerate perturbations of protein structure as the mechanism of anaesthetic action. *Nature* 276:775–79

63. Pringle, M. J., Brown, K. B., Miller, K. W. 1981. Can the lipid theories of anesthesia account for the cutoff in anesthetic potency in homologous series of alcohols? *Mol. Pharmacol.* 19:49–55

64. Chin, J. H., Goldstein, D. B. 1977. Effects of low concentrations of ethanol on the fluidity of spin-labeled erythrocyte and brain membranes. *Mol. Pharmacol.* 13:435–41

65. Chin, J. H., Goldstein, D. B. 1981. Membrane-disordering action of ethanol: Variation with membrane cholesterol content and depth of the spin label probe. *Mol. Pharmacol.* 19:425–31

66. Goldstein, D. B., Chin, J. H. 1981. Disordering effect of ethanol at different depths in the bilayer of mouse brain membranes. *Alcoholism (NY)* 5:256–58

67. Huang, C.-H. 1977. A structural model for the cholesterol-phosphatidylcholine complexes in bilayer membranes. *Lipids* 12:348–56

68. Goldstein, D. B., Chin, J. H., Lyon, R. C. 1982. Ethanol disordering of spin-labeled mouse brain membranes: Correlation with genetically determined ethanol sensitivity of mice. *Proc. Natl. Acad. Sci. USA* 79:4231–33

69. Pesce, A. J., Rosén, C.-G., Pasby, T. L., 1971. *Fluorescence Spectroscopy. An Introduction for Biology and Medicine.* New York: Dekker. 247 pp.

70. Stubbs, G. W., Litman, B. J., Barenholz, Y. 1976. Microviscosity of the hydrocarbon region of the bovine retinal rod outer segment disk membrane determined by fluorescent probe measurements. *Biochemistry* 15:2766–72

71. Klausner, R. D., Kleinfeld, A. M., Hoover, R. L., Karnovsky, M. J. 1980. Lipid domains in membranes. Evidence derived from structural perturbations induced by free fatty acids and lifetime heterogeneity analysis. *J. Biol. Chem.* 255:1286–95

72. Jacobson, K., Wobschall, D. 1974. Rotation of fluorescent probes localized within lipid bilayer membranes. *Chem. Phys. Lipids* 12:117–31

73. Shinitzky, M., Dianoux, A.-C., Gitler, C., Weber, G. 1971. Microviscosity and order in the hydrocarbon region of micelles and membranes determined with fluorescent probes. I. Synthetic micelles. *Biochemistry* 10:2106–13

74. Papahadjopoulos, D., Jacobson, K., Poste, G., Shepherd, G. 1975. Effects of local anesthetics on membrane properties. I. Changes in the fluidity of phospholipid bilayers. *Biochim. Biophys. Acta* 394:504–19

75. Harris, R. A., Schroeder, F. 1982. Effects of barbiturates and ethanol on the physical properties of brain membranes. *J. Pharmacol. Exp. Ther.* 223:424–31

76. Cherenkevich, S. N., Vanderkooi, J. M., Holian, A. 1982. The lipid integrity of

membranes of guinea pig alveolar macrophages studied by nanosecond fluorescence decay of 1,6-diphenyl-1,3,5-hexatriene: The influence of temperature and benzyl alcohol. *Arch. Biochem. Biophys.* 214:305–10

77. Kutchai, H., Cooper, R. A., Forster, R. E. 1980. Erythrocyte water permeability. The effects of anesthetic alcohols and alterations in the level of membrane cholesterol. *Biochim. Biophys. Acta* 600:542–52

78. Kutchai, H., Chandler, L. H., Geddis, L. M. 1980. Effects of anesthetic alcohols on membrane transport processes in human erythrocytes. *Biochim. Biophys. Acta* 600:870–81

79. Zavoico, G. B., Kutchai, H. 1980. Effects of n-alkanols on the membrane fluidity of chick embryo heart microsomes. *Biochim. Biophys. Acta* 600:263–69

80. Harris, R. A., Schroeder, F. 1981. Ethanol and the physical properties of brain membranes. Fluorescence studies. *Mol. Pharmacol.* 20:128–37

81. Hirata, F., Axelrod, J. 1978. Enzymatic methylation of phosphatidylethanolamine increases erythrocyte membrane fluidity. *Nature* 275:219–20

82. Chauhan, V. P. S., Sikka, S. C., Kalra, V. K. 1982. Phospholipid methylation of kidney cortex brush border membranes. Effect on fluidity and transport. *Biochim. Biophys. Acta* 688:357–68

83. Goldstein, D. B., Brett, P. B. 1983. Role of membrane fluidity in events mediated by phospholipid methyltransferases. *J. Neurochem.* 41:S51A (Abstr.).

84. Nhamburo, P. T., John, G. R., Littleton, J. M. 1982. Alterations in phospholipid methylation in rat brain synaptosomal membranes produced by ethanol in vitro and in vivo. *Biochem. Pharmacol.* 31:3936–38

85. Jain, M. K., Wu, N. Y.-M., Wray, L. V. 1975. Drug-induced phase change in bilayer as possible mode of action of membrane expanding drugs. *Nature* 255:494–96

86. Hill, M. W. 1974. The effect of anaesthetic-like molecules on the phase transition in smectic mesophases of dipalmitoyllecithin. I. The normal alcohol up to C=9 and three inhalation anaesthetics. *Biochim. Biophys. Acta* 356:117–24

87. Kamaya, H., Kaneshina, S., Ueda, I. 1981. Partition equilibrium of inhalation anesthetics and alcohols between water and membranes of phospholipids with varying acyl chain-lengths. *Biochim. Biophys. Acta* 646:135–42

88. Mountcastle, D. B., Biltonen, R. L., Halsey, M. J. 1978. Effect of anesthetics and pressure on the thermotropic behavior of multilamellar dipalmitoylphosphatidylcholine liposomes. *Proc. Natl. Acad. Sci. USA* 75:4906–10

89. Trudell, J. R., Payan, D. G., Chin, J. H., Cohen, E. N. 1975. The antagonistic effect of an inhalation anesthetic and high pressure on the phase diagram of mixed dipalmitoyl-dimyristoylphosphatidyl-choline bilayers. *Proc. Natl. Acad. Sci. USA* 72:210–13

90. MacDonald, A. G. 1978. A dilatometric investigation of the effects of general anaesthetics, alcohols and hydrostatic pressure on the phase transition in smectic mesophases of dipalmitoyl phosphatidylcholine. *Biochim. Biophys. Acta* 507:26–37

91. Galla, H.-J., Trudell, J. R. 1980. Asymmetric antagonistic effects of an inhalation anesthetic and high pressure on the phase transition temperature of dipalmitoyl phosphatidic acid bilayers. *Biochim. Biophys. Acta* 599:336–40

92. Lee, A. G. 1976. Interactions between phospholipids and barbiturates. *Biochim. Biophys. Acta* 455:102–08

93. Houslay, M. D., Dipple, I., Gordon, L. M. 1981. Phenobarbital selectively modulates the glucagon-stimulated activity of adenylate cyclase by depressing the lipid phase separation occurring in the outer half of the bilayer of liver plasma membranes. *Biochem. J.* 197:675–81

94. Lee, A. G. 1976. Interactions between anesthetics and lipid mixtures. Normal alcohols. *Biochemistry* 15:2448–54

95. Hill, M. W. 1975. Partition coefficients of some anaesthetic-like molecules between water and smectic mesophases of dipalmitoylphosphatidylcholine. *Biochem. Soc. Trans.* 3:149–52

96. Rowe, E. S. 1981. Membrane:buffer partition coefficient for ethanol in dimyristoylphosphatidylcholine. *Alcoholism (NY)* 5:259–63

97. Rowe, E. S. 1982. The effects of ethanol on the thermotropic properties of dipalmitoylphosphatidylcholine. *Mol. Pharmacol.* 22:133–39

98. Jain, M. K., Wu, M. N. 1977. Effect of small molecules on the dipalmitoyl lecithin liposomal bilayer III. Phase transition in lipid bilayer. *J. Membr. Biol.* 34:157–201

99. Eliasz, A. W., Chapman, D., Ewing, D. F. 1976. Phospholipid phase transitions. Effects of n-alcohols, n-monocarboxylic acids, phenylalkyl alcohols and quarter-

nary ammonium compounds. *Biochim. Biophys. Acta* 448:220–30

100. Hill, M. W., Bangham, A. D. 1975. General depressant drug dependency: A biophysical hypothesis. *Adv. Exp. Med. Biol.* 59:1–9

101. Sinensky, M. 1974. Homeoviscous adaptation—A homeostatic process that regulates the viscosity of membrane lipids in *Escherichia coli. Proc. Natl. Acad. Sci. USA* 71:522–25

102. Henriques, V., Hansen, C. 1901. Vergleichende Untersuchungen über die chemische Zusammensetzung des thierischen Fettes. *Skand. Arch. Physiol.* 11:151–56

103. Littleton, J. M., John, G. 1977. Synaptosomal membrane lipids of mice during continuous exposure to ethanol. *J. Pharm. Pharmacol.* 29:579–80

104. Waring, A. J., Rottenberg, H., Ohnishi, T., Rubin, E. 1981. Membranes and phospholipids of liver mitochondria from chronic alcoholic rats are resistant to membrane disordering by alcohol. *Proc. Natl. Acad. Sci. USA* 78:2582–86

105. Chin, J. H., Goldstein, D. B. 1983. Effects of alcohols on membrane fluidity and lipid composition. In *Membrane Fluidity in Biology*, Vol. III, eds. R. C. Aloia, J. M. Boggs. New York: Academic. In press

106. Chin, J. H., Parsons, L. M., Goldstein, D. B. 1978. Increased cholesterol content of erythrocyte and brain membranes in ethanol-tolerant mice. *Biochim. Biophys. Acta* 513:358–63

107. Johnson, D. A., Lee, N. M., Cooke, R., Loh, H. H. 1979. Ethanol-induced fluidization of brain lipid bilayers: Required presence of cholesterol in membranes for the expression of tolerance. *Mol. Pharmacol.* 15:739–46

108. Smith, T. L., Gerhart, M. J. 1982. Alterations in brain lipid composition of mice made physically dependent to ethanol. *Life Sci.* 31:1419–25

109. Smith, T. L., Vickers, A. E., Brendel, K., Gerhart, M. J. 1982. Effects of ethanol diets on cholesterol content and phospholipid acyl composition of rat hepatocytes. *Lipids* 17:124–28

110. Wing, D. R., Harvey, D. J., Hughes, J., Dunbar, P. G., McPherson, K. A., et al. 1982. Effects of chronic ethanol administration on the composition of membrane lipids in the mouse. *Biochem. Pharmacol.* 31:3431–39

111. Lyon, R. C., Goldstein, D. B. 1983. Changes in synaptic membrane order associated with chronic ethanol treatment in mice. *Mol. Pharmacol.* 23:86–91

112. Daniels, C. K., Goldstein, D. B. 1982. Movement of free cholesterol from lipoproteins or lipid vesicles into erythrocytes. Acceleration by ethanol in vitro. *Mol. Pharmacol.* 21:694–700

113. Chin, J. H., Goldstein, D. B. 1977. Drug tolerance in biomembranes. A spin label study of the effects of ethanol. *Science* 196:684–85

114. Johnson, D. A., Lee, N. M. Cooke, R., Loh, H. H. 1980. Adaptation to ethanol-induced fluidization of brain lipid bilayers: Cross-tolerance and reversibility. *Mol. Pharmacol.* 17:52–55

115. Perlman, B. J., Goldstein, D. B. 1983. Ethanol and sodium valproate disordering of membranes from chronic ethanol treated mice. *Fed. Proc.* 42:2123 (Abstr.)

116. Johnson, D. A., Friedman, H. J., Cooke, R., Lee N. M. 1980. Adaptation of brain lipid bilayers to ethanol-induced fluidization. Species and strain generality. *Biochem. Pharmacol.* 29:1673–76

Ann. Rev. Pharmacol. Toxicol. 1984. 24:65–83

CHANGES IN VASCULAR SMOOTH MUSCLE REACTIVITY DURING DEVELOPMENT

Sue Piper Duckles and William Banner, Jr.

Departments of Pharmacology and Pediatrics, University of Arizona College of Medicine, Tucson, Arizona 85274

THE SCOPE OF THE REVIEW

Our understanding of the numerous factors that control vascular smooth muscle tone in the adult has advanced considerably in the last ten years. Salient points to emerge from the considerable amount of work done on the subject include a remarkable heterogeneity in vascular smooth muscle reactivity among different vascular beds and among different species and the variation in mechanisms and intensity of adrenergic control of different blood vessels (1). This explosion of knowledge about factors controlling blood vessel tone has only recently led investigators to explore in detail the way these mechanisms might change at different ages. A few exploratory studies have been done that point the way toward more intensive analysis.

This review has two purposes. The first is to summarize what is currently known about variations in factors that control vascular smooth muscle tone in the first few weeks of life. The second is to highlight methodological considerations that must be taken into account in order to optimize future studies in this area.

This review will focus on alterations in reactivity of vascular smooth muscle to neuronal influences and circulating substances during the first few weeks of life. The emphasis will be on in vitro studies because this approach allows one to study vascular smooth muscle reactivity without interference from reflex effects, differences in pharmacokinetics, etc. This does not imply that in vivo studies are not important or useful. Studies in vitro allow one to distinguish

65

0362-1642/84/415–0065$02.00

specific mechanisms that may be changing during growth. A basic knowledge of these mechanisms should make possible an improved design for in vivo studies in order to determine the physiological and pathological importance of changes in vascular smooth muscle reactivity. Indeed, a general overview of the in vivo approach is also included here.

This review will not deal with the dramatic changes in the cardiovascular system that occur at the time of birth and shortly thereafter. This aspect has recently been reviewed (2). Nor will we deal with studies of the factors that influence differentiation of smooth muscle or factors that determine the extent and pattern of innervation. Further information on these aspects can be found in several other reviews (3–5).

SPECIES VARIATION

Significant species differences in vascular smooth muscle reactivity have been defined in a single vascular bed (6, 7). However, more critical for studies of development are the differences in relative maturity at birth among various species. In the commonly used laboratory species this ranges from animals born in a highly developed state, such as guinea pigs and sheep, through pigs, dogs, and cats, to animals born in a highly immature state—rabbits and rats (8, 9). Thus, the age of the animal per se does not provide a good index of the stage of development when making comparisons between species. Throughout this review the age referred to is postnatal age unless otherwise specified.

Several researchers have claimed that pigs and dogs provide the closest model to the newborn human in terms of the stage of cardiovascular development (10–13). Indeed, a model of cerebral intraventricular hemorrhage, one of the most prevalent causes of morbidity and mortality in premature infants (14), has been developed in the newborn beagle (15).

THE GENERAL SCHEME OF ADRENERGIC NERVOUS SYSTEM ONTOGENY

From studies of the development of adrenergic nervous control of various organs a general principle can be derived: the function of the post-synaptic component can generally be demonstrated before the presynaptic elements are fully functional (16). Aspects of this process can be gleaned from studies on the vasculature and the general principle appears applicable to blood vessels. However, comprehensive studies are not yet available. Therefore, it is worthwhile to review the sequence of developmental events as they occur in a much more carefully studied tissue. The careful work of Slotkin's group, with its primary emphasis on the development of autonomic control of the heart, provides an important model for studies of developmental changes in other organs.

Heart

At birth, activation of β-adrenergic receptors with isoproterenol produces both an increase in rate and force of contraction of the rat heart (17). However, responses to stimulation of sympathetic nerves, as tested using tyramine to release adrenergic transmitter, are small in the newborn and increase steadily over the first week of life (18). This increased responsiveness to adrenergic nerve activation can be correlated with development of the capacity of adrenergic nerves to accumulate norepinephrine by an active uptake mechanism (18). Cardiac norepinephrine content also increases steadily over the first two weeks of life (19).

It has been suggested that the key factor involved in the development of sympathetic neurotransmission is maturation of neurotransmitter synaptic vesicles, the organelle involved in storage and release of transmitter (20). This has been demonstrated both morphologically (20) and by measuring accumulation and content of norepinephrine.

While functional adrenergic nerves appear to be present in the heart of rats by one week of age, these nerves do not appear to be active either tonically or to play a role in reflex effects until a later stage of development. Treatment with the ganglionic blocker chlorisondamine does not affect heart rate in animals one week of age or younger, although heart rate is lowered by chlorisondamine in rats eleven days of age (17). In adult rats, administration of the vasodilator hydralazine causes a depletion of cardiac norepinephrine levels by reflex activation of sympathetic nerves. This effect of hydralazine cannot be seen in rats until fourteen days of age (19), nor does hydralazine evoke reflex tachycardia before fourteen days of age (21). Thus, immaturity of reflex activation must reside either in the afferent or sensory limb of this reflex or within the central nervous system itself.

The ability of the enzyme ornithine decarboxylase to respond to β-adrenergic activation of the heart has been used to trace the development of cardiac adrenergic control systems. The enzyme ornithine decarboxylase has a rather short turnover time, so its activity can alter rapidly (22, 23). Since this enzyme is sensitive to a number of specific hormones and neurotransmitters, it can provide a very sensitive index of responsiveness of an organ to direct or indirect stimuli. Thus, activity of ornithine decarboxylase has been used as an index of functional development of the peripheral nervous system (24).

In the first five days of life, administration of isoproterenol to rats increases ornithine decarboxylase activity, but administration of nicotine, which acts through adrenergic nerves, does not affect ornithine decarboxylase activity until animals are older than six days of age (25). In addition, insulin-induced hypoglycemia, which stimulates ornithine decarboxylase activity in the adult rat heart by reflex sympathetic activation, has no effect in the neonatal rat heart until eight days of age (26). This confirms the immaturity of sympathetic control of the heart in rats younger than one week.

Adrenal Medulla

Maintenance of cardiovascular function in the newborn may be more dependent on activity of the adrenal medulla than is true of the adult. In adrenalectomized newborn puppies, ability to maintain responsiveness of the heart to repeated and prolonged sympathetic stimulation is reduced in comparison to sham-operated dogs (27).

In addition, mechanisms of responsiveness of the adrenal medulla in immature animals appear to be unique. In the immature sheep and calf, hypoxia produces an adrenal medullary discharge, primarily of norepinephrine, which is not dependent on an intact splanchnic innervation (28). In the sheep, this unique response disappears before birth, while in the less mature newborn calf it is present until 24 hours after birth.

The time course of development of adrenal medullary control mechanisms has been explored most intensively in the rat (20). Stimulation of the splanchnic nerve of the newborn rat does not produce a response in the adrenal. Furthermore, insulin-induced hypoglycemia, which in the adult produces sympathetic activity, does not cause release of adrenal medullary catecholamines from the newborn rat. However, direct activation of the adrenal medulla by nicotine, which activates cholinergic receptors in the organ itself, does cause release of catecholamines in the neonatal rat. Thus, the limiting factor in the development of adrenergic control of this organ is not development of reactivity of the organ itself but rather development of splanchnic nerve function.

Vascular Smooth Muscle

Much less work has been done on the development of adrenergic control of vascular smooth muscle than of the heart. The situation is further complicated by the marked heterogeneity among different vascular beds of mechanisms controlling blood vessel tone. Those studies that have been done suggest that the same general principle elaborated above applies to vascular smooth muscle: the capability of vascular smooth muscle to respond to circulating substances develops before functional adrenergic nerves are present (29). Thus, the fetal lamb carotid artery contracts in vitro to norepinephrine before responses to adrenergic nerve stimulation can be detected. By a gestational age of 115–130 days responses to adrenergic nerve stimulation can be detected, but their magnitude continues to increase until 140–150 days of gestational age. Thus, in the lamb, which is born in a highly developed state, development of blood vessel reactivity predates establishment of functional adrenergic nerve connections.

BLOOD VESSELS

Adrenergic Innervation

There are a number of different approaches to assessing the density or functional capacity of sympathetic innervation. These include histological assessment using catecholamine fluorescence (30, 31); measurement of cocaine-sensitive accumulation of ^{3}H-norepinephrine (32) or an unmetabolized analog, ^{3}H-metaraminol (33, 34); and measurement of endogenous norepinephrine content and assessment of activities of catechol-o-methyl transferase and monoamine oxidase, enzymes that metabolize norepinephrine. The unique localization of adrenergic nerves to the adventitia and advential-medial border of blood vessels makes it difficult to determine what is the most appropriate index for evaluating the density of adrenergic innervation. Since the adrenergic nerve plexus approaches a two-dimensional form, comparisons based on tissue weight may be misleading if the smooth muscle cell layer differs greatly in thickness, as may be true at different stages of growth. The best solution to this problem is to include more than one index of nerve density. A histochemical approach using quantitative image analysis has proved particularly productive (35).

In the rabbit at one week before birth adrenergic nerves appear straight, smooth, and faintly fluorescent in the blood vessel wall, with few varicose swellings (35). By one day before birth, the number of nerves has increased markedly and more varicosities can be seen. A period of rapid nerve growth in the large arteries then occurs until one day after birth, with large increases in number of varicosities in the carotid, renal, and femoral arteries.

The time of development of adrenergic innervation varies considerably among blood vessels. The femoral artery has almost reached the adult level of varicosity number by one day after birth. Smaller arteries, such as the mesenteric artery and the basilar artery, have very sparse nerve plexuses at one day after birth, and adrenergic nerves in these vessels show a rapid growth period between one day after birth and six weeks of age.

Similar conclusions about the developmental pattern of vascular adrenergic innervation can be drawn from other studies. In the rat portal vein, development of the two layers of muscle characteristic of this tissue can be observed at four days after birth. At this point, adrenergic nerves are restricted to the outer layer of the vessel wall. For the next two weeks adrenergic nerve fibers penetrate through the outer longitudinal muscle layer to establish a two-dimensional plexus between the two muscle layers (36).

Studies of three rat arteries, the tail, superficial epigastric, and saphenous, show patterns of nerve development similar to what was found in the rabbit (37). A comparison of rabbit and guinea pig renal arteries shows a decline in adrenergic nerve density in the guinea pig renal artery from birth to four weeks, while rabbit renal arteries continue to gain in adrenergic nerve density for up to six months (35, 38).

These differences in time course of nerve development have been primarily studied in large arteries and it is difficult to extrapolate from this to true resistance vessels. Despite this limitation, such studies make it clear that at least three phases of nerve growth can be distinguished (35). The first phase involves outgrowth of new axons, which in the rabbit may take place either before or after birth. In the second phase of growth, regions of intense fluorescence appear along the nerve. This presumably corresponds to development of transmitter synthesis and storage capacity. This is followed by a period of rapid growth and differentiation of adrenergic nerve varicosities. In large arteries of the rabbit, this takes place shortly after birth, but in many blood vessels this period may extend for several weeks after birth.

In Vitro Studies

MECHANICAL PROPERTIES   Changes that occur in the structure and mechanics of arteries during development have been reviewed previously (39). In some specialized vessels, for example the pulmonary artery, the time of birth produces profound specific changes in structure and function, including a slight thickening and a decline in mechanical stiffness. In most vessels, however, development is associated with a marked thickening of the vessel wall and progressively increasing mechanical stiffness.

The structure of the rat aorta has been carefully studied during development (40). During the first ten to fifteen weeks of life, the rat aorta increases in length to correspond with a rapid increase in total body weight and crown rump length. The bulk of cell division in the rat aorta as measured by autoradiographic incorporation of ^{3}H-thymidine occurs during the first weeks of life in the thoracic segment and during the first eighteen days in the abdominal segment. Total DNA and RNA content of the developing rat aorta increases markedly in the first five weeks of life, although when expressed as a function of dry weight there is a marked decrease in both DNA and RNA content (41). This corresponds to a decrease in number of cells per unit dry weight during growth; thus, there is a decrease in cellularity of the entire aorta during the first month of life. Both collagen and elastin, as total amounts and when expressed per unit dry weight, show increases during development in the rat aorta (41). The amount of collagen continues to increase up to fifteen weeks of age, while elastin content per unit dry weight reaches a peak by eighteen days of life and then shows a progressive decline to twenty-two weeks of age.

Similar results were found in a study of the dog carotid artery (42). Collagen content as a function of wet weight increased from two to twenty-eight weeks of age, while elastin content increased slightly from two to seven weeks and then declined to reach a constant level by twenty-eight weeks. This corresponds to an increase in collagen-to-elastin ratio between seven and twenty-eight weeks of life.

Analysis of extracellular and intracellular water and electrolyte contents shows that in the canine carotid artery there is a decrease in total water content, primarily due to a decrease in extracellular water space as measured by distribution of ^{60}CO-EDTA (42–44). Intracellular water space does not change during development. Total electrolyte content of the canine aorta and carotid artery, including sodium, potassium, chloride, magnesium, and calcium, also declines in the first few weeks of life (43, 44). In addition, with increasing age, efflux of $^{42}K^+$ slows in both the canine aorta and carotid artery.

The effect of these developmental changes in structure and connective tissue content on mechanical properties of large blood vessels has also been studied (42, 43). Because of the rapid alteration in tissue diameter during growth, in order to compare mechanical properties of vessels from animals of different ages diameter at each pressure is normalized by dividing by the diameter at zero pressure. Passive tangential stress-strain curves are shifted progressively with increasing age so that for a given normalized external diameter the passive tangential stress is increased in older animals. This has been shown for canine iliac, renal, carotid, and mesenteric arteries, and aorta. These changes have been interpreted as indicating an increase in arterial wall stiffness with age, corresponding to a decrease in cellularity and increase in connective tissue content.

SMOOTH MUSCLE RESPONSIVENESS   Several different approaches can be used for investigating vascular smooth muscle responsiveness in the tissue bath: vessel segments can be perfused or isometric or isotonic contractions can be measured using ring segments or strips (45). For determination of receptor characteristics in vascular smooth muscle, isometric recording is widely used. Effects of drugs or transmitter substances added to the bath can be determined, or nerves in the vessel wall can be stimulated using transmural electric pulses (46).

For studies of isometric contraction, the resting tension placed on the vessel is critical, since the active force developed is dependent on the passive force applied to the tissue (39). In order to maintain vessels of different sizes or mechanical properties at the same point on the length tension curve, these should all be studied at the optimum resting tension. This is defined as the resting tension at which active contractile responses are maximized.

Once the appropriate resting tension for a given vessel is determined, one must then decide how to control for changes in structure, orientation of smooth muscle cells, etc. In this regard, a measure of contractile ability that is not specific for a single receptor mechanism has been useful. For example, activation with a high concentration of potassium has been used as a non-specific contractile stimulus. If one wishes to examine changes in responsiveness to activation of a specific receptor type, for example the β-adrenergic receptor, then it is important to select experimental conditions that involve activation of that receptor alone, without interference from other mechanisms (47). Methods for analysis of dose-response data and for determination of receptor characteristics using smooth muscle responses have been reviewed (48).

In the last ten years powerful radioligand binding methods have been developed that make it possible to look at characteristics of receptors themselves (49). While these techniques are extremely useful, one should remember that they give little indication of alterations in the multiple processes involved in receptor-contraction coupling.

β-*Adrenergic stimulation*   One of the best defined age-dependent alterations in vascular smooth muscle reactivity is the change in magnitude of the β-adrenergic response (50). In both rabbit and rat aorta, as well as several other arteries, β-adrenergic relaxation declines with advancing age. For example, in rabbit aorta isoproterenol-induced relaxation declines from 56–70 days of age, so that in aortae from animals three to five years of age there is no relaxation response to isoproterenol (51, 52). This age-related change has been shown to be altered by variation in diet (53). Aortae from rats fed a restricted diet (60% of amount consumed by controls) showed a greater decline in the magnitude of β-adrenergic relaxation than aortae from control rats.

Since the magnitude of drug-induced relaxation depends on the level of initial smooth muscle tone, it is important in such studies to use equivalent levels of contraction in vessels from animals of different ages (54). One way to demonstrate specificity of alterations in relaxation magnitude is to use several different drugs that act by different mechanisms to produce relaxation. For example, if a specific change in β-adrenergic stimulation occurs, then relaxation responses to nitroglycerin, nitrite, or papaverine should not change (51, 54). Studies of the rat aorta showed that when the level of smooth muscle tone was equated on the basis of percent maximal tension, the magnitude of nitroglycerin-induced relaxation was not constant. Only when a similar level of grams force was maintained did the nitroglycerin-induced relaxation remain constant in aortic strips from animals of different ages.

Closer examination of the first few weeks of life shows that β-adrenergic mechanisms are not fully developed in the newborn. In aortic strips from rabbits 1–2 days old, only small relaxations to isoproterenol are seen, and these reach a maximal level by one month of age. In contrast, the magnitude of relaxation to sodium nitrite or papaverine stays constant at all ages. Relaxation responses to adenosine also show an age-related decline, so that aortae from rabbits 360 days old show very little relaxation response to this substance (55).

α-*Adrenergic stimulation*   The magnitude of β-adrenergic relaxation changes with age, and many substances, such as norepinephrine, that stimulate α-adrenergic receptors also activate β-adrenergic receptors. Therefore, in many studies where β-adrenergic responses are not blocked it is difficult to draw conclusions about changes in α-adrenergic mechanisms per se. For example, it has been shown that the β-adrenergic antagonist propranolol potentiates responses to norepinephrine in aortae from immature (2–12 days) rabbits, but to a much lesser extent in aortae from rabbits 90 days of age (55). Thus, the much greater β-adrenergic relaxation present in aortae from young animals has a greater impact on responses to norepinephrine than in aortae from older animals, where there is much less β-adrenergic response.

A more fundamental problem in the interpretation of many studies is that no control of the profound changes in blood vessel size and mechanics is included. Since in some cases data are not normalized to the maximum contractile response of the tissue, it is difficult to decide whether increased responses to α-adrenergic stimulation are due to growth of the vessel or to a relative increase in development of α-adrenergic responsiveness.

In most studies, however, there appears to be an increase in maximal responses to norepinephrine in the first few weeks of life when these are corrected for the contractile ability of the tissue. In canine iliac, carotid, renal, and mesenteric arteries, vessels from animals younger than two weeks of age showed smaller responses to α-adrenergic stimulation relative to responses to KCl compared to adults (43). However, in the canine aorta one study showed no change in α-adrenergic responsiveness with age (56). In fetal sheep, the maximum response to norepinephrine as a percent of maximum response to serotonin increases when animals 115–130 days of gestation are compared to fetuses at 140–150 days (29).

When sensitivity to α-adrenergic stimulation is examined, there is much more disagreement among studies. In several studies no change in the norepinephrine EC_{50} (concentration for 50% of the maximal response) has been noted [sheep fetus (29), sheep ear artery (57), guinea pig and rabbit renal arteries (38), rat portal vein (58)]. However, a decrease in EC_{50} for both norepinephrine and phenylephrine has been found in the canine aorta and for norepinephrine in the sheep carotid (56, 59). In guinea pig and rabbit renal arteries, there was no difference in norepinephrine EC_{50} when newborn and adult animals were compared. However, the slope of the concentration-response curve was different. At low concentrations the newborn guinea pig renal artery was more sensitive to norepinephrine than the adult, while the adult rabbit renal artery was more sensitive than the newborn at low norepinephrine concentrations (38). The phentolamine pA_2, an estimate of the antagonist dissociation constant, did not change for the sheep ear artery from animals of five age groups ranging from 110 day-old fetuses to adults (57).

Examination of the rabbit mesenteric and intestinal microvasculature showed no change in the ability of norepinephrine to produce arteriolar constriction from day 23 of gestation to the adult (60). However, the duration of the response was longer in older fetuses and the adult.

Responses to adrenergic nerve stimulation show clear-cut developmental changes that correspond to the growth of adrenergic nerves during this time period. In the sheep ear artery and carotid artery, responses to nerve stimulation show a progressive increase from 110 days of gestation to the adult (29, 57). Newborn rabbit renal arteries also have a relatively smaller response to nerve stimulation than vessels from the adult (38). Responses to nerve stimulation have also been studied using tyramine, which releases transmitter from adrenergic nerves, showing a similar pattern of development of adrenergic responsiveness (56, 58).

Significant species differences have been highlighted in studies of the portal vein (8). The newborn guinea pig portal vein responds as well as the adult's to nerve stimulation, while the newborn rat portal vein does not contract to nerve stimulation. Intermediate are portal veins of rabbits and cats, which do have a small response to nerve stimulation that becomes much larger in the adult.

Other vasoactive substances   There is considerable variability in the developmental profile of other types of vasoactivity. For example, the spontaneous activity seen in the portal vein is present at birth in the guinea pig but absent in the newborn rabbit and cat (8). In the rat portal vein, spontaneous activity does not develop until 15–20 days of age (58).

Responses to serotonin show a decrease in EC_{50} during development in the sheep carotid artery (29, 59), but no change in the sheep ear artery (57). The maximal response to serotonin declined in the sheep carotid artery from 250% of the norepinephrine response at 53–90 days gestation to 112% at 140–150 days (57). In the rabbit aorta, the maximal contractile response to serotonin declined relative to the norepinephrine response from 5 to 360 days of age (55).

The EC_{50} for angiotensin was shown to be higher in the newborn sheep carotid artery than in the adult (59), while responses to vasopressin did not change during development in the sheep ear artery (57). The EC_{50} for acetylcholine did not change with age in the rat portal vein (58).

In Vivo Studies

In some species, depending on the state of maturity at birth, reflex responses of the vasculature mediated by adrenergic nerves may be incompletely developed in the newborn. In other species, however, responses may be indistinguishable from the adult. In pigs, fully integrated vascular responses to reflex activation of the adrenergic nervous system are not fully developed until two weeks of age (61, 62).

In the mature-at-birth sheep, the magnitude of neurohumoral control was assessed by the change in blood pressure produced by α-adrenergic blockade with phenoxybenzamine or ganglionic blockade with trimethaphan. Responses to blockade of neurohumoral control were greater in the term fetus than in the neonate and declined with age to the adult (63), suggesting more intense sympathetic control of blood pressure in the term fetus and newborn than in the adult.

In the dog, on the other hand, some studies seem to demonstrate that vascular responses to adrenergic nerve stimulation are not fully developed in the newborn. Sympathetic nerve stimulation of the isolated perfused hindquarters of the newborn dog produced a vasodilator response that was blocked by atropine. Not until two weeks of age was a vasoconstrictor response to nerve stimulation seen (64). Bilateral carotid occlusion produced an increase in blood pressure in newborn dogs, although the magnitude of this increase was smaller than that in dogs ten days old or in adults (65). In contrast, though, the indirectly acting adrenergic agonist tyramine produced similar pressor effects in newborn and adult dogs (66).

Arterial blood pressure in the newborn is low and increases progressively to the adult level in a number of species that have been studied (65, 67, 68). This makes it difficult to decide how to compare blood pressure responsiveness in animals of different ages, since the absolute amount of change in blood pressure produced by a given stimulus would be expected to alter just on the basis of differences in resting blood pressure. To circumvent this problem, some authors have expressed changes as percent of resting blood pressure.

Despite these difficulties in interpretation of in vivo data, studies of responses to adrenergic drugs confirm conclusions reached from in vitro studies. In the newborn pig, higher doses of isoproterenol are necessary to produce a fall in systemic blood pressure, and for a given dose of isoproterneol there was a smaller decrease in resistance as calculated from femoral and carotid arterial flows (69). Thus, in pigs β-adrenergic responsiveness of vascular smooth muscle is apparently still developing during the second postnatal week. Intravenous injections of isoproterenol also had much smaller effects on blood pressure in the term fetus of the sheep than in the adult (63).

Confounding effects of differences in drug disposition and metabolism are illustrated by the study of Boatman et al (64). Injections of epinephrine and norepinephrine produced similar increases in pressure in the isolated perfused hindquarters of the dog at all ages studied. However, the effective concentration of the drug was less in the adult due to its much larger size. These authors, therefore, concluded that newborn dogs were much less sensitive to adrenergic drugs than the adult. In addition, they noted that the duration of the response in the newborn was much longer than in the adult and suggested that there are differences in metabolism of adrenergic agonists perhaps related to immaturity of adrenergic nerves. In another study of the dog, there was no change in blood pressure response to norepinephrine, although, again, the response duration was longer in the newborn than in the adult (66).

In newborn pigs, higher doses of norepinephrine were necessary to produce a significant change in blood pressure compared to adults (69). In addition, the absolute magnitude of blood pressure change was greater in the adult, although the significance of this observation is difficult to interpret.

Studies of blood pressure in the sheep show no significant alteration in maximal responses to norepinephrine with age (63). However, comparison of dose response curves to norepinephrine indicate that the term fetus showed considerably less sensitivity to norepinephrine than the neonate.

Examination of blood pressure responses to angiotensin in the lamb showed no alterations in the newborn lamb from birth to 60 days of age, even though baseline blood pressure rose progressively (70). In these animals, maintained on a carefully monitored sodium intake, the rise in arterial pressure with age could not be accounted for by a change in vascular sensitivity to angiotensin.

To this date, most in vivo studies have focused on changes in systemic blood pressure. However, as shown by morphological and in vitro studies, there are significant differences among vascular beds in the rat of maturation of adrenergic mechanisms. Therefore, it will be important in future studies to carefully analyze regional variations in vascular adrenergic mechanisms.

CLINICAL CORRELATES

From the clinician's standpoint, a major impetus to understanding the way in which the vascular system develops is the important role that this system plays in the adaptation of the newborn to the extrauterine environment. With advances taking place in the management of the pulmonary components of hyaline membrane disease, the major clinical challenges facing us in the care of premature and full-term infants are vascular disorders of adaptation. Three disorders in which the vasculature appears to play a major role are persistent fetal circulation, intraventricular hemorrhage, and necrotizing enterocolitis.

Persistent Fetal Circulation

The transition occurring at the moment of birth is the single most dramatic physiologic event in the life of a human (71). In those few seconds the pattern of circulation must change from one based on placental transfer of oxygen to one allowing pulmonary exchange of gases. These changes are primarily vascular in origin, resulting in vasodilation of the pulmonary vessels and constriction of the umbilical arteries. They are uniquely characteristic of the infant born after 37 weeks' gestation. At younger ages, or in cases where the birth process is complicated by severe asphyxia, these vascular transitions may not occur or may be altered. This abnormal circulatory state has been termed persistent fetal circulation and is manifest primarily as pulmonary hypertension and failure of the ductus arteriosus to close (72).

During the normal birth process, at the instant of the first breath the resistance in the pulmonary vasculature drops dramatically and the ductus arteriosus closes. The mediators of this process have not been defined, although the compounds most commonly implicated are the prostaglandins. Evidence for a partial role of prostaglandins in "first-breath" vasodilation has been described (73). However, the failure of indomethacin to completely inhibit the "first-breath" effect suggests that other mediators may also be involved.

Following an acute episode of asphyxia, the normal pulmonary vasodilation associated with the "first breath" fails (72). While factors such as hypoxia and systemic acidemia have been implicated as contributing factors, the cellular or chemical mediators that cause pulmonary vasoconstriction to persist have not been identified. In the preterm infant, unknown chemical mediators associated with prematurity and hyaline membrane disease may contribute to decreased pulmonary blood flow.

The various approaches to treatment of this disorder further underline our lack of basic information as to etiology. Tolazoline is one frequently recommended drug for persistent fetal circulation (74). This drug has histaminergic, α-adrenergic, and cholinergic properties (75). In some species, the vasodilator properties of tolazoline have been attributed to stimulation of histamine type 1 and 2 receptors (76), while in other species it has been suggested that the efficacy of this drug is related to α-adrenergic antagonism (77). Without some basic understanding of the mechanisms involved in the human neonatal response to a drug such as tolazoline, it will be impossible to predict or design drug regimens that would be most efficacious in treating this disorder.

Intraventricular Hemorrhage

Until the 36th week of gestation in the human infant, there exists an area in the brain at the level of the caudate nucleus that is referred to as the subependymal germinal matrix layer (78). This layer gives rise to cells that migrate out and further develop the neuronal elements of the central nervous system. In its role as a center of growth, this area is richly supplied with a network of capillary blood vessels. Thus, the premature infant has a unique vascular structure that is absent at full-term normal birth. On the basis of cumulative evidence (79–81), it appears that this vascular bed is predisposed to hemorrhage into the ventricular system when subjected to asphyxial conditions followed by surges of cerebral blood flow. In a prospective study (82), evidence of hemorrhage in the subependymal area was present in 78% of all premature infants admitted into an intensive-care nursery. This process of acute hemorrhage is associated with a high incidence of nonobstructive hydrocephalus as well as focal and global neurologic deficits.

Because of the severity of this problem, much effort has been directed toward an understanding of the etiology of these acute hemorrhages. In an animal model (83), intraventricular hemorrhage can be produced by asphyxia, hypertension (secondary to catecholamine infusion), and infusions of substances causing an increase in plasma volume and/or osmolality. This has led investigators (84) to speculate that autoregulation may not be intact in the normal premature newborn. Based on work using xenon washout in premature infants, it has been suggested that flow to the premature infant's brain is pressure passive, with only very limited autoregulatory capabilities. This evidence has led Volpe (85) to hypothesize that the richly vascularized subependymal germinal matrix layer has a poorly developed supportive structure and is injured by hypoxia and hypoperfusion. Following this injury, any pressure-passive surges in blood flow to the area result in rupture of the capillary and precapillary vessels.

It is apparent that if cerebral blood flow is indeed pressure passive in the neonate, then events that alter the systematic arterial blood pressure may have a dramatic effect on the central nervous system. Thus, infants with cardiovascular compromise on the basis of hyaline membrane disease and secondary pulmonary vasoconstriction or altered blood flow pathways (such as through a ductus arteriosus) may also have associated intraventricular hemorrhage.

In addition, the implications for therapeutic intervention are great. The use of vasoactive substances that have no effect on the cerebral blood vessels but cause increases in peripheral resistance and pressure may be deleterious to the newborn. Current efforts to minimize the incidence of intraventricular hemorrhage have all centered around elimination of high-risk situations (86). These attempts, while perhaps able to decrease the incidence of this problem, fail to address the underlying etiology of either a lack of or a failure of the cerebral autoregulatory mechanisms. Only by understanding the mechanisms associated with control of cerebral blood flow in the neonate can reasonable therapeutic choices be made in emergency situations requiring aggressive support of vital signs.

Necrotizing Enterocolitis

A third clinical entity of major concern in neonatal intensive care units is necrotizing enterocolitis. While the exact etiologic role of vascular smooth muscle in this disorder is not clear, epidemiologic evidence points to cardiovascular disorders as a major risk factor (87). This is primarily a disease of premature infants; the majority weigh less than 2.5. kg at birth and have a gestational age of less than 38 weeks (88). For all neonatal intensive care units across the United States, an average of about 3000 deaths per year may occur as a results of this disorder (89).

Cardiovascular risk factors associated with the development of necrotizing enterocolitis include cyanotic congenital heart disease, patent ductus arteriosus, umbilical artery catheterization, and exchange transfusion (87). In addition, it has been recognized that unique cardiovascular reflexes present in the perinatal period may contribute to hypoperfusion states for the mesenteric circulation. It has been noted that asphyxiated newborn infants develop bradycardia and an increase in lactate concentration in the blood (90). These responses are similar to the so-called diving reflex, a phenomenon observed in the diving seal where the heart rate drops and the renal, mesenteric, and peripheral circulations are vasoconstricted to maintain maximal blood flow to the central nervous system (91). This similarity has led to speculation that the normal diving reflex may lead to mesenteric ischemia, particularly in the preterm infant who is asphyxiated.

In infants with cyanotic congential heart disease or vascular shunts causing rapid runoff of arterial circulation (such as patent ductus arteriosus), this mesenteric ischemia may be further exaggerated. In a similar manner, emboli associated with procedures such as umbilical artery catheterization may also cause mesenteric ischemia. If one accepts mesenteric ischemia as a primary event in the development of necrotizing enterocolitis, it follows that ischemic breakdown of the mucosal defense barriers may contribute to invasion of bacteria and further breakdown of the gut endothelium.

From an empirical standpoint, the prevention of necrotizing enterocolitis should involve prevention of asphyxial states and, thus, the avoidance of the diving-seal phenomenon. In addition, care should be taken to prevent other vascular embolic events, such as those associated with use of indwelling catheters. This provides us with a minimal clinical base from which to operate, however. Without an understanding of the underlying mechanisms involved in local regulation of the vascular responses of the mesenteric bed, it is impossible to rationally treat infants who have been exposed to asphyxial episodes. Basic research should be directed at an understanding of the effects of endogenous and exogenous vasoactive compounds in order to optimize and restore blood flow to critical areas in the asphyxiated neonate.

ACKNOWLEDGMENTS

Dr. Duckles is an Established Investigator of the American Heart Association with funds provided in part by the Arizona Affiliate.

Literature Cited

1. Bevan, J. A., Bevan, R. D., Duckles, S. P. 1980. Adrenergic regulation of vascular smooth muscle. In *Handbook of Physiology, Section 2, Cardiovascular System: Vascular Smooth Muscle*, ed. D. F. Bohr, A. P. Somlyo, H. V. Sparks, 2:515-66. Bethesda, Md: Am. Physiol. Soc. 686 pp.
2. Heymann, M. A., Iwamoto, H. S., Rudolph, A. M. 1981. Factors affecting changes in the neonatal systemic circulation. *Ann. Rev. Physiol.* 43:371–83
3. Hendry, I. A. 1976. Control in the development of the vertebrate sympathetic nervous system. In *Reviews of Neuroscience*, ed. S. Ehrenpreis, I. J. Kopin, 2:149–94. New York: Raven. 270 pp.
4. Black, I. B. 1978. Regulation of autonomic development. *Ann. Rev. Neurosci.* 1:183–214
5. Burnstock, G. 1981. Development of smooth muscle and its innervation. In *Smooth Muscle*, ed. E. Bulbring, A. F. Brading, A. W. Jones, T. Tomita, pp. 431–57. Austin: Univ. Tex. Press. 563 pp.
6. Duckles, S. P., Lee, T. J.-F., Bevan, J. A. 1977. Cerebral arterial responses to nerve stimulation in vitro. Species variation in the constrictor and dilator components. In *Neurogenic Control of the Brain Circulation*, ed. C. Owman, L. Edvinsson, pp. 133–142. New York: Pergamon. 510 pp.
7. Duckles, S. P. 1979. Neurogenic dilator and constrictor responses of pial arteries in vitro. Differences between dogs and sheep. *Circ. Res.* 44:482–90
8. Stage, D., Ljung, B. 1978. Neuroeffector maturity of portal veins from newborn rats, rabbits, cats and guinea pigs. *Acta Physiol. Scand.* 102:218–23
9. Buckley, N. M., Gootman, P. M., Yellin, E. L., Brazeau, P. 1979. Age-related cardiovascular effects of catecholamines in anesthetized piglets. *Circ. Res.* 45:282–92
10. Haworth, S. G., Hislop, A. A. 1981. Adaptation of the pulmonary circulation to extra-uterine life in the pig and its relevance to the human infant. *Cardiovas. Res.* 15:108–19
11. Ment, L. R., Duncan, C. C., Stewart, W. B. 1983. Local cerebral blood flow and metabolism alterations in the newborn beagle puppy model of intraventricular hemorrhage, In *Concepts in Pediatric Neurosurgery*, ed. A. J. Raimondi, 3:108–24. Basel: Karger. 224 pp.
12. Book, S. A., Bustad, L. K. 1974. The fetal and neonatal pig in biomedical research. *J. Anim. Sci.* 38:997–1002
13. Glauser, E. M. 1966. Advantage of piglets as experimental animals in pediatric research. *Exp. Med. Surg.* 24:181–90
14. Volpe, J. J. 1981. Current concepts in neonatal medicine. Neonatal intraventricular hemorrhage. *N. Engl. J. Med.* 304:886–91
15. Goddard, J., Lewis, R. M., Armstrong, D. L., Zeller, R. S. 1980. Moderate, rapidly induced hypertension as a cause of intraventricular hemorrhage in the newborn beagle model. *J. Pediatrics* 96:1057–60
16. Pappano, A. J. 1977. Ontogenetic development of autonomic neuroeffector transmission and transmitter reactivity in embryonic and fetal hearts. *Pharmacol. Rev.* 29:3–33
17. Seidler, F. J., Slotkin, T. A. 1979. Presynaptic and postsynaptic contributions to ontogeny of sympathetic control of heart rate in the preweanling rat. *Brit. J. Pharmacol.* 65:431–34
18. Bareis, D. L., Slotkin, T. A. 1980. Maturation of sympathetic neurotransmission in the rat heart. I. Ontogeny of the synaptic vesicle uptake mechanism and correlation with development of synaptic function. Effects of neonatal methadone administration on development of synaptic vesicles. *J. Pharmacol. Exp. Ther.* 212:120–25
19. Seidler, F. J., Slotkin, T. A. 1981. Development of central control of norepinephrine turnover and release in the rat heart: Responses to tyramine, 2-deoxyglucose and hydralazine. *Neuroscience* 6:2081–86
20. Slotkin, T. A., Smith, P. G., Lau, C., Bareis, D. L. 1980. Functional aspects of development of catecholamine biosynthesis and release in the sympathetic nervous system. In *Biogenic Amines in Development*, ed. H. Parvez, S. Parvez, pp. 29–48. New York: Elsevier/North Holland. 735 pp.
21. Bartolome, J., Mills, E., Lau, C. Slotkin, T. A. 1980. Maturation of sympathetic neurotransmission in the rat heart. V. Development of baroreceptor control of sympathetic tone. *J. Pharmacol. Exp. Ther.* 215:596–600
22. Russell, D. H., Snyder, S. H. 1968. Amine synthesis in rapidly growing tissues: Ornithine decarboxylase activity in regenerating rat liver, chick embryo and

various tumors. *Proc. Natl. Acad. Sci. USA* 60:1420–27

23. Russell, D. H., Snyder, S. H. 1969. Amine synthesis in regenerating rat liver: Extremely rapid turnover of ornithine decarboxylase. *Mol. Pharmacol.* 5:253–62

24. Slotkin, T. A. 1979. Ornithine decarboxylase as a tool in development neurobiology. *Life Sci.* 24:1623–30

25. Bartolome, J., Lau, C., Slotkin, T. A. 1977. Ornithine decarboxylase in developing rat heart and brain: Role of sympathetic development for responses to autonomic stimulants and the effects of reserpine on maturation. *J. Pharmacol. Exp. Ther.* 202:510–18

26. Bareis, D. L., Slotkin, T. A. 1978. Responses of heart ornithine decarboxylase and adrenal catecholamines to methadone and sympathetic stimulation in developing and adult rats. *J. Pharmacol. Exp. Ther.* 205:164–74

27. Erath, H. G., Boerth, R. C., Graham, T. P. Jr. 1982. Functional significance of reduced cardiac sympathetic innervation in the newborn dog. *Am. J. Physiol.* 243:H20–H26

28. Comline, R. S., Silver, M. 1966. The development of the adrenal medulla of the foetal and newborn calf. *J. Physiol.* 183:305–40

29. Su, C., Bevan, J. A., Assali, N. S., Brinkman, C. R. 1977. Development of neuroeffector mechanisms in the carotid artery of the fetal lamb. *Blood Vessels* 14:12–24

30. Falck, B., Hillarp, N.-A., Thieme, G., Torp, A. 1962. Fluorescence of catecholamines and related compounds condensed with formaldehyde. *J. Histochem. Cytochem.* 10:348–54

31. Cowen, T., Burnstock, G. 1980. Quantitative analysis of the density and pattern of adrenergic innervation of blood vessels. *Histochemistry* 66:19–34.

32. Su, C., Duckles, S. P., Florence, V. 1977. Uptake of ³H-norepinephrine in rabbit mesenteric blood vessels. *Blood Vessels* 14:65–76

33. Hermann, W., Graefe, K.-H. 1977. Relationship between the uptake of ³H metaraminol and the density of adrenergic innervation in isolated rat tissues. *Naunyn-Schmiedeberg's Arch. Pharmacol.* 296:99–110

34. Duckles, S. P. 1980. Comparison of ³H-norepinephrine and ³H-metaraminol accumulation as indices of adrenergic nerve density in rabbit blood vessels. *Eur. J. Pharmacol.* 67:355–61

35. Cowen, T., Haven, A. J., Wen-Qin, C., Gallen, D. D., Franc, F., Burnstock, G.

1982. Development and aging of perivascular adrenergic nerves in the rabbit. A quantitative fluorescence histochemical study using image analysis. *J. Autonomic Nerv. Syst.* 5:317–36

36. Lundberg, J., Ljung, B., Stage, D., Dahlstrom, A. 1976. Postnatal ontogenic development of the adrenergic innervation pattern in the rat portal vein. *Cell Tissue Res.* 172:15–27

37. Todd, M. E. 1980. Development of adrenergic innervation in rat peripheral vessels: A fluorescence microscopic study. *J. Anatomy* 131:121–33

38. Gallen, D. D., Cowen, T., Griffith, S. G., Haven, A. J. Burnstock, G. 1982. Functional and non-functional nerve-smooth muscle transmission in the renal arteries of the newborn and adult rabbit and guinea pig. *Blood Vessels* 19:237–46

39. Dobrin, P. B. 1978. Mechanical properties of arteries. *Physiol. Rev.* 58:397–460

40. Berry, C. L., Looker, T., Germain, J. 1972. The growth and development of the rat aorta. I. Morphological aspects. *J. Anat.* 113:1–16

41. Looker, T., Berry, C. L. 1972. The growth and development of the rat aorta. II. Changes in nucleic acid and scleroprotein content. *J. Anat.* 113:17–34

42. Cox, R. H., Jones, A. W., Fischer, G. M. 1974. Carotid artery mechanics, connective tissue and electrolyte changes in puppies. *Am. J. Physiol.* 227:563–68

43. Cox, R. H., Jones, A. W., Swain, M. L. 1976. Mechanics and electrolyte composition of arterial smooth muscle in developing dogs. *Am. J. Physiol.* 231:77–83

44. Cox, R. H. 1981. Potassium efflux and chemical content of canine arteries during growth and development. *IRCS Med. Sci.* 9:820–21

45. Daniel, E. E., Paton, D. M., eds. 1975. *Methods in Pharmacology: Smooth Muscle, Vol. 3.* New York: Plenum. 731 pp.

46. Duckles, S. P., Silverman, R. W. 1980. Transmural nerve stimulation of blood vessels in vitro: A critical examination. *Blood Vessels* 17:53–57

47. Furchgott, R. F. 1972. The classification of adrenoceptors. In *Catecholamines*, ed H. Blaschko, E. Muscholl, pp. 283–335 New York: Springer-Verlag. 1040 pp.

48. Tallarida, R. J., Jacob, L. S. 1979. *The Dose-Response Relation in Pharmacology.* New York: Springer-Verlag 207 pp.

49. Williams, L. T., Lefkowitz, R. J. 1978. *Receptor Binding Studies in Adrenergic*

Pharmacology. New York: Raven. 151 pp.

50. Fleisch, J. H. 1980. Age-related changes in the sensitivity of blood vessels to drugs. Pharmacol. Ther. 8:477–87

51. Fleisch, J. H., Maling, H. M., Brodie, B. B. 1970. β-receptor activity in aorta. Variations with age and species. Circ. Res. 26:151–62

52. Fleisch, J. H., Hooker, C. S. 1976. The relationship between age and relaxation of vascular smooth muscle in the rabbit and rat. Circ. Res. 38:243–49

53. Herlihy, J. T., Yu, B. P. 1980. Dietary manipulation of age-related decline in vascular smooth muscle function. Am. J. Physiol. 238:H652–55

54. Cohen, M. L., Berkowitz, B. A. 1974. Age-related changes in vascular responsiveness to cyclic nucleotides and contractile agonists. J. Pharmacol. Exp. Ther. 191:147–55

55. Hayashi, S., Toda, N. 1978. Age-related changes in the response of rabbit isolated aortae to vasoactive agents. Br. J. Pharmacol. 64:229–37

56. Gray, S. D. 1977. Reactivity of neonatal canine aortic strips. Biol. Neonate 31:10–14

57. Wyse, D. G., Van Petten, G. R., Harris, W. H. 1977. Responses to electrical stimulation, noradrenaline, serotonin and vasopressin in the isolated ear artery of the developing lamb and ewe. Can. J. Physiol. Pharmacol. 55:1001–06

58. Ljung, B., Stage, D. 1975. Postnatal ontogenetic development of neurogenic and myogenic control in the rat portal vein. Acta Physiol. Scand. 94:112–27

59. Gray, S. D. 1976. Effect of angiotensin II on neonatal lamb carotid arteries. Experientia 32:350–51

60. Fehn, P. A., McCuskey, R. S. 1971. Response of the fetal mesenteric microvascular system to catecholamines. Microvas. Res. 3:104–09

61. Reddy, G. D., Gootman, N., Buckley, N. M., Gootman, P. M., Crane, L. 1974. Regional blood flow changes in neonatal pigs in response to hypercapnia, hemorrhage and sciatic nerve stimulation. Biol. Neonate 25:249–62

62. Buckley, N. M., Gootman, P. M., Gootman, N., Reddy, G. D., Weaver, L. C., Crane, L. A. 1976. Age-dependent cardiovascular effects of afferent stimulation in neonatal pigs. Biol. Neonate 30:268–79

63. Woods, J. R. Jr., Dandavino, A., Murayama, K., Brinkman, C. R. III, Assali, N. S. 1977. Autonomic control of cardiovascular functions during neonatal development and in adult sheep. Circ. Res. 40:401–07

64. Boatman, D. L., Shaffer, R. A., Dixon, R. L., Brody, M. J. 1965. Function of vascular smooth muscle and its sympathetic innervation in the newborn dog. J. Clin. Invest. 44:241–46

65. Gauthier, P., Nadeau, R. A., De Champlain, J. 1975. The development of sympathetic innervation and the functional state of the cardiovascular system in newborn dogs. Can. J. Physiol. Pharmacol. 53:763–76

66. Privitera, P. J., Loggie, J. M. H. Gaffney, T. E. 1969. A comparison of the cardiovascular effects of biogenic amines and their precursors in newborn and adult dogs. J. Pharmacol. Exp. Ther. 166:293–98

67. Gootman, P. M., Gootman, N., Turlapaty, P. D. M. V., Yao, A. C., Buckley, B. J., Altura, B. M. 1981. Autonomic regulation of cardiovascular function in neonates. In Development of the Autonomic Nervous System. Ciba Found. Symp. 83, pp. 70–93. London:Pitman Medical

68. Fisher, D. J., Heymann, M. A., Rudolph, A. M. 1982. Regional myocardial blood flow and oxygen delivery in fetal, newborn and adult sheep. Am. J. Physiol. 243:H729–31

69. Buckley, N. M., Gootman, P. M., Yellin, E. J., Brazeau, P. 1979. Age-related cardiovascular effects of catecholamines in anesthetized piglets. Circ. Res. 45:282–92

70. Wilson, T. A., Kaiser, D. L., Wright, E. M., Peach, M. J., Carey, R. M. 1981. Ontogeny of blood pressure and the renin-angiotensin-aldosterone system. Sequential studies in the newborn lamb. Circ. Res. 49:416–23

71. Nelson, N. M. 1975. The onset of respiration. In Neonatology: Pathophysiology and Management of the Newborn, ed. G. Avery, pp. 76–97. Philadelphia: Lippincott. 1136 pp.

72. Rudolph, A. M. 1980. High pulmonary vascular resistance after birth. I. Pathophysiologic considerations and etiologic classification. Clin. Pediatr. 19:585–90

73. Leffler, C. S., Tyler, T. L., Cassin, S. 1978. Effect of indomethacin on pulmonary vascular response to ventilation of fetal goats. Am. J. Physiol. 234:346–51

74. Tooley, W. J., Phibbs, R. H. 1975. Delivery room management of the newborn. See Ref. 71, pp. 111–26

75. Ahlquist, R. P., Huggins, R. A., Woodbury, R. A. 1947. The pharmacology of

benzyl-imidazoline (Priscol). *J. Pharmacol. Exp. Ther.* 89:271–88

76. Goetzman, B. W., Milstein, J. M. 1979. Pulmonary vasodilator action of tolazoline. *Pediat. Res.* 13:942–44

77. Tucker, A., Brown, D. T., Greenlees, K. H. 1982. Pulmonary and systemic vascular actions of tolazoline in anesthetized dogs. *Ped. Pharmacol.* 2:231–43

78. Volpe, J. J. 1979. Intracranial hemorrhage in the newborn: current understanding and dilemmas. *Neurology* 29:632–35

79. Lou, H. C., Skov, H., Pedersen, H. 1979. Low cerebral blood flow: A risk factor in the neonate. *J. Pediatr.* 95:606–09

80. Lou, H. C., Lassen, N. A., Tweed, W. A., Johnson, G., Jones, M., Palahniuk, R. J. 1979. Pressure passive cerebral blood flow and breakdown of the blood-brain barrier in experimental fetal asphyxia. *Acta Paediatr. Scand.* 68:57–63

81. Wigglesworth, J. S., Pape, K. E. 1978. An integrated model for haemorrhagic and ischaemic lesions in the newborn brain. *Early Hum. Dev.* 212:179–99

82. Papile, L., Burstein, J., Burstein, R., Koffler, H. 1978. Incidence and evolution of subependymal and intraventricular hemorrhage. *J. Pediatr.* 92:529–34

83. Goddard, J., Lewis, R. M., Alcala, H., Zeller, R. S. 1980. Intraventricular hemorrhage: An animal model. *Biol. Neonate* 37:39–52

84. Lou, H. C., Lassen, N. A., Friis-Hansen, B. 1970. Impaired autoregulation of cerebral blood flow in the distressed newborn infant. *J. Pediatr.* 94:118–21

85. Volpe, J. J. 1979. Cerebral blood flow in the newborn infant: Relation to hypoxic-ischemic brain injury and periventricular hemorrhage. *J. Pediatr.* 94:170–73

86. Lou, H. C., Lassen, N. A., Friis-Hensen, B. 1979. Is arterial hypertension crucial for the development of cerebral hemorrhage in premature infants? *Lancet* 1:1215–17

87. Touloukian, R. J. 1980. Etiologic role of the circulation. In *Neonatal Necrotizing Enterocolitis,* ed. E. G. Brown, A. Y. Sweet, pp. 41–56. New York: Grune & Stratton. 203 pp.

88. Brown, E. G., Sweet, A. Y. 1982. Neonatal necrotizing enterocolitis. *Pediatr. Clin. North Am.* 29:1149–70

89. Ryder, R. W., Shelton, J. D., Gwinan, M. E. 1980. Necrotizing enterocolitis: A prospective multicenter investigation. *Am. J. Epidemiol.* 112:113–23

90. James, L. S. 1959. Biochemical aspects of asphyxia at birth. In *Adaptation to Extrauterine Life: Report of the 31st Ross Conference on Pediatric Research,* ed. T. K. Oliver, Jr. pp. 66–71. Columbus: Ross Lab. 94 pp.

91. Scholander, P. E. 1963. The master switch of life. *Sci. Am.* 209:92–105

Ann. Rev. Pharmacol. Toxicol. 1984. 24:85–103

PHARMACOKINETICS OF PCBs

H. B. Matthews

National Institute of Environmental Health Sciences, P.O. Box 12233, Research Triangle Park, North Carolina 27709

R. L. Dedrick

Biomedical Engineering and Instrumentation Branch, National Institutes of Health, Building 13, Room 3W13, Bethesda, Maryland 20205

INTRODUCTION

Polychlorinated biphenyls (PCBs) are the products of varying degrees of chlorination of the biphenyl molecule (Figure 1). Given 10 available positions for chlorination, 209 different chlorinated biphenyls (PCB congeners) are possible. These compounds are named according to their positions and degrees of chlorination, i.e. a biphenyl molecule having chlorine atoms at the 2 and 5 positions of each ring (Figure 1) is named 2,5,2',5'-tetrachlorobiphenyl.PCBs were first synthetized over one hundred years ago (1), and commercial production of PCBs in the US began in 1929 (2). Commercial PCB formulations do not consist of a single chlorinated biphenyl but are complex mixtures of chlorinated biphenyls named according to the percent weight accounted for by chlorine. For example, Aroclor® 1248 contains 48 percent by weight of chlorine and several dozen individual chlorinated biphenyls. Because of their desirable physical properties, PCBs have been widely used in a diverse number of commercial products, including heat transfer agents, hydraulic fluids, plasticizers, adhesives, cutting oils, and inks. However, due to their dielectric properties, thermal stability, and nonflammability, PCBs were used most extensively in electrical capacitors and transformers (3). Annual use of PCBs in the US peaked at approximately 85 million pounds in 1970. After 1970, the use of PCBs in the US declined, but it is estimated that almost one billion pounds had been sold up to that date (2).

Given the volume of PCBs used and the period of time during which they were used, the safety record for these compounds was relatively uneventful.

85

0362-1642/84/415-0085$02.00

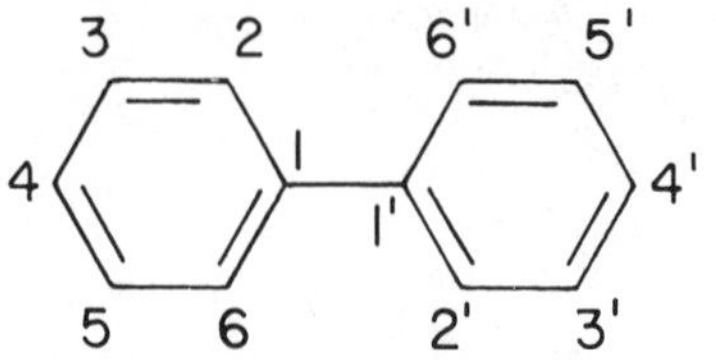

Figure 1   Biphenyl

For a number of years, reports and concern regarding the health effects of PCBs were restricted to workers in direct contact with the compounds in the course of their production or use (4–7). Possibly because they were present as diverse mixtures rather than as one or two individual compounds, PCBs were not recognized as environmental contaminants until 1966 (8). Once their presence had been pointed out and the methods for their detection perfected, PCB contamination was found to be worldwide and in virtually every type of biological sample assayed. The first incident in which PCBs were recognized as the causative agent in the intoxication of the general public occurred in 1968 in Japan, when a PCB mixture used in the cooling system of a rice oil plant leaked into rice oil subsequently consumed by over 1600 persons (9, 10). A similar incident occurred in Taiwan in 1979 (11). The PCB formulation involved in the Japanese incident and to a lesser extent in the Taiwanese incident contained a number of chlorinated dibenzofurans (11, 12). Therefore, it is not known to what extent the diverse symptoms observed in the exposed individuals were due to PCB intoxication or were due in part to the very much more toxic chlorinated dibenzofuran contaminants.

Studies of PCB toxicity in laboratory animals indicate that sensitivity to physiological intoxication by these compounds varies widely with species. Laboratory rats are largely resistant to intoxication by PCBs (13, 14), whereas rhesus monkeys are quite sensitive (15, 16). Human sensitivity to intoxication by PCBs appears to be related to the source of exposure. Numerous industrial exposures have resulted in relatively mild symptoms, primarily chloracne, whereas exposure in the Yusho incident resulted in a number of diverse and marked symptoms of intoxication (9, 10, 17). Studies of PCB carcinogenicity in laboratory animals have resulted in mixed conclusions. A bioassay of Aroclor 1254 for possible carcinogenicity by the National Cancer Institute concluded that this PCB formulation was not carcinogenic (18). However, the results of several other studies indicate that PCBs may be carcinogenic to laboratory animals (19–21).

Tissue Distribution

Due to the incidents of human poisoning and widespread environmental contamination, the production and use of PCBs has virtually ceased worldwide. However, concern regarding PCBs remains, due to their lingering existence in products manufactured prior to their discontinued use and their bioaccumulation and persistence in higher animals and the environment. Since PCBs may be very persistent in tissues of higher animals, knowledge of the pharmacokinetics of these chemicals was and is an essential complement to an assessment of health effects likely to result from long-term, low-dose exposure to these compounds. However, classical pharmacokinetic modeling of PCB disposition in higher animals has been complicated by the existence of PCBs as complex mixtures and by the variable capacity of different animal species to metabolize and clear these compounds. Therefore, most pharmacokinetic studies of PCBs have concentrated on establishing the basic parameters that determine their absorption, tissue distribution, metabolism, and clearance.

The lipid solubility of PCBs promotes passive absorption of these compounds from the aqueous environment of the intestine across the more lipophilic cell membranes of the intestine wall (22–25); the concentration gradient favors partition across the cells into blood. Once absorbed, PCBs are rapidly transported by the blood to all tissues. Transport in blood is apparently achieved by nonspecific association of PCBs with both blood cells and plasma proteins (26–28). Distribution of PCBs in plasma is apparently determined primarily by partition among the various proteins according to lipid solubility and concentration. Similarly, the partition of PCBs between blood and tissues is determined by lipid content and concentration gradient. Therefore, initial distribution of PCBs to tissues is largely determined by the volume, affinity, and rate of perfusion of the tissue in question.

The initial distribution of PCBs is determined by biophysical factors such as tissue volume, tissue/blood partition ratios, absorption to proteins, and perfusion rate, and is therefore similar in all species studied (24–31). Liver and muscle are the primary early depots because liver is highly perfused and has some affinity for these compounds, and muscle is by far the largest tissue volume. However, since PCBs are highly lipid-soluble compounds, they have a higher affinity for lipid-rich tissues, particularly adipose tissue, and a slower process of redistribution begins simultaneously with initial distribution. Therefore, these compounds are eventually most concentrated in adipose tissue and skin (24, 32), and a dynamic equilibrium of PCB concentrations is established among all tissues for each PCB homolog.

The interrelationship between PCB concentrations in all tissues is illustrated by the flow diagram in Figure 2 (33). At equilibrium, a change in the PCB concentration or tissue volume of any one tissue will result in a corresponding change in all tissues. For example, if the concentration of a PCB in liver is decreased by metabolism and excretion, then the concentration of that PCB in all tissues will be decreased proportionally. If another PCB cannot be metabolized and excreted, then that homolog will be concentrated in adipose tissue but not isolated there. PCBs that are concentrated in adipose tissue are still

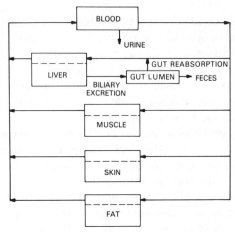

Figure 2   Flow diagram for pharmacokinetic model of chlorinated biphenyls. Source: Lutz et al (33)

circulated to all other tissues by the blood, and the exposure of each tissue is proportional to the respective tissue/blood ratios and the concentration in the major tissue depots, e.g. adipose tissue. The result is that the PCB congeners that can be cleared are depleted from all tissues and those that can not be cleared persist.

Examples of clearance of some PCB congeners and retention of others have been seen, though sometimes not recognized, in reports of human and animal samples in which the PCB profile of the samples did not match the profile of the mixture to which the organism was exposed. Documented examples have been provided by Bush et al (34), who demonstrated that the composition of Aroclor 1254 changed as it passed through the hen and the rat. Chen et al (35) reported that PCB residues in tissues of humans exposed in the Taiwan rice oil incident were preferentially depleted of homologs with adjacent unsubstituted carbon atoms at the 3 and 4 positions. Therefore, it follows that the concentration of an individual PCB in tissues of exposed animals and humans will be a function of level and duration of exposure, the ability of the exposed organism to clear the given PCB, and the time period following exposure.

Metabolism

Polychlorinated biphenyls are highly lipophilic molecules that are virtually insoluble in water. On the other hand, all biological excretory mechanisms are polar systems that involve intimate contact of aqueous fluids with cell membranes containing the usual complement of proteins and lipids. For this reason, intact PCBs are not readily excreted. Even if they were to enter the excretory systems of kidney or liver they would partition from the aqueous media into the more lipophilic membranes and from these membranes back into blood according to the concentration gradient. Some passive elimination occurs, but PCBs are excreted to an appreciable extent only after they are metabolized and conjugated to form more polar molecules.

The metabolism of all 209 chlorinated biphenyls has not been studied, but enough of these compounds have been studied to permit general conclusions about the mechanisms involved. Metabolism of chlorinated biphenyls is achieved primarily by the hepatic mixed-function oxidases and is strongly directed by the phenyl rings and the position(s) of chlorination (36). The presence of the biphenyl linkage directs metabolism to the ends of the molecule, so that the major metabolite of biphenyl is 4-hydroxybiphenyl. However, lesser amounts of 2- and 3-hydroxybiphenyl are also detected (37). The 2- and 4-hydroxybiphenyl metabolites are believed to be formed preferentially by mixed-function oxidases utilizing cytochromes P-448 and P-450 respectively, and the formation of each is thought to involve an arene oxide intermediate. However, 3-hydroxybiphenyl is believed to be formed by direct insertion of a hydroxyl group (37). Arene oxides are believed to be the reactive intermediates that account for hepatic toxicity or even carcinogenicity associated with many chemicals (38, 39). Arene oxides are also believed to be involved in covalent binding of PCBs (40). However, arene oxides have not yet been shown to account for PCB hepatotoxicity or carcinogenicity (41).

Chlorination deactivates the carbon atoms of the biphenyl molecule and directs metabolism to the unchlorinated positions. For example, the presence of a single chlorine atom on 4-chlorobiphenyl directs metabolism exclusively to the unchlorinated ring to yield a single major metabolite, 4-hydroxy-4'-chlorobiphenyl, in all species studied (41–45). However, PCB metabolism becomes more complex as the degree of chlorination increases. These compounds are readily metabolized as long as chlorination is restricted to one ring (46, 47), but metabolism may be greatly restricted when both rings are chlorinated (48). Several investigators have provided evidence that the critical factor to PCB metabolism is the availability of adjacent unsubstituted carbon atoms on at least one of the rings, preferably at the 3,4-positions (24, 32, 49). The presence of adjacent unsubstituted carbon atoms facilitates the formation of arene oxide intermediates that subsequently yield the 2- or 4-hydroxylated metabolites. Metabolism by the insertion mechanism at the 3 position proceeds much more slowly and in most cases is not a major factor in PCB metabolism (32, 48).

Biphenyl metabolites are readily conjugated and excreted and with few exceptions are not persistent in tissues. The major exception is the persistence of sulfur-containing metabolites of certain PCBs in the bronchial mucosa (50–53). Recent work indicates that these metabolites are products of glutathione reaction with arene oxide intermediates formed in PCB metabolism.

These glutathione conjugates are excreted in bile, subsequently metabolized by intestinal microbes, reabsorbed from the intestine, and preferentially accumulated in bronchial mucosa (53). The mechanism(s) that account for the affinity of these products for bronchial mucosa and the toxicological significance of this accumulation are as yet unknown, but the amount of the total PCB dose involved is relatively small.

While most studies of PCB metabolism have used the laboratory rat, PCB metabolism has been studied in a number of other species as well. The ability of various types of animals to metabolize PCBs increases in the order of fish < birds < mammals. However, the mechanisms involved appear to be similar in all species studied. That is, the primary metabolites formed by all species are hydroxylated biphenyls most probably formed primarily by hepatic mixed-function oxidases. Therefore, degree and position of chlorination play a major role in the rate of PCB metabolism by all species. The importance of adjacent unsubstituted carbon atoms observed in rats may be even more important in species with less capacity for PCB metabolism. Studies of PCB metabolism by fish indicate a minimal capacity to metabolize these compounds and then only those homologs having adjacent unsubstituted carbon atoms in the 3–4 positions (29, 54, 55). Birds have a greater capacity to metabolize PCBs than fish, but less than most mammalian species (29, 34). Even among mammals the capacity to metabolize PCBs varies greatly with species. Studies of the same PCB homologs in a number of species indicate that dogs metabolize these compounds most rapidly, followed by rats and mice, whereas monkeys metabolize these compounds relatively slowly (57–61). A study of PCB metabolism by human hepatic microsomes indicates that PCB metabolism by humans may be slow relative to other species (62). However, since PCBs are not readily excreted prior to metabolism, it is assumed that humans can metabolize these compounds in vivo because both Jensen (63) and Chen (35) have observed that PCB residues in human tissues are deficient in homologs having adjacent unsubstituted carbon atoms. That is, the more easily metabolized PCB homologs are apparently metabolized and excreted by humans, whereas the others tend to persist.

The net effect of PCB metabolism is the same for all species. Those homologs that can be metabolized will be metabolized to more polar compounds and excreted. Those homologs that can not be readily metabolized will be retained in the body and concentrated in tissues having the highest triglyceride content. The distribution of PCBs to all tissues is proportional to the respective tissue/blood ratios. Therefore, the concentration of a given PCB homolog in any tissue at any time will be determined by the level of exposure, the ability of the given species to metabolize that particular homolog, and time.

Elimination

In the present context, elimination is differentiated from excretion by the fact that excretion implies active processes involving specialized mechanisms located primarily in kidney and liver. Elimination of PCBs by higher animals is passive and coincidental to the passage of other substances from the body. Furthermore, excretion of PCBs is minimal prior to metabolism to more polar compounds, but these compounds are eliminated as unmetabolized parent compounds in association with any substance that may pass from the body. Due to their high lipid solubility, PCBs are most concentrated in substances that have a high lipid content and have been detected in the oils on hair of humans and animals (64). However, the major routes for PCB elimination are substances having the greatest volume and/or lipid content, e.g. milk, eggs, and fetuses, and are thereby restricted to females. Elimination by these routes arouses greater concern because of the possible threat to the young.

Elimination of PCBs in milk varies greatly with the species involved, due to differences in volume and lipid content of the milk produced. However, the basic mechanisms involved are the same for all species. Lipid in milk consists predominantly of triglycerides that originate both from circulating lipids in blood and de novo synthesis in the mammary gland (65). Since PCBs in the body are in dynamic equilibrium with all tissues, the creation of a new lipid depot with the beginning of lactation results in passive movement of PCBs from blood to milk and a corresponding movement of PCBs from all tissues to blood to maintain their respective tissue/blood ratios. A favorable gradient for passive transport of PCBs from blood to milk is maintained by continued synthesis and secretion of milk lipid. Vodicnik & Lech (66–69) have provided excellent examples of the role milk can play in PCB elimination in their comparative studies of PCB elimination in lactating and virgin mice. In these studies, lactating mice transferred most of the body burden to their nursing young in a period of 20 days, whereas the body burden of the virgin animals remained essentially constant. Other studies have demonstrated that PCB elimination in milk by cattle and humans is proportional to the level of exposure, and in the case of cattle accounted for 11–12% of the daily dose consumed (70, 71). In the Yusho incident, at least one infant received a toxic dose of PCBs solely as a result of nursing (72). However, the volume and lipid content of human milk is relatively low compared to that of other species, and there is no evidence that lactation has significantly reduced the PCB body burden of humans.

Eggs, particularly egg yolks, represent another concentration of newly synthesized lipids that may serve as a route for PCB elimination. Unmetabolized PCBs have been detected in the eggs of fish (73), turtles (74), and wild birds (75), as well as in the eggs of domestic fowl used in laboratory studies of

PCB clearance (56). Bush et al (56) studied the fate of Aroclor 1254 in chickens and observed that the concentration of PCBs in egg yolk increased as the body burden increased and decreased when Aroclor administration was discontinued. They also observed that the poorly metabolized PCB homologs were more concentrated in egg yolk than those congeners more readily metabolized and excreted. Steady-state levels have not been predicted in birds, but in a study of the closely related polybrominated biphenyls in chickens, Fries et al (76) demonstrated that elimination in eggs equaled dietary intake in approximately 63 days. In summary, eggs, like milk, represent a depot of newly synthesized lipid that can account for the elimination of significant concentrations of PCBs. Elimination of PCBs in eggs is greatest in domestic fowl, which produce the largest number of eggs. However, wild fowl that produce eggs only once a year may accumulate high body burdens of PCBs and therefore may be more likely to have concentrations in their eggs that would endanger their young.

Polychlorinated biphenyls are relatively small, highly lipophilic molecules that readily cross cell walls; therefore, the placenta offers the fetus little protection from these compounds. However, the fetus, as opposed to milk and eggs, is lean relative to maternal tissues. Therefore, even though an equilibrium is established in which PCBs are partitioned between all tissues, including placenta and blood, PCBs are not concentrated in fetal tissues. Nevertheless, the fetus is exposed (9, 77, 78), and in the case of the Yusho incident children born to mothers who consumed PCB-containing rice oil exhibited signs of intoxication (9). However, Vodicnik et al (66, 68, 69) demonstrated that concentration and elimination of PCBs in the mouse fetus were minimal when compared to those in milk.

PHARMACOKINETIC MODELING

Relatively little work has been conducted on pharmacokinetic modeling of PCBs. Mathematical analyses have for the most part been confined to regression analysis of tissue burdens or excretion rates to characterize their time course in an objective way. These analyses have been primarily descriptive and have provided little insight into the underlying physiologic and biochemical mechanisms involved. We believe that a pharmacokinetic model that places individual physiologic processes and biochemical interactions in quantitative perspective more accurately reflects the mechanisms involved. Therefore, such a model has been used to study several PCBs in the rat (33) and the mouse (58). The present review concentrates on a description of that model.

The pharmacokinetic model is described by the flow diagram in Figure 2, which contains the tissues that account for most of the body burden of PCBs and their metabolites. The mathematical model consists of a set of differential equations that are mass balances on each chemical species in each compartment. These have been described in detail (33), so only two illustrative examples are cited here. For a tissue in which metabolism may occur, such as the liver, the mass balance takes the form

$$\frac{d}{dt}(V_L C_L) = Q_L \left[C_B - \frac{C_L}{R_L} \right] - K_m \frac{C_L}{R_L} \qquad\qquad 1.$$

where t = time
V = tissue volume or mass
C = concentration
Q = blood flow rate
K_m = metabolic clearance
R = equilibrium tissue-to-blood distribution ratio

and the subscripts L and B refer to liver and blood respectively. For a compartment in which metabolism is neglected, such as adipose tissue, the mass balance takes the form

$$\frac{d}{dt}(V_A C_A) = Q_A \left[C_B - \frac{C_A}{R_A} \right] \qquad\qquad 2.$$

The product of the tissue volume and the tissue concentration, which equals the amount of PCB in the tissue, has been written in the derivative to allow for the fact that the volume may not be constant on a time scale relevant to the pharmacokinetics of the very slowly cleared PCBs.

An important concept incorporated in Equations 1 and 2 is flow limitation. It is assumed that the PCB in blood leaving any tissue is in equilibrium with the tissue. This assumption has not been explored thoroughly; however, it is known that PCBs leave the blood and enter tissues very rapidly. For example, following intravenous (i.v.) administration, more than half a single dose of 2,4,5,2',5'-pentachlorobiphenyl is removed from blood of rats within two minutes and only 6% can be accounted for in blood at 10 minutes (79). Further, pharmacokinetic simulations based on flow limitation have generally been satisfactory with the important exception of the skin, for which the intercompartment transport parameter had to be reduced by a factor of ten. The limiting factor for skin has not yet been determined.

The blood flow rates and tissue volumes for a 250-gram(g) rat are shown in Table 1; distribution coefficients and kinetic parameters are shown in Table 2 for four PCB congeners: 4-chloro-, 4,4'-dichloro-,2,4,5,2',5'-pentachloro- and 2,4,5,2',4',5'-hexachlorobiphenyl (1-CB, 2-CB, 5-CB, and 6-CB) (33). These two tables illustrate the following important points.

1. The compartment sizes and blood flows are independent of the chemical being modeled. With the exception of effective skin blood flow, all can be

Table 1 Compartment sizes and perfusion rates for a 240-g male Sprague-Dawley rat[a]

Compartment	Volume	Blood flow
	ml	ml/min
Blood	22.5	
Gut lumen	14	
Muscle	125	7.5
Liver	10	16
Skin	40	(0.5)[b]
Adipose tissue	17.5	0.4

[a]Source: Lutz et al (33)
[b]Effective blood flow; see text

measured by methods that do not depend on pharmacokinetic observations. Further, the model can be applied to other animal species by the appropriate choice of tissue sizes and blood flow rates.

2. The tissue-to-blood distribution coefficients show the expected change resulting from metabolism. The parent compounds are lipophilic and tend to concentrate in tissues, while the metabolite (here taken to be a single species

Table 2 Tissue/blood distribution ratios[a]

Compartment	Parent				Metabolite			
	1-CB	2-CB	5-CB	6-CB	1-CB	2-CB	5-CB	6-CB
Blood	1	1	1	1	1	1	1	1
Gut lumen	1	1	1	1	1	1	1	1
Muscle	1	2	1	4	0.14	0.40	0.10	0.30
Liver	1	3	6	12	2	5	2	4
Skin	10	10	7	30	0.25	0.30	0.10	2
Adipose	30	70	70	400	0.40	0.60	0.40	2

Kinetic Parameters				
Rate constant	1-CB	2-CB	5-CB	6-CB
Metabolic clearance, K_m, ml/min	10.0	2.0	0.39	0.045
Kidney clearance, K_k, ml/min	0.20	0.133	0.033	0.030
Biliary clearance, K_B, ml/min	0.20	0.35	0.30	0.30
Gut reabsorption, K_G, min^{-1}	0.00016	0.00016	0.00016	0.00016
Fecal transport, K_F, min^{-1}	0.0008	0.0008	0.0008	0.0008

[a]Source: Lutz et al (33)

representative of all metabolites) shows a pattern more characteristic of water-soluble materials.

3. There is a great range in the metabolic clearances (K_m). The K_m for 1-CB is 10 ml/min, which represents a significant fraction of the 16 ml/min liver blood flow resulting in a substantial extraction of this compound during a single pass through the liver. The K_m value for 6-CB is only 0.045 ml/min, or less than 1/200 of that for 1-CB. Since the analysis of Lutz et al (33), evidence has suggested that most of the 6-CB cleared by the rat is unchanged material (48, 80, 81). The value of 0.045 ml/min, therefore, represents a total body clearance, most of which may be accounted for by passive transport from blood to intestinal contents (82, 83). The actual metabolic clearance of 6-CB could be an order of magnitude lower than the value shown in Table 2.

Figures 3 and 4 show model simulations resulting from numerical solution of the complete set of differential equations with the parameters chosen for 1-CB and compare these with experimental data of radioactivity derived from 1-CB. These simulations show the important role of skin and fat in mediating the pharmacokinetics of the compound. Parent material enters these tissues with the blood early in the time scale. The tissues serve as reservoirs from which

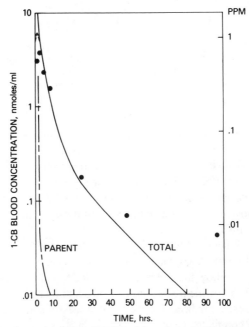

Figure 3   1-CB blood concentration as a function of time after a single i.v. dose of 0.6 mg/kg in the rat. Points represent experimental data for total 1-CB. Simulations are given for total equivalents (——) and parent 1-CB (– – –). Beyond 10 hours, total concentration in blood is composed almost entirely of metabolite. Source: Lutz et al (33)

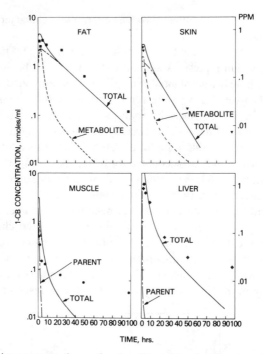

Figure 4   1-CB tissue concentration as a function of time after a single i.v. dose of 0.6 mg/kg in the rat. Points represent experimental data for total 1-CB in the tissues. In each figure, total equivalent concentration (——), metabolite concentration (– – –), and parent concentration (– – –) are shown. Source: Lutz et al (33)

1-CB can reenter the blood and be distributed to the other tissues. Parent material disappears very rapidly from the blood, muscle, and liver. The discrepancy between the model simulations and the data at longer times shows that a small fraction of the radioactivity, typically about 1% of peak concentrations, is behaving kinetically very differently from the mobile metabolite. The nature of this slow component is unknown, but it may reflect covalent binding in these tissues (40).

The pharmacokinetics of the very slowly metabolized 6-CB (Figure 5) show a pattern very different from that of 1-CB. The concentrations in the liver and muscle are able to follow the concentration in the blood quite well after a short redistribution phase, while 6-CB continues to accumulate in skin for about one day and in fat for several days. The transient processes can be assessed without solution of the complete set of differential equations. A characteristic time scale (T) for the movement of a chemical between blood and tissue is seen for constant parameters in Equations 1 and 2 to have the form

$$T = \frac{RV}{Q} \qquad\qquad 3.$$

or the physiologic volume of distribution of the tissue (RV) divided by the blood flow rate (Q). For 6-CB in the rat, T ranges from $(12)(10)/16 = 7.5$ minutes in the liver to $(400)(17.5)/0.4 = 17,500$ min or 12 days in the fat. As noted above, therefore, the 6-CB concentration in liver can follow that in the blood quite closely, while the concentration in fat shows a considerable lag relative to that in blood.

The total physiologic volume of distribution, V_D, of the 250-g rat may be obtained by summing the RV terms for all compartments.

$$V_D = \sum RV \qquad\qquad 4.$$

Performing the indicated arithmetic for 6-CB yields a value of $V_D = 8856$ ml or 35 l/kg, of which fat contributes 79% and skin 14%.

The characteristic time scale for elimination from the animal is

$$\frac{V_D}{K_m} = \frac{8856}{0.045} = 196,800 \text{ minutes}$$

or 4.5 months.

The long time scale involved in studies of very slowly metabolized PCBs introduces an additional complication, because growth of young experimental animals cannot be ignored. Growth of the rat (33) and swine (31) has been shown to be the major factor responsible for declining adipose tissue concentrations of 6-CB in the absence of a similar decrease in body burden. The relative importance of growth and elimination can be inferred from a one-compartment model of the rat

$$\frac{d}{dt}(V_D C_B) = -K_m C_B \qquad\qquad 5.$$

Equation 5 may be rearranged to

$$\frac{1}{C_B}\frac{dC_B}{dt} = -\frac{1}{V_D}\frac{dV_D}{dt} - \frac{K_m}{V_D} \qquad\qquad 6.$$

which states that the relative rate of change in concentration is equal to the negative of the sum of the fractional growth rate of V_D and the total body clearance per unit volume of distribution. If we take the growth rate as 0.017

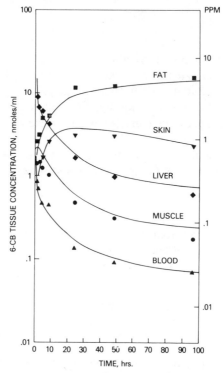

Figure 5   6-CB tissue concentration as a function of time for 96 hours after a single i.v. dose of 0.6 mg/kg in the rat. Source: Lutz et al (33)

day $^{-1}$ (33) and compare this with $K_m/V_D = 0.007$ day $^{-1}$, we see that growth of the 250-g rat is more than twice as important as elimination in reducing adipose tissue concentration. This figure is conservative, because the growing rat substantially increases the fraction of its body mass that is fat relative to lean tissues. For this reason, the rate of growth of 6-CB volume of distribution considerably exceeds the growth rate of the rat.

A consequence of the effect of growth on C_B is a finite total excretion based on extrapolation of excretion rate (% dose/day) curves to infinite time. It has been observed by Matthews & Anderson (24) and confirmed by Muhlebach & Bickel (81) that less than 20% of 6-CB would ever be excreted based on long-term pharmacokinetic studies. This limitation appears to be a consequence of Equation 5. The excretion rate would be

$$K_T = \frac{K_m C_B}{\text{dose}}$$ 7.

or proportional to C_B if K_m is constant. Support for the proportionality between K_f and C_B is provided by the starvation experiments of Wyss et al (80). Since C_B decreases more rapidly than elimination alone would suggest in the growing rat, extrapolation of excretion to infinite time remains less than the dose.

Pharmacokinetic studies of PCB congeners have provided considerable insight into the determinants of their uptake, accumulation, and disposition. Pharmacokinetic modeling of PCB disposition offers the best opportunity to extrapolate knowledge gained with laboratory animals to predict the disposition of these compounds in other species, including humans. Most of the data presented in Tables 1 and 2 are available or could be generated for other laboratory species. However, work with a number of species has demonstrated that one parameter basic to any pharmacokinetic model, metabolic clearance (K_m), varies greatly with species (54–61). Therefore, meaningful extrapolation of laboratory data to other species is dependent on determining the K_m for the species of interest. In the case of man, reliable prediction of PCB disposition will depend on development of an in vitro method for the determination of this parameter.

SUMMARY

The pharmacokinetics of PCBs are complicated by numerous factors, not the least of which is the existence of up to 209 different chlorinated biphenyls. Whereas all PCB congeners are highly lipophilic and most are readily absorbed and rapidly distributed to all tissues, PCBs are cleared from tissues at very different rates, and the same congeners may be cleared at different rates by different species. With the exception of special situations in which PCBs may be passively eliminated in lipid sinks, e.g. milk or eggs, clearance is minimal prior to metabolism to more polar compounds. Rates of PCB metabolism vary greatly with species and with the degree and positions of chlorination. Mammals metabolize these compounds most rapidly, but even among mammalian species rates of metabolism vary greatly. In all species studied, the more readily metabolized chlorinated biphenyls have adjacent unsubstituted carbon atoms in the 3–4 positions. Congeners that do not have adjacent unsubstituted carbon atoms may be metabolized very slowly and are therefore cleared very slowly. Those PCBs not readily cleared concentrate in adipose tissue. A physiologic pharmacokinetic model best illustrates how the concentrations of PCBs in all tissues approach equilibrium with the blood and with one another. Thus, the model illustrates how a depot of PCBs in any tissue, e.g. adipose tissue, will result in exposure of all tissues in proportion to the respective tissue/blood ratios and the body burden. The disposition of a number of PCBs in the rat has been accurately described by a physiologic model, and the model has been extrapolated to predict the disposition of these same PCBs in the mouse (58). Therefore, the physiologic pharmacokinetic model is believed to offer the best opportunity to extrapolate data obtained with laboratory animals to predict the disposition of PCBs in other species, including man. Most of the parameters of a model of PCB disposition in man are available or could be estimated. The major limitation to the construction of such a model is the absence of accurate estimates of metabolic clearance of individual PCBs by man. Accurate estimates of metabolic clearance depend on development of suitable in vitro methods to accurately predict clearance in vivo.

Literature Cited

1. Griefs. 1867. Erzetzung des Wasserstoffs durch Stickstoff in organischen Verbindungen. Tetrazodiphenyl-Verbindungen. *J. Prakt. Chem.* 101:91–94
2. Interdepartmental Task Force on PCBs. 1972. *PCBs and the Environment.* Com-72-10419, Springfield, Va., Nat. Techn. Inf. Serv., pp. 5, 11
3. US Environmental Protection Agency. 1976. *PCBs in the United States. Industrial Use and Environmental Distribution,* PB-252 012, Springfield, Va., Nat. Tech. Inf. Serv., pp. 4–5, 34–35, 54–57, 198–210, 322–34
4. Drinker, C. K., Warren, M. F., Bennett, G. A. 1937. The problem of possible systemic effects from certain chlorinated hydrocarbons. *J. Ind. Hyg. Toxicol.* 19:283–311
5 Greenburg, L., Mayers, M. R., Smither, A. R. 1939. The systemic effects resulting from exposure to certain chlorinated hydrocarbons. *J. Ind. Hyg. Toxicol.,* 21:29–38
6. Schwartz, L., Burlow, F. A. 1942. Chloracne from cutting oils. *US Public Health Rep.* 57:1747–52
7. Meigs, J. W., Albom, J. J., Kartin, B. L. 1954. Chloracne from an unusual exposure to Aroclor. *J. Am. Med. Assoc.* 154:1417–18
8. Anon. 1966. Report of a new chemical hazard. *New Sci.* 32:612
9. Kuratsune, M., Yoshimura, T., Matsuzaka, J., Yamaguchi, A. 1972. Epidemiologic study on Yusho, a poisoning caused by ingestion of rice oil contaminated with a commercial brand of polychlorinated biphenyls. *Environ. Health Perspect.* 1:119–28
10. Urabe, H., Koda, H., Asahi, M. 1979. Present state of Yusho patients. *Ann. NY Acad. Sci.* 320:273–76

11. Chen, P. H., Chang, K. T., Lu, Y. D. 1981. Polychlorinated biphenyls and polychlorinated dibenzofurans in the toxic rice-bran oil that caused PCB poisoning in Taichung. *Bull. Environ. Contam. Toxicol.* 26:489–95
12. Nagayama, J., Kuratsune, M., Masuda, Y. 1976. Determination of chlorinated dibenzofurans in kanechlors and "Yusho oil." *Bull. Environ. Contam. Toxicol.* 15:9–13
13. Allen, J. R., Abrahamson, L. J. 1973. Morphological and biochemical changes in the liver of rats fed polychlorinated biphenyls. *Arch. Environ. Contam. Toxicol.* 1:265–80
14. Allen, J. R., Carstens, L. A., Abrahamson, L. J. 1976. Response of rats exposed to polychlorinated biphenyl for fifty-two weeks. I. Comparison of tissue levels of PCB and biological changes. *Arch. Environ. Contam. Toxicol.* 4:404–19
15. Allen, J. R. 1975. Response of the nonhuman primate to polychlorinated biphenyl exposure. *Fed. Proc.* 34:1675–79
16. Allen, J. R., Norback, D. H. 1976. Pathological responses of primates to polychlorinated biphenyl exposure. In *Proc. Natl. Conf. Polychlorinated Biphenyls, Chicago, 1975.* EPA-560/6–75–004, pp. 43–49. Washington DC: EPA 471 pp.
17. IARC Monographs on the Evaluation of the Carcinogenic Risk of Chemicals to Humans. *Polychlorinated Biphenyls,* 18:59–66, 80–83. Lyon: Int. Agency Res. Cancer
18. National Cancer Institute. 1975. *Bioassay of Aroclor 1254 for Possible Carcinogenicity,* CAS No. 27323–18–8, NCI-CG-TR-38, DHEW Publ. No. (NIH) 78–838. Washington DC: US Dept. Health, Education and Welfare. 62 pp.

19. Ito, N., Nagasaki, H., Arai, M., Makiura, S., Sugihara, S., Hirao, K. 1973. Histopathological studies on liver tumorigenesis induced in mice by technical polychlorinated biphenyls and its promoting effect on liver tumors induced by benzene hexachloride. *J. Natl. Cancer Inst.* 51:1637–46

20. Ito, N., Nagasaki, H., Makiura, S., Arai, M. 1974. Histopathological studies on liver tumorigenesis in rats treated with polychlorinated biphenyls. *Gann* 65: 545–49

21. Kimbrough, R. D., Squire, R. A., Linder, R. E., Strandberg, J. D., Montali, R. J., Burse, V. W. 1975. Induction of liver tumors in Sherman strain female rats by polychlorinated biphenyl Aroclor 1260. *J. Natl. Cancer Inst.* 55:1453–59

22. Albro, P. W., Fishbein, L. 1972. Intestinal absorption of polychlorinated biphenyls in rats. *Bull. Environ. Contam. Toxicol.* 8:26–31

23. Berlin, M., Gage, J. C., Holm, S. 1975. Distribution and metabolism of polychlorinated biphenyls. *Int. Symp. Proc., Vol. 2: Recent Advances in the Assessment of the Health Effects of Environmental Pollution, Paris, June 24–28*, pp. 895–902. 2522 pp.

24. Matthews, H. B., Anderson, M. W. 1975. Effect of chlorination on the distribution and excretion of polychlorinated biphenyls. *Drug Metab. Dispos.* 3:371–80

25. Gage, J. C., Holm, S. 1976. The influence of molecular structure on the retention and excretion of polychlorinated biphenyls by the mouse. *Toxicol. Appl. Pharmacol.* 36:555–60

26. Maliwal, B. P., Guthrie, F. E. 1982. *In vitro* uptake and transfer of chlorinated hydrocarbons among human lipoproteins. *J. Lipid Res.* 23:474–79

27. Vomachka, M. S., Vodicnik, M. J., Lech, J. J. 1983. Characteristics of 2,4,5,2',4',5'-hexachlorobiphenyl distribution among lipoproteins *in vitro*. *Toxicol. Appl. Pharmacol.* In press

28. Matthews, H. B., Surles, J. R., Carver, J. G., Anderson, M. W. 1983. Halogenated biphenyl transport by blood components. *Fund. Appl. Toxicol.* In press

29. Hutzinger, D., Nash, D. M., Safe, S., DeFreitas, A. S. W., Norstrom, R. J., Wildish, D. J., Zitko, V. 1972. Polychlorinated biphenyls: Metabolic behavior of pure isomers in pigeons, rats and brook trout. *Science* 178:312–14

30. Hsu, I. C., VanMiller, J. P., Seymour, J. L., Allen, J. R. 1975. Urinary metabolites of 2,5,2',5'-tetrachlorobiphenyl in

31. the non-human primate. *Proc. Soc. Exp. Biol. Med.* 150:185–88

31. Hansen, L. G., Welborn, M. E. 1977. Distribution, dilution and elimination of polychlorinated biphenyl analogs in growing swine. *J. Pharmacol. Sci.* 66: 497–501

32. Matthews, H. B., Tuey, D. B. 1980. The effect of chlorine position on the distribution and excretion of four hexachlorobiphenyl isomers. *Toxicol. Appl. Pharmacol.* 53:377–88

33. Lutz, R. J., Dedrick, R. L., Matthews, H. B., Eling, T. E., Anderson, M. W. 1977. A preliminary pharmacokinetic model for several chlorinated biphenyls in the rat. *Drug Metab. Dispos.* 5:386–96

34. Bush, B., Baker, F. D., Tumasonis, C. E., Fu-Chun, L., Houck, C. L. 1975. Modification of the homolog and isomer composition of a polychlorinated biphenyl mixture during passage through two biological systems. See Ref. 23, pp. 879–85

35. Chen, P. H., Luo, M. L., Wong, C. K., Chen, C. J. 1982. Comparative rates of elimination of some individual polychlorinated biphenyls from the blood of PCB-poisoned patients in Taiwan. *Food Chem. Toxicol.* 20:417–25

36. Matthews, H. B. 1982. Aryl halides. In *Metabolic Basis of Detoxication*, ed. W. B. Jacoby, J. R. Bend, S. Cardwell, pp. 51–68. New York: Academic. 375 pp.

37. Billings, R. E., McMahon, R. E. 1978. Microsomal biphenyl hydroxylation: The formation of 3-hydroxybiphenyl and biphenyl catechol. *Mol. Pharmacol.* 14:145–54

38. Miller, E. C. 1978. Some current perspectives on chemical carcinogens in humans and experimental animals: Presidential address. *Cancer Res.* 38:1478–96

39. Hanzlik, R. P. 1982. Effects of substituents on reactivity and toxicity of chemically reactive intermediates. *Drug Metabol. Rev.* 13:207–34

40. Morales, N. M., Matthews, H. B. 1979. *In vivo* binding of 2,3,6,2',3',6'-hexachlorobiphenyl and 2,4,5,2',4',5'-hexachlorobiphenyl to mouse liver macromolecules. *Chem. Biol. Interact.* 27: 99–110

41. Weltman, R. H., Norback, D. H. 1983. Lack of hepatocarcinogenic activity after 2,3,6,2',3',6'-hexachlorobiphenyl (HCB) exposure in Sprague-Dawley rats. *Toxicologist* 3:401

42. Safe, S., Hutzinger, O., Jones, D. 1975. The mechanism of chlorobiphenyl metabolism. *J. Agric. Food Chem.* 23:851–53

43. Safe, S., Platonow, N., Hutzinger, O. 1975. Metabolism of chlorobiphenyls in the goat and cow. *J. Agric. Food. Chem.* 23:259–61

44. Safe, S., Ruzo, L. O., Jones, D., Platonow, N. S., Hutzinger, O. 1975. The metabolism of 4-chlorobiphenyl in the pig. *Can. J. Physiol. Pharmacol.* 53: 392–96

45. Safe, S., Jones, D., Kohli, J., Ruzo, L. O., Hutzinger, O., Sundstrom, G. 1976. The metabolism of chlorinated aromatic pollutants by the frog. *Can. J. Zool.* 54:1818–23

46. Goto, M., Sugiura, K., Hattori, M., Miyagawa, T., Okamura, M. 1974. Metabolism of 2,3-dichlorobiphenyl-^{14}C and 2,4,6-trichlorobiphenyl-^{14}C in the rat. *Chemosphere* 5:227–32

47. Goto, M., Sigiura, K., Hattori, M., Miyagawa, T., Okamura, M. 1974. Metabolism of 2,3,4,5,6-tetrachlorobiphenyl-^{14}C and 2,3,4,5,6-pentachlorobiphenyl-^{14}C in the rat. *Chemosphere* 5:233–38

48. Kato, S., McKinney, J. D., Matthews, H. B. 1980. Metabolism of symmetrical hexachlorobiphenyl isomers in the rat. *Toxicol. Appl. Pharmacol.* 53:389–98

49. Berlin, M., Gage, J. C., Holm, S. 1974. Distribution and metabolism of polychlorobiphenyls. See Ref. 23, pp. 895–902

50. Mio, T., Sumino, K., Mizutani, T. 1976. Sulfur-containing metabolites of 2,5,-2',5'-tetrachlorobiphenyl, a major component of commercial PCBs. *Chem. Pharm. Bull.* 24:1958–60

51. Mizutani, T. 1978. Identification of sulfur-containing metabolites of 2,4,2',4'-tetrachlorobiphenyl in mice. *Bull. Environ. Contam. Toxicol.* 20:219–26

52. Bergman, A., Brandt, I., Jansson, B. 1979. Accumulation of methylsulfonyl derivatives of some bronchial-seeking polychlorinated biphenyls in the respiratory tract of mice. *Toxicol. Appl. Pharmacol.* 48:213–20

53. Bergman, A., Biessmann, A., Brandt, I., Rafter, J. 1982. Metabolism of 2,4,5-trichlorobiphenyl: Role of the intestinal microflora in the formation of bronchial-seeking methylsulphone metabolites in mice. *Chem. Biol. Interact.* 40:123–31

54. Melancon, M. J., Lech, J. J. 1976. Isolation and identification of a polar metabolite of tetrachlorobiphenyl from bile of rainbow trout exposed to ^{14}C-tetrachlorobiphenyl. *Bull. Environ. Contam. Toxicol.* 15:181–88

55. McKim, J. M., Heath, E. M. 1983. Dose determinations for waterborne 2,5,2',5'-[^{14}C]-tetrachlorobiphenyl and related pharmacokinetics in two species of trout (Salmo gairdneri and Salvelinus fontinalis): A mass-balance approach. *Toxicol. Appl. Pharmacol.* 68:177–87

56. Bush, B., Tumasonis, C. F., Baker, F. D. 1974. Toxicity and persistence of PCB homologs and isomers in the avian system. *Arch. Environ. Contam. Toxicol.* 2:195–211

57. Sipes, I. G., Slocumb, M. L., Perry, D. F., Carter, D. E. 1980. 4,4'-dichlorobiphenyl: Distribution, metabolism, and excretion in the dog and the monkey. *Toxicol. Appl. Pharmacol.* 55:554–63

58. Tuey, D. B., Matthews, H. B. 1980. Use of a physiological compartmental model for the rat to describe the pharmacokinetics of several chlorinated biphenyls in the mouse. *Drug Metab. Dispos.* 8:397–403

59. Abdel-Hamid, F. M., Moore, J. A., Matthews, H. B. 1981. Comparative study of 3,4,3',4'-tetrachlorobiphenyl in male and female rats and female monkeys. *J. Toxicol. Environ. Health* 7:181–91

60. Sipes, I. G., Slocumb, M. L., Perry, D. F., Carter, D. E. 1982. 2,4,5,2',4',5'-hexachlorobiphenyl: Distribution, metabolism, and excretion in the dog and the monkey. *Toxicol. Appl. Pharmacol.* 65:264–72

61. Sipes, I. G., Slocumb, M. L., Chen, H-S. G., Carter, D. E. 1982. 2,3,6,2',3',6'-hexachlorobiphenyl: Distribution, metabolism, and excretion in the dog and the monkey. *Toxicol. Appl. Pharmacol.* 62:317–24

62. Schnellmann, R. G., Putnam, C. W., Sipes, I. G. 1983. Metabolism of 2,2',3,3',6,6'-hexachlorobiphenyl and 2,2',4,4',5,5'-hexachlorobiphenyl by human hepatic microsomes. *Biochem. Pharmacol.* In press

63. Jensen, S., Sundstrom, G. 1974. Structure and levels of most chlorobiphenyls in two technical PCB products and in human adipose tissue. *Ambio* 3:70–76

64. Matthews, H. B., Domanski, J. J., Guthrie, F. E. 1976. Hair and its associated lipids as an excretory source for chlorinated hydrocarbons. *Xenobiotica* 6:425–29

65. Bauman, D. E., Davis, C. I. 1974. Biosynthesis of milk fat. In *Lactation,* ed. B. L. Larson, V. R. Smith, 2: pp. 31–75. New York: Academic. 458 pp.

66. Vodicnik, M. J., Lech, J. J. 1980. The transfer of 2,4,5,2',4',5'-hexachlorobiphenyl to fetuses and nursing offspring. I. Disposition in pregnant

and lactating mice and accumulation in young. *Toxicol. Appl. Pharmacol.* 54: 293–300

67. Vodicnik, M. J., Elcombe, C. R., Lech, J. J. 1980. The transfer of 2,4,5,-2',4',5'-hexachlorobiphenyl to fetuses and nursing offspring. II. Induction of hepatic microsomal monooxygenase activity in pregnant and lactating mice and their young. *Toxicol. Appl. Pharmacol.* 54:301–10

68. Vodicnik, M. J., Lech, J. J. 1982. The transfer of 3,4,5,3',4',5'-hexachlorobiphenyl (6-CB) from mothers to fetuses and nursing offspring. *Toxicologist.* 2:136

69. Vodicnik, M. J. 1983. The effect of pregnancy and lactation on the elimination of ^{14}C-2,4,2',4'-tetrachlorobiphenyl (4-CB). *Toxicologist* 3:161

70. Takeshita, R., Suzuki, M., Hayashi, M. 1974. Transference of polychlorinated biphenyls in human adipose tissue to human milk. *J. Hyg. Chem.* 20:256–65

71. Willett, L. B. 1975. Excretory behavior of polychlorinated biphenyls in lactating cows fed normal and thyroprotein containing rations. *J. Dairy Sci.* 58:765

72. Yoshimura, T. 1974. Epidemiological study on Yusho babies born to mothers who had consumed oil contaminated by PCB. *Fukuoka Acta Med.* 65:74–80

73. Johnson, L. G., Morris, R. I. 1974. Chlorinated insecticide residues in the eggs of some freshwater fish. *Bull. Environ. Contam. Toxicol.* 11:503–10

74. Thompson, H. P., Runkin, P. W., Johnson, D. W. 1974. Polychlorinated biphenyls and p,p' DDE in green turtle eggs from Ascension Island, South Atlantic Ocean. *Bull. Environ. Contam. Toxicol.* 11:399–406

75. Koivusaari, J., Laamanen, A., Nuuja, I., Palokangas, R., Vihko, V. 1972. Concentrations of some environmental chemicals in the eggs of the white-tailed eagle in the Quarken area of the Gulf of Bothnia. *Work Environ. Health* 9:44–45

76. Fries, G. F., Cecil, H. C., Bitman, J., Lillie, R. J. 1976. Retention and excretion of polybrominated biphenyls by hens. *Bull. Environ. Contam. Toxicol.* 15:278–82

77. Polishak, Z. W., Wasserman, D., Wasserman, M., Cuses, S., Ron, M. 1977. Organochlorine compounds in mother and fetus during labor. *Environ. Res.* 13:278–84

78. Lucier, G. W., McDaniel, O. S., Schiller, C. M., Matthews, H. B. 1978. Structural requirements for the accumulation of PCB metabolites in the fetal intestine. *Drug Metab. Dispos.* 6:584–90

79. Matthews, H. B., Anderson, M. W. 1975. The distribution and excretion of 2,4,2,2',5'-pentachlorobiphenyl in the rat. *Drug Metab. Dispos.* 3:211–19

80. Wyss, P. A., Muhlebach, S., Bickel, M. H. 1982. Pharmacokinetics of 2,2',4,4',5,5'-hexachlorobiphenyl (6-CB) in rats with decreasing adipose tissue mass. I. Effects of restricting food intake two weeks after administration of 6-CB. *Drug Metab. Dispos.* 10:657–61

81. Muhlebach, S., Bichel, M. H. 1981. Pharmacokinetics in rats of 2,4,5,-2',4',5'-hexachlorobiphenyl: An unmetabolizable lipophilic model compound. *Xenobiotica* 11:249–57

82. Yoshimura, H., Yamamoto, H. 1975. A novel route of excretion of 2,4,3',4'-tetrachlorobiphenyl in rats. *Bull. Environ. Contam. Toxicol.* 13:681–88

83. Bungay, P. M., Dedrick, L. L., Matthews, H. B. 1981. Enteric transport of chlordecone (Kepone®) in the rat. *J. Pharmacokin. Biopharm.* 9:309–41

Ann. Rev. Pharmacol. Toxicol. 1984. 24:105–120

ANTIADRENERGIC ANTIHYPERTENSIVE DRUGS: THEIR EFFECT ON RENAL FUNCTION

Keevin N. Bernstein and Daniel T. O'Connor

Department of Medicine, University of California-San Diego, and Veterans Administration Medical Center, San Diego, California 92161

INTRODUCTION

Since Richard Bright's first intimation of the link between renal and cardiovascular disease, investigators have debated the relationship between the renal vasculature and hypertension. Although it appears that essential hypertension precedes and induces morphologic microvascular disease in the kidney, functional vascular abnormalities may precede not only the onset of morphologic changes, but the onset of clinical hypertension as well (1, 2).

It is unusual to find a normal renal arterial tree devoid of dynamic abnormalities in vascular tone in hypertension patients (3). Numerous studies have demonstrated functional abnormalities in vascular tone in all categories of hypertensive patients, ranging from pre-hypertensives (4) (normotensive offspring of hypertensive patients) to established hypertensives (2, 5–11). In established hypertensives, renal vascular resistance (RVR) (5, 6) is typically increased along with decreased renal plasma flow (RPF) (7–10). Not only have these changes in RPF and RVR been demonstrated early in the majority of young hypertensives (2), but even hypertensives with normal renal vascular tone at rest have exaggerated responses to exogenous vasodilators (1). Lastly, RPF of normal offspring of hypertensive parents differs from that of other normotensive subjects (4). All these changes may occur with relative preservation of glomerular filtration rate (GFR).

Enhanced renal blood flow (RBF) variability in hypertensive patients (1, 2), asymmetry of perfusion between paired hypertensive kidneys, and ameliora-

105

0362-1642/84/415-0105$02.00

tion of increased RVR by vasodilators (2) all support the concept of functional, rather than fixed, renal hemodynamic abnormalities in hypertension (3).

α-Adrenergic participation may be an important factor in the generation of abnormal renal vascular tone and reactivity in early essential hypertensives (1). In laboratory animals, direct electrical stimulation of efferent renal nerves results in reduction of RBF and GFR; these changes are abolished by α-adrenergic blockade with phentolamine or phenoxybenzamine (11). Although its actions are still controversial, endogenous norepinephrine appears to constrict the afferent arterioles preferentially, decreasing both GFR and RBF, while angiotensin II constricts the efferent arteriole, maintaining glomerular hydrostatic pressure and thus GFR (12, 13). While α-adrenergic tone is important in maintaining renal vascular tone in non-basal states, the β-adrenergic system may also participate by regulating renin release (11).

Functional abnormalities in the adrenergic system resulting in dynamic reduction in RBF with preservation of GFR may occur in early hypertensives (1–3). Studies by Hollenberg et al (1) indicate an exaggerated increase in RBF in response to α blockade with phentolamine in early hypertensives versus normotensives, while patients with advanced nephrosclerosis have a reduced response consistent with fixed structural lesions (1).

Although drug therapy has significantly reduced the morbidity and mortality in moderate and severe hypertension (14), and only recently has been demonstrated to benefit mild hypertension (15), adverse drug reactions may negate any potential therapeutic effect. If patients with early essential hypertension have adrenergically mediated and reversible renal vascular abnormalities, the use of adrenergic antihypertensive agents may affect RBF. Such drugs may, in theory, either potentiate or ameliorate the renal vascular abnormalities, perhaps either hastening or preventing the progression of fixed nephrosclerotic changes.

In this paper, we will review the effects of commonly used adrenergic antihypertensive agents on renal hemodynamics and GFR, with a major emphasis on β blockers.

DRUGS INTERACTING WITH α-ADRENERGIC RECEPTORS (Table 1)

α-Adrenoceptor Agonists

CLONIDINE   Clonidine is an α_2 agonist whose hypotensive action is generally thought to be the result of its direct agonist effect on central adrenergic receptors that increase baroreceptor sensitivity, inhibit sympathetic outflow, and perhaps increase parasympathetic outflow to the heart. In addition, it may act on peripheral α_2 receptors to decrease norepinephrine release, and, in large

Table 1   Effect of oral α adrenergic drugs on renal hemodynamics[a]

Drug	Author	GFR	RBF	RVR	FF	Number of patients	Duration
Clonidine	Onesti (18)	↔	↔	↔	NR	7	acute
	Cohen (19)	↔	↔	↓	↔	13	1 month
	Thananopavorn (20)	↔	↔	↔	↔	16	1 week
α-methyl dopa	Mohammed (25)	↔	↔	NR	NR	8	10 days
	Grabie (23)	↓	↔	NR	NR	10	8 days
	Sannerstedt (26)	↔	↔	NR	NR	11	—
	Cruz (24)	↓	↔	↔	↓	6	12 days
Guanabenz	Bosanac (27)	↓	↓	NR	NR	8	acute
	Bosanac (27)	↔	↔	NR	NR	8	3 days
	O'Connor (28)	↔	↔	↓	↔	10	5–7 weeks
Prazosin	Maxwell (30)	↔	↔	NR	NR	4	acute
	Koshy (31)	↔	↔	NR	NR	14	8 weeks
	Preston (32)	↔	↔	↓	↔	10	1 month

[a] ↔ no change; ↑ increased; ↓ decreased; NR: not reported.
GFR: glomerular filtration rate; RBF: renal blood flow; RVR: renal vascular resistance; FF: filtration fraction.

doses, may even stimulate post synaptic α_1 receptors, paradoxically elevating blood pressure (16).

In dogs (17), intrarenal arterial administration of clonidine not only decreased RBF without affecting GFR but increased blood pressure, while intravenous administration decreased RBF without affecting either GFR or blood pressure. This may be explained by the fact that clonidine acts predominantly at post-synaptic α receptors in the former instance, while acting in addition at presynaptic and central sites in the latter instance (17).

However, human studies have shown that neither acute nor chronic oral clonidine disturbs RBF and in fact may decrease RVR in hypertensive patients (18, 19). Onesti et al (18) reported that acute oral clonidine reduced mean arterial pressure (MAP) without affecting RBF or GFR in seven hypertensive patients. In addition, it preserved RBF and GFR despite an acute reduction in MAP that occurred with upright posture. Cohen et al (19) reported that in 13 hypertensive patients, chronic (one month) oral clonidine reduced MAP and RVR without affecting RBF or GFR. More recently, Thananopavorn et al (20) reported similar findings in 16 essential hypertensives. Thus, it appears that oral clonidine in humans, unlike parenteral clonidine in animals, decreases RVR to preserve RBF.

Both Campese et al (21) and Thananopavorn et al (20) found a correlation between the reduction in MAP and plasma free catecholamines during clonidine therapy, while Cohen et al (19) found a correlation between reduced RVR and plasma renin activity (PRA), perhaps an indirect marker of sympathetic activity, suggesting that clonidine reduces RVR by inhibiting sympathetic outflow or renin angiotensin vasoconstrictor tone.

α-METHYL DOPA   Although α-methyl dopa's hypotensive actions were initially thought to reflect its role as a false transmitter, its major action is now generally considered to be as a central α agonist (22), perhaps via its metabolite α-methylnorepinephrine.

Grabie et al (23) and Cruz et al (24) reported studies assessing the effects of α-methyl dopa on renal hemodynamics in patients with normal baseline GFR. They both found a preservation of RPF, but with a reduction in GFR and filtration fraction (FF). This suggests that α-methyl dopa may act at the efferent arteriole to preserve RPF but at the expense of decreasing GFR, perhaps by decreasing glomerular capillary hydrostatic pressure.

In contrast, Mohammed et al (25) reported a preservation of both GFR and RPF in six hypertensive patients with mild renal impairment. Sannerstedt et al (26) also reported a preservation of RPF and GFR in 11 hypertensive patients. However, all six of those patients with baseline GFR greater than 100 ml/min had a reduction in GFR.

Although all these studies were relatively short-term (less than 10 days), they suggest that patients with normal baseline renal hemodynamics may be susceptible to a functional decrement in GFR, while those with baseline renal impairment may be relatively resistant to these dynamic changes. Longer-term studies are required to determine if these functional changes persist.

GUANABENZ   Guanabenz is a recently released central α agonist. One study by Bosanac et al (27) reported a decrease in RPF and GFR in eight hypertensive patients after acute oral guanabenz therapy. However, after three days of guanabenz monotherapy, the GFR and RBF returned to baseline. O'Connor et al (28) reported that guanabenz during chronic (5–7 weeks) therapy in 10 hypertensive patients not only preserved RPF and GFR but reduced RVR. Although the reduced RVR did not correlate with the hypotensive effect, and thus was not paramount to its hypotensive action, it may be important in preserving RBF despite a reduction in systemic perfusion pressure.

α-Adrenoceptor Antagonists

There are currently two orally administered peripheral α antagonists commercially available.

PHENOXYBENZAMINE   Phenoxybenzamine, an α_2 blocker, is used almost exclusively for management of hypertension in patients with pheochromocytoma. There are no recent published studies evaluating its long-term effects on renal hemodynamics.

PRAZOSIN   Prazosin, a post-synaptic α_1 adrenergic blocking vasodilator (29), is widely used in essential hypertension.

Maxwell (30) reported that acute intravenous and acute and chronic oral prazosin had no effect on GFR or RBF in essential hypertensive patients. Subsequent chronic studies done by Koshy et al (31), Preston et al (32), and O'Connor et al (33) confirmed these findings while demonstrating a reduction in RVR (32, 33). Since prazosin reduced RVR without affecting filtration (32, 33), it may act directly on the afferent arteriole to reduce afferent and total RVR, perhaps via post-synaptic α_1 blockade in the afferent arteriole. This is consistent with the observation that the endogenous sympathetic neurotransmitter and α agonist norepinephrine modulates RVR chiefly at the afferent arteriole.

Summary of α-Adrenergic Drugs

Although it is impossible to draw definitive conclusions from a limited number of short-term studies, it appears that peripheral α-adrenergic antagonists preserve renal hemodynamics, while central α-agonists have varying effects. Both acute and chronic clonidine preserve renal hemodynamics. Chronic guanabenz preserves renal hemodynamics, while acute guanabenz does not. In contrast, α-methyl dopa appears to decrease GFR despite preservation of RPF in non-azotemic patients, while renal hemodynamics in patients with nephrosclerosis are unaffected by α-methyl dopa. Pharmacologic properties that account for differences between these α agonists are not readily apparent.

β-ADRENOCEPTOR ANTAGONISTS (Table 2)

The β-adrenergic system may influence renal perfusion and GFR through its effects on cardiac output, renin release, and β-mediated vasodilation (34). β blockade suppresses cardiac output and inhibits β-mediated vasodilation. Both these effects could impair renal perfusion. On the other hand, most β blockers inhibit renin release with a resultant decrease in local angiotensin II production, which may increase renal perfusion and perhaps GFR. In addition, renin suppression could alter sodium and potassium balance because of reduced aldosterone release. Therefore, the net effect of β blockers on renal function is often difficult to predict.

The variable effects of individual β blockers (35) on cardiac output (36) and renin release (37), as well as variability in such properties as cardioselectivity (35, 37, 38), hydrophilicity (38), and intrinsic sympathomimetic activity (35), may result in different effects on RPF and GFR.

Table 2   Effect of various β blockers on renal hemodynamics[a]

Drug	Author	GFR	RBF	RVR	FF	Number of patients	Duration
Propranolol	Wilkinson (45)	↓15%*	NR	NR	NR	15	2 months
	Bauer (72)	↔[†]	↓15%[††]	↔	↔	14	5–6 months
	Ibsen (46)[b]	↓13%**	NR	NR	NR	19	4 months
	Falch (48)[c]	NR	↓20%[§]	NR	NR	13	8 months
	O'Connor (49)[d]	↓12%*	↓15%[††]	↑	↔	15	1 month
	Falch (47)	NR	↓13%	NR	NR	11	2 weeks
	Bauer (50)[f]	↓27%[†]	↓20%[††]	NR	↔	8	—
	Danesh (55)	↔	↔	↔	↔	7	5 weeks
Atenolol	Dreslinski (57)	↔*	↔[§]	NR	NR	10	4 weeks
	Wilkinson (45)	↔*	NR	NR	NR	17	2 months
	Falch (56)	NR	↔[§]	NR	NR	13	4 months
Nadolol	O'Connor (51)[d]	↔[†]	↔[††]	↔	↔	10	6 weeks
	Textor (52)[d]	↔[§]	↔	↔	NR	15	4 weeks
	Textor (53)	↔[§]	↔	↔	NR	13	2 months
	Britton (54)[e]	NR	↓31%[§]	NR	NR	6	2–4 weeks
	Danesh (55)	↔	↑18%[§]	↓	↓	7	5 weeks
Metoprolol	Sugino (59)	↔*	↔[††]	↔	↔	9	5–7 weeks
Pindolol	Wainer (44)	↔[†]	↔[††]	↔	NR	10	6 months
	Wilcox (58)	↔	↔	NR	—	—	—
Acebutolol	Dreslinski (60)	↔*	↓18%[§]	NR	NR	11	4 weeks

[a]* clearance of creatinine; ** clearance of ^{51}Cr-EDTA; † clearance of inulin; †† clearance of paraaminohippurate; § clearance of orthoiodohippurate; NR: not reported. GFR: glomerular filtration rate; RBF: renal blood flow; RVR: renal vascular resistance; FF: filtration fraction.
[b]GFR improved two months after withdrawal of drug
[c]RBF decreased progressively: 11% at one month, 21% at eight months
[d]inverse correlation between baseline RBF and RBF change
[e]When separated into high/low baseline cardiac output and RBF, those with high cardiac output and RBF had a decrease in RBF of 41%
[f]Normotensive subjects

   All of the following studies were done on non-azotemic essential hypertensive patients unless otherwise noted.

Acute Parenteral β Blockers

Acute intravenous β blockers suppress cardiac output but increase systemic vascular resistance (SVR). Except in high-renin hypertension, baseline MAP remains unchanged (39). As SVR decreases toward or below baseline values with chronic therapy, a reduction in MAP occurs (39). The elevated SVR is believed to be the result of unopposed α-mediated vasoconstriction after acute intravenous β blockade (39). The mechanism for the reduction in SVR with chronic therapy remains unclear. A similar phenomenon appears to occur in the renal vasculature. In studies using Xenon washout to determine RPF, Sullivan et al (40) found a 14% reduction in RPF with an increased RVR following intravenous propranolol, while Foley et al (41) found a similar decrement with intravenous cardioselective metoprolol. In contrast, Foley et al found a 13% increment in RPF with nadolol (41). Hollenberg et al (42), using a Xenon washout technique, also found a RPF increment (26%) in response to intravenous nadolol. Using paraaminohippurate (PAH) clearance, Wainer et al (43) found that intravenous pindolol, a β blocker that differs from others in that it has intrinsic sympathomimetic activity (ISA), decreased GFR without affecting RPF. This decrement in GFR returned to baseline with chronic therapy in these same patients. Lastly, Zech et al (44) demonstrated a 16% reduction in RBF with intravenous atenolol, a cardioselective hydrophilic β blocker. The studies by Foley et al (41), Sullivan et al (40), and Wainer et al (43) reported no change in MAP following parenteral β blockers, while Hollenberg et al (42) and Zech et al (44) did not report blood pressure.

Thus, it appears that all β blockers reported except nadolol impair renal hemodynamics with acute parenteral administration. Since blood pressure did not change in these studies, the increased RVR that occurred is likely analogous to the increased SVR that occurs with parenteral β blockers—unopposed α-adrenergic vasoconstriction. The one exception is nadolol, which increased RPF in two separate studies. The mechanism by which intravenous nadolol increases RPF is presently unknown.

Chronic Oral β Blockers

Although acute parenteral β blockers reduce RBF, the potential long-term effect on renal hemodynamics is more important clinically during chronic oral therapy. In seven studies (33, 45–49, 55) of oral propranolol therapy, GFR was determined in five studies (33, 45, 46, 49, 55), with four reporting reductions in mean GFR ranging from 10–27% (33, 45, 46, 49). RBF was determined in five studies (33, 47, 48, 49, 55), with four (33, 47, 48, 49) finding a mean decrement ranging from 13–26%. In only one study (55) was propranolol shown to preserve GFR and RBF. In one other often-quoted study, Bauer (50) demonstrated a reduction in both GFR and RBF in normotensives. RBF returned to baseline two months following cessation of therapy. While creatinine clearance also returned to normal, the decrement in inulin clearance persisted. However, since these were normotensive subjects, the findings may not be relevant to a consideration of propranolol's effect on renal hemodynamics in hypertensives, since normal baseline hemodynamics differ from those of hypertensive patients (1).

Renal hemodynamic studies on the other β blockers with differing pharmacologic properties have had variable results.

Nadolol, a noncardioselective β blocker that is considerably less lipophilic than propranolol (36, 39), did not decrease mean GFR or RBF in five separate studies (51–55). In fact, it actually increased RBF in two studies, by 18% and 31% respectively (54, 55).

Atenolol, whose properties are similar to nadolol's except for its cardioselectivity, did not affect GFR or RBF in three studies (45, 56, 57).

Two separate studies (44, 58) reported that pindolol, which differs from propranolol in that it lacks membrane-stabilizing activity (MSA) but has ISA, did not reduce GFR or RBF.

Metoprolol, which is cardioselective but lacks MSA, ISA, and hydrophilicity, did not affect RBF or GFR in one study (59).

Finally, acebutolol, a β blocker not presently available in the USA, in a single study reduced RBF without affecting GFR (60). Acebutolol is one of three β blockers (acebutolol, alprenolol, oxyprenolol) that share MSA with propranolol. Alprenolol was assessed in one study (61), but the results are not easily interpretable, since the study was done while the majority of patients were on hydralazine. There are no published studies on renal hemodynamic effects of oxprenolol.

PATHOPHYSIOLOGY OF VARIABLE EFFECTS OF β BLOCKERS UPON THE RENAL CIRCULATION

Systemic Hemodynamics

Since RBF accounts for 20% of cardiac output (62), any drug that reduces cardiac output would be expected to reduce RPF and thus GFR. This relationship has been previously described (63). However, even though all β blockers reduce cardiac output, not all of them reduce RBF. The observation that some β blockers do not reduce RBF suggests that suppression of cardiac output is not pivotal in the reduction of RBF, or that certain β blockers contain intrinsic properties that preserve autoregulation of renal perfusion in the face of altered systemic hemodynamics. For example, intravenous doses of propranolol insufficient to reduce cardiac output or heart rate have been shown to reduce renal perfusion (64). The altered intrarenal hemodynamics may be a function of intrinsic pharmacologic properties of the β blocker.

While cardiac output reduction may be instrumental in reducing renal perfusion during acute parenteral β blocker administration, these effects on renal hemodynamics may be overcome by chronic renal perfusion autoregulation.

Plasma Volume

Intravascular volume contraction might contribute to impaired renal perfusion. Tarazi et al (65) demonstrated an 8% mean reduction in plasma volume with chronic propranolol monotherapy. However, more recent studies have noted neither contraction nor expansion of plasma volume (46, 48, 49, 57, 59, 66,

67). Thus, volume depletion alone cannot be considered a factor in reducing renal perfusion during β blockade.

Pharmacologic Properties (Table 3)

CARDIOSELECTIVITY β_2 adrenergic receptors have been demonstrated in the renal vasculature. Blockade of these vasodilatory receptors may result in unopposed α-adrenergic vasoconstriction. It has been proposed that propranolol-induced renal hemodynamic changes could be secondary to unopposed α-adrenergic renal vasoconstriction (33, 49). This is partially supported by the fact that atenolol and metoprolol, cardioselective β blockers, preserve RBF (45, 56, 57, 59). However, nadolol, a non-cardioselective β blocker, has been repeatedly demonstrated not only to preserve RBF but actually to augment RBF. Thus, although cardioselectivity may be important, it is not the only factor influencing RBF.

ISA   β blockers with ISA might be expected to spare the effects of unopposed α-adrenergic vasoconstriction. This may be why pindolol preserves GFR and RBF (44, 58). However, nadolol, which preserves RBF, is not only non-cardioselective but also lacks ISA. In addition, acebutolol has ISA but has been reported to reduce renal perfusion (60).

HYDROPHILICITY   Hydrophilic β blockers, as determined by low partition between octanol and water (38), have difficulty crossing cellular membranes. Thus, unlike lipophilic β blockers, they are not metabolized by the liver, are excreted unchanged by the kidney, reach most compartments of the body with relative difficulty, and have long plasma half lives (38). The most hydrophilic β blockers, atenolol and nadolol, have both been demonstrated to preserve RBF. Whether and how this preservation of RBF is related to hydrophilicity is not established. In contrast, some lipophilic β blockers, such as pindolol and metoprolol, preserve renal perfusion (44, 58, 59), while the lipophilic β blocker propranolol diminishes RBF (49).

MEMBRANE-STABILIZING ACTIVITY   Propranolol and acebutolol are the β blockers that most consistently reduce RPF during chronic oral monotherapy (49, 60). In addition, both have MSA (Table 3), although the renal perfusion effects of other β blockers with MSA have not been determined. However, MSA, also known as a local anesthetic effect or quinidine-like effect, does not seem to occur at β-blocker doses used for hypertension (35). Since MSA has no known effects on renal perfusion or autoregulation, it cannot be definitively implicated in RBF decrements.

Table 3 Pharmacologic properties of various β blockers[a]

Agent	Cardioselectivity	ISA[b]	MSA	Hydrophilicity
Propranolol	−	−	+	−
Nadolol	−	−	−	+
Atenolol	+	−	−	+
Metoprolol	+	−	−	−
Pindolol	−	+	−	−
Timolol	−	−	−	−
Acebutolol	+	+	+	−

[a] + present; − absent
[b]ISA: intrinsic sympathomimetic activity; MSA: membrane stabilizing activity.

Renal Vasoactive Hormones

RENIN-ANGIOTENSIN SYSTEM   In sodium-depleted states, the renin system—via angiotensin II—tends to decrease RBF (13). Therefore, suppression of renin might tend to increase RBF. However, despite propranolol's well-described inhibition of renin release (66, 67), it decreases RBF. In addition, there has been no correlation between suppression of plasma renin activity and change in RBF (43, 49, 56, 57, 60).

KALLIKREIN-KININ SYSTEM   Urinary kallikrein is produced in the distal renal tubule and cleaves kininogen to yield kinins—vasodilatory peptides. Evidence suggests that in man, renal kallikrein-kinin system activity correlates with RBF (68, 69) and may modulate RVR. It is of interest that black hypertensives are both poorly responsive to propranolol (70) and deficient in renal kallikrein excretion (68, 69), suggesting a relationship between the two. O'Connor & Preston (49) reported a reduction in urinary kallikrein excretion with propranolol monotherapy, while kallikrein measured by the same technique did not change with nadolol monotherapy (51). Although there was not a significant correlation between change in RBF and change in urinary kallikrein excretion during propranolol therapy, the study does suggest that reduction in kallikrein may play some role in the RBF decrement by interfering with a possible compensatory vasodilator system.

Patient Characteristics

PATIENT SELECTION   Two reported crossover studies allowed for control of patient selection variables. In one (55), nadolol statistically enhanced RBF. Following a washout period of six weeks, propranolol did not affect RBF. However, there was no significant difference between RBF after nadolol and RBF after propranolol. Since this is the only study reporting preservation of RBF with propranolol, it suggests that patient selection may be important in demonstrating these changes.

On the other hand, Wilkinson et al (45) conducted a similar study comparing the effects of atenolol and propranolol on GFR. They found that atenolol preserved GFR while propranolol decreased it, with a significant difference between GFR on propranolol versus atenolol. Although they did not measure RBF, based upon other studies the altered GFR is presumably a reflection of altered renal hemodynamics. Thus, patient selection is not the only important factor governing renal response to β blockade.

AGE   Although it is known that RBF decreases with age (9), even in normotensives, none of the β blocker studies correlated the renal hemodynamic changes with age. The importance of this factor thus remains unknown.

PRETREATMENT RBF   Until recently, most investigators have overlooked the potential relationship between baseline RBF and altered RBF induced by β blockers. As suggested by Hollenberg's study (1), patients with more advanced nephrosclerotic changes are relatively impervious to dynamic changes induced by antiadrenergic drugs. O'Connor and Preston (49) demonstrated an inverse correlation between baseline RBF and RBF decrement in response to propranolol; i.e. those patients with the highest pretreatment RBF had the greatest fall in RBF on treatment. O'Connor et al found a similar correlation in reevaluating their data in patients studied while on nadolol (71), as well as a similar correlation in Textor's published data on nadolol (71). However, a similar correlation was not found by Sugino et al in patients studied while on metoprolol (59), nor by Bauer (72) in propranolol-treated hypertensives.

In addition, although Britton et al (54) reported an increase in mean RBF in essential hypertensives treated with nadolol, when they divided the patients into those with high and low baseline cardiac output and mean RBF they found that those with high baseline values had a decrement in RBF (41%) while those with low baseline values had a mean increment in RBF (31%).

Since other investigators have not routinely assessed this correlation, it is not possible to comment on whether differences in pretreatment renal function may account for changes seen with propranolol in other studies. Nonetheless, it appears that pretreatment RBF may be an important predictor of renal perfusion impairment after propranolol (49).

UNDERLYING RENAL INSUFFICIENCY   Although Warren et al (73) reported marked deterioration in renal function in three azotemic patients after β blockade, the risk may have been overemphasized (74). The paucity of similar reports in the literature suggests it is a rare occurrence. This is consistent with the notion (49) that patients with advanced nephrosclerosis are relatively protected from the dynamic alterations in renal perfusion induced by propranolol.

NEPHROTOXICITY   There is no evidence that propranolol or other β blockers are nephrotoxic. In the studies cited above, when both GFR and RBF were measured the decrement in GFR was commensurate with the decrement in RBF. None of our patients whose GFR decreased with propranolol (49) had any evidence of renal parenchymal disease (i.e. urinary cells, casts, or proteinuria).

Clinical Importance

One limitation of all the studies cited is the duration of therapy. The longest study period was eight months, which is far shorter than the natural history of hypertension or its usual duration of treatment. Although one study (48) demonstrated a progressive decrement in RBF while on propranolol, decreasing by 11% at one month and a further 10% at eight months, the cumulative data are insufficient to determine the role, if any, of propranolol in hastening the progression of nephrosclerosis.

Despite the reduction of both RBF and GFR, the clinical impact of propranolol on renal function remains unclear since the usual clinical indices of renal function, blood urea nitrogen and serum creatinine concentrations, do not change with therapy (33, 49). Longer-term studies are needed to determine if RBF and GFR decrements after propranolol could progress toward azotemia.

The reversibility of propranolol's effects on renal hemodynamics has yet to be determined conclusively. Ibsen et al (46) reported an improvement in GFR with cessation of therapy. Bauer et al (50) found a persistent decrease in inulin clearance in normotensives after cessation of propranolol; on the other hand, Bauer et al (72) found a persistent decrease in renal blood flow two weeks after cessation of propranolol in hypertensives.

The use of vasodilators in concert with β blockers may confer renal hemodynamic protection, although once again the data is limited. Falch et al (47) reported that the addition of propranolol to hydralazine did not reduce RBF, but following cessation of hydralazine, RBF did decrease.

There is insufficient data to indicate whether factors such as chronicity of hypertension, concomitant use of other medications, dose of β blockers, duration of therapy, or intravascular volume status confer protection or predispose patients to β-blocker–induced decrements in renal hemodynamics.

Although there is one report of profound renal functional deterioration after propranolol (73), preexisting renal insufficiency might actually confer protection against the dynamic changes induced by propranolol in these patients, who would be expected to have the least reactive renal vasculatures (49). Perhaps the patients we should be most concerned with are early hypertensives with intact renal vascular reactivity. Nonetheless, we would not proscribe the use of propranolol in such patients (74). However, if a patient's renal function deteriorates without apparent cause on propranolol therapy, one may consider changing therapy to another β blocker or to another category of drug altogether.

SUMMARY

Peripheral α antagonists not only preserve renal hemodynamics, but decrease RVR and maintain renal perfusion autoregulation in the face of decreased systemic perfusion pressures. On the other hand, central α agonists appear to have variable effects. Clonidine preserves RBF and GFR both acutely and chronically, guanabenz decreases RBF acutely but not chronically, and α-methyl dopa preserves RBF but decreases GFR.

β blockers also have variable effects on RBF: the most-often–studied β blocker, propranolol, has reduced RBF by 10–20% while other commonly used β blockers, such as nadolol and metoprolol, may preserve RBF. This may reflect propranolol's inability to maintain renal perfusion autoregulation in the face of decreased systemic blood pressure. This failure of propranolol is not completely understood but may be a function of its lack of cardioselectivity or ISA (49). It is also possible that inhibition of renal vasodilators such as the kallikrein-kinin system plays a role (49).

Finally, it appears that patients with normal renal vascular tone may be at highest risk to suffer decrements in RBF with β blockers. Perhaps most importantly, the clinical impact of propranolol's effect on renal function is unclear, since the reductions in GFR have not in general been sufficient to produce azotemia.

Acknowledgments

Supported by the Veterans Administration, the National Institutes of Health (HL-25,457), the National Kidney Foundation, and the American Heart Association. Dr. O'Connor is an Established Investigator of the American Heart Association. We appreciate the collaboration of the following investigators in our studies of renal perfusion in hypertension: Drs. Richard A. Stone, Arthur R. Olshan, John A. Mitas, Irving M. Cohen, Sanford E. Warren, Anna P. Barg, Coleman P. Mosley, Kenneth L. Duchin, Richard A. Preston, Eric H. Sasso, Gerald R. Sugino, and Ronald P. Frigon. We appreciate the technical assistance of Justine Cervenka, Gail Levine, and Annie Chen, and the secretarial support of Marta Zekan-Czoka. Dr. Bernstein is a fellow of the National Kidney Foundation.

118   BERNSTEIN & O'CONNOR

Literature Cited

1. Hollenberg, N. K., Adams, D. F., et al. 1975. Renal vascular tone in essential and secondary hypertension. *Medicine* 54:29
2. Hollenberg, N. K., Borucki, L. J., Adams, D. F. 1978. Renal vasculature in early essential hypertension: Evidence for a pathogenic role. *Medicine* 57:167
3. Hollenberg, N. K., Adams, D. F. 1976. The renal circulation in hypertensive disease. *Am. J. Med.* 60:773
4. Bianchi, G., Cusi, D., Gatti, M., et al. 1979. A renal abnormality as a possible cause of essential hypertension. *Lancet* 1:173
5. Pederson, E. B. 1976. Renal hemodynamic and plasma renin in patients with essential hypertension. *Clin. Sci. Mol. Med.* 50:409
6. Gomez, D. M. 1951. Evaluation of renal resistence with special reference to changes in essential hypertension. *J. Clin. Invest.* 30:1143
7. Logan, A. G., Velasquez, M. T., Cohen, I. M. 1973. Renal cortical blood flow, cortical function, and cortical blood volume in hypertensive subjects. *Circulation* 47:1306
8. Lowenstein, J., Steinmetz, P. R., Effros, R. M., et al. 1967. The distribution of intrarenal blood flow in normal and hypertensive man. *Circulation* 35:250
9. deLeeuw, P. W., Kho, T. L., Falke, H. E., Birkenhager, W. H., Wester, A. 1978. Hemodynamic and endocrinological profile of essential hypertension. *Acta Medical Scand.* 1978 (Suppl. 622):9–86
10. Warren, S. E., O'Connor, D. T., Cohen, I. M., Mitas, J. A. 1981. Renal hemodynamics during longterm antihypertensive therapy. *Clin. Pharmacol. Ther.* 29:310
11. Kopp, U. C., Dibona, G. F. 1982. The functions of renal nerves. *Kidney* 15:17
12. Moss, N. G. 1982. Renal function and renal afferent and efferent nerve activity (editorial). *Am. J. Physiol.* 243:F425
13. Navar, L. G., Marsh, D. J., Blantz, R. C., et al. 1979. Intrinsic control of renal hemodynamics. *Fed. Proc.* 41:3022
14. Hypertension Detection and Follow-up Program Cooperative Group. 1979. Five year findings of the Hypertension Detection and Follow-up Program. *J. Am. Med. Assoc.* 242:2562
15. Hypertension Detection and Follow-up Program Cooperative Group. 1982. The effects of treatment on mortality in mild hypertension. *N. Engl. J. Med.* 307:976
16. Itskovitz, H. D. 1980. Clonidine and the kidney. *J. Cardiovasc. Pharmacol.* 2(Suppl.1):547

17. Chrysant, S. G., Lavendar, A. P. 1975. Direct renal hemodynamic effects of clonidine. *Arch. Int. Pharmacodyn. Ther.* 218:207
18. Onesti, G., Schwartz, A. B., et al. 1971. Antihypertensive effect of clonidine. *Circ. Res.* 28(Suppl.II):II53
19. Cohen, I. M., O'Connor, D. T., et al. 1979. Reduced renovascular resistance by clonidine. *Clin. Pharmacol. Ther.* 26:572
20. Thananopavorn, C., Golub, M. S., Eggena, P. 1982. Clonidine, a centrally acting sympathetic inhibitor, as monotherapy for mild to moderate hypertension. *Am. J. Cardiol.* 49:153
21. Campese, V. M., Romoff, M., et al. Role of sympathetic nerve inhibition and body sodium-volume state in antihypertensive action of clonidine in essential hypertension. *Kidney Int.* 18:351
22. Henning, M., Van Zweitin, P. A. 1968. Central hypotensive effect of alpha methyl dopa. *J. Pharm. Pharmacol.* 20:409
23. Grabie, M., Nussbaum, P., et al. 1980. Effects of methyl dopa on renal hemodynamics and tubular function. *Clin. Pharmacol. Ther.* 27:522–27
24. Cruz, F., O'Neill, W. M., et al. 1981. Effects of labetolol and methyl dopa on renal function. *Clin. Pharmacol. Ther.* 30:57
25. Mohammed, S., Hanenson, I. B., et al. 1968. The effects of alpha methyl dopa on renal function in hypertensive patients. *Am. Heart J.* 76:21
26. Sannerstedt, R., Bojs, G., Garnauskas, E., Werko, L. 1963. Alpha methyl dopa in arterial hypertension. Clinical, renal and hemodynamic studies. *Acta Med. Scand.* 174:53
27. Bosanac, P., Dubb, P., et al. 1976. Renal effects of guanabenz: A new antihypertensive agent. *J. Clin. Pharmacol.* 17:631
28. O'Connor, D. T., Mosley, C., et al. 1982. Guanabenz selectively reduces renal vascular resistance in essential hypertension. *Kidney Int.* 21:191 (Abstr.)
29. Colucci, W. S. 1982. Alpha adrenergic receptor blockade with prazosin. *Ann. Int. Med.* 97:67
30. Maxwell, M. H. 1975. Effects of prazosin on renal function and fluid electrolyte metabolism. *Postgrad. Med.* (SI):36–41
31. Koshy, M. C., Mickley, D., et al. 1977. Physiologic evaluation of a new antihypertensive agent: Prazosin HCl. *Circulation* 55:533
32. Preston, R. A., O'Connor, D. T., Stone, R. A. 1979. Prazosin and renal hemody-

namics: Arteriolar vasodilation during therapy of essential hypertension in man. *J. Cardiovasc. Pharmacol.* 1:277

33. O'Connor, D. T., Preston, R. A., Sasso, E. H. 1979. Renal perfusion changes during treatment of essential hypertension: Prazosin vs. propranolol. *J. Cardiovasc. Pharmacol.* 1:S38(Suppl.)

34. Weber, M. A., Drayer, J. I. M. 1980. Renal effects of beta adrenoceptor blockade. *Kidney Int.* 18:686

35. Frishman, W. H. 1981. Beta-adrenoceptor antagonists. New drugs and new indications. *N. Engl. J. Med.* 305:500

36. Svensson, A., Gubrandsson, T., Sivertsson, R., Hansson, L. 1982. Hemodynamic effects of metoprolol and pindolol. A comparison in hypertensive patients. *Br. J. Clin. Pharmacol.* 13(Suppl. 2):2595

37. Buhler, F. R., Burkart, F., Lutold, B. E. 1975. Antihypertensive beta blocking action as related to renin and age. A pharmacologic tool to identify pathogenic mechanisms in essential hypertension. *Am. J. Cardiol.* 36:653

38. Cruickshank, J. M. 1980. The clinical importance of cardioselectivity and lipophilicity in beta blockers. *Am. Heart. J.* 100:160

39. Hansson, L., Zweifler, A. J., Julius, S., Hunyor, S. N. 1974. Hemodynamic effects of acute and prolonged beta adrenergic blockade in essential hypertension. *Acta Med. Scand.* 196:27

40. Sullivan, J. M., Adams, D. F., Hollenberg, N. K. 1976. Beta adrenergic blockade in essential hypertension: Reduced renin despite renal vasoconstriction. *Circ. Res.* 39:537

41. Foley, J., Penner, B., Fury, H. 1981. Short term renal hemodynamic effects of nadolol and metoprolol in normotensive and hypertensive subjects. *Clin. Pharmacol. Ther.* 29:245 (Abstr.)

42. Hollenberg, N. K., Adams, D. F., McKinstry, D. N. 1979. Adrenoceptor blocking agents and the kidney. Effect of nadolol and propranolol on renal circulation. *Brit. J. Clin. Pharmacol.* 7(Suppl. 2):2195

43. Wainer, E., Boner, G., Rosenfeld, J. B. 1980. Effects of pindolol on renal function. *Clin. Pharmacol. Ther.* 28:575

44. Zech, P., Pozet, N., Labeeuw, M., et al. 1975. Acute renal effect of new beta blockers on renal function. *Kidney Int.* 8:132 (Abstr.)

45. Wilkinson, R., Stevens, I. M., Pickering, M., et al. 1980. A study of the effects of atenolol and propranolol on renal function in patients with essential hypertension. *Brit. J. Clin. Pharmacol.* 10:51

46. Ibsen, H., Sederberg-Olsen, P. 1973. Changes in glomerular filtration rate during longterm treatment with propranolol in patients with arterial hypertension. *Clin. Sci.* 44:129

47. Falch, D. K., Odegaard, A. E., Norman, N. 1978. Renal plasma flow and cardiac output during hydralazine and propranolol treatment in essential hypertension. *Scand. J. Clin. Lab. Invest.* 38:143

48. Falch, D. K., Odegaard, A. E., Norman, N. 1979. Decreased renal plasma flow during propranolol treatment in essential hypertension. *Acta Med. Scand.* 205:91

49. O'Connor, D. T., Preston, R. A. 1982. Urinary kallikrein activity, renal hemodynamics, and electrolyte handling during chronic beta blockade with propranolol in hypertension. *Hypertension* 4:742

50. Bauer, J. H., Brooks, G. S. 1979. The long term effect of propranolol therapy on renal function. *Am. J. Med.* 66:405

51. O'Connor, D. T., Barg, A. P., Duchin, K. L. 1982. Preserved renal perfusion during treatment of essential hypertension with the beta blocker nadolol. *J. Clin. Pharmacol.* 22:187

52. Textor, S. C., Fouad, F. M., Bravo, E. L. 1982. Redistribution of cardiac output to the kidney during oral nadolol administration. *N. Engl. J. Med.* 307:601

53. Textor, S. C., Fouad, F. M., Tarazi, R. C., Bravo, E. L. 1981. Nadolol and cardiac hemodynamics. *R. Soc. Med., Int. Congr. Symp.* 37; p. 71

54. Britton, K. E., Gruenewald, S. M., Nimmon, C. C. 1981. Nadolol and renal hemodynamics. *R. Soc. Med., Int. Congr. Symp.* 37; p. 77

55. Danesh, B. J. Z., Brunton, J. 1981. Nadolol and renal hemodynamics. *R. Soc. Med., Int. Congr. Symp.* 37; p. 87

56. Falch, D. K., Ovist, P. A., et al. 1979. Central and renal circulation, electrolytes, body weight, plasma aldosterone, and renin during atenolol treatment in essential hypertension. *Curr. Ther. Res.* 26:813

57. Dreslinski, G. R., Messerli, F. H., et al. 1982. Hemodynamics, biochemical and reflexive changes produced by atenolol in hypertension. *Circulation* 65:1365, (Abstr.); 1981 *Clin. Pharmacol. Ther.* 23:241

58. Wilcox, C. S., Lewis, P. S., et al. 1981. Renal function, body fluid composition, renin, aldosterone and norepinephrine during treatment of hypertension with

pindolol. *J. Cardiovasc. Pharmacol.* 3:598

59. Sugino, G., Barg, A. P., O'Connor, D. T. 1983. Renal perfusion is preserved during cardioselective beta blockade with metoprolol in hypertension. *Am. J. Kidney Dis.* In press

60. Dreslinski, G. R., Aristimuno, G. G., Messerli, F. H., et al. 1979. Effects of beta blockade with acebutolol on hypertension, hemodynamics, and fluid volume. *Clin. Pharmacol. Ther.* 26:562

61. Pederson, E. B., Mogensen, C. E. 1976. Effect of antihypertensive treatment on urinary albumin excretion, glomerular filtration rate, and renal plasma flow in patients with essential hypertension. *Scand. J. Clin. Lab. Invest.* 36:231

62. Beeuwker, R., Ichikawa, I., Brenner, B. M. 1982. Renal circulation. In *The Kidney*, ed. B. M. Brenner, F. C. Rector, p. 249. Philadelphia: W. B. Saunders. 2nd ed.

63. Nies, A. S., McNeil, A. S., Schrier, R. W. 1971. Mechanisms of increased sodium reabsorption during propranolol administration. *Circulation* 44:596

64. Carriere, S. 1969. The effect of norepinephrine, isoproterenol and adrenergic blockers upon the intrarenal distribution of blood flow. *Can. J. Physiol. Pharmacol.* 47:199

65. Tarazi, R. C., Frohlich, E. D., Dustan, H. P. 1971. Plasma volume changes with longterm beta adrenergic blockade. *Am. Heart J.* 82:770

66. Buhler, F. R., Laragh, J. H., Baer, L., et al. 1972. Propranolol inhibition of renin secretion. *N. Engl. J. Med.* 287:1209

67. Hollifield, J. W., Sherman, K., Vanderzwagg, R., Shand, D. G. 1976. Proposed mechanisms of propranolol's antihypertensive effect in essential hypertension. *N. Engl. J. Med.* 295:68

68. Warren, S. E., O'Connor, D. T. 1980. Does a renal vasodilator system mediate racial differences in essential hypertension? *Am. J. Med.* 69:425

69. Levy, S. B., Lilley, J. J., Frigon, R. P., Stone, R. A. 1977. Urinary kallikrein and plasma renin activity as determinants of renal blood flow. *J. Clin. Invest.* 60:129

70. Humphreys, G. S., Devlin, D. G. 1968. Ineffectiveness of propranolol in hypertensive Jamaicans. *Brit. Med. J.* 1:601

71. O'Connor, D. T. 1983. Renal blood flow during nadolol administration (letter). *N. Engl. J. Med.* 308:49

72. Bauer, J. H. 1983. Effects of propranolol therapy on renal function and body fluid composition. *Arch. Int. Med.* 143:927–31

73. Warren, D. J., Wainson, C. P., Wright, N. 1974. Deterioration in renal function after beta blockade with chronic renal failure and hypertension. *Brit. Med. J.* 2:193

74. Mitas, J. A., O'Connor, D. T., Stone, R. A. 1978. Hypertension in renal insufficiency: A major therapeutic problem. *Postgrad. Med.* 64:113–20

Ann. Rev. Pharmacol. Toxicol. 1984. 24:121–46

THE COUPLING OF THE NEURONAL MUSCARINIC RECEPTOR TO RESPONSES

M. McKinney and E. Richelson

Departments of Psychiatry and Pharmacology, Mayo Foundation, Rochester, Minnesota 55905

MUSCARINIC RECEPTORS

Introduction

Muscarinic acetylcholine receptors are plasma membrane proteins that bind the neurotransmitter acetylcholine and by their conformational changes elicit specific biological events within cells. They are pharmacologically defined by their binding selectivity for a specific class of drugs, among which are the agonists muscarine and oxotremorine and the various atropine-like antagonists. Muscarinic receptors mediate various types of responses in cardiac muscle, in numerous smooth muscles, in exocrine glands, throughout the peripheral and central nervous system, and in some kinds of cultured nerve cells. Usually two or three subtypes of muscarinic receptors exist, distinguished by their relative binding affinity for agonists (1). Though the types of biological responses among these tissues are varied, the respective proteins that bind the agonist appear to be similar or identical in binding properties and molecular size. It is probably their coupling to unique tissue-specific effectors that gives rise to varied responses.

Responses mediated by muscarinic receptors are slow in onset and development and thus are distinctly different from nicotinic responses, but like nicotinic responses they can desensitize. In the brain, where the muscarinic receptor is the predominant cholinergic receptor, its activation can lead to either excitation or inhibition of neurons (2). In the cerebral cortex, for example, pyramidal cells become depolarized from decreases in potassium (K^+) conductance (3),

121

0362-1642/84/415-0121$02.00

while in the ventral thalamus inhibitory responses are encountered (4). In cardiac muscle, hyperpolarization results from increases in K^+ conductance (2). In a tissue where there are no action potentials, the parotid gland, muscarinic receptors trigger calcium (Ca^{+2}) influx from a neurotransmitter-sensitive pool, probably located in plasma membrane binding sites, that then mediates secretion of amylase (5). An apparently separate but Ca^{+2}-dependent response in this gland is K^+ efflux (6). Muscarinic receptors in smooth muscle can cause either contraction or relaxation or can modulate spontaneously contracting muscle (7). K^+ efflux in smooth muscle may also be a separate response. In many tissues with muscarinic receptors there are often additional responses of a biochemical nature. The stimulation of guanylate cyclase (8–14) and/or the inhibition of adenylate cyclase (12, 13, 15–21) is often observed; these responses are often dependent upon the presence of Ca^{+2} in the extracellular medium. The metabolism of phospholipids is sometimes a consequence of muscarinic activation (22–24) and there are some recent data implicating arachidonic acid metabolism (25, 26). Most of these biochemical responses have been observed to desensitize (27–29).

Many of the responses cited conveniently occur in "neuron-like" murine neuroblastoma cells (for example, clone N1E-115), and thus these cells have been extensively employed as model systems to study the function of the muscarinic receptor. Studies of the muscarinic receptors of neuroblastoma provide valuable supplementary information to studies of the receptor in the nervous system. Neuroblastoma systems are particularly useful for asking questions at the molecular level, where such approaches are very difficult with in vivo systems.

Memory is one example of a brain function in which more knowledge of muscarinic processes at the molecular level would be useful. According to current thought, memory involves cholinergic systems innervating the cerebral cortex and hippocampus (30). Muscarinic receptors are probably involved in mediating this input. Antimuscarinic agents, apparently by blocking these receptors, can cause memory processing impairments similar to those seen in the aged (31). A possible pathologic correlate of pharmacologic blockade of cholinergic input to these muscarinic receptors is Alzheimer's disease, where a profound lesion of the basal forebrain source of cholinergic innervation of the cerebral cortex and hippocampus apparently leads to deficits in cognitive function (32). As this disease progresses, the patient loses his ability to process recent memory. In the later stages deterioration in general cognitive function occurs; in the terminal phase there is profound dementia. The exact changes that occur in the muscarinic receptor system in response to the absence of cholinergic input and to subsequent administration of drugs in substitution or precursor therapy are not known. There is some information from binding studies with homogenates of human brain indicating up-regulation (33), but the details of the biochemical response of the receptor to denervation are not known. Conceivably, such basic knowledge, much of which is coming from studies of receptors in cultured cells, could contribute to successful drug therapy for Alzheimer's dementia and perhaps other brain disorders that have a component of dementia or memory dysfunction. The advantages of studying the muscarinic receptor of intact N1E-115 cells have been exemplified by the finding that many psychotherapeutic agents, including antidepressants and neuroleptics (34) and local anesthetics (35), mediate effects at these receptors [blockade of guanosine cyclic monophospate (cGMP) formation (36)].

The Biochemical Nature of the Receptor

The muscarinic receptor can be solubilized from membranes and studied in extracts with high-affinity reversible ligands or with irreversible alkylating ligands, but because of its instability and low abundance the receptor has not been purified. Several proteins with muscarinic binding sites were detached from membranes of rat brain with high salt concentrations; the putative receptor had a molecular weight of only 30,000 daltons (37). More recently, the receptor was affinity labeled, solubilized with detergents, and studied by SDS gel electrophoresis (38, 39). The receptor from rat brain and smooth muscle had an estimated molecular weight of 80,000 daltons and migrated as a single band (38). Affinity labeling was largely prevented by atropine, which indicates the receptor's muscarinic nature. The affinity-labeled receptor of mouse cerebral cortex, where the low-affinity receptor is prevalent, had a molecular weight of 86,000 daltons (39). Affinity labeling of the muscarinic receptor in the mouse brain stem, where there are mostly high-affinity receptors, revealed both 86,000 and 180,000 dalton proteins. Mild alkaline hydrolysis converted these proteins into 40,000 dalton fragments. It was suggested that the low-affinity receptor was a dimer and the high-affinity receptor was a tetramer of 40,000-dalton, covalently coupled subunits. This was supported by the apparent interconversion of sites by a guanosine triphosphate (GTP) analog or by manganese (Mn^{+2}), which are known to have such effects on binding to mouse brain muscarinic receptors (40, 41).

The brain receptor has been shown by lesion experiments to be located for the most part post-synaptically. A small fraction of the binding sites are tentatively identified as pre-synaptic in cortex (42) and hippocampus (43), where there is also physiological evidence for their presence (44). After subcellular fractionation of the brain tissue, the muscarinic receptor is found in the synaptosomes (45). In autoradiographic experiments, receptors can be visualized over cell bodies or dendritic fields of neurons (46). Thus, binding studies of the brain can be expected to provide information about synaptically located receptors. In general, antagonists bind to a single class of sites with rank order of affinities that correlate very well with their potencies in the blockade of cholinergic function in intact tissues (47). However, occupancy curves for agonists are multiphasic, with Hill slopes less than unity, and their Scatchard transforms are concave upward (48–50). This phenomenon is due to the presence of multiple independent binding sites for agonists, which sometimes can apparently be induced to interconvert in vitro. It was shown in rat cortex that the low Hill slopes for agonists were not due to negative cooperativity by using an affinity alkylating agent to partially occlude sites before performing binding with carbachol (48). Though there has been some evidence indicating cooperativity in the binding of the receptor in the pituitary (51), the brain itself has generally been found to possess independent agonist sites (48, 50). Studies with iterative computer methods for analyzing binding data have shown that two agonist sites (high- and low-affinity) predominate in brain and heart, and that another one of higher affinity ("super-high") is also present in low concentrations in the brain (52). In the brain, the proportions of these sites vary with region but a substantial number of muscarinic agonists bind to these three sites in a given brain region in virtually the same ratios of capacities (52). Agonists do not seem to induce multiple-site phenomena in vitro; thus, it would be expected that these more-or-less fixed-capacity multiple binding sites in some way reflect functional heterogeneity. N1E-115 cells possess low- and high-affinity agonist sites (53).

Since a single receptor protein of 86,000 daltons (or a multiple of it) is able to produce multiphasic binding, the most parsimonious explanation for this apparent heterogeneity is that it is attributable to differences in the receptor's conformation, perhaps to its chemical modification, or to its coupling with another protein (54). The affinity-labeling data cited above, for example, suggest that heterogeneity results from the covalent intercoupling of subunits. Guanyl nucleotides (GTP, etc) have an effect on agonist binding to the muscarinic receptor that is similar to that seen with the β-adrenergic receptor: agonist occupancy curves are shifted to the right (40, 41, 55, 56). This GTP effect is variable with brain region: the brain-stem receptors show a substantial shift similar to that observed in the heart (55), but cortical receptors display little or no change in the dose with which the agonist inhibits [^{3}H]-antagonist binding by 50% (IC_{50}).

Computer analyses of these effects have indicated that heart or brain-stem high-affinity sites are possibly being converted into low-affinity sites (40, 54). By analogy with the β-adrenergic receptor, this suggests that the low-affinity site, at least in the brain-stem, is coupled to responses. It has been shown that incubating synaptosomes under phosphorylating conditions partially inhibits this rightward shift, though the receptor itself is not phosphorylated (57). Other agents, such as certain metal ions, apparently have been able to change the proportions of sites seen in broken-cell preparations (41, 54). Although these observations are suggestive of regulatory mechanisms in vivo, the physiological meaning for multiple agonist binding sites in the brain remains unclear. It is possible that either receptors are coupled to different effectors for unique responses or that multiple sites are features of a regulatory mechanism involving a single effector. It is also possible that heterogeneity is an artifact of homogenization. The effects of GTP on binding to the brain-stem receptor is evidence in favor of genuine functional differences between these sites.

When the neuronal muscarinic receptor is solubilized with detergents, its agonist-binding heterogeneity disappears (58). The solubilized receptor-detergent complex binds carbachol with a binding affinity very much like that of the low-affinity agonist site in the membrane. If the coupling is disrupted by digitonin solubilization, this would mean that the high-affinity form is the coupled receptor. But this presumes that the conformations of the membrane-bound and solubilized receptor are the same. A body of physiological evidence suggests that the low-affinity membrane-bound receptor of a variety of tissues is coupled to responses:

1. Birdsall et al have found that the equilibrium binding constants for agonists at the brain low-affinity agonist site (K_L) correlate roughly with the potencies of these agonists for contraction of smooth muscle when spare receptors are accounted for (48).
2. The negative chronotropic response of chick atria in vitro correlates with the occupancy of the low-affinity receptor of this tissue (59).
3. The dose of carbachol effective for 50% down-regulation of the receptor of intact heart cells in culture is at a value typical of K_L in brain or neuroblastoma (60).
4. The half-maximal dose for carbachol's stimulation of K^+ efflux of these heart cells and its desensitization is in the range of the neuronal K_L (60).
5. In N1E-115 cells the dose for half-maximal cGMP response (ED_{50}) for several agonists correlates almost exactly with the K_L for these agonists and not their K_H (equilibrium dissociation constant for the high-affinity site) (61). However, the N1E-115 muscarinic inhibition of prostaglandin E_1–stimulated adenosine cyclic monophosphate (cAMP) formation correlates with K_H (62).
6. In synaptosomal preparations of cerebral cortex the dose-response for muscarinic mediation of phosphatidylinositol turnover correlates with K_L (63). With N1E-115 the turnover of phosphatidylinositol has an ED_{50} for carbachol at 10μM, a concentration in at least tenfold excess of K_H (28).
7. In slices of the rat striatum, Hanley & Iversen showed that for the formation of cGMP by various muscarinic agonists the ED_{50}'s were near their K_L's (9).

Thus, there is considerable evidence that the low-affinity agonist site is a "functional" site in vivo. However, as has been noted (1), in a given tissue the ED_{50}'s for stimulation of various responses can differ widely. Thus, there may well be responses coupled to the high-affinity or super-high-affinity receptors. A good example of this is the muscarinic receptor of pancreatic acini, where amylase secretion seems to involve high-affinity receptors (64). It is not yet known if the agonist binding sites are located on the same or different neurons in brain tissue, but high- and low-affinity sites do appear to be differentially distributed in cortical cell layers (65). N1E-115 cells possess both predominant agonist sites in the same proportion as those in whole rat cerebral cortex (53).

The binding of antagonists by the muscarinic receptor has sometimes appeared multiphasic. Pirenzepine has been shown to bind to multiple sites in the brain as well as in other tissues (66); it labels two sites in human cerebral cortex in the same approximate proportions as the rat cortical high- and low-affinity receptors (67). In synaptosomes of the cortex of cat brain, [^{3}H]-quinuclidinyl benzilate (^{3}H-QNB) was observed to associate to two sites in roughly the same proportion as the two predominant agonist sites (68). In the adenohypophysis there seem to be two antagonist sites (69). In frog heart, two antagonist sites for ^{3}H-QNB are thought to correlate with two agonist sites for oxotremorine, and interconversion of these sites appears to be effected by guanine nucleotides (70). The meaning of multiple antagonist sites remains elusive and somewhat controversial. One possible explanation for binding heterogeneity with antagonists is that, under the appropriate conditions, it reflects the coupling phenomenon, as agonists appear to. It is not a general finding in brain tissue. There has been one report of two antagonist sites in N1E-115 and NG108-15 neuroblastoma cells (71).

The brain muscarinic receptor apparently has a sulfhydryl group that is important for its conformation (72, 73). Alkylation of receptors in membranes with N-ethylmaleimide (NEM), which is selective for sulfhydryl groups, seems to convert the agonist binding sites into a higher affinity state (74, 75). However, the opposite effect with NEM has also been observed in brain (76). The inconsistency of NEM effects as observed in brain tissue requires a conservative view of the value of NEM in site conversion. The degree of chemical modification of the sulfhydryls of the brain receptor can be varied by the presence of ligands at the binding site and, with agonists at least, this is due to an induced conformational change (77). Reducing agents like dithiothreitol can decrease the binding of an antagonist or agonist to the brain receptor (72, 75); this is suggestive of the importance of a disulfide bond in the conformation of the protein.

Most metal ions do not affect binding except at high concentrations (78). Ca^{+2} ions at physiological concentrations do not change binding, but the lanthanides, which are antagonists at Ca^{+2}-binding sites, affect muscarinic binding (78, 79) and also affect mediation of cGMP formation in N1E-115 cells. Transitional metal ions affect receptor binding in rat (78) and mouse (41) cerebral cortex and cGMP formation in N1E-115 cells (80, 81). Mn^{+2}, nickel ions (Ni^{+2}), and cobalt ions (Co^{+2}) seem to convert mouse low-affinity sites to high-affinity sites, which is interesting in light of the ability of Mn^{+2} and Ni^{+2} to stimulate cGMP formation in N1E-115 cells (80, 81). The effects of these ions could be due to their action at receptor sulfhydryl groups, which seem to be important for the receptor's conformation, or at Ca^{+2} binding sites on the receptor or on neighboring phospholipids. Ca^{+2} has been shown to bind to acidic phospholipids (82) and this is affected by phenytoin, which is a blocker of Ca^{+2}-dependent cGMP formation in N1E-115 cells (83). It has been found that very high monovalent metal ion concentrations will obscure differences in binding affinities of the high- and low-affinity sites in cortex (54); it may be then that sites within a given region are identical polypeptides with various conformations as dictated by their ionic environment. However, in a study of the effects of metals on antagonist binding to the rat brain receptor, Ikeda et al found that the effect of metal ions at high concentrations was different, even opposite, for forebrain and brainstem areas (74). These workers suggested that the concept of a single receptor protein with two conformational states of differing agonist binding affinities, with relative proportions of the states being a function of brain region, could not fully explain this particular effect of metals (74).

The phospholipids of the membrane may act on the receptor to affect its conformation. Exogenous phosphatidylserine, phospatidic acid, and phosphatidylinositol enhance ^{3}H-QNB binding to the receptor in homogenates (84). The types of fatty acyl groups in the phospholipids are probably also important, since exogenous unsaturated but not saturated fatty acids, or treatment of the membranes with phospholipase A, will inhibit ^{3}H-QNB binding (84). The effect of changing the lipid environment of the receptor on agonist binding has not been investigated, but it is possible that lipids are involved in the mechanism of agonist-induced regulation of the receptor. The type and concentration of unsaturated lipids present in the membrane phospholipids are known to be important in plasma membrane processes; for example, the growth of PC12 pheochromocytoma cells with various unsaturated fatty acids in the media changes the composition of the membrane phospholipid acyl groups and profoundly affects opiate receptor binding (85); exogenous arachidonic acid reduces γ-aminobutyric acid and glutamate uptake and Na^+/K^+-ATPase activity in brain slices and synaptosomes (86). Membrane fluidity, a function of lipid composition, is important in muscarinic processes, as can be seen by the effect of temperature on carbachol-stimulated cGMP formation in N1E-115 cells: receptor-mediated cyclic GMP formation and the desensitization and resensitization of the effect will not occur below 21°C, which is in the vicinity of the transition temperature for lipid bilayers (87).

MOLECULAR CONSEQUENCES OF RECEPTOR ACTIVATION

Changes in Electrical Properties of the Cell

Slow depolarization of the plasma membrane is commonly observed in the central nervous system (CNS) in response to iontophoresis of muscarinic agonists (2). This raises the level of excitability of the neuron and slowly increases spontaneous firing. This is in contrast to the rapid depolarization and increased firing rate elicited by an agent like glutamate.

Particularly well-studied is the muscarinic response of the pyramidal cells of cerebral cortex, where there is a typical slowing of firing for about 5–10 seconds, followed by a long period of increased firing rate caused by gradual depolarization (3). These excitatory effects of acetylcholine have been shown to be mediated by a decrease in the resting membrane conductance for K^+ and by a partial inactivation of voltage-sensitive K^+ channels that repolarize the cell (3). The action of acetylcholine on cortical neurons is blocked by the metabolic inhibitor dinitrophenol (DNP), which does not inhibit the stimulation of these cells by glutamate except in high doses (88). This indicates that the post-synaptic muscarinic action in vivo involves metabolic processes. The ionic basis for inhibitory responses, such as those found in the thalamus, is not known.

There is some evidence that Ca^{+2} is necessary for muscarinic effects on K^+ conductance in the CNS. Barium ion (Ba^{+2}), which is Ca^{+2}-like, excites cortical neurons in a way similar to acetylcholine, by reduction in K^+ conductance, and these neurons also usually respond to acetylcholine (89). It is possible that Ba^{+2} substitutes for Ca^{+2} in some Ca^{+2}-dependent process; Ba^{+2} and Sr^{+2} can substitute for Ca^{+2} in the muscarinic stimulation of cGMP formation in rat ductus deferens (90) and Ba^{+2} can pass through Ca^{+2} channels (91). A role for internal Ca^{+2} in modulation of K^+ conductance has been shown in spinal motor neurons, where intracellular injection of Ca^{+2} increases the K^+ conductance (92) and injection of EGTA blocks K^+ conductance (93).

Differentiated N1E-115 cells can generate action potentials and the voltage-dependent sodium ion (Na^+), K^+, and Ca^{+2} channels of these cells have been shown to be very similar to other well-characterized neuronal channels (94). The voltage-sensitive Ca^{+2} channel is relatively weak and is blocked by Co^{+2}, Mn^{+2}, or the lanthanides (95). Activation of this channel by increasing the external K^+ concentration to a depolarizing level can cause cGMP formation in N1E-115 cells (96). N1E-115 cells have another K^+ channel that is triethylamine(TEA)-resistant and Ca^{+2}-dependent, which can give rise to a prolonged after-hyperpolarization (AHP) (97). Activation of muscarinic receptors of N1E-115 cells, in addition to causing cGMP formation, also causes the cells to become hyperpolarized (98). Neurotransmitter-mediated cGMP formation, which occurs in both differentiated and undifferentiated cells, is a Ca^{+2}-dependent process. However, it is not due to activation of voltage-sensitive Ca^{+2} channels. Carbachol's stimulation of cGMP formation is additive to cGMP formation mediated by high K^+ depolarization (96). Thus, to mediate the hyperpolarization the neurotransmitter receptor and the action potential may be indirectly operating the same TEA-insensitive Ca^{+2}-dependent K^+ channels, both by separate Ca^{+2}-mediated pathways. This idea of separate Ca^{+2} channels is supported by the finding that the dihydropyridines inhibit cGMP formation mediated via the voltage-sensitive Ca^{+2} channel but do not inhibit the neurotransmitter-stimulated cGMP formation (R. M. Snider, E. Richelson, unpublished information). It is thus conceivable that there are additional steps between Ca^{+2} influx and the effect on these delayed K^+ channels in N1E-115 cells. These steps may be the stimulation of guanylate cyclase and some cGMP-dependent action on K^+ channels, perhaps the phosphorylation of the K^+ channel by a cGMP-dependent protein kinase.

A role for cGMP in membrane events in the muscarinic activation of cortical neurons has been implicated by recent experiments. When cyclic GMP is iontophoresed on to cortical pyramidal cells an increase in their firing rate follows (99). Intracellular injection of cGMP into cortical pyramids causes an increase in membrane resistence and increased firing identical to that caused by acetylcholine when it is iontophoresed on to the same cell extracellularly (100). In these carefully controlled experiments, blockade of acetylcholine effects but not cGMP effects by atropine showed that the receptor involved was muscarinic. To draw a parallel, then, perhaps Ca^{+2}-dependent K^+ channels in both the brain and in N1E-115 cells mediate the muscarinic electrical responses, either excitatory or inhibitory, contingent upon or in parallel with cGMP formation. Supportive of the contingent involvement of cGMP is the finding that N1E-115 cells will hyperpolarize when cGMP is added to the medium (98).

The hypothesis that cGMP is the mediator of neuronal muscarinic-linked ionic events via direct activation of the cyclase by Ca^{+2} passing in through channels is complicated somewhat by the recent finding that N1E-115 cells loaded with the Ca^{+2}-sensitive photoprotein aequorin (101) do not emit light when stimulated with carbachol (E. Richelson, R. M. Snider, M. McKinney, C. Forray, submitted for publication), indicating the absence of a rise in intracellular free Ca^{+2}. The preloaded cells will emit light when stimulated by high K^+ or with the ionophore X537A, however. Ca^{+2} influx into the cytosolic pool then may not be a consequence of neuronal muscarinic stimulation (105). A messenger other than Ca^{+2} may be interposed between receptor and cyclase (see below). This additional step may explain the odd voltage-dependence of the N1E-115 delayed K^+ channel (95, 97).

If cGMP formation is not involved in ionic events, one must consider alternative functions in neural tissue; it is interesting to note in this context that cGMP has been shown to be involved in memory at the cellular level in sympathetic ganglia (103), although in mammals it has not yet been possible to show a direct link between cGMP and changes in membrane conductance (104). Cylic GMP thus may not in general mediate the voltage changes in nervous tissue typically seen with muscarinic agents, but in both cortical neurons and N1E-115 cells it appears that a rise in intracellular cGMP concentration does by an obscure mechanism lead to membrane conductance changes.

Biochemical Responses

PHOSPHOLIPID METABOLISM   Acetylcholine, acting at muscarinic receptors, is one of the many agents that can stimulate the phosphatidylinositol (PI) cycle (22–24). Several lines of evidence support a role for the PI cycle in neurotransmitter action in the CNS (24); much of this evidence concerns muscarinic action. Although the metabolism of PI and the less prevalent polyphosphoinositides (PPI) is stimulated by brain muscarinic receptors and Ca^{+2} seems to be required for this, it is not yet certain whether neurotransmitter-stimulated Ca^{+2} influx is the required Ca^{+2} event. This aspect of the hypothesis of the PI cycle (Ca^{+2} gating) remains unsettled.

Muscarinic-mediated PI metabolism in brain tissue has been demonstrated in vivo and in vitro (with synaptosomes or slices) by the incorporation of ^{32}P-phosphoric acid into PI, PPI, and phosphatidic acid (PA), and by release of [^3H]*myo*inositol phosphate from PI (24). In a typical study, carbachol was shown to stimulate the release of inositol-phosphate(s) 5.4–8.3× over basal in slices of cortex, striatum, hypothalamus, and hippocampus (24). Removal of the predominant cholinergic input to the hippocampus by a fornix lesion does not affect muscarinic-mediated PI turnover in hippocampal synaptosomes (105), while direct lesion of intrinsic hippocampal neurons with the neurotoxin ibotenic acid does reduce synaptosomal PI turnover (106). This is good evidence that synaptosomal PI turnover is located post-synaptically.

The agonist stimulation of the synaptosomal PI cycle does not require Ca^{+2} in the medium, but added EGTA will block it (107). This has been interpreted to mean that an endogenous store of Ca^{+2}, perhaps plasma membrane–bound, is available as a source for the effect of the neurotransmitter. The divalent cation ionophore A23187 will stimulate a similar synaptosomal PI turnover and this is not blocked by atropine (108). Submaximal levels of A23187 and acetylcholine added together cause a synergistic effect. It has thus been supposed that calcium influx occurs with both types of stimulation. The hypothesis of a common pathway of Ca^{+2} influx preceding the PI cycle is supported by the blockade of the effect of both agents by EGTA. However, although influx of Ca^{+2} as caused by A23187 is sufficient to elicit PI labeling, it is not necessary to suppose that the receptor causes influx. The muscarinic receptor may or may not use the same mechanism to stimulate the cycle. This can be seen in the situation cited above, where the cGMP response of N1E-115 cells can be elicited by both ionophore X537A and by carbachol, yet Ca^{+2} transport can be measured only with the ionophore. The mechanism of neurotransmitter stimulation of the synaptosomal PI cycle then may also not require transport of Ca^{+2} to the inside in the same way an ionophore does.

Agranoff et al have recently refined their study of the synaptosomal muscarinic receptor by comparing agonist occupancy curves with PI dose-response curves (63). Full but not partial muscarinic agonists bound to two sites, with the majority of sites (65%) in the low-affinity conformation. Carbachol's dose-response curve, however, was nearly monophasic with an ED_{50} of 109 μM, quite close to the K_D for the low-affinity site (77 μM). The conclusion is that the low-affinity agonist site of cerebral cortex mediates the synaptosomal PI turnover. By analogy with the hippocampal studies cited above, these findings in the cortex probably reflect a post-synaptic localization for the response.

Mn^{+2} is generally regarded as a Ca^{+2}-channel blocker in neural tissue. However, it modulates the PI cycle in synaptosomes (109) by increasing incorporation of inositol into PI. Mn^{+2} will inhibit the PI labeling by [^{3}H]inositol evoked by the muscarinic receptor. The mechanism of Mn^{+2} stimulation may involve a stimulation of the PI cycle by stimulating PI synthesis (24, 109). This is one example of a mechanism of stimulating the PI cycle that probably involves neither Ca^{+2} influx nor a stimulation of PI turnover. Mn^{+2} alone transiently increases cGMP formation in N1E-115 cells and with prolonged incubation it will inhibit carbachol-mediated cGMP formation (80, 81). This is an interesting parallel with the effects of Mn^{+2} on the synaptosomal PI cycle, suggesting that Mn^{+2} and the neurotransmitter may activate a common pathway for the stimulation of cGMP synthesis. One implication is that the muscarinic receptor may mediate the cGMP response by stimulating the PI cycle, and this is supported by the recent finding that N1E-115 muscarinic receptors mediate PI turnover (28).

As with the cGMP response, the PI turnover response of N1E-115 cells desensitizes (28). Ca^{+2} in the medium is not required for carbachol to stimulate labeling of PI in N1E-115 cells. As Ca^{+2} can be absent from the medium and the cGMP response will also still desensitize, this is a feature common to these two responses. The half-maximal PI response of N1E-115 cells occurs at 10 μM. This implies that the N1E-115 PI cycle and cGMP response are both stimulated by the low-affinity receptor and that desensitization of the two responses might be by the same mechanism, perhaps at a point in the PI cycle.

In smooth muscle cells, where there is a Ca^{+2}-dependent muscarinic-mediated cGMP response, exogenous PA will cause contraction with a time course similar to that of carbachol (111). PA has been proposed as the mediator of the presynaptic Ca^{+2} influx that causes neurotransmitter release (112).

Studies such as these implicate PA as a Ca^{+2} ionophore. PA could then be a candidate link between the PI cycle and the other responses of N1E-115 if it acts to carry Ca^{+2} inside. Exogenous PA will cause $^{45}Ca^{+2}$ uptake and cGMP formation in N1E-115 cells (110), and it will evoke the emission of light when the cells are preloaded with the photoprotein aequorin (R. M. Snider, personal communication). However, the guanylate cyclase is a soluble enzyme in N1E-115 cells (113) and is probably not directly activated by Ca^{+2}, so there is a question as to what intracellular agent stimulates the cyclase.

In platelets, the stimulation of the PI cycle by thrombin causes PI to be metabolized by a phospholipase C (PLC) and a phospholipase A_2 (PLA_2) (114). Diacylglycerol is formed, which is phosphorylated to PA, while arachidonic acid is released. The arachidonate release is probably dependent upon the operation of the PI cycle because protease inhibitors, which inhibit the PLC, block the release and metabolism of arachidonate (115). Since the PLA_2 is a Ca^{+2}-dependent enzyme, one possible mode of its activation by the PI cycle could be by transport of Ca^{+2} into its vicinity, perhaps by chelation to headgroups of acidic phospholipids (e.g. PA), which could be generated locally by receptor activation of the PI cycle. A complex of Ca^{+2}-PA is electrically neutral and although phospholipids do not normally flip-flop, a Ca^{+2} electrochemical gradient can apparently supply the necessary energy for this in smooth muscle (111) and in synaptosomes (112) in a Pressman chamber (116). Arachidonic acid metabolism has been recently implicated in the N1E-115 neurotransmitter-mediated cGMP response: thrombin will stimulate cGMP-formation in these cells with a Ca^{+2}-dependence and a time course similar to that of the neurotransmitter (117).

CYCLIC NUCLEOTIDE RESPONSES

Muscarinic stimulation of cyclic GMP in brain tissue and neuroblastoma cells   The formation of cGMP, discussed above in several contexts, is a common response to muscarinic activation (14). By analogy with what is known of cAMP, a second messenger role for cGMP has been postulated (118). Protein phosphorylation by cGMP-dependent protein kinases can be demonstrated in smooth muscle (119); cGMP-dependent protein phosphorylation has been shown to occur in mammalian brain (where a 23,000-dalton protein is phosphorylated), but a link to the muscarinic receptor has not been shown (120). In primary cultures of rat cerebellum, long-term exposure to carbachol causes phosphorylation of proteins (121) but we do not know whether this is mediated by cGMP or not. cGMP is certainly a good indicator of neuronal muscarinic activation, but specifically what types of physiological responses it mediates is unclear. When its level is increased in cortical neurons or in N1E-115 cells it can lead to changes in membrane resistence but by unknown mechanisms.

Levels of cGMP in various areas of the brain are elevated with systemic administration of oxotremorine, a muscarinic agonist (12). Immunohistochemical reactions to cGMP in nervous tissue have shown that it is present in neurons and glial cells in the caudate-putamen (122), in neurons and glial cells in the cerebellum (123), and in neurons of the superior cervical ganglion (8). Slices of brain tissue form cGMP when incubated with muscarinic agonists (9, 10), though the degree of response is never very large, presumably because only a small fraction of the neurons in the slice are cholinoceptive.

The dose-response curves for agonists in slices of rat striatum have Hill slopes closer to unity than their occupancy curves, and the ED_{50} for carbachol and arecholine are near their dissociation constants at the low-affinity receptor (9). Ca^{+2} at a physiological level is required and the Ca^{+2} dependence appears similar to that for muscarinic responses in N1E-115 cells. In this study of the striatum, cAMP was also elevated by muscarinic agonists and the formation of both nucleotides was blocked by atropine. It is not known whether the muscarinic stimulation of cGMP was direct or involved interneurons, but the cAMP response could also be blocked by a dopamine antagonist, indicating that cAMP was formed after dopamine release stimulated by the muscarinic agonist. This illustrates some of the complexities in interpreting the results of experiments with brain slices. In a study of the septo-hippocampal pathway, electrical stimulation of the medial septum caused elevated cGMP levels in the hippocampus, but this was not blocked by systemic administration of scopolamine (124). As there is a cholinergic component to this pathway, these data do not support a post-synaptic role for cGMP in the brain, which is demonstrable in the superior cervical ganglion (8). Thus, the evaluation of a link between the muscarinic receptor and cGMP in the brain is not simple.

N1E-115 cells display many of the properties of neurons, including the possession of neurotransmitter receptors, the formation of cyclic nucleotides with stimulation of these receptors, and the possession of voltage-sensitive ion channels that can operate action potentials (125). N1E-115 muscarinic receptors mediate a marked rise in intracellular cGMP and an inhibition of neurotransmitter-stimulated cAMP formation (13, 35). NG108–15 hybrid neuroblastoma-glioma cells have muscarinic receptors that inhibit cAMP formation and are capable of acting on a guanine nucleotide binding protein (15, 18). Thus, these two cell lines provide useful model systems to ask questions about cyclic nucleotide responses to muscarinic activation that pertain to responses in the brain.

Coupling and cyclic GMP response in N1E-115 cells   Two types of agonist binding sites exist in membranes prepared from homogenates of N1E-115 cells, with dissociation constants for carbachol of 50 μM (K_L) and 0.1 μM (K_H) (53). The dose-response curve for carbachol-mediated cGMP formation via the muscarinic receptor has an ED_{50} at about 70 μM, not too far from the K_L (27, 34, 35). The Hill coefficient for muscarinic stimulation of cGMP is of unity or greater value, while the agonist binding Hill coefficient is always less than unity due to the presence of multiple sites. The ED_{50} for agonist desensitization of the receptor is also close to the ED_{50} for cGMP stimulation (126). All this taken together suggests that two sites are involved in binding, while only one, probably the low-affinity site, is involved in the stimulation of cGMP formation and its desensitization. This seems to be a parallel with the synaptosomal PI response discussed above.

Increasing the Ca^{+2} concentration from 1.8 mM to 10 mM increases the potency of carbachol's cGMP stimulation while not affecting its binding (79); this presumably reflects an action of the ion at the putative effector, which mediates the stimulation with an absolute requirement for Ca^{+2}. The lanthanides, which are classical Ca^{+2} antagonists, block this effector (79), possibly by competition with Ca^{+2} at sites of its action, because increasing the Ca^{+2} concentration can overcome the depression of V_{MAX} by the lanthanides. Lanthanides also decrease the ED_{50} for carbachol, suggesting that these ions have a separate effect on receptor-effector coupling. As discussed above, Mn^{+2} can induce cGMP formation in the presence of Ca^{+2}, with a time course similar to that of the neurotransmitters (80). This is probably an action on the coupling mechanism, because Mn^{+2} does not affect [³H]-QNB binding to the N1E-115 receptor and probably does not enter the cell. Verapamil will block both muscarinic- and Mn^{+2}-mediated cGMP formation, apparently by blockade of Ca^{+2}-channels, and this agent will displace [³H]-QNB from the receptor (81). These data taken together support a concept of muscarinic receptors as physically coupled to Ca^{+2}-effectors. These effectors could be Ca^{+2}-channels, but because neurotransmitter-stimulated Ca^{+2} influx is not observable, it is preferable to refer to them as Ca^{+2}-effectors. The concept of precoupled receptors (i.e. that they exist coupled in both the basal and stimulated states) is also supported by an experiment that showed that desensitization of the muscarinic and histamine receptors has an additive inhibition on Mn^{+2}-mediated cGMP formation (80). Thus, the mobile receptor hypothesis (127) (which presumes that receptors are uncoupled in the basal state) may not apply to the initial cGMP response in N1E-115 cells. These cells might change the proportion of pre-coupled receptors in the regulation of this response, however, and in this sense the latter hypothesis may apply (126). The coexistence of precoupled and uncoupled N1E-115 receptors may also explain multiple agonist binding sites if coupling to a channel affects the conformation of the receptor (54, 78). This is the more probable situation if binding studies reveal a constant ratio of sites with a range of full agonists, as is observed in cortical membranes (52). This would mean that the receptors are pre-coupled. However, it has not yet been rigorously shown that binding in homogenates accurately reflects the conformations of the receptor in intact cells.

Calcium translocation and the cyclic GMP response in N1E-115 cells   All the agents that stimulate cGMP formation in N1E-115 cells require Ca^{+2} to be present in the medium. However, as noted above, Ca^{+2} transport is not measurable during neurotransmitter stimulation of cGMP formation. Macroscopic Ca^{+2} translocation thus does not occur with the neurotransmitters. Yet Ca^{+2} must be present on the outside of the cells for cGMP to be formed intracellularly, and Ca^{+2} is somehow involved in the muscarinic receptor-effector coupling mechanism. It appears that subsequent to agonist binding, a transmembrane event not involving Ca^{+2} flux into the cytosol per se is catalyzed by the presence of Ca^{+2}. This implies the involvement of Ca^{+2} located in the plasma membrane pool that is accessible to extracellular free Ca^{+2}. Such a concept of Ca^{+2} movement has been proposed for the "filling phase" of muscarinic receptor-stimulated Ca^{+2} fluxes in parotid acinar cells (128).

High K^+ (110 mM) in the medium, X537A, and PA all translocate Ca^{+2} inside and stimulate cGMP formation with a profile containing a rise to a peak and a return to basal levels. Ca^{+2} influx with these agents is very rapid but the time course of the subsequent cGMP formation is slower, even slower than that seen with carbachol or histamine (E. Richelson, R. M. Snider, M. McKinney, C. Forray, submitted for publication). First, this suggests that the calcium dependence of the action of the neurotransmitter to stimulate cGMP formation is somehow vectorial. Second, it suggests that an additional time-dependent process is involved. As was suggested above, Ca^{+2} may be chelated by head groups of phospholipid moities locally generated by the PI cycle, possibly PA, which then bind to and activate proteins within the membrane or activate an internal membrane-associated protein such as the enzyme phospholipase A_2 or diglyceride lipase, which releases another messenger. This would satisfy the vectorial and possibly the temporal constraint. Another possibility is that a Ca^{+2}-PA complex is the effective substrate for the PLA_2. The metabolism of PA by the muscarinic-stimulated PI cycle in N1E-115 cells has recently been shown (28), and its independence of Ca^{+2} might be taken as supportive of a role for a PI cycle product in some type of neurotransmitter-linked Ca^{+2} translocation. In any case, because of lack of evidence of transport into the cytosol, such a mechanism requires that the internal Ca^{+2} concentration does not change, so Ca^{+2} remains in a bound state or is released in minute quantities. It is thus hypothesized that the effector coupled to the receptor uses Ca^{+2} to mediate the release of another messenger (possibly arachidonic acid; see below) that can enter the cytosol and that effects stimulation of guanylate cyclase (102). The function of the effector (which may be the PI cycle) is to bring Ca^{+2} into the vicinity of this "activator," which actually releases the messenger (see Figure 1).

According to this hypothesis, Mn^{+2} is able to bypass the receptor and, by acting on the effector, directly trigger the Ca^{+2}-dependent membrane event leading to cGMP formation. This action is not specific to the muscarinic receptor; Mn^{+2} also activates the effector of the histamine receptor (80, 81). As Mn^{+2} is able to modulate the PI cycle in synaptosomes, Mn^{+2} may modulate the PI cycle in N1E-115 cells, which then leads to translocation of Ca^{+2} into the vicinity of the activator, followed by the stimulation of cGMP formation in these cells.

Implications from the time course of cyclic GMP formation   Upon receptor-linked stimulation of cGMP formation in N1E-115 cells, the levels of the cyclic nucleotide rise rapidly, typically to 5- to 15-fold over basal levels (13, 35). This is followed by a rapid return of cGMP levels to the basal value. The time to the peak varies with the stimulant (carbachol, histamine, thrombin) but usually lasts between 30–60 seconds. This temporal profile has been observed in other systems.

Considering muscarinic receptor stimulation, the climb to the peak is the result of turning on the membrane event R→E→A (see Figure 1). This peak

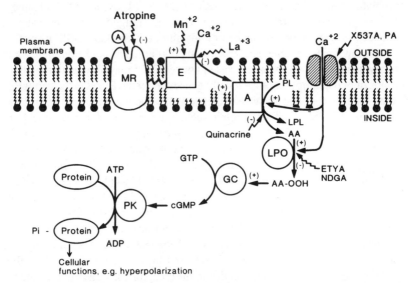

Figure 1   Hypothetical scheme for molecular events involved in muscarinic-receptor mediated cGMP response in neurons. MR: muscarinic receptor; Ⓐ: agonist; Ⓐ: activator; Ⓔ: effector; X537A: ionophore; PA: phosphatidic acid; PL: phospholipids; LPL: lysophospholipids; AA: arachidonic acid; ETYA: eicosatetraynoic acid; NDGA: nordihydroguairetic acid; AA-OOH: hydroperoxide of arachidonic acid; GC: guanylate cyclase; PK: protein kinase. For explanation, see text.

concentration is hyperbolically dependent upon the neurotransmitter concentration and is thus proportional to occupancy of some receptor subtype. Therefore, the neurotransmitter, by its binding to the receptor, effects the rapid stimulation of the guanylate cyclase to a high and constant velocity. This distinctive temporal profile implies that the guanylate cyclase is an allosteric enzyme and that its activating ligand is released subsequent to binding of the agonist. The sharpness of the peak at 30 seconds means that a turning-off event occurs: near the peak the activating process ceases and the removal of cGMP begins or takes over. In the absence of phosphodiesterase inhibition the cGMP levels decline hyperbolically. Isobutylmethylxanthine, a phosphodiesterase inhibitor, flattens the decline, indicating that phosphodiesterase is involved in the removal process (13). Lowering the temperature also prolongs the decline and shifts the peak to the right; thus, either the phosphodiesterase is temperature-sensitive or the turning-off process is a membrane event dependent on membrane fluidity (87).

The profiles of cGMP levels during stimulation of cGMP by K^+, Mn^{+2}, and PA also contain the rapidly declining phases (80, 96, 110). Thus, because these agents probably do not activate receptors directly, the turn-off event must be downstream of the receptor.

Activating mechanism   By a calcium-dependent process, thrombin, a PLA_2 stimulant in platelets, stimulates cGMP formation in N1E-115 cells (117). This implicates membrane-derived fatty acids, possibly arachidonic acid, in this response. Quinacrine, an inhibitor of PLA_2, blocks thrombin-, histamine-, and carbachol-mediated cGMP formation in these cells (117; M. McKinney, R. M. Snider, E. Richelson, unpublished information). Lipoxygenase (LPO) inhibition with nordihydroguairetic acid or eicostetraynoic acid also blocks cGMP formation; it is unlikely that these agents have a direct effect on the receptor. Indomethacin, which blocks the cycloxygenase that synthesizes prostaglandins, has no effect on carbachol- or thrombin-mediated cGMP formation. The effects of the inhibitors suggest that the receptor causes the release of arachidonic acid and that the lipoxygenase produces a metabolite that stimulates the guanylate cyclase.

The guanylate cyclase of guinea pig myometrium can be activated by arachidonate metabolites in broken cell preparations (22), and the guanylate cyclase in rat ductus deferens is stimulated by the muscarinic receptor through a lipoxygenase metabolic pathway (25). Guanylate cyclase in other tissues can be activated by unsaturated fatty acids and their derivatives (129, 130). Recently the platelet guanylate cyclase has been shown to be activated by membrane-derived arachidonate (130a). Since the initial product formed by lipoxygenase is a hydroperoxide and since hydroperoxide metabolites of arachidonate were most effective in stimulating guanylate cyclase in most of the above studies, it is expected that the activating agent in N1E-115 will turn out to be a transient arachidonate hydroperoxide. Since the PI cycle is stimulated in N1E-115 cells by the muscarinic receptor and because this cycle has been implicated in the activation of PLA_2 in other systems, it is reasonable next to examine the requirement for PI turnover in cGMP responses and determine if the activation of PLA_2 in N1E-115 cells is the mechanism of generating an intracellular messenger for the muscarinic receptor. It is likely that the PLA_2 and lipoxygenase of N1E-115 cells are Ca^{+2}-dependent, as they are in other systems (131, 132); exactly how Ca^{+2} reaches these enzymes to activate them must await detailed biochemical studies.

Turnoff of cGMP formation could be due to a cessation of PLA_2 activity. The cessation of activity could be due to feedback inhibition of free arachidonate or one of its metabolites on the Ca^{+2}-transport mechanism or on PLA_2. Alternatively, PLA_2 may turn off simply because of a local depletion of its substrate or because of product inhibition by the lyso-phospholipids.

Cyclic AMP and a role for the high-affinity muscarinic binding site of N1E-115 cells   The possibility of a physiologic response mediated by the high-affinity receptor is supported by the muscarinic inhibition of prostaglandin E_1-stimulated adenylate cyclase activity in N1E-115 cells analogous to that seen in NG108–15 cells. In experiments in which the same cells were assayed for both stimulation of cGMP and inhibition of prostaglandin E_1-stimulated cAMP formation, there was a separation of the ED_{50}'s for these two responses by nearly two orders of magnitude (62). The ED_{50}'s for the effects are 50 μM for cGMP stimulation and 1 μM for cAMP inhibition. These are remarkably close to the dissociation constants for the two sites. The receptor-mediated inhibition of adenylate cyclase in NG108–15 by opiates, α-adrenergic agents, and muscarinic agents is likely to be by stimulation of a GTPase activity that results in the dissociation of the guanyl nucleotide protein from the adenylate cyclase (133). Muscarinic receptor interaction with a guanyl nucleotide protein is suggested by the effects of muscarinic agonists on the β-adrenergic-receptor-mediated cAMP formation in canine cardiac membranes (134) and by the effects of GTP on brain and heart muscarinic receptor binding (40, 41, 55, 56). Thus, for N1E-115 muscarinic receptors the high-affinity agonist subtype could be mediating an effect on the coupling of the prostaglandin E_1 receptor to guanine nucleotide proteins by causing hydrolysis of GTP and subsequent decoupling of the putative guanyl nucleotide protein from adenylate cyclase. The presence of isobutylmethylxanthine does not prevent the muscarinic inhibition, which means that hydrolysis by phosphodiesterase is not stimulated via the muscarinic receptor to cause the cAMP reduction (S. Stenstrom, E. Richelson, unpublished information). Since prostaglandin E_1 will also stimulate cGMP formation in N1E-115 cells and this is additive to carbachol's stimulation (13), a simple shuttling mechanism of a putative guanine nucleotide regulatory protein is difficult to envision.

Short-term desensitization of neuroblastoma muscarinic responses Attenuation of N1E-115 cGMP and PI responses occurs upon prolonged incubation of these cells with muscarinic agonists (27, 28). Because these effects occur in minutes, it is referred to as short-term desensitization. With desensitization, the dose-response curve for carbachol-mediated cGMP formation shifts to the right and the maximum is depressed, with increasing times of preincubation with the agonist (27). If the cells are then incubated without agonist present, they will gradually become increasingly responsive to another challenge. These processes will not occur below 21°C, which probably means that membrane fluidity is required (87). Desensitization will occur without Ca^{+2} ions in the medium, indicating that cGMP formation is not required for it to occur, which is further support for the hypothesis that desensitization is a membrane event. Additionally, the process is dose-dependent (126). A candidate site for the event(s) then is the receptor itself. Antagonist binding to the muscarinic receptor of N1E-115 cells is not changed by desensitization, but recently it has been shown that the binding of agonists is affected by desensitization (62). The dissociation constants for all three agonist sites are increased during desensitization, perhaps accounting for the rightward shift in dose-response curves.

Histamine H_1 receptors and muscarinic receptors of N1E-115 cells do not cross-desensitize more than 15%; this specific desensitization is evidence for a change in the receptor protein or a protein coupled to it. Because these receptors both trigger cGMP responses in a Ca^{+2}-dependent fashion, it is possible that they use the same types of effectors. Mn^{+2}, an agent which can mediate cGMP formation without a neurotransmitter present, will inhibit histamine- and carbachol-mediated cGMP formation. This inhibition by Mn^{+2} is similar to the attenuation seen in desensitization. If the cells are desensitized to either histamine or carbachol, the cGMP response mediated by Mn^{+2} is reduced by about half. Mn^{+2} does not affect receptor binding, as observed with [^{3}H]-QNB. The site of the action of Mn^{+2} is likely then to be on the effector to which receptors couple. The Ca^{+2} dependence of Mn^{+2}-mediated cGMP formation also supports this. Additionally, and most importantly, the simultaneous desensitization of these two receptors has almost additive inhibitory effects on the Mn^{+2} stimulation (80). This strongly suggests that each receptor is coupled to a dedicated effector and that desensitization occurs not only at the receptor but also at the effector or at the mechanism of their coupling. What kind of change occurs in the effector or on the coupling mechanism cannot be addressed until more is understood about what role Ca^{+2} ions have in generating the intracellular messenger; i.e. how the effector functions. Initial effort might be best directed at discerning if the PI cycle and arachidonic acid metabolism are involved. It should be kept in mind that the PI response to the muscarinic receptor of N1E-115 cells also displays short-term desensitization (28).

Resensitization is a slower process and is not dependent on the agonist concentration used to desensitize (87, 127). The dose-response curves for resensitized cells shift inversely to the direction of shift with desensitization, suggesting that the process is a simple reversal. Its slowness suggests continuous enzymatic action; a conformational change might be expected to occur more quickly. Though one may suspect changes in covalent bonds, such as disulfide bond formation, there is no direct evidence as yet of this phenomenon. Sulfhydryl agents do affect muscarinic receptor binding in brain homogenates; some have suggested that the muscarinic receptor shifts between agonist states with N-ethylmaleimide treatment or with the transitional metals.

The muscarinic receptors of NG108–15 neuroblastoma-glioma cells also desensitize; they become less able to inhibit the prostaglandin E_1-mediated cAMP response (29). This desensitization is specific to the muscarinic receptor, since α-adrenergic receptors or opiate receptors can still inhibit prostaglandin E_1-mediated cAMP formation. The GTP coupling proteins, extracted from desensitized NG108-15, were still able to stimulate cAMP in another, coupling-protein-deficient cell, so it is likely that it is the receptor or its ability to act on the GTP protein that has been affected by desensitization. Somehow desensitization has caused the receptor to lose its effect on the GTPase. It is not yet known whether desensitization occurs with the N1E-115 muscarinic receptor-mediated inhibition of prostaglandin E_1-stimulated cAMP formation.

ACKNOWLEDGMENTS

R. M. Snider and C. Forray are thanked for stimulating discussion and the use of unpublished results. Support has been from the Mayo Foundation and U.S.P.H.S. grants MH27692 and AM07147-E.

Literature Cited

1. Birdsall, N. J. M., Hulme, E. C. 1976. Biochemical studies on muscarinic acetylcholine receptors. *J. Neurochem.* 27:7–16
2. Krnjevic, K. 1974. Chemical nature of synaptic transmission in vertebrates. *Physiol. Rev.* 54:418–540
3. Krnjevic, K., Pumain, R., Renaud, L. 1971. The mechanism of excitation by acetylcholine in the cerebral cortex. *J. Physiol.* 215:247–68
4. Ben-Ari, Y., Dingledine, R., Kanazawa, I., Kelly, J. S. 1976. Inhibitory effects of acetylcholine on neurones in the feline nucelus reticularis thalami. *J. Physiol.* 261:647–61
5. Putney, J. W. 1977. Muscarinic, alpha-adrenergic and peptide receptors regulate the same calcium influx sites in the parotid gland. *J. Physiol.* 268:139–49
6. Putney, J. W. 1978. Role of calcium in the fade of the potassium release response in the rat parotid gland. *J. Physiol.* 281:383–94
7. Bolton, T. B. 1979. Cholinergic mechanisms in smooth muscle. *Br. Med. Bull.* 35:275–83
8. Kebabian, J. W., Steiner, A. L., Green-

gard, P. 1975. Muscarinic cholinergic regulation of cyclic guanosine 3', 5'-monophosphate in autonomic ganglia: Possible role in synaptic transmission. *J. Pharmacol. Exp. Ther.* 193:474–88

9. Hanley, M. R., Iversen, L. L. 1978. Muscarinic cholinergic receptors in rat corpus striatum and regulation of guanosine cyclic 3', 5'-monophosphate. *Mol. Pharmacol.* 14:246–55

10. Ferrendelli, J. A., Steiner, A. L., McDougal, J. R., Kipnis, D. M. 1970. The effect of oxotremorine and atropine on cGMP and cAMP levels in mouse cerebral cortex and cerebellum. *Biochem. Biophys. Res. Commun.* 41:1061–67

11. George, W. J., Polson, J. B., O'Toole, A. B., Goldberg, N. D. 1970. Elevation of guanosine 3', 5'-cyclic phosphate in rat heart after perfusion with acetylcholine. *Proc. Natl. Acad. Sci. USA* 66:398–403

12. Lenox, R. J., Kant, G. J., Meyerhoff, J. L. 1980. Regional sensitivity of cyclic AMP and cyclic GMP in rat brain to central cholinergic stimulation. *Life Sci.* 26:2201–9

13. Matsuzawa, H., Nirenberg, M. 1975. Receptor-mediated shifts in cGMP and cAMP levels in neuroblastoma cells. *Proc. Natl. Acad. Sci. USA* 72:3472–76

14. Lee, T.-P., Kuo, J. F., Greengard, P. 1972. Role of muscarinic cholinergic receptors in regulation of guanosine 3':5'-cyclic monophosphate content in mammalian brain, heart muscle, and intestinal smooth muscle. *Proc. Natl. Acad. Sci. USA* 69:3287–91

15. Nathanson, N. M., Klein, W. L., Nirenberg, M. 1978. Regulation of adenylate cyclase activity mediated by muscarinic acetylcholine receptors. *Proc. Natl. Acad. Sci. USA* 75:1788–95

16. Palmer, G. C., Chronister, R. B., Palmer, S. J. 1980. Cholinergic agonists and dibutyryl cyclic guanosine monophosphate inhibit the norepinephrine-induced accumulation of cyclic adenosine monophosphate in the rat cerebral cortex. *Neurosci.* 5:319–22

17. Walker, J. B., Walker, J. P. 1973. Neurohormonal regulation of adenylate cyclase activity in rat striatum. *Brain Res.* 54:386–90

18. Lichtshtein, D., Boone, G., Blume, A. 1979. Muscarinic receptor regulation of NG108–15 adenylate cyclase: Requirement for Na$^+$ and GTP. *J. Cyclic Nucleotide Res.* 5:367–75

19. Gross, R. A., Clark, R. B. 1977. Regulation of adenosine 3'5'-monophosphate

content in human astrocytoma cells by isproterenol and carbachol. *Mol. Pharmacol.* 13:242–50

20. Traber, J., Fischer, K., Buchen, C., Hamprecht, B. 1975. Muscarinic response to acetylcholine in neuroblastoma X glioma hybrid cells. *Nature* 255:558–60

21. Olianas, M. C., Onali, P., Neff, N. H., Costa, E. 1982. Adenylate cyclase activity of synaptic membranes from rat striatum. *Mol. Pharmacol.* 23:393–98

22. Mitchell, R. H., Kirk, C. J., Jones, L. M., Downes, C. P., Creba, J. A. 1981. The stimulation of inositol lipid metabolism that accompanies calcium mobilization in stimulated cells: Defined characteristics and unanswered questions. *Phil. Trans. R. Soc. London Ser. B* 296:123–37

23. Hawthorne, J. N., Pickard, M. R. 1979. Phospholipids in synaptic function. *J. Neurochem.* 32:5–14

24. Downes, C. P. 1982. Receptor-stimulated inositol phospholipid metabolism in the central nervous system. *Cell Calcium* 3:413–28

25. Leiber, D., Harbon, S. 1982. The relationship between the carbachol stimulatory effect on cyclic GMP content and activation by fatty acid hydroperoxides of a soluble guanylate cyclase in the guinea pig myometrium. *Mol. Pharmacol.* 21:654–63

26. Spies, C., Schultz, K. D., Schultz, G. 1980. Inhibitory effects of mepacrine and eicosatetraynoic acid on cyclic GMP elevations caused by calcium and hormonal factors in rat ductus deferens. *Naunyn-Schmiedeberg's Arch. Pharmacol.* 311:71–77

27. Richelson, E. 1978. Densensitization of muscarinic receptor-mediated cyclic GMP formation by cultured nerve cells. *Nature* 272:366–68

28. Cohen, N. M., Schmidt, D. M., McGlennen, R. C., Klein, W. L. 1983. Receptor-mediated increases in phosphatidylinositol turnover in neuron-like cell lines. *J. Neurochem.* 40:547–54

29. Green, D. A., Clark, R. B. 1982. Specific muscarinic-cholinergic desensitization in the neuroblastoma-glioma hybrid NG108–15. *J. Neurochem.* 39:1125–31

30. Drachman, D. A. 1977. Memory and cognitive function in man: Does the cholinergic system have a specific role? *Neurol.* 27:783–90

31. Drachman, D. A., Leavitt, J. 1974. Human memory and the cholinergic system. *Arch. Neurol.* 30:113–21

32. Coyle, J. T., Price, D. L., DeLong, M.

R. 1983. Alzheimer's disease: A disorder of cortical cholinergic innervation. *Science* 219:1184–90

33. Nordberg, A., Larsson, C., Adolfsson, R., Alatuzoff, I., Winblad, B. 1983. Muscarinic receptor compensation in hippocampus of Alzheimer patients. *J. Neural Transm.* 56:13–19

34. Richelson, E., Divinetz-Romero, S. 1977. Blockade by psychotropic drugs of the muscarinic acetylcholine receptor in cultured nerve cells. *Biol. Psychiatry* 12:771–85

35. Richelson, E., Prendergast, F. G., Divinetz-Romero, S. 1978. Muscarinic receptor-mediated cyclic GMP formation by cultured nerve cells—Ionic dependence and effects of local anesthetics. *Biochem. Pharmacol.* 27:2039–48

36. Richelson, E., El-Fakahany, E. 1981. The molecular basis of neurotransmission at the muscarinic receptor. *Biochem. Pharmacol.* 30:2887–91

37. Alberts, P., Bartfai, T. 1976. Muscarinic acetylcholine receptor from rat brain. *J. Biol. Chem.* 251:1543–47

38. Birdsall, N. J. M., Burgen, A. S. V., Hulme, E. C. 1979. A study of the muscarinic receptor by gel electrophoresis. *Br. J. Pharmacol.* 66:337–42

39. Avissar, S., Amitai, G., Sokolovsky, M. 1983. Oligomeric structure of muscarinic receptors is shown by photoaffinity labeling: Subunit assembly may explain high- and low-affinity agonist states. *Proc. Natl. Acad. Sci. USA* 80:156–59

40. Sokolovsky, M., Gurwitz, D., Galron, R. 1980. Muscarinic receptor binding in mouse brain: Regulation by guanine nucleotides. *Biochem. Biophys. Res. Commun.* 94:487–92

41. Gurwitz, D., Sokolovsky, M. 1980. Agonist-specific reverse regulation of muscarinic receptors by transition metal ions and guanine nucleotides. *Biochem. Biophys. Res. Commun.* 96:1296–304

42. McKinney, M., Coyle, J. T. 1982. Regulation of neocortical muscarinic receptors: Effects of drug treatment and lesions. *J. Neurosci.* 2:97–106

43. Aguilar, J. S., Jerusalinsky, D., Stockert, M., Medina, J. H., DeRobertis, E. 1982. Localization of hippocampal muscarinic receptors after kainic acid lesion of CA3 and fimbria-formix transection. *Brain Res.* 247:335–40

44. Szerb, J. C. 1978. Characterization of presynaptic muscarinic receptors in central cholinergic neurons. In *Symposium on Cholinergic Mechanisms and Psychopharmacology,* ed. D. Jenden, pp. 49–60. New York: Plenum. 885 pp.

45. Yamamura, H. I., Snyder, S. H. 1974. Muscarinic cholinergic binding in rat brain. *Proc. Natl. Acad. Sci. USA* 71:1725–29

46. Kuhar, M. J., Yamamura, H. I. 1976. Localization of cholinergic muscarinic receptors in rat brain by light microscopic radioautography. *Brain Res.* 110:229–43

47. Hulme, E. C., Birdsall, N. J. M., Burgen, A. S. V., Mehta, P. 1978. The binding of antagonists to brain muscarinic receptors. *Mol. Pharmacol.* 14:737–50

48. Birdsall, N. J. M., Burgen, A. S. V., Hulme, E. C. 1978. The binding of agonists to brain muscarinic receptors. *Mol. Pharmacol.* 14:723–36

49. Kloog, Y., Egozi, Y., Sokolovsky, M. 1979. Characterization of muscarinic acetylcholine receptors from mouse brain: Evidence for regional heterogeneity and isomerization. *Mol. Pharmacol.* 15:545–58

50. Ellis, J., Hoss, W. 1980. Analysis of regional variations in the affinities of muscarinic agonists in the rat brain. *Brain Res.* 193:189–98

51. Henis, Y. I., Galron, R., Avissar, S., Sokolovsky, M. 1982. Interactions between antagonist-occupied muscarinic binding sites in rat adenohypophysis. *FEBS Lett.* 140:173–76

52. Birdsall, N. J. M., Hulme, E. C., Burgen, A. 1980. The character of the muscarinic receptors in different regions of the rat brain. *Proc. R. Soc. London Ser. B* 207:1–12

53. Strange, P. G., Birdsall, N. J. M., Burgen, A. S. V. 1978. Ligand-binding properties of the muscarinic acetylcholine receptor in mouse neuroblastoma cells. *Biochem. J.* 172:495–501

54. Birdsall, N. J. M., Berrie, C. P., Burgen, A. S. V., Hulme, E. C. 1980. Modulation of the binding properties of muscarinic receptors: Evidence for receptor-effector coupling. In *Receptors for Neurotransmitters and Peptide Hormones,* ed. G. Pepeu, M. J. Kuhar, S. J. Enna, pp. 107–16. New York: Raven

55. Berrie, C. P., Birdsall, N. J. M., Burgen, A. S. V., Hulme, E. C. 1979. Guanine nucleotides modulate muscarinic receptor binding in the heart. *Biochem. Biophys. Res. Commun.* 87:1000–5

56. Ehlert, F. J., Roeske, W. R., Rosenberger, L. B., Yamamura, H. I. 1980. The influence of guanyl-5'-yl imidodiphosphate and sodium on muscarinic receptor binding in the rat brain and longitudinal muscle of the rat ileum. *Life Sci.* 26:245–52

57. Burgoyne, R. D. 1983. Regulation of the muscarinic acetylcholine receptor: Effects of phosphorylating conditions on agonist and antagonist binding. *J. Neurochem.* 40:324–31

58. Hurko, O. 1978. Specific [^{3}H]quinuclidinyl benzilate binding activity in digitonin-solubilized preparations from bovine brain. *Arch. Biochem. Biophys.* 190:434–45

59. Halvorsen, S. W., Nathanson, N. M. 1981. *In vivo* regulation of muscarinic acetylcholine receptor number and function in embryonic chick heart. *J. Biol. Chem.* 256:7941–48

60. Galper, J. B., Dziekan, L. C., Miura, D. S., Smith, T. W. 1982. Agonist-induced changes in the modulation of K$^+$ permeability and beating rate by muscarinic agonists in cultured heart cells. *J. Gen. Physiol.* 80:231–56

61. Strange, P. G., Birdsall, N. J. M., Burgen, A. S. V. 1977. Occupancy of muscarinic acetylcholine receptors stimulates a guanylate cyclase in neuroblastoma cells. *Biochem. Soc. Trans.* 5:189–91

62. McKinney, M., Stenstrom, S., Richelson, E. 1983. Effect of short-term desensitization on muscarinic receptor binding in intact murine neuroblastoma cells (clone N1E-115). *Abstr. Soc. Neurosci.* 9:581

63. Fisher, S. K., Klinger, P. D., Agranoff, B. W. 1982. Muscarinic agonist binding and phospholipid turnover in brain. *J. Biol. Chem.* 258:7358–63

64. Larose, L., Dumont, Y., Asselin, J., Morisset, J., Poirier, G. G. 1981. Muscarinic receptor of rat pancreatic acini: [^{3}H]QNB binding and amylase secretion. *Eur. J. Pharmacol.* 76:247–54

65. Wamsley, J. K., Zarbin, M. A., Birdsall, N. J. M., Kuhar, M. J. 1980. Muscarinic cholinergic receptors: Autoradiographic localization of high and low affinity agonist binding sites. *Brain Res.* 200:1–12

66. Hammer, R., Berrie, C. P., Birdsall, N. J. M., Burgen, A. S. V., Hulme, E. C. 1980. Pirenzepine distinguishes between different subclasses of muscarinic receptors. *Nature* 283:90–92

67. Caulfield, M. P., Straughan, D. W., Cross, A. J., Crow, T., Birdsall, N. J. M. 1982. Cortical muscarinic receptor subtypes and Alzheimer's disease. *Lancet* 2:1277

68. Aguilar, J. S., Salas, P. J. I., DeRobertis, E. 1982. Cholinergic muscarinic receptor in synaptosomal membranes: Heterogeneity of binding sites for L-[^{3}H]quinuclidinyl benzilate. *Mol. Pharmacol.* 22:304–9

69. Avissor, S., Egozi, Y., Sokolovsky, M. 1981. Biochemical characterization and sex dimorphism of muscarinic receptors in rat adenohypophysis. *Neuroendocrinology* 32:303–9

70. Burgisser, E., Delean, A., Lefkowitz, R. J. 1982. Reciprocal modulation of agonist and antagonist binding to muscarinic cholinergic receptor by guanine nucleotide. *Proc. Natl. Acad. Sci. USA* 79:1732–36

71. Burgermeister, W., Klein, W. L., Nirenberg, M., Witkop, B. 1978. Comparative binding studies with cholinergic ligands and histrionicotoxin at muscarinic receptors of neural cell lines. *Mol. Pharmacol.* 14:751–67

72. Hedlund, B., Bartfai, T. 1979. The importance of thiol- and disulfide groups in agonist and antagonist binding to the muscarinic receptor. *Mol. Pharmacol.* 15:531–44

73. Aronstam, R. S., Abood, L. G., Hoss, W. 1978. Influence of sulfhydryl reagents and heavy metals on the functional state of muscarinic acetylcholine receptor in rat brain. *Mol. Pharmacol.* 14:575–86

74. Ikeda, S. R., Aronstam, R. S., Eldefrawi, M. E. 1980. Nature of regional and chemically-induced differences in the binding properties of muscarinic acetylcholine receptors from rat brain. *Neuropharmacology* 19:575–85

75. Aronstam, R. S., Eldefrawi, M. E. 1979. Reversible conversion between affinity states for agonists of the muscarinic acetylcholine receptor from rat brain. *Biochem. Pharmacol.* 28:701–3

76. Korn, S. J., Martin, M. W., Harden, T. K. 1983. N-ethylmaleimide-induced alteration in the interaction of agonists with muscarinic cholinergic receptors of rat brain. *J. Pharmacol. Exp. Ther.* 224:118–26

77. Vauguelin, G., Andre, C., Debacker, J.-P., Laduron, P., Strosberg, A. D. 1982. Agonist-mediated conformational changes of muscarinic receptors in rat brain. *Eur. J. Biochem.* 125:117–24

78. Birdsall, N. J. M., Burgen, A. S. V., Hulme, E. C., Wells, J. W. 1979. The effects of ions on the binding of agonists and antagonists to muscarinic receptors. *Br. J. Pharmacol.* 67:371–77

79. El-Fakahany, E., Richelson, E. 1980. Effects of lanthanides on muscarinic acetylcholine receptor function. *Mol. Pharmacol.* 19:282–90

80. El-Fakahany, E., Richelson, E. 1980. Involvement of calcium channels in short-

term desensitization of muscarinic receptor-mediated cyclic GMP formation in mouse neuroblastoma cells. *Proc. Natl. Acad. Sci. USA* 77:6897–6901

81. El-Fakahany, E., Richelson, E. 1983. Effect of some calcium antagonists on muscarinic receptor-mediated cyclic GMP formation. *J. Neurochem.* 40:705–10

82. Chweh, A. Y., Leslie, S. W. 1981. Enhancement of $^{45}Ca^{2+}$ binding to acidic lipids by barbiturates, diphenylhydantoin, and ethanol. *J. Neurochem.* 36:1865–67

83. Study, R. E. 1980. Phenytoin inhibition of cyclic guanosine 3':5'-monophosphate (cGMP) accumulation in neuroblastoma cells by calcium channel blockade. *J. Pharmacol. Exp. Ther.* 215:575–81

84. Aronstam, R. S., Abood, L. G., Baumgold, J. 1977. Role of phospholipids in muscarinic binding by neural membranes. *Biochem. Pharmacol.* 26:1689–95

85. McGee, R., Kenimer, J. G. 1982. The effects of exposure to unsaturated fatty acids on opiate receptors, prostaglandin E_1 receptors and adenylate cyclase activity of neuroblastoma X glioma hybrid cells. *Mol. Pharmacol.* 22:360–68

86. Chan, P. H., Kerlan, R., Fishman, R. A. 1983. Reductions of gamma-aminobutyric acid and glutamate uptake and $(Na^+ + K^+)$-ATPase activity in brain slices and synaptosomes by arachidonic acid. *J. Neurochem.* 40:309–16

87. El-Fakahany, E., Richelson, E. 1980. Temperature dependence of muscarinic acetylcholine receptor activation, desensitization and resensitization. *J. Neurochem.* 34:1288–95

88. Godfraind, J. M., Kawamura, H., Krnjevic, K., Pumain, R. 1971. Actions of dinitrophenol and some other metabolic inhibitors on cortical neurons. *J. Physiol.* 215:199–222

89. Krnjevic, K., Pumain, R., Renaud, L. 1971. Effects of Ba^{2+} and tetraethylammonium on cortical neurons. *J. Physiol.* 215:223–45

90. Schultz, G., Hardman, J. G., Schultz, K., Baird, C. E., Sutherland, E. W. 1973. The importance of calcium ions for the regulation of guanosine 3':5'-cyclic monophosphate levels. *Proc. Natl. Acad. Sci. USA* 70:3889–93

91. Kostyuk, P. G. 1980. Calcium ionic channels in electrically excitable membrane. *Neurosci.* 5:945–59

92. Krnjevic, K., Lisiewicz, A. 1972. Injections of calcium ions into spinal motoneurones. *J. Physiol.* 225:363–90

93. Krnjevic, K., Puil, E., Werman, R. 1978. EGTA and motoneuronal after-potentials. *J. Physiol.* 275:199–223

94. Moolenaar, W. H., Spector, I. 1977. Ionic currents in cultured mouse neuroblastoma cells under voltage-clamp conditions. *J. Physiol.* 278:265–86

95. Moolenaar, W. H., Spector, I. 1979. The calcium action potential and a prolonged calcium dependent after-hyperpolarization in mouse neuroblastoma cells. *J. Physiol.* 292:297–306

96. Study, R. E., Breakfield, X. O., Bartfai, T., Greengard, P. 1978. Voltage-sensitive calcium channels regulate guanosine 3'5'-cyclic monophosphate levels in neuroblastoma cells. *Proc. Natl. Acad. Sci. USA* 75:6295–99

97. Moolenaar, W. H., Spector, I. 1979. The calcium current and the activation of a slow potassium conductance in voltage-clamped mouse neuroblastoma cells. *J. Physiol.* 292:307–23

98. Wastek, G. J., Lopez, J. R., Richelson, E. 1980. Demonstration of a muscarinic receptor-mediated cyclic GMP-dependent hyperpolarization of the membrane potential of mouse neuroblastoma cells using [^{3}H]tetraphenylphosphonium. *Mol. Pharmacol.* 19:15–20

99. Stone, T. W., Taylor, D. A., Bloom, F. E. 1975. Cyclic AMP and cyclic GMP may mediate opposite neuronal responses in rat cerebral cortex. *Science* 187:845–46

100. Swartz, B. E., Woody, C. D. 1979. Correlated effects of acetylcholine and cyclic guanosine monophosphate on membrane properties of mammalian neocortical neurons. *J. Neurol.* 10:465–88

101. Snider, R. M., Richelson, E., Blinks, J. R. 1981. *Abstr. Soc. Neurosci.* 8:124

102. Richelson, E., Snider, R. M., McKinney, M., Forray, C. 1983. Neurotransmitter receptor-mediated cyclic GMP formation: A new hypothesis implicating the involvement of phospholipase A_2 and arachidonic acid metabolites. *Abstr. Soc. Neurosci.* 9:458

103. Libet, B., Kobayashi, H., Tanaka, T. 1975. Synaptic coupling into the production and storage of a neuronal memory trace. *Nature* 258:155–57

104. Frey, E. A., McIsaac, R. J. 1981. A comparison of cyclic guanosine 3':5'-monophosphate and muscarinic excitatory responses in the superior cervical ganglion of the rat. *J. Pharmacol. Exp. Ther.* 218:115–21

105. Fisher, S. K., Boast, C. A., Agranoff, B. W. 1980. The muscarinic stimulation of phospholipid labeling in the hippocampus is independent of its cholinergic input. *Brain Res.* 189:284–88

106. Fisher, S. K., Frey, K. A., Agranoff, B. W. 1981. Loss of muscarinic receptors and of stimulated phospholipid labeling in ibotenate treated hippocampus. *J. Neurosci.* 1:407–13

107. Fisher, S. K., Agranoff, B. W. 1980. Calcium and the muscarinic synaptosomal phospholipid labeling effect. *J. Neurochem.* 34:1231–40

108. Fisher, S. K., Agranoff, B. W. 1981. Enhancement of the muscarinic stimulation of phospholipid labeling effect by the ionophore A23187. *J. Neurochem.* 37: 968–77

109. Yandrasitz, J. R., Segal, S. 1979. The effect of $MnCl_2$ on the basal and acetylcholine-stimulated turnover of phosphatidylinositol in synaptosomes. *FEBS Lett.* 108:279–82

110. Ohsako, S., Deguichi, T. 1981. Stimulation by phosphatidic acid of calcium influx and cyclic GMP synthesis in neuroblastoma cells. *J. Biol. Chem.* 256: 10945–48

111. Salmon, D. M., Honeyman, T. W. 1980. Proposed mechanism of cholinergic action in smooth muscle. *Nature* 284:344–47

112. Harris, R. A., Schmidt, J., Hitzemann, B. A., Hitzemann, R. J. 1981. Phosphatidate as a molecular link between depolarization and neurotransmitter release in the brain. *Science* 212:1290–91

113. Amano, E., Nakane, M., Deguchi, T. 1979. Guanylate cyclase in neuroblastoma N1E-115 cells: Presence of endogenous activator. *J. Cyclic Nucleotide Res.* 5:135–44

114. Lapetina, E. G., Billah, M. M., Cuatrecasas, P. 1981. The phosphatidylinositol cycle and the regulation of arachidonic acid production. *Nature* 292:367–69

115. Walenga, R., Vanderhoek, J. Y., Feinstein, M. B. 1980. Serine esterase inhibitors block stimulus-induced mobilization of arachidonic acid and phosphatidylinositide-specific phospholipase C activity in platelets. *J. Biol. Chem.* 255:6024–27

116. Tyson, C. A., Zande, H. V., Green, D. E. 1976. Phospholipids as inophores. *J. Biol. Chem.* 251:1326–32

117. Snider, R. M., Richelson, E. 1983. Thrombin stimulates cyclic GMP formation in murine neuroblastoma cells (clone N1E-115). *Science* 217:566–67

118. Beam, K., Greengard, P. 1976. Cyclic nucleotides, protein phosphorylation and synaptic function. *Cold Spring Harbor Symp. Quant. Biol.* 30:157–68

119. Casnellie, J. E., Greengard, P. 1974. Guanosine 3':5'-cyclic monophosphate-dependent phosphorylation of endogenous substrate proteins in membranes of mammalian smooth muscle. *Proc. Natl. Acad. Sci. USA* 71:1891–95

120. Schlichter, D. J., Casnellie, J. E., Greengard, P. 1978. An endogenous substrate for cGMP-dependent protein kinase in mammalian cerebellum. *Nature* 223:61–62

121. Burgoyne, R. D., Pearce, B. 1981. Muscarinic acetylcholine receptor regulation and protein phosphorylation in primary cultures of rat cerebellum. *Dev. Brain Res.* 2:55–63

122. Ariano, M. A., Martus, A. I. 1981. Ultrastructural localization of cyclic GMP and cyclic AMP in rat striatum. *J. Cell. Biol.* 91:287–92

123. Chan-Palay, V., Palay, S. L. 1979. Immunocytochemical localization of cyclic GMP: Light and electron microscope evidence for involvement of neuroglia. *Proc. Natl. Acad. Sci. USA* 76:1485–88

124. Segal, M., Guidotti, A. 1981. Cyclic GMP in rat hippocampus: Regulation by the septo-hippocampal pathway. *Neuropharmacology* 20:1129–33

125. Richelson, E. 1976. Use of tissue culture to study cholinergic function. In *Biology of Cholinergic Function*, ed. A. M. Goldberg, I. Hanin, pp. 451–84. New York: Raven. 716 pp.

126. Liu-Chen, L.-Y., Richelson, E. 1983. Evidence for a cyclic model for the short-term desensitization of muscarinic receptor-mediated cyclic GMP formation by murine neuroblastoma cells. *J. Neurochem.* Submitted for publication

127. Cuatrecasas, P. 1974. Membrane receptors. *Ann Rev. Biochem.* 43:169–214

128. Poggioli, J., Putney, J. W. 1982. Net calcium fluxes in rat parotid acinar cells. *Pfluegers Arch.* 392:239–43

129. Glass, D. B., Frey, W. II, Carr, D. W., Goldberg, N. D. 1977. Stimulation of human platelet guanylate cyclase by fatty acids. *J. Biol. Chem.* 252:1279–85

130. Goldberg, N. D., Graff, G., Haddox, M. K., Stephenson, J. H., Glass, D. B., Moser, M. E. 1978. Redox modulation of splenic cell soluble guanylate cyclase activity: Activation by hydrophilic and hydrophobic oxidants represented by ascorbic and dehydroascorbic acids, fatty acid hydroperoxides, and prostaglandin endoperoxides. In *Advances in Cyclic Nucleotide Research*, ed. W. J. George,

L. J. Ignamo, pp. 101–30. New York: Raven

130a. Genzer, R., Hamet, P., Ross, A. H., Lawson, J. A., Hardman, J. G. 1983. Calcium-induced release from platelet membranes of fatty acids that modulate soluble guanylate cyclase. *J. Pharmacol. Exp. Ther.* 226:180–86

131. Billah, M. M., Lapetina, E. G., Cuatrecasas, P. 1980. Phospholipase A_2 and phospholipase C activities of platelets. *J. Biol. Chem.* 255:10227–31

132. Jakschik, B. A., Sun, F. F., Lee, L.-H., Steinhoff, M. M. 1980. Calcium stimulation of a novel lipoxygenase. *Biochem. Biophys. Res. Commun.* 95:103–10

133. Koski, G., Klee, W. A. 1981. Opiates inhibit adenylate cyclase by stimulating GTP hydrolysis. *Proc. Natl. Acad. Sci. USA* 78:4185–89

134. Watanabe, A. M., McConnaughey, M. M., Strawbridge, R. A., Fleming, J. W., Jones, L. R., Besch, H. R. 1978. Muscarinic cholinergic receptor modulation of β-adrenergic receptor affinity for catecholamines. *J. Biol. Chem.* 253:4833–36

Ann. Rev. Pharmacol. Toxicol. 1984. 24:147–74

IMMUNOSTIMULATION: SYNTHETIC AND BIOLOGICAL MODULATORS OF IMMUNITY

H. Hugh Fudenberg and H. D. Whitten

Department of Basic and Clinical Immunology and Microbiology, Medical University of South Carolina, Charleston, South Carolina 29425

INTRODUCTION

In 1960 the immune system was an enigma to scientists, and treatments for immunological abnormalities sometimes reflected this lack of knowledge. Infants born with enlarged thymuses were often treated with thymic irradiation, for example. In 1961 and 1962, however, it was demonstrated (1–3), first in the chicken, that the immune system consists of two limbs, one comprised of thymus-derived lymphocytes (T cells), the other of cells that in birds derive from the bursa of Fabricius and in mammals that originate in the fetal liver and migrate to the bone marrow during early intrauterine life (B cells). By 1968, this had been documented in man; however, methods of identifying B and T cell subpopulations and enumerating them in human peripheral blood and tissues have been developed only in the last 10 years.

During the past decade it has become evident that circulating immunologically virgin B cells develop an antigen-specific antibody (membrane receptor) upon exposure to a given antigen. This stimulated B cell gradually differentiates and then produces large amounts of specific antibody molecules to the given antigen; these antibodies are secreted from the cell and exported into the serum, where quite specifically they bind the antigen, activate the complement system, and kill the "foreign" cell. Since these molecules are transported via the circulation, this limb of the immune system is termed *humoral* immunity. The humoral immune system is responsible for protection against the classic microorganisms—meningococcus, streptococcus, pneumococcus, etc. Prophylaxis is attained by vaccination with the appropriate antigen at subinfect-

147

ing doses to stimulate the development of memory cells able to produce rapidly large amounts of specific antibody when the organism is reencountered later in the environment.

Upon antigen exposure, the T cell also acquires surface membrane-specific receptors. The exact nature of these receptors is still controversial; however, they appear to be unrelated in structure to any antibody molecule (4). Furthermore, T cells do not secrete classical antibody. Instead, the cells become activated and are morphologically transformed into entities with the appearance of leukemic lymphoblasts; during and after this blast transformation they appear to participate directly in a variety of protective pathways, collectively termed *cell-mediated immunity*. T cells can be identified by their ability to form rosettes with sheep erythrocytes. This arm of the immune system is responsible for resistance to protozoal, parasitic, fungal, and most viral infections. Delayed cutaneous hypersensitivity (skin test) reactions are mediated by T cells, as are reactions to genetically foreign tissues such as skin and kidney grafts. Some T cells when activated can kill foreign cells with which they come into contact by a process termed *cellular cytotoxicity;* this is an important mechanism for destroying malignant cells. Although T cells do not secrete antibody, they do make a wide variety of small information-carrying molecules with either antigen-specific or nonspecific effects on foreign cells and, interestingly, on other cells of the immune system. These informational molecules are collectively termed *mediators of cellular immunity* (MCI) or *lymphokines* (Table 1).

In the past decade our knowledge of the immune system has expanded enormously. The above classification is much more complicated than originally supposed, especially with regard to the cell-mediated immune system. We know now that T cells account for at least 80% of the lymphocytes present in normal human peripheral blood, and several functional classes and subclasses of T cells have been identified. These include, in addition to the cytotoxic T cells described above, regulatory T cells that regulate the functions of both B cells and other T cells. Helper T cells can increase antibody production by B cells, and different types of suppressor T cells exist that are collectively capable of an impressive variety of regulatory functions, including generalized suppression of immunoglobulin synthesis (5), suppression of the synthesis of a single class of immunoglobulin (e.g. only IgA), suppression of the synthesis of a single-antibody specificity (e.g. antibody against Epstein-Barr virus) (6), suppression of cell-mediated immune functions (e.g. mixed leukocyte reactivity of T cells) (7), suppression of B and helper T cell division, and others. It is increasingly apparent that each of these regulatory functions is mediated by a distinct subpopulation of T lymphocytes.

Additionally, at least two other cell types present in the peripheral circulation have a crucial impact on immune function. Some mononuclear cells lack the typical surface markers of either T or B cells and are termed *null* cells. These

Table 1 Mediators of cellular immunity elaborated by sensitized lymphocytes after addition of antigen[a]

Factor	Heuristic explanation of roles of some factors
Skin permeability factor	Dilutes capillaries in the skin, making it easier for cells involved in the immune response to reach foreign substances (antigens) that have entered the body tissue
Chemotactic factors for macrophages	Attract macrophages (which engulf and destroy foreign cells or parasites, or break them into pieces small enough for the immune system to handle)
Macrophage migration inhibitory factor (MIF)	Prevents macrophages from migrating away from the foreign cells while they are being engulfed
Macrophage activating factor (same as MIF?)	Prevents macrophages from migrating away from the foreign cells while they are being engulfed
Chemotactic factors for other leukocytes (neutrophils, eosinophils, basophils, lymphocytes)	Attract other blood cells which break down and release enzymes that attack viruses, protein, etc
Granulocytic migration inhibitory factor (LIF)	Prevents those cells from moving away
Growth inhibitory factors (clonal inhibitory factor, proliferation inhibitory factor)	Prevent "transformed" (cancer) cells or foreign organisms from dividing and thus increasing in mass
Lymphocytotoxin (toxic for all cells other than lymphocytes)	Kills transformed cells and foreign organisms
Osteoclast activating factor	Activates bone-destroying cells
Collagen synthesizing factor	Stimulates synthesis of collagen
Interferon	Inhibits, at least in animals, the growth of viruses, both those that cause cancer and those that do not
Mitogenic factor(s) for lymphocytes	Causes lymphocytes to divide and thus start the process over again—i.e. this is an amplication mechanism
Interleukin 2 (TCGF)	T-cell growth factor that allows T cells to be grown in continuous tissue culture and causes proliferation of T cells
Dialyzable leukocyte extract (transfer factor)	DLE-transfer factor; transfers delayed hypersensitivity (see text)

[a]Nearly 100 different mediators have been tentatively identified in studies of lymphocytes in cell culture (11). It appears that many of these substances might be isolated and perhaps used for the therapy of a number of different diseases. However, further basic research is required.

cells (or a subpopulation of cells) are the effectors of a cytotoxic mechanism termed *antibody-dependent cell-mediated cytotoxicity* (ADCC) that appears to be an important defense against the growth of malignant cells (8). Another null subset, the so-called natural killer (NK) cell, seems even more important in protecting against malignancies. These NK cells, unlike ADCC cells, do not need antibody to kill target tumor cells (82). A fourth, the monocyte-macrophage series, is regarded by many as one of the most important components of the immune system and has many functions. For example, macrophages and monocytes (MΦ) engulf and "process" an organism with many antigens (epitopes) into smaller bits, and present antigens on their surfaces to T and B cells; like T cells, they secrete a variety of soluble mediators involved in immunoregulation, including both helpers (9) and suppressors (10) of immune functions. Interestingly, monocytes have functional subsets (e.g. suppressor monocytes); even neutrophils and eosinophils have been shown to be capable of ADCC and NK activity in vitro. Our understanding of their in vivo role in the immunoregulatory panorama is still in its infancy.

The above summary, although necessarily incomplete due to space limitations, provides an indication of the complexity of the human immune system. Each of the two arms, humoral and cellular, is now known to have many hands and each hand many fingers. Further, the two arms are not viewed as distinct entities, since they interact extensively within a complex regulatory network. For instance, the list of soluble mediators (MCI) produced by immunocytes (Table 1) has grown to over 100 named factors (11), including antigen-specific and nonspecific activities, helper and suppressor factors, factors restricted and nonrestricted for histocompatibility antigens, and factors acting on B cells, T cells, macrophages, neutrophils, tumor cells, virus-infected cells, basophils, eosinophils, osteoclasts, and even vascular epithelium.

Clearly, further investigation is required before a clear picture of this complex system emerges. Nevertheless, within the scope of the limited knowledge available, applications to clinical situations have been possible. In particular, experimental approaches to immunotherapy have developed recently along several important lines. Many biological and synthetic immunostimulants, adjuvants, and drugs with specific or nonspecific effects on immunocytes are now being investigated, and new immunomodulators are being developed in many countries. Although most are still restricted to a few research centers, others are used widely in the therapy of a variety of disorders. Recent findings of immune defects in cancer have stimulated widespread interest in the development of immunomodulators that will be effective as adjuncts in the treatment of malignancies, and some promising results have been reported (12).

The various immunomodulators now in use undoubtedly act at different points in the immune spectrum, but the exact target cell has been identified in only a very few instances (Table 2). Obviously, a need exists for development of agents that can selectively inhibit or enhance one specific class or subclass of immunocytes: e.g. increase suppressor T cells in systemic lupus erythematosus (13), decrease antigen-specific suppressor T cells in various malignancies (14), or increase natural cell activity in leukemia (15). At present, we can classify immunotherapeutic approaches generally as (a) nonspecific systemic immunostimulation, (b) adjuvant contact therapy, (c) active specific immunotherapy, and (d) adoptive transfer of immunity. These agents can also be classified as active on the humoral immune system, the cellular immune system, or both. Some agents employed and the results obtained in clinical trials are described briefly herein. In general, each immunotherapeutic agent is more effective when the amount of antigen (whether bacterium, virus, fungus, tumor cells, etc) in the patient is small, the bulk having been removed by appropriate antibiotics in the case of infectious agents, or the primary tumor having been removed by surgery when immunotherapy is used as an adjunct (or to prevent clinical metastases) in cancer immunotherapy.

SPECIFIC ACTIVE IMMUNOTHERAPY

In recent clinical trials, cancer patients have been treated with injections of purified tumor-associated antigens to bolster their specific antitumor immunity. The purified antigens were isolated from tumor cell surfaces by sophisticated biochemical and/or biophysical separation procedures (16, 17). Administration of purified lung tumor antigen in Freund's adjuvant by Stewart, Hollinshead, and co-workers to 28 patients with stage I lung cancer following surgical removal of the lung tumors resulted in a significant increase in survival (18). The experimental group received monthly injections of soluble antigen homogenized in Freund's complete adjuvant for three months without other therapy, whereas the third group received monthly chemotherapy followed by tumor antigen immunotherapy for three months. Eighty-three percent of the patients in both the immunotherapy and chemoimmunotherapy groups were still alive after four years, compared with only 49% in the control group, who received chemotherapy alone. The immunotherapy did not appear to prolong survival in stage II or stage III patients, indicating the importance of minimizing the antigenic burden (tumor) before immunotherapy, as stated above. However, in this trial no control was included for Freund's adjuvant alone. Thus, it is possible that the apparent beneficial effects may have been due to nonspecific adjuvant immunostimulation rather than to specific antitumor immunity against the lung tumor antigen. Additional trials in a larger number of lung cancer patients have been initiated, and trials in colonic cancer, malignant melanoma, and other types of cancer patients have just been instigated; a Freund's adjuvant alone group also will be included (A. C. Hollinshead,

Table 2 Some immunomodulators of therapeutic interest

Category	Example	Possible mode of action	Reference
Specific Active			
1. Tumor-associated (specific) antigens	Lung cancer, osteogenic sarcoma	Stimulates cell-mediated anti-tumor immunity	16–18
			113
2. Killed, virus- or enzyme-treated	Neuraminidase, viral xenogenization	Increases antigenicity of tumor epitopes	19, 20
			23, 25, 26
3. Cytotoxic drugs coupled to antitumor antibodies	Adriamycin, chlorambucil	Antibodies bring cytotoxic drug to tumor cells	35, 36
Adoptive Transfer			
Non-Specific			
1. Gamma globulin	Cohn Fraction II	Restores antibody levels in general	5
2. Isolated complement components	C2, 4, etc	Restores deficient complement level	12, 28
Antigen-Specific			
1. Immune-RNA	Allogeneic RNA	Stimulates cell-mediated anti-tumor immunity	34
	Xenogeneic RNA		32
2. Transfer factor	Dialyzable leukocyte extracts (DLE)	Increases T cell-specific immunity	54, 56
3. Monoclonal antibodies	Neuroblastoma, melanoma, leukemia osteosarcoma	Specific cytotoxicity	28–37
Non-Antigen–Specific			
1. Adjuvant (microbial)	BCG,	Stimulation of CMI and reticulo-endothelial system	58–60
	C. parvum,		68
	Bestatin		69
2. Thymic hormones	Facteur thymique serique	Stimulates differentiation and maturation of T cell precursors	2
	thymopoietin		9, 73
	thymosin		113
3. Anti-viral substance	Interferon	Stimulates natural killer cell and anti-viral activity	76–78
4. Chemically synthesized	Levamisole	Restores CMI	83, 85
	NPT 15392	Stimulates T and NK cells	113
	Methisoprinol	Increases CMI limb	98
	MVE	Stimulates immunocyte function	97
	NPT 16416	Thymic hormone-like effects	113
	Azimexon	T and B cell stimulation	113
5. Ig-derived	Tuftsin	Stimulates macrophage function	112

personal communication). In addition to the use in treatment of lung cancer, its efficacy in preventing lung cancer in high-risk individuals (heavy smokers, for example) merits exploration.

Another approach to specific active immunotherapy in cancer patients is the use of killed or modified tumor cells. Animal experiments demonstrate that pretreatment of tumor cells with the neuraminidase enzyme increases their immunogenicity. Many tumor cells are surrounded by a sialomucin coat, the glycocalix, which may protect from immunological attack. Neuraminidase treatment removes sialic acid and increases tumor cell antigenicity and susceptibility to cytotoxic antibody and complement. Heightened immunogenicity of neuraminidase-treated cells was demonstrated by their ability to induce antitumor immunity when injected into isogeneic animals (19). Consequently, a trial has been undertaken in human patients with acute myeloblastic leukemia (20) and other malignancies. These patients received multiple intradermal injections of neuraminidase-treated myeloblasts in combination with chemotherapy. Although trials of this nature as yet are not finalized, the preliminary results are encouraging. Significant increases in remission duration have been achieved. In a group of 85 acute myelocytic leukemia (AML) patients in which 41 received chemoimmunotherapy using neuraminidase-treated myeloblasts and another 45 were treated with chemotherapy alone, 24% of the patients in the chemotherapy group are in complete remission. This compares with 49% in complete remission in the group who received neuraminidase-treated myeloblasts. Fifty-eight percent of the patients in the immunotherapy group are alive, compared to 29% in the chemotherapy group. Considerable improvement in cell-mediated immunity occurred among AML patients immunized with neuraminidase-treated myeloblasts as measured by conversion to positive to at least three recall antigens: mumps, candida, and varidase. Thus, a progressive restoration of lymphocyte function in AML patients with this type of immunotherapy is apparent (21). In another trial, patients with lung cancer received injections of neuraminidase-treated tumor cells after surgical removal of their tumors and had longer remissions than controls who were treated only by surgery (22). However, side effects (especially high fevers) are common; indeed, thermal activation of monocytes, NK cells, etc, may be important precipitating factors in the immunity. Also, pretreatment of tumor cells with some viruses has led to cell modification and increased immunogenicity in animals (23). Preliminary trials with virus-treated tumor cells are being undertaken in humans. The induction of virally associated neoantigens (VAA) on tumor cells following artificial infection has been referred to as antigenic conversion (24), heterogenization (25), or viral xenogenization (26). It may be feasible to cause viral infection of an existing human tumor to xenogenize it, thereby causing immune-mediated tumor regression without surgical removal. Probably the nonlytic virus would have to be focused or concentrated into the tumor tissue very rapidly. One method of attaining this might be attaching tumor-specific antibody chemically to the virus. Also, diethylaminoethyl-D (DEAE-D) can attach foreign elements to the cell surface due to change in the negative charge induced on the tumor cells. Virally infected liposomes might also be employed for producing foreign antigens on tumor cells. The future of specific active immunotherapy will depend on the isolation, characterization, and purification of those tumor cell-surface–associated or specific antigens that can be used to bolster immunological attack. Sufficient quantities of these antigens must be prepared for immunotherapy and immune monitoring.

We anticipate that specific active immunotherapy, particularly in cancer, will continue to receive careful study. For example, one form of possible treatment currently under investigation is the use of cytotoxic drugs coupled to antitumor antibodies, especially monoclonal (hybridoma) antibodies. In animals this technique has been shown to cause specific destruction of some tumor cells, presumably because the drug is delivered directly to the tumor site (27). Promising results have been reported in animal osteosarcoma models using purified antiosteosarcoma antibodies coupled to adriamycin (28). Similarly, radiolabeled anti-CEA (carcinoembryonic antigen) is being used in clinical trials for both early radiologic diagnosis and therapy of human lung cancer metastases (29).

ADOPTIVE TRANSFER OF IMMUNITY

Like specific active immunotherapy, adoptive transfer of immunity is intended to increase the patient's immune response to a specific antigen. In this case, however, the aim is to transfer such immunity from the donor to the recipient. In the case of humoral immunodeficiencies or isolated complement component deficiencies, the use of fresh frozen plasma or purified gamma globulin (Cohn fraction II) has become a standard therapeutic method (30). More recently, attempts have been made to develop techniques for the transfer of cell-mediated immunity from donors with normal or elevated levels demonstrable by in vitro assays to patients with either broad-spectrum or antigen-selective (i.e. one organism) cell-mediated immune defects. (Presumably these are due to rare immune response genes and are thus genetically determined defects.) To date, two such biologic agents have been used for clinical trials in humans: immune RNA and dialyzable leukocyte extracts (transfer factor).

Immune RNA

In recent years, several studies have produced evidence for a beneficial therapeutic effect of immune RNA (I-RNA) in animals with tumors. For example, after surgical extirpation of B16 melanoma isografts in C57BL/6 mice, administration of xenogeneic I-RNA prevented the fatal pulmonary metastases that inevitably developed in other murine tumors; the same effect has been shown in rats and guinea pigs (31). There are two potential sources of I-RNA for cancer immunotherapy in human patients: allogeneic I-RNA derived from lymphocytes of cured cancer patients, and xenogeneic I-RNA derived from animals specifically immunized with neoplastic cells from the tumor-bearing patient or from another patient with a tumor of identical histologic type. However, repeated removal of lymphocytes from patients in remission theoretically could produce deficient cell-mediated immunity and consequent exacerbation of the disease; furthermore, there is evidence that tumor-specific immunity in such patients diminishes or disappears after several disease-free years. Therefore, initial clinical trials have employed xenogeneic (animal) I-RNA, an approach that also eliminates the problems of donor selection and availability. Two methods have been used for administering I-RNA to cancer patients: injecting it parenterally, and incubating the patient's peripheral blood lymphocytes with I-RNA in vitro and returning them to the patient intravenously.

In a phase-I trial reported by Pilch et al (32), 35 cancer patients (15 malignant melanoma, 12 hypernephroma, and 8 others) were injected with I-RNA extracts from the spleens and lymph nodes of sheep that had received three-weekly intradermal injections of viable tumor cells in complete Freund's adjuvant. No significant local or systemic toxicity was noted, pain at the site of injection was minimal, and no evidence of local irritation or febrile, allergic, or anaphylactoid reactions was recorded. The immune status of the recipients was monitored by in vitro cytotoxicity testing, and in some patients significant increases in tumor-specific cytotoxicity were observed. Clinical improvement or stabilization of the disease occurred in 17 of the 35 patients treated. The same investigators later reported promising results in nonrandomized trials of I-RNA therapy for advanced renal cell carcinoma (J. A. Mannick, personal communication). The regression of pulmonary metastases suggests that this approach to adoptive immunotherapy is ready for more broad clinical development. These preliminary results indicate that I-RNA may prove to be a valuable immunotherapeutic agent, particularly in view of the apparent absence of adverse side effects. Trials by others, not yet fully reported, suggest that immune RNA will be of value in patients with hypernephroma (33).

It has also been reported that lymphoid and myeloid cells from tumor-bearing mice, when transferred into normal syngeneic mice, imparted information that resulted in the production of tumor-specific cytotoxic cells by the recipients (34). Similar results have been reported recently in experiments using tumor-sensitized xenogeneic cells (i.e. from other species, such as rats). The production of tumor-specific cytotoxic cells in the recipients may involve the transfer of information by I-RNA in the injected cells and suggests that xenogeneic cells eventually might prove useful for passive immunotherapy of human tumors.

One of the most exciting prospects for future adoptive immunotherapy in humans may be the utilization of cell hybridization-cell cloning methodology. Because the use of interleukin 2 (T-cell growth factor) insures the ability to generate continuously proliferating clones of cytotoxic T cells, these autologous cells could be administered repeatedly in therapy. Passive immunotherapy (serotherapy), in which purified xenogeneic antibodies have been coupled to drugs or radioactive isotopes, has been used to increase contact with the tumor. Antibody coupled to chlorambucil (35) and [131]I (36) have been used to treat malignant melanoma and hepatoma respectively. With the development of human myeloma-lymphocyte hybridomas, the use of the cloned B-cell populations that produce highly specific high-titer monoclonal antibody against tumor-associated (or specific) antigens make this form of passive immunotherapy particularly promising. Monoclonal antibodies have been developed for therapeutic use against colorectal carcinoma, neuroblastoma, malignant melanoma, leukemias, and lymphomas (37). Also, studies with monoclonal antibodies directed against tumor-associated antigens have recently been utilized in therapeutic trials (e.g. inoperable pancreatic carcinoma) with dramatic results (37a). The clinical experiences in humans with acute lymphocytic leukemia and B-cell lymphoma demonstrate the necessity of selecting target antigens that do not undergo antigenic modulation on the tumor-cell surface and, as important, the need to select patients with minimal tumor burden and circulating tumor antigen. To date, however, the ultimate usefulness of these reagents in therapy is unknown.

Dialyzable Leukocyte Extracts (Transfer Factor)

In normal subjects, injection of dialyzable leukocyte extracts (DLE) has been shown to *transfer* both skin-test reactivity (delayed hypersensitivity) and the ability to produce various mediators of cellular immunity, such as macrophage migration inhibitory factor (MIF) and leukocyte migration inhibitory factor (LIF), in the presence of the same antigen(s) to which the donor of the leukocytes responded (38). The transfer factor prepared by the dialysis method originally described by Lawrence in 1955 (39) is in fact a crude DLE preparation and has been shown to contain approximately 160 separate moieties. Consequently, DLE is the current designation for such preparations, and the term *transfer factor* (TF) or *dialyzable transfer factor* (TFd) is now reserved for the component(s) with antigen-specific activity (40). Studies from our laboratory (41) have indicated that the TF activity in DLE resides in two distinct nucleopeptides of molecular weight 2000–2500 containing both RNA and protein but not DNA, and structural models of these putative moieties have been proposed (40). Crude DLE preparations contain both nonspecific immunomodulatory (adjuvant) activity and one or more inhibitory activities in addition to the TF components (42, 43).

The mode(s) of action of the antigen-specific moieties in DLE remain undetermined. TF may act on a naive stem cell to induce specificity for an antigen or group of antigens or, alternatively, may assist in the recruitment of specific antigen-sensitive cells. On the other hand, the adjuvant moieties in DLE appear to act nonspecifically by enhancing the preexisting reactivity of the recipient's lymphocytes. DLE is a readily available nonantigenic substance that can be lyophilized and stored indefinitely without loss of potency. It does not transmit infectious disease, has no HLA antigens, and causes no serious side effects. It does not produce graft-versus-host reactions nor transfer humoral immunity, an advantage that could be important for cancer immunotherapy in avoiding immunological enhancement—a mechanism by which antitumor antibodies may coat the tumor cells, interact via immune complexes with T cells, and exclude cytotoxic T cells from interacting with tumor-cell antigenic sites.

Various in vitro tests can be used for assessing the immune status of donors, testing DLE preparation activity, and monitoring recipients [reviewed in (38)]. These include induction of enhanced chemotaxis, increased intracellular cyclic nucleotides, augmented antigen and mitogen responses, and increased formation of active T-cell rosettes (44), either by untreated lymphocytes from patients with low levels in vivo or by trypsinized normal lymphocytes. Recent studies by several groups (45–47) showed that the leukocyte migration inhibition (LMI) assay in agarose, which measures the production of LIF, can be used to measure both nonspecific and antigen-specific effects of DLE in vitro, and this is currently the method of choice for clinical applications. It should be emphasized that careful selection of donors, testing of DLE activity (both specificity and potency), and monitoring of recipients by immunological tests are essential for optimal clinical efficacy regardless of the type of disorder being treated.

DLE has received widespread clinical use [reviewed in (48)]. Although few clinical trials have been double-blind, the results obtained in some viral, fungal, and other diseases have been striking. DLE was first applied as a therapeutic and prophylactic agent in patients with Wiskott-Aldrich syndrome (49), an X-linked deficiency of cellular immunity in which death invariably occurred before age 20. Impressive results were obtained in more than half the treated patients; it was demonstrated later that the patients who responded favorably constituted a subgroup of this syndrome characterized by a defect in monocyte receptors for IgG (50). Other genetically determined immune deficiencies treated successfully with DLE include severe combined immunodeficiency disease, ataxia telangiectasia, genetically determined antigen-selective defects with recurrent infections, recurrent shingles and refractory cytomegalovirus, candida infection, and others (48). Conflicting results reported by several different investigators probably reflect the different methods for selecting donors, preparing the DLE, and monitoring the recipients. In addition, it is likely that, as in the case of Wiskott-Aldrich syndrome, different subgroups of patients classified within a given syndrome may respond differently to the same therapy.

A number of infectious (viral, fungal, and mycobacterial) and parasitic diseases (i.e. especially diseases due to agents handled by T cells) also have been treated with DLE (48). In viral infections, dramatic improvements have been reported by our group and others in disseminated vaccinia, measles, pneumonia, congenital *Herpes simplex, Herpes zoster,* cytomegalovirus, and other infections treated with antigen-specific DLE. In fungal infections, clinical improvement after reduction of the antigenic load has been reported in disseminated mucocutaneous candidiasis, disseminated coccidioidomycosis, and disseminated histoplasmosis refractory to conventional antifungal therapy. Several mycobacterial diseases refractory to the usual antibiotics and associated with antigen-selective defects in cell-mediated immunity, such as miliary tuberculosis, lupus vulgaris, and progressive BCG *(Mycobacterium bovis)* infection refractory to standard therapy, also have been treated successfully with DLE. Recently, human transfer factor therapy (administered orally) was seen to cause a remarkable clearing of pruitic and plaque lesions in a patient with *Psoriasis vulgaris* that had been recalcitrant to any other treatment (51). One of the few well-controlled double-blind clinical trials of DLE has been reported in the parasitic disease chronic cutaneous leishmaniasis (52). The results indicated both clinical efficacy and antigenic specificity of DLE prepared from donors with demonstrable in vitro cell-mediated immunity *Leishmania* antigens. In patients with persistent cutaneous leishmaniasis, administration of more than 100 units of specific DLE over a one-year period was usually required for complete eradication of the lesions (53).

At present it is impossible to reach any conclusion about the potential of DLE in the treatment of malignancies. A significant problem is the selection of appropriate leukocyte donors. As previously mentioned, antitumor immunity in cured patients is usually short-lived, and removal of their lymphocytes theoretically may lead to increased susceptibility to recurrence. However, it has been found that some 25–50% of the household contacts of cancer patients have specific cell-mediated immunity against the tumor type present in the patient (54), and these healthy individuals often prove to be suitable donors. For example, in one trial of DLE in osteosarcoma, the tumor in which this agent has been studied most extensively, five of seven patients were treated for 18–24 months after surgical removal of their primary tumor (and in two patients with lung metastases) with antigen-specific DLE prepared from the leukocytes of household contacts with specific cell-mediated reactivity against osteosarcoma cells in vitro (55). The patients did not receive any other therapy after surgery. All five of the recipients at last report have been in remission for more than five years, a highly significant advance over historical controls (56). DLE has been given also in breast carcinoma, malignant melanoma, and alveolar cell carcinoma with reported clinical and immunological improvement in some cases (48).

NONANTIGEN-SPECIFIC IMMUNOTHERAPY

Most of the immunomodulating agents in clinical use are administered with the intent of general stimulation (or suppression) of the patient's immune system, without attempting to direct the activity of the modulated cell toward a given antigen. These nonantigen-specific immunotherapeutic agents can be divided roughly into two groups, those requiring a functional immune system and those with effects only or primarily on a suppressed immune system. In the first group, particulate adjuvants such as BCG or *Corynebacterium parvum* are generally most effective in patients capable of mounting normal immune responses. These two adjuvants have been utilized for both nonspecific immunostimulation and adjuvant contact chemotherapy in cancer patients. Agents with restorative effects, such as levamisole and thymosin (or other thymic hormones), are in the second group and seem to act by conferring temporary immune competence in patients with suppressed immunity. They apparently have little or no effect when administered to patients with a normal immune apparatus.

Of particular importance is the development of synthetic compounds with immunotherapeutic applications. Due to space limitations, only a few of these synthetic drugs (increasing daily in number) are discussed below. Many other agents have been or are being tested as nonspecific immunomodulators, including microbial extracts (some of which apparently increase suppressor cell activity) (57), vitamin A and several of its analogs, tilorone, L-fucose, synthetic polynucleotides (poly A-U, poly I-C), lynestrenole, thiabendazole, tolazoline, lentinen, schizophyllan, picibanil, bestatin, and others.

Bacillus Calmette-Guérin (BCG)

BCG is a viable attenuated strain of *Mycobacterium bovis* obtained by progressive reduction of virulence in a culture medium enriched with beef bile. This nonspecific immunostimulant is thought to act by stimulating the reticuloendothelial system, but this effect may be secondary to T-cell activation and mediator production. BCG also stimulates natural killer cells, which can nonspecifically kill malignant cells. Some investigators believe that BCG also cross-reacts immunologically with hepatoma, melanoma, and leukemic cells, a finding which might account for some of its apparently specific effects on these tumors. Nonviable extracts of BCG have also been shown to be immunostimulatory and to inhibit tumor growth in animals, as have smaller molecules such as the monomeric subunit of the peptidoglycan component of the cell wall. The smallest active compound derived from BCG thus far identified is muramyl dipeptide (MDP), which is an effective nonspecific adjuvant of macrophage activation in mice but not in humans. A synthetic analog of muramyl dipeptide, SM-1213, is also under investigation. In addition, the methanol-extractable residue of phenol-treated BCG (MER-BCG) has been employed in some preliminary oncologic trials in humans, and the results appear promising for solid tumors, acute leukemias, and perhaps melanomas, especially in conjunction with chemotherapy to reduce the antigen burden.

Various routes of administration have been employed for BCG immunotherapy, including intradermal injection, oral administration, intravenous injection, intralesional injection, and intrapleural administration in lung-cancer patients after primary tumor resection. The most widely used method of administration is scarification, where about 10^8 viable organisms are applied to an area of the upper arm or upper thigh after a series of incisions about 2 mm deep have been made either with a needle or with a Heaf gun. After weekly scarifications with BCG, some patients show an absence of cutaneous reactivity to the treatment. Other tests indicate that they usually become immunosuppressed and therapy must be discontinued for a month or more, only to be resumed when immune function is restored. In addition, BCG therapy sometimes may have dangerous side effects, usually consisting of a severe hypersensitivity reaction and shock. Rarely patients have died after intralesional therapy. Complications of BCG therapy administered by scarification or with the Heaf gun are mild, and no fatalities have been reported.

The effectiveness of BCG has been shown most dramatically in trials using the scarification technique for therapy of malignant melanoma (58). Preliminary results, especially in patients with only local regional involvement, appear very encouraging provided BCG is given near the tumor site. In patients with stage IV melanoma, the combination of chemotherapy and BCG (chemoimmunotherapy) produced more remissions, longer remissions, and longer survival than chemotherapy alone (59). It has been reported that increases in urinary lysozyme excretion and active T cells are valid indicators of clinical improvement in such patients after BCG therapy, and that no improvement is seen if such increases are absent (60).

The first clinical trial of BCG was reported by Mathé and co-workers in patients with acute lymphocytic leukemia (61). A small group of patients received chemotherapy and irradiation of the central nervous system to induce complete clinical remission, followed by either BCG immunotherapy, BCG in combination with irradiated allogeneic tumor cells, or no immunotherapy. The duration of the immunotherapy was five years. Patients receiving weekly doses of BCG by scarification, either with or without specific immunotherapy (tumor cells), appear to have responded best, since 7 out of 20 such patients are still in remission 17 years after initiation of treatment. The majority of the BCG-treated patients who suffered relapse did so before 100 days, indicating that the number of tumor cells left after chemo- and radiotherapy in these patients was greater than the maximum able to be controlled by immunotherapy. In a later trial with a newer chemotherapy regimen and with cranial irradiation rather than total central nervous system radiotherapy, the median survival duration was increased to 10 years (62). However, these results could not be confirmed by English or American investigators using different therapeutic regimens and different sources of BCG. [The French BCG (Pasteur strain) is alive, non-lyophilized, and has more activity than the British (Glaxo) or American (Tice) strains, which are killed and/or lyophilized. Therefore, the French BCG has produced the best clinical results.]

Preliminary trials of BCG therapy have been conducted also in acute and chronic myelogenous leukemia, lymphoma, breast cancer, head and neck tumors, and colon cancer with promising results, but all of these observations will require confirmation. In lung cancer, a 1977 study suggested that intra-pleural BCG injection after surgical removal of bronchial carcinoma decreased the incidence of relapse (63). Later studies in malignant melanoma (64) and lung cancer (65) suggest that intralesional immunotherapy of the primary malignant lesions is feasible and can lead to increased survival. BCG has been used intravesically with documented beneficial results in bladder carcinoma (66). However, for most human clinical cancer studies in which a benefit was seen, there is another report that negates this, so that BCG effectiveness thus far must be said to be equivocal. In contrast, in adult acute myelogenous leukemias, either alone or in combination with an allogeneic irradiated tumor cell vaccine, BCG therapy has provided prolongation of survival, remission, or both (67).

Corynebacterium parvum

C. parvum, a gram-positive bacterium, is a systemic adjuvant used for im-munotherapy as a heat-killed and formaldehyde-treated suspension, given orally or injected parenterally either directly into the lesion or at a distant site. It appears that C. parvum, like BCG, induces macrophage activation; paradox-ically, it appears to depress T-cell function, especially that of splenic T cells. Many clinical trials with C. parvum are under way and claims have been made of increased duration of remissions in lung cancer and in metastatic breast cancer when the agent is used in conjunction with chemotherapy. Recent study in mice indicate that a synergistic effect is produced when C. parvum adminis-tration precedes chemotherapy with cyclophosphamide, but when the order of administration is reversed (cyclophosphamide followed by C. parvum) the antitumor effects of the adjuvant are delayed and toxic side effects are increased (68). Such studies are clearly of major importance for the development of optimal chemoimmunotherapeutic protocols for human neoplasias. Although C. parvum can cause tumor regression after intralesional injection, and in one human study induced regression of lung metastatic nodules in diverse sites with disseminated cancers in 40% of cases, its toxicity and lack of major activity in most cases seem to preclude further use in human cancer.

The major drawback to the use of *C. parvum* for immunotherapy is its sometimes serious toxic effects. Fever up to 40°C, headache, and vomiting may follow its administration, and some patients have developed mild hypertension and/or peripheral vasoconstriction. For these reasons, we avoid it.

Bestatin

Bestatin, a metabolite dipeptide of *Streptomyces olivoreticuli,* potentiates both humoral and cell-mediated immune responses in vivo and in vitro (69) and has been effective therapeutically in controlling the metastasizing murine ESb-lymphoma. Bestatin seems to induce a macrophage-mediated tumoricidal activity even in nude mice. Oral administration to cancer patients has augmented NK activity and increased the T cells in the peripheral blood. Furthermore, Bestatin seems to induce the release of interleukin 2 from lymphocytes and to impede the turnover of lymphocyte membrane structures (70). A plethora of other augmenting agents of microbial origin and/or their components, too numerous to mention here in detail, are the subjects of extensive experimentation. Whether these agents eventually will find a niche in the clinicians' immunomodulating repertoire is unknown. For instance, Yamamura (71) employed the cell-wall skeleton of *Nocardia rubra* clinically to control malignant effusions of the pleura with considerable effectiveness. Although serious side effects were encountered, lung-cancer remission was considerably prolonged in a randomized trial. Another immunostimulating agent derived from the edible Japanese mushroom *Lentinus edodes* is a purified polysaccharide extract called lentinan (LNT). This agent in preliminary trials produced significant life prolongation in patients with advanced or recurrent cancers of the breast, stomach, and colon-rectum (72).

Thymic Hormones

Immunotherapeutic applications of thymic factors have received increasing attention in recent years, and a detailed description of clinical results and chemical studies can be found in the proceedings of several excellent symposia devoted to this topic (2, 9, 73). Many factors with thymic-hormone–like activity have been isolated and described, including thymosin, facteur thymique serique (FTS), and thymopoietin. Thymosin, a mixture of seven different peptides with different biological activities and the most widely studied of the thymic hormones, promotes T-cell differentiation and also may have other effects on cell-mediated immunity. The other thymic hormones appear to be comparable in activity yet different in structure. Although animal experiments have shown little or no toxicity, reactions to thymosin have been reported in a few patients [see for example (74)], presumably to bovine-specific antigens since bovine thymosin is used generally for immunotherapy. Thus, thymosin should not be given to patients with histories of severe milk allergies; in our laboratory, patients receiving repeated injections are monitored by skin testing with the thymosin itself. A number of laboratories have isolated these different thymic hormones, and some of the fractions have been purified, sequenced, and chemically synthesized. In fact, thymosin has been biologically synthesized with the use of recombinant DNA.

Thymic factors have been used most extensively in patients with acquired or congenital T-cell defects, and dramatic improvements have been reported in some instances. In some patients with congenital T-cell deficiency, combined therapy using both thymosin and DLE appears to be beneficial, even though thymosin or DLE alone is without effect. Thymus extracts also are being tried in some autoimmune diseases such a systemic lupus erythematosus, since it appears that they can induce the differentiation of null cells into suppressor T cells in patients with apparent deficiencies in suppressor activity and, conversely, can cause a reduction in suppressor activity (or an increase in helper activity) in some hypogammaglobulinemic patients. Thymosin increases the percentage of T cells in vitro in some cancer patients. In clinical trials with thymus extracts for the treatment of solid tumors, clinical improvement appears to occur only in those patients who show such an in vitro response. In one controlled study, patients with lung oat cell carcinoma treated with multiple chemotherapy and thymosin demonstrated increased survival (113); however, at this point it is still too early to evaluate the efficacy of thymic hormones in cancer immunotherapy. To date, more than 300 cancer patients have been treated for periods up to four years with thymosin fraction 5 or thymosin and consequent therapy in phase I or II protocols. In one study, thymosin significantly prolonged survival in patients who showed eradication of all detectable disease by chemotherapy. The median survival for thymosin and chemotherapy was 500 days compared to 240 days for chemotherapy and placebo (75). It will be important to synthesize each component of the thymic hormones (Thymosin fraction 5 contains at least 20 different peptides), and test each component separately for immunomodulating effects in animal models before ultimately meaningful clinical trials in humans.

Interferon

Interferon, originally described and characterized as a specific antiviral substance, is now receiving widespread attention as a possible antitumor agent. Interferon preparations derived from pooled buffy coat cells of normal human blood donors currently are being tested in cancer patients. However, most of the early work with interferon has been done with preparations of dubious purity. For example, crude interferon preparations from human buffy coat cells probably contain less than 0.5% interferon. Virus-induced type I interferons are proteins or glycoproteins of molecular weight between 15,000 and 40,000. The major effect of the active ingredient in interferon appears to be the potentiation and stimulation of natural killer cell activity (76).

A clinical trial of interferon was begun in 1971 in Sweden, using a crude preparation to treat patients with osteosarcoma. Twenty-eight patients received daily injections of 3×10^6 units of leukocyte interferon, followed by three injections per week for 17 months. Although the tumor load was reduced by surgical extirpation or irradiation before immunotherapy, no other therapy was used. The results indicated that after two and a half years the incidence of pulmonary metastases in the interferon treatment group was about 50% of that in concurrent controls, and the mortality rate was less than 50% of that for controls (77). Strander and co-workers in Stockholm also have treated patients with several other types of neoplasia (78). Preliminary results indicated some beneficial effects in patients with Hodgkin's disease, multiple myeloma, laryngeal papilloma, condyloma acuminata, and osteogenic sarcoma following surgical amputation. Partially purified human leukocyte interferon was used to treat these patients daily for a two-year period. Compared to groups of non-randomized concurrents and historical controls, significant prolongation of disease-free survival was noted. In 1979, the same workers using interferon saw complete or partial remissions in multiple myeloma (79), and others accomplished a 30% complete and partial remission rate in patients with metastatic breast cancer, non-Hodgkin's lymphoma, multiple myeloma (80), and partial regressions of both malignant melanoma and gastric carcinoma (81). The excitement surrounding interferon relates to the fact that it is a natural mediator molecule (produced in response to viral infection) that has shown antitumor activating potential in humans. The results of a handful of recent National Cancer Institute-sponsored trials have reported that, while interferon is not a cancer panacea, it indeed can counter some human cancers. Of 81 who received pure interferon made by recombinant DNA techniques, nine patients demonstrated a decrease in tumor size. In another study, 52 patients with various unresponsive cancers were treated and seven experienced tumor regression (82). Although these meager results were phase I trials in which dosage and administration schedules were being assessed, the use of sufficient quantities of pure (recombinant DNA) interferon preparations in the near future should afford a critical appraisal of its efficacy. Others have reported promising results in a few patients with cervical cancer, basal cell carcinoma, breast cancer, non-Hodgkin's lymphoma, and neuroblastoma. As already stated, however, the interferon preparations used in the earliest trials were extremely heterogeneous, containing less than 1% of interferon in an uncharacterized mixture of other leukocyte products, including, in our hands, many mediators of cellular immunity and TF as gauged by in vitro tests. Results now being obtained with preparations of greater purity seem to indicate far fewer beneficial effects. Indeed, we believe that trials on cancer with more highly purified interferon will show that the beneficial effects of interferon preparations were due to the contaminants, i.e. other mediators of cellular immunity, including TF, present in the buffy coat extracts, rather than to interferon itself, and that purified leukocyte interferon will be only a weak immunomodulator (fibroblasts also make an interferon that is slightly different from leukocyte interferon).

CHEMICALLY SYNTHESIZED IMMUNOMODULATORS

Levamisole

Levamisole is a synthetic derivative of tetramisole that has been used extensively as a veterinary anthelmintic drug. It immunopotentiates the graft-versus-host reaction in experimental rats and in some animal diseases causes an apparent increase in host resistance to tumor cells. It acts on the cellular limb of the immune system and can restore impaired cell-mediated immune responses to normal levels but fails to hyperstimulate the normal functioning immune system (83). Thus, it shows true immunomodulator activity. Recent studies suggest that a metabolite of levamisole, DL-2-oxo-3-(2-mercapto-ethyl)-5-phenylimidazolidine, is the compound active on the immune system (84). The primary mechanism of action of levamisole may be to facilitate the participation of monocytes in the cellular immune response (85), apparently by enhancing monocyte chemotaxis (86). In addition, it has been reported to increase DNA synthesis of T lymphocytes and to augment their proliferative responses to mitogens, as well as their production of mediators of cellular immunity in vitro (87). NPT-16416, an immunomodulating levamisole-like purine, has been shown to have thymic hormone effects. It increases "active" T cell rosettes in human peripheral blood, augments by 30% lymphokine-induced macrophage proliferation, and induces the maturation of murine prothymocytes. It also demonstrates a restorative effect on the deficient E-rosetting capacity of peripheral blood lymphocytes of rheumatoid arthritics.

In humans, levamisole has been reported to restore delayed hypersensitivity reactions in anergic cancer patients and to be of some benefit in the treatment of aphthous stomatitis, rheumatoid arthritis, systemic lupus erythematosus, viral diseases, chronic staphylococcal infections, and breast cancer. In a placebo-controlled study of levamisole immunotherapy in resectable lung cancer, Amery (88) reported that both disease-free intervals and survival times were increased in patients who received the drug in three-day courses beginning three days prior to surgical removal of the tumor and courses every two weeks for two years. Thereafter, with adequate doses patients showed 25% versus 50% relapses and 15% versus 44% deaths respectively when compared to controls. Also, the number of hematogenous metastases was diminished significantly. However, in the last few years, several in-depth studies of levamisole in patients with bronchogenic carcinoma, both alone and in conjuction with other therapy (e.g. BCG), were unable to demonstrate a therapeutic benefit. Indeed, in some cases the treated groups responded less favorably than the untreated (12, 89). Conflicting or negative data regarding the ameliorative effects of levamisone have been reported in breast cancer (90), colon cancer (91), head and neck cancer (92), melanoma (93), and leukemia (94). The reasons for these overall disappointing results are uncertain but may relate to the degree of tumor burden. With the emergence of more refined methods of detecting neoplasia in the early stages, levamisole may find a place in the oncological regimen.

Levamisole has a variety of side effects, and patients may complain of nausea, flu-like malaise, and cutaneous rashes that disappear after cessation of therapy. The most serious side effect is a granulocytopenia that is reversed upon therapy termination, but white cell counts should be monitored in patients taking the drug for prolonged periods. Interestingly, levamisole has been shown to suppress the formation of anti-DNA antibody in nude mice (95) and in high concentrations to produce suppression rather than augmentation of human T-cell mitogenic responses in vitro (96). Thus, clinical trials in patients should include careful immune monitoring to ensure that the immune system is stimulated rather than suppressed.

Maleic Anhydride-Divinyl Ether

MVE is a copolymer that has been studied extensively in animals for immunoregulatory capabilities. This compound and a series of similar polymers are reported to have anti-tumor activity through regulation of T, B, macrophage, and NK cell functions; they have been shown to possess antiviral activity, induce interferon, and act as adjuvants to tumor cell and viral vaccines (97). The early copolymers had extensive toxicity, but recently developed copolymer products have led to an enthusiastic reappraisal of this type of immunostimulant. Currently, phase-I cancer trials are under way with MVE-2 and preliminary results in humans affirm the animal studies.

Methisoprinol (Inosiplex) (Isoprinosine)

Methisoprinol (ISO), the p-acetamidobenzoic acid salt of N,N-dimenthyl-amino-2-propanol:inosine complex (3:1 molar ratio), is a synthetic immunomodulatory drug recently approved for clinical use in the United States. It appears to be effective in a wide variety of viral diseases. ISO increases cell-mediated immune functions in vitro, such as T-cell proliferative responses to antigens or mitogens, active T rosette formation, and macrophage activation. It also increases active T-cell levels in vivo in patients with low levels before treatment (98).

In vitro experiments have shown that ISO inhibits the replication of both DNA and RNA viruses in tissue culture, including *Herpes simplex,* adenovirus, and vaccinia (DNA viruses), and poliovirus, influenzae types A and B, rhinovirus, ECHO, and Eastern equine encephalitis (RNA viruses). Toxicological, teratogenicity, and carcinogenicity studies have demonstrated that ISO is safe, well tolerated, and remarkably free of side effects, even upon prolonged administration. It contains an inosine moiety, a naturally occurring purine in lymphocytes, that is metabolized via normal biochemical pathways to uric acid.

ISO potentiates cell-mediated immune responsiveness in vivo (103), and a major factor in its effectiveness against viral infections appears to be its ability to prevent the depression of cell-mediated immunity shown to occur during viral infection and to persist for four to six weeks thereafter (44). It may prove useful as an adjunct in cancer therapy as well, since there is considerable evidence for a viral etiology of some types of malignancies in humans (99), and since cancer cells produce immunosuppressive factors (100) that might be counteracted by the immunoenhancing effects of ISO. ISO has been shown to enhance production of interleukin 2, and its structure probably helps to increase the general metabolic availability of inosine. A synergistic effect with NPT 15392 was noted on mitogen stimulation, induction of suppressor-cell activity in vitro, and suppression of mixed lymphocyte reactivity; an increase of 63% over controls was achieved in lymphocyte lymphotoxin production in 60 *Herpes simplex* patients (101). Although little evaluation of ISO has been done yet in cancer patients, it has been extensively studied in a hamster model (102). Recently, in 47 human patients with primary tumors (26 lung carcinoma, 14 breast carcinoma, and 7 melanoma), ISO restored to normal all three parameters tested, including ConA-induced lymphocyte proliferation, NK cell activity, and monocyte chemotaxis (103).

The clinical efficacy of ISO has been well documented in double-blind trials; for example, ISO produces a striking decrease in both the duration of infection and severity of symptoms in a whole host of viral diseases, including influenza virus infections (104), rhinovirus infections (105), *Herpes labialis* and *Herpes progenitalis* (106), *Herpes zoster* (107), viral hepatitis (108), rubella (109), and viral otitis (E. Berthaux, unpublished observation, 1978). Of particular interest are the results of ISO therapy in subacute sclerosing panencephalitis (SSPE), a progressive disease due to a chronic measles virus infection that results in complete debilitation and eventual death of the patient. ISO has been reported to halt the progression of SSPE when given in stages I and II of the disease in 80% of the patients provided it is administered for at least six months (111). Indeed, ISO is the only agent to date with documented beneficial effects in SSPE patients. The mechanism of action is unknown, but it appears to prevent virus-induced and cancer-induced immunosuppression.

NPT 15392

This hypoxanthine analogue is a relatively new heterocyclic immuno-stimulating compound that possesses neutrophil, T-cell, and NK stimulatory properties. Its structure is related to inosine and its action to methisoprinol. It augments human T-cell mitogen stimulation by PHA or ConA, lymphokine-induced macrophage proliferation, and suppressor T-cell induction. When 20 cancer patients were treated with 0.4 or 0.7 mg of NPT 15392 every three days for 10 days, the numbers of blood T cells, percentages of E rosettes, and autologous T rosettes were increased; furthermore, a decrease in the OKT4+ T-cell subpopulation also was observed. This drug is appealing particularly since it has virtually no adverse side effects. Another related synthetic com-pound belonging to the 2-cyanaziridines is Azimexon. This agent, although active mainly on T-lymphocytes in normals, has been shown to have a B-cell activation effect on the deficient immune system in chronic lymphocytic leukemia. No clinical side effects have been reported and the patients demon-strated significant improvements in testing for in vitro cell-mediated immunity and IgM and IgG immunoglobulin synthesis. Therapeutic effects have been noticed in arthritis and tumor systems, with increases in suppressor T-cell activity and concomitant decreases in T helper cell activity. One exciting aspect of this drug is that it seems to diminish markedly the chemotherapy-induced immunosuppression seen with other neoplastic drugs, such as cyclophospha-mide. While it reduces their toxicity, it induces leukocytosis and reconstitutes the nuclear cellular components of the bone marrow.

Tuftsin

Tuftsin is a biological naturally occurring tetrapeptide with remarkable im-munostimulating capability. It is generated in the serum by two enzymatic cleavages from the parent molecule, a cytophilic immunoglobulin, and repre-sents amino-acid residues 289 through 292 of the constant region of the IgG heavy chain. Tuftsin accentuates a number of activities associated with the macrophage and neutrophil, including motility, phagocytosis, immunogenic functions, augmentation of antibody production, bactericidal activity, and antitumor effects in animal systems (112). This naturally occurring immuno-potentiator shows tremendous promise as an antineoplastic agent. It is antici-pated that clinical cancer trials in humans soon will be attempted.

CONCLUSION

The above review provides an indication of the rapid progress made in recent years in the development of immunostimulating agents for the treatment of human disease. As stated earlier, the clinical effects of these other immuno-modulators are generally more favorable in patients with a minimal antigenic burden; this is the rationale for the use of these agents in combination with chemotherapy, radiotherapy, and/or surgery, particularly in cancer patients, an approach termed chemoimmunotherapy or immunochemotherapy. Furthermore, most of the immunotherapeutic agents now employed for cancer therapy are more effective against lymphoid malignancies than other types of cancers: for example, acute lymphatic leukemia responds far better to immunotherapy than does acute myelogenous leukemia, and lymphomas respond better than solid tumors (colon, breast, etc).

It may be also that combinations of immunomodulators will prove more effective than single agents. It can be envisioned that once the mechanisms of action of the various drugs and biologicals are known in detail, specific combinations can be used in sequence to produce a desired clinical result, such as ISO to combat viral infection, followed by DLE to provide prophylaxis against future infection with the same virus in a patient with a genetically determined antigen-specific defect in cell-mediated immunity against that particular viral agent. Studies of the type described above with *C. parvum* and levamisole should provide valuable insights into the possibilities of this sort of approach.

Finally, in regard to synthetic immunostimulants, rapid advances are accruing in the development of many new agents. Second- and third-generation compounds related to ISO and other chemically synthesized immunomodulators (e.g. azimexone) are already under investigation, and it is anticipated that future research will provide both further insights into the nature and mechanisms of action of such compounds and increasing clinical benefits to patients who receive immunotherapy.

ACKNOWLEDGMENT

We thank Nancy Butler and Linda Paddock for excellent secretarial assistance. The research for this paper was supported in part by US Public Health Service grant AI-18727–08. Publication no. 633 from the BCIM of the MUSC.

Literature Cited

1. Miller, J. F. A. P. 1961. Immunological function of the thymus. *Lancet* 2:748–49
2. Warner, N. L., Szenberg, A., Burnet, F. M. 1962. The immunological role of different lymphoid organs in the chicken. I. Dissociation of immunological responsiveness. *Aust. J. Exp. Biol. Med. Sci.* 40:373–88
3. Good, R. A., Dalmasso, A. P., Martinez, C., Archer, O. K., Pierce, J. C., Papermaster, B. W. 1962. The role of the thymus in development of immunologic capacity in rabbits and mice. *J. Exp. Med.* 116:733–96
4. Williamson, A. R. 1982. Genes coding for T lymphocyte receptors. *Immunol. Today* 3:68–72
5. Waldmann, T. A., Durm, M., Broder, S., Blackman, M., Blaese, R. M., Strober, W. 1974. Role of suppressor T-cells in pathogenesis of common variable hypogammaglobulinemia. *Lancet* 2: 609–13
6. Benjamin, D. C. 1975. Evidence for specific suppression in the maintenance of immunological tolerance. *J. Exp. Med.* 141:635–46
7. Engleman, E. G., McMichael, A. J.,

Batey, M. E., McDevitt, H. O. 1978. A suppressor T cell of the mixed lymphocyte reaction in man specific for the stimulating alloantigen. *J. Exp. Med.* 147:137–46

8. Haller, O., Hansson, M., Kiessling, R., Nigzell, H. 1977. Role of nonconventional natural killer cells in resistance against syngeneic tumor cells *in vivo. Nature* 270:609–11

8a. Tsang, K. Y., Fudenberg, H. H., Pan, J. F., Gnagy, M. J., Bristow, C. B. 1983. An *in vitro* study on the effects of isoprinosine on immune responses in cancer patients. *Int. J. Pharmacol.* In press

9. Unanue, E. R. 1978. The regulation of lymphocyte functions by the macrophage. *Immunol. Rev.* 40:227–55

10. Laughter, A. H., Lidsky, M. D., Twomey, J. J. 1979. Suppression of immunoglobulin synthesis by monocytes in health and in patients with systemic lupus erythematosus. *Clin. Immunol. Immunopathol.* 14:435–40

11. Cohen, S., Pick, E., Oppenheim, J. J., eds. 1979. *Biology of the Lymphokines,* p. 611. New York: Academic. 656 pp.

12. Mihich, E., ed. 1982. *Immunological Approaches to Cancer Therapeutics,* p. 587. New York: Wiley. 587 pp.

13. Raveche, E. S., Steinberg, A. D. 1979. Lymphocytes and lymphocyte functions in systemic lupus erythematosus. *Sem. Hematol.* 16:344–70

14. Herberman, R. B. 1974. Cell-mediated immunity to tumor cells. *Adv. Cancer Res.* 19:207–63

15. Ono, A., Amos, D. B., Koren, H. S. 1977. Selective cellular natural killing against human leukemic T cells and thymus. *Nature* 266:546–48

16. Hollinshead, A. C., Jaffurs, W. T., Alpert, L. K., Harris, J. E., Herberman, R. B. 1974. Isolation and identification of soluble skin-reactive membrane antigens of malignant and normal human breast cells. *Cancer Res.* 34:2961–68

17. Kamiyama, M., Hashim, G. A., Kyriakidis, G., Fitzpatrick, H. F. 1980. A tumor-associated antigen isolated from human breast adenocarcinoma. *Clin. Immunol. Immunopathol.* 16:151–65

18. Stewart, T. H. M., Hollinshead, A., Harris, J., Raman, S., Belanger, R., Crepeau, A., Crook, A., Hirte, W., Hooper, D., Klaassen, D., Rapp, E., Sachs, H. 1977. Survival study of specific active immunochemotherapy in lung cancer. In *Neoplasm Immunity: Solid Tumor Therapy,* ed. R. G. Crispen, pp.

37–48. Philadelphia: Franklin Institute Press

19. Simmons, R. L., Rios, A., Lundgren, G., Ray, P. K., McKhann, C. F., Haywood, G. R. 1971. Immunospecific regression of methylcholanthrene fibrosarcoma with the use of neuraminidase. *Surgery* 70:38–46

20. Sedlacek, H. H., Seiler, F. R. 1978. Spontaneous mammary tumor in mongrel dogs. A relevant model to demonstrate tumor therapeutical success by application of neuraminidase-treated tumor cells. *Cancer Immunol. Immunother.* 5:153–61

21. Bekesi, J., Holland, J. F., Robog, J. P. 1982. Immunotherapy trials with neuraminidase-modified tumor cells. In *Immunological Approaches to Cancer Therapeutics,* ed. E. Mihich, pp. 441–85. New York: John Wiley and Sons. 587 pp.

22. Fudenberg, H. H., Wybran, J. 1980. Experimental immunotherapy. In *Basic and Clinical Immunology,* ed. H. H. Fudenberg, D. P. Stites, J. L. Caldwell, J. V. Wells, pp. 722–36. Los Altos, Calif: Lange Medical Publications. 3rd ed. 782 pp.

23. Gillette, R., Boone, C. W. 1976. Augmented immunogenicity of tumor cell membrane produced by surface budding viruses: Parameters of optimal immunization. *Int. J. Cancer* 18:216–22

24. Stuck, B., Old, L. J., Boyse, E. A. 1964. Antigenic conversion of established leukemias by an unrelated leukemogenic virus. *Nature* 202:1016–18

25. Hamburg, V. P., Svet-Moldavsky, G. J. 1964. Artificial heterogenization of tumors by means of herpes simplex and polyoma virus. *Nature* 203:772–73

26. Kobayashi, H. 1979. Viral xenogenization of intact tumors. 1979. *Adv. Canc. Research,* 30:279–99

27. Zaharko, D. S., Przybylski, M., Oliverio, V. T. 1979. Binding of anticancer drugs to carrier molecules. *Meth. Cancer Res.* 16:347–80

28. Yoshioka, M., Kanda, M., Irie, H. 1980. 4th International Congress of Immunology

29. Goldenberg, D. M., Kim, E. E., DeLand, F. H., Bennett, S., Primus, F. J. 1980. Radioimmunodetection of cancer with radioactive antibody to carcinoembryonic antigen. *Cancer Res.* 40:2984–92

30. Stiehm. E. R., Vaerman, J.-P., Fudenberg, H. H. 1966. Plasma infusions in immunologic deficiency states: Meta-

bolic and therapeutic studies. *Blood* 28:918–37

31. Cohen, E. P. , ed. 1976. *Immune RNA.* Boca Raton, Fla: CRC Press

32. Pilch, Y. H., Kern, D. H. 1976. Immune RNA and tumor immunity. See Ref. 31, p. 71

33. Deleted in proof

34. Fisher, B., Wolmark, N., Saffer, E. A. 1979. Cellular cytotoxicity and serum inhibition in normal mice following transfer of xenogeneic tumor-sensitized cells. *Cancer Res.* 39:4772–76

35. Ghose, T., Norvell, S. T., Guclu, A. 1972. Immunochemotherapy of cancer with chlorambucil carrying antibody. *Br. Med. J.* 3:495–99

36. Order, S. E., Klein, J. L., Ettinger, E., Adereson, P., Siegelman, S., Leichner, P. 1980. Phase I-II study of radiolabeled antibody integrated in the treatment of primary hepatic malignancies. *Int. J. Radiat. Oncol. Bio. Phys.* 6:703–10

37. Colcher, D., Hand, P., Nuti, M., Sehlon, J. 1981. A spectrum of monoclonal antibodies reactive with human mammary tumor cells. *Proc. Natl. Acad. Sci. USA* 78:3199–203

37a. Sears, H. F., Mattis, J., Herlyn, D., Hayry, P., Atkinson, B., Ernst, C., Steplewski, Z., Koprowski, H. 1982. Phase I clinical trial of monoclonal antibody treatment of gastrointestinal tumors. *Lancet* 1:762–65

38. Fudenberg, H. H., Wilson, G. B., Goust, J. M., Nekam, K., Smith, C. L. 1980. Dialyzable leukocyte extracts (transfer factor): A review of clinical results and immunological methods for donor selection, evaluation of activities and patient monitoring. See Ref. 73, pp. 391–421

39. Lawrence, H. S. 1955. The transfer in humans of delayed skin sensitivity to streptococal M substance and to tuberculin with disrupted leucocytes. *J. Clin. Invest.* 34:219–30

40. Wilson, G. B., Fudenberg, H. H. 1983. Is controversy about "transfer factor therapy" nearing an end? *Immunol. Today.* 4:157–61

41. Wilson, B. G., Paddock, G. V., Fudenberg, H. H. 1980. Effects of dialyzable leukocyte extracts with transfer factor activity on leukocyte migration in vitro. V. Antigen-specific lymphocyte responsiveness can be initiated by two structurally distinct polyribonucleotides. *Thymus* 2:257-76

42. Wilson, G. B., Fudenberg, H. H., Jonsson, H. T. Jr., Smith, C. L. 1980. Effects of dialyzable leukocyte extracts with transfer factor activity on leukocyte migration in vitro. IV. Two distinct effects of DLE on leukocyte migration can be produced by prostaglandin. *Clin. Immunol. Immunopathol.* 16:90–102

43. Wilson, G. B., Smith, C. L., Fudenberg, H. H. 1979. Effects of dialyzable leukocyte extracts with transfer factor activity on leukocyte migration in vitro. III. Characterization of the antigen-independent migration inhibition factor in DLEs as a neutrophil immobilizing factor. *J. Allerg. Clin. Immunol.* 64:56–66

44. Wybran, J., Fudenberg, H. H. 1973. Thymus-derived rosette forming cells in various human disease states: Cancer, lymphoma, bacterial and viral infections, and other diseases. *Clin. Invest.* 52:1026–32

45. Wilson, G. B., Fudenberg, H. H., Horsmanheimo, M. 1979. Effects of dialyzable leukocyte migration in vitro. I. Antigen-dependent inhibition and antigen-independent inhibition and enhancement of migration. *J. Lab. Clin. Med.* 93:800–18

46. Borkowsky, W., Lawrence, H. S. 1979. Effects of human leukocyte dialysates containing transfer factor in the direct leukocyte migration inhibition (LMI) assay. *J. Immunol.* 123:1741–48

47. Sirianni, M. C., Fiorilli, M., Pana, A., Pezzella, M., Aiuti, F. 1979. *In vitro* transfer of specific reactivity to cytomegalovirus and *Candida* to cord blood leukocyte with dialyzable leukocyte extracts. *Clin. Immunol. Immunopathol.* 14:300–06

48. Arala-Chaves, M. P., Horsmanheimo, M., Goust, J. M., Fudenberg, H. H. 1978. Biological and clinical aspects of transfer factor. In *Immunological Engineering,* ed. D.W. Jirsch, p. 35. London: MTP. 361 pp.

49. Levin, A. S., Spitler, L. E., Stites, D. P., Fudenberg, H. H. 1970. Wiskott-Aldrich syndrome, a genetically determined cellular immunologic deficiency: Clinical and laboratory responses to therapy with transfer factor. *Proc. Natl. Acad. Sci. USA* 67:821–28

50. Spitler, L. E., Levin, A. S., Stites, D. P., Fudenberg, H. H., Pirofsky, B., August, C. S., Stiehm, E. R., Hitzig, W. H., Gatti, R. A. 1972. The Wiskott-Aldrich syndrome. Results of transfer factor therapy. *J. Clin. Invest.* 51:3216–24

51. Schwartz, R. A., Jeter, W. S. 1981. Oral administration of human dialyzable

transfer factor in a patient with Psoriasis. *Arch. Dermatol.* 117:3–4

52. Sharma, M., Firouz, R., Ala, F., Momtaz, A. 1979. Transfer factor therapy in human cutaneous leishmania infection (CLI): A double blind study. In *Immune Regulators in Transfer Factor,* ed. A. Khan, C. H. Kirkpatrick, N. O. Hill, p. 563. New York: Academic

53. Sharma, M., Anaraki, F., Ala, F. 1979. Preliminary results of transfer factor therapy of persistant cutaneous leishmania infection. *Clin. Immunol. Immunopathol.* 12:183–90

54. Byers, V. S., Levin, A. S., Hackett, A. J., Fudenberg, H. H. 1975. Tumor-specific cell mediated immunity in household contacts of cancer patients. *J. Clin. Invest.* 55:500–13

55. Levin, A. S., Byers, V. S., Fudenberg, H. H., Wybran, J., Hackett, A. J., Johnston, J. O., Spitler, L. E. 1975. Osteogenic sarcoma: Immunologic parameters before and during immunotherapy with tumor-specific transfer factor. *J. Clin. Invest.* 55:487–99

56. Byers, V. S., Le Cam, L., Levin, A. S., Johnston, J. O., Hackett, A. J. 1979. *Cancer Immunol. Immunother.* 6:243

57. Arala-Chaves, M. P., Higerd, T. B., Porto, M. T., Munoz, J., Goust, J. M., Fudenberg, H. H., Loadholt, C. B. 1979. Evidence for the synthesis and release of strongly immunosuppressive, noncytotoxic substances by *Streptococcus intermedius. J. Clin. Invest.* 64:871–83

58. Morton, D. L., Eilber, F. R., Joseph, W. L., Wood, W. C., Trahan, E., Ketcham, H. S. 1970. Immunological factors in human sarcomas and melanoma. *Ann. Surg.* 172:740–47

59. Gutterman, J. U., Mavligit, G., Gottlieb, J. A., Burgess, M. A., McBride, C. M., Einhorn, L., Freireich, E. J., Hersh, E. M. 1974. Chemotherapy of disseminated malignant melanoma with dimethyl triazeno imidazode carboxamide and Bacillus Calmette Guerin. *N. Eng. J. Med.* 291:592–97

60. Lieberman, R., Fudenberg, H. H. 1979. Effects of BCG on lysozyme and "active" T cells in patients with malignant melanoma: A preliminary study. *Clin. Immunol. Immunopathol.* 12:191–203

61. Máthe, G., Vassal, F., Delgado, M., Pouillart, P., Belpomme, D., Hayat, M., Schwartzenberg, L., Amiel, J. L., Misset, J. L., Musset, M., Jasmin, C. 1976 *Cancer Immunol. Immunother.* 1:77–87

62. Máthe, G. 1976. *Cancer Active Immunotherapy. Immunoprophylaxis and*

Immunorestoration. Berlin: Springer. 405 pp.

63. Holmes, E. C., Ramming, K. P., Mink, J., Coulson, W. F., Morton, D. L. 1977. A new method of immunotherapy for lung cancer. *Lancet* 2:586–87

64. Mastrangelo, M. J., Sulit, H. L., Prehn, L. M., Bornstein, R. S., Yarbro, J. W., Prehn, R. T. 1976. Intralesional BCG in the treatment of metastatic malignant melanoma. *Cancer* 37:684–92

65. Holmes, E. C., Rummey, K. P., Bein, M. E., Coulson, W. F. 1979. Intralesional BCG immunotherapy of pulmonary tumors. *J. Thor. Card. Surg.* 77:362–68

66. Terry, W. D., D. Windhorst, eds. 1978. *Immunotherapy of Cancer: Present Status of Trials in Man.* New York: Raven

67. Powles, R. L. 1974. Immunotherapy for acute myelogenous leukemia using irradiated and unirradiated leukemia cells. *Cancer* 34:1558–62

68. Scott, M. T. 1979. Analysis of the principles underlying chemoimmunotherapy of mouse tumors. 1: Treatment with cyclophosphamide followed by Corynebacterium-parvum. *Cancer Immunol. Immunother.* 6:107–12

69. Blomgren, H. 1980. Bestatin: A new immunomodulator. *Int. J. Immunopharmacol.* 2:166

70. Blomgren, H. 1982. Immunomodulation by bestatin in the human. *Int. J. Pharmacol.* 4:360

71. Yamamura, Y. Immunotherapy of lung cancer with oil-attached cell wall skeleton. See Ref. 66, p. 173

72. Taguchi, T., Furue, H., Kimura, T., Kondoh, T., Hattori, T., Itoh, I., Ogawa, N. 1982. Life span prolongation effects of Lentinan on patients with advanced or recurrent colo-rectal cancer. *Int. J. Pharmacol.* 4:272

73. Aiuti, F. A., Wigzell, H., eds. *Thymus, Thymic Hormones, and T Lymphocytes.* London: Academic

74. Bamzai, A. K., Kretschmer, R. R., Rothberg, R. M., Gotoff, S. P. 1979. Thymosin-induced leukocyte histamine release reaction in an infant with DiGeorge syndrome. *Clin. Immunol. Immunopathol.* 14:70–76

75. Lipson, D. S., Chretien, P. B., Makuch, R., Kenady, D. E., Cohen, M. H. 1979. Thymosin immunotherapy in patients with small cell carcinoma of the lung. *Cancer* 43:863–70

76. Zarling, J. M., Eskra, L., Borden, E. C., Horoszewicz, J., Carter, W. A. 1979. Activation of human natural killer cells cytotoxic for human leukemia cells by

purified interferon. *J. Immunol.* 123:63–70

77. Strander, H. 1978. Anti-tumor interferon and its possible use as an anti-neo-plastic agent in man. *Texas Rep. Biol. Med.* 35:429–35

78. Strander, H. 1977. Interferons: Antineoplastic drugs? *Blut* 35:277–88

79. Mellstedt, H., Bjorkholm, M., Johansson, B., Ahre, A., Holm, G., Strander, H. 1979. Interferon therapy in myelomatosis. *Lancet* 1:245–47

80. Gutterman, J., Yap, Y., Buzdar, A., Alexanian, R., Hersh, E. M., Cadanillas, F., Greenberg, S. 1979. Leukocyte interferon induced tumor regression in patients with breast cancer and B cell neoplasm. *Proc. Am. Assoc. Cancer. Res.* 20:167

81. Priestman, T. J. 1980. Initial evaluation of human lymphoblastoid interferon in patients with advanced malignant disease. *Lancet* 2:113–18

82. Treichel, J. A. 1982. Interferon: More anti-cancer response. *Sci. News* 121:310

83. Symoems, J., Rosenthal, M. 1977. Levamisole in the modulation of the immune response: The current experimental and clinical state. *J. Reticuloendothel. Soc.* 21:175–221

84. Van Ginckel, R., De Brabander, M. 1979. The influence of a levamisole metabolite (DL-2-OXO-3-[2-mercaptoethyl]-5-phenylimidazolidine) on carbon clearance in mice. *J. Reticulonendothel. Soc.* 25:125–31

85. Kazura, J. W., Negendank, W., Guerry, D., Schreiber, A. D. 1979. Human monocyte-lymphocyte interaction and its enhancement by levamisole. *Clin. Exp. Immunol.* 35:258–68

86. Pike, M. C., Daniels, C. A., Snyderman, R. 1977. Influenza-induced depression of monocyte chemotaxis: Reversal by levamisole. *Cell. Immunol.* 32:234–38

87. Whitcomb, M. E., Merluzzi, V. J., Cooperband, S. R. 1976. The effect of levamisole on human lymphocyte mediator production *in vitro*. *Cell. Immunol.* 21:272–77

88. Amery, W. K. 1978. Final results of a multicenter placebo-controlled levamisole study of resectabel lung cancer. *Cancer Treat. Rep.* 62:1677–83

89. Borden, E. C., Crowley, J., Davis, T. E., Wolberg, W. H., Grouernan, D. 1980. Levamisole: Effects in primary and recurrent colorectal carcinoma. In *Proceedings of Second International Conference on Immunotherapy of Cancer Bethesda, Md.* ed. W. D. Terry

90. Paterson, A. H. G., Nutting, M., Takats,

L., Edwards, A. M., Schinnour, D., McClellard, A. 1980. Chemoimmunotherapy with levamisole in metastatic breast carcinoma. *Cancer Clin. Trials* 3:5–10

91. Bedikian, A. Y., Valdeviesco, M., Mavligit, G., Burgess, M. A., Rodrequez, V., Boder, G. P. 1978. Sequential chemoimmunotherapy of colorectal cancer. *Cancer* 42:2169–76

92. Wanebo, H. J., Hilal, E. Y., Pinsky, C. M., Strong, E. W., Mike, V., Hirshaut, Y., Oettgen, H. F. 1978. Randomized trial of levamisole in patients with squamous cancer of the head and neck: A preliminary report. *Cancer Treat. Rep.* 62:1663–69

93. Spitler, L. E., Sagebial, R. 1980. A randomized trial of levamisole versus placebo as adjuvant therapy in malignant melanoma. *N. Engl. J. Med.* 303:1143–47

94. Chang, P., Wiernek, P. H., Schiffer, C. A., Lichtenfield, J. L. 1978. Levamisole, cytosinearabinoside, and daurorubicin therapy of acute nonlymphocytic leukemia. *Proc. Am. Soc. Clin. Oncol.* 19:370–78

95. Ogita, T., Hayakawa, T., Horiuchi, Y., Mizushima, Y. 1979. Effect of levamisole on the autoantibody formation. *Int. Arch. Allerg. Immunol.* 59:222–26

96. Sampson, D. 1978. Immunopotentiation and tumor inhibition with levamisole. *Cancer Treat. Rep.* 62:1623–25

97. Pavlidis, N. A., Schultz, R. M., Chirigos, M. A., Leutzeler, J. 1978. Effect of maleic anhydride-divinyl ether copolymers on experimental M109 metastases and macrophage tumoricidal functions. *Cancer Treat. Rep.* 62:1817–22

98. Friedman, H., Cole, R., Morin, A. 1980. Increased active T cells after isoprinosine. Immunological evidence for a viral etiology certain malignant tumor. *Int. J. Immunopharmacol.* 2:153–64

99. Fudenberg, H. H., Byers, V., Levin, A. S. 1975. Immunological evidence for a viral etiology of certain malignant tumors. In *Perspectives in Virology IX,* ed. M. Pollard, pp. 153–64. New York: Academic

100. Kamo, I., Friedman, H. 1977. Immunosuppression and the role of suppressive factors in cancer. *Adv. Cancer Res.* 25:271–321

101. Bradshaw, L. J., Summer, H. L. 1977. *In vitro* studies on cell-mediated immunity in patients treated with inosiplex for herpes virus infection. *Ann. NY Acad. Sci.* 284:190–96

102. Tsang, K. Y., Pan, J. F., Fudenberg, H.

H. 1983. Treatment of osteosarcoma in an animal model with osteosarcoma specific dialyzable leukocyte extracts. In preparation
103. Deleted in proof
104. Betts, R. F., Douglas, R. G. Jr., George, S. D., Rinehart, C. J. 1978. ISO in influenza virus infections. *78th Ann. Meet. Am. Soc. Microbiology, Las Vegas, Nevada, May 1978.*
105. Waldman, R. H., Ganguly, R. 1977. ISO in rhino virus infections. Therapeutic efficacy of Inosiplex (Isoprinosine) in rhino virus infection. *Ann. NY Acad. Sci.* 284:153–60
106. Bradshaw, L. J., Summer, H. L. 1977. *In vitro* studies on cell-mediated immunity in patients treated with Inosiplex for herpes virus infection. *Ann. NY Acad. Sci.* 284:190–96
107. Laude, J., LeSound, B., Rancurel, G., Doumerc, S., Moulias, R. 1980. Isoprinosine trial in Herpes zoster. Effects on

delayed cutaneous hypersensitivity. *Int. J. Immunopharmacol.* 2:195
108. Calonghi, G. F., Suerl, L., Cadeo, G. P., Del Massa, M. 1979. Viral hepatitis *Convegno Internazionale sulla Isoprinosina: Roma,* p. 75
109. Silva Baeza, J., de Luna Solano, J. L. 1973. *El Medico* 23:57
110. Deleted in proof
111. Huttenlocher, P. R., Mattson, R. H. 1979. Isoprinosine in subacute sclerosing panencephalitis. *Neurology* 29:763: 71
112. Najjar, V. A. 1978. Molecular basis of familial and acquired phagocytosis deficiency involving the tetrapeptide, Tuftsin. *Exp. Cell. Biol.* 46:114–26
113. Chretien, P. B., Lipson, S. D., Makach, R. W., Kenady, D. E., Coehn, M. H. 1979. Effects of thymosin *in vitro* in cancer patients and correlation with clinical course after thymosin immunotherapy. *Ann. NY Acad. Sci.* 332:148–59

Ann. Rev. Pharmacol. Toxicol. 1984. 24:175–97

THE ROLE OF ENDOTHELIUM IN THE RESPONSES OF VASCULAR SMOOTH MUSCLE TO DRUGS

Robert F. Furchgott

Department of Pharmacology, Downtown Medical Center, State University of New York, Brooklyn, New York 11203

INTRODUCTION

Several years ago we accidentally discovered that relaxation of isolated preparations of arteries (rings, transverse strips, or helical strips) by acetylcholine (ACh) was strictly dependent on the presence of endothelial cells on the intimal surface of the preparations (1–3). This discovery helped resolve the paradox that ACh, a potent vasodilator of arteries in vivo, often produced no relaxation or even contraction of isolated preparations of arteries in vitro (4, 5). Apparently those isolated preparations that had failed to relax had had their endothelial cells unintentionally rubbed off during the course of their preparation for experiments. This discovery also led to the finding that a number of other agents, including some but not all of the most potent known endogenous vasodilators, also require endothelial cells to produce relaxation in isolated arteries. A number of laboratories are now engaged in research on various aspects of the endothelium-dependent relaxation of blood vessels by various agents. This review attempts to bring together the more important findings in this new area of research. A fuller description of early experimental results in this area obtained by the author and others is available in another recent review (6). The reader is also referred to that review for a discussion of a postulated role for endothelial cells in mediating or facilitating contractions of some blood vessels under special conditions.

175

0362-1642/84/415-0175$02.00

RELAXATION OF ARTERIES BY ACETYLCHOLINE

The Requirement for Endothelial Cells and the Lack of Involvement of Prostaglandins

That endothelial cells are required for relaxation by ACh was first suggested when it was found that precontracted rings or strips prepared from the descending thoracic aorta of the rabbit (henceforth referred to as rabbit aorta) would not relax in response to ACh if their intimal surfaces had been rubbed during the making of the preparation—either unintentionally, as must have been the usual case in earlier work with helically cut strips, or intentionally (1–3, 5). When care was taken not to rub the intimal surface of the aorta on foreign surfaces or on itself during the entire procedure of preparing and mounting, the rings and strips uniformly gave excellent relaxation in response to ACh. Typical records of ACh-induced relaxation of aortic preparations precontracted to moderate levels of tone by norepinephrine are shown in Figure 1. Figure 1 also illustrates the complete loss of the relaxation response in preparations after their intimal surfaces have been rubbed. That the loss of capacity to relax in response to ACh was the result of removing endothelial cells during the rubbing was clearly demonstrated using both scanning electronmicroscopy and en face microscopy after silver staining (2, 3).

The en face examination of preparations immediately after pharmacological experiments showed that those preparations giving excellent relaxation (as in

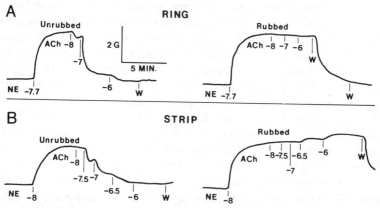

Figure 1   Relaxation by acetylcholine (ACh) of a ring (A) and a transverse strip (B) of rabbit thoracic aorta, and lack of relaxation by ACh after the intimal surfaces had been rubbed to remove endothelial cells. Concentrations of drugs added to the Krebs solution in the muscle chambers are expressed as logarithms of cumulative molar concentrations. NE is norepinephrine, and W indicates washout of the muscle chamber. Rings were mounted on L-shaped hooks, and transverse strips were mounted with specially designed clips. [From (3), used with the permission of Raven Press.]

Figure 1) usually had about 60 to 80% of their endothelial cells still present, that preparations with only a few percent of these cells remaining still gave moderate relaxation, but that preparations completely free of these cells gave no relaxation at all. It was also shown with rabbit aorta that complete removal of endothelial cells enzymatically by collagenase pretreatment also resulted in complete loss of the relaxation response to ACh (2). Although initial studies were on the rabbit aorta, we and others soon found that endothelial cells were required for relaxation by ACh in isolated arteries from all mammalian species tested, including rabbit (2), dog (2, 3, 7, 8), cat (3, 9), guinea pig (2), rat (2, 10), pig (11), cow (12), and man (13).

Although a number of other agents in addition to ACh were subsequently found to require the presence of endothelial cells for eliciting relaxation of isolated arteries (see later sections), the removal of endothelial cells did not interfere with relaxations produced by isoproterenol, sodium nitrite, glyceryl trinitrate, sodium azide (2), sodium nitroprusside (14), papaverine (8, 9), and prostaglandins such as PGE_2 and PGI_2 (8, 15). Removal of endothelial cells also did not interfere with relaxation by adenosine and adenylic acid in rabbit aorta (16) and dog femoral artery (7) but did reduce the degree of relaxation produced by those agents in pig aorta (11). Photorelaxation of rabbit aorta (17) had no endothelial-cell requirement (2), nor did relaxation of dog femoral artery by the addition of KCl after a period of exposure to K^+-free solution (7).

Very early in the work with ACh on rabbit aorta, we ruled out the possibility that an endothelium-derived prostaglandin serves as a mediator of relaxation. Not only did PGI_2, PGE_2, and a variety of other prostaglandins fail to produce relaxation of this artery, but the cyclooxygenase inhibitors indomethacin and aspirin did not interfere with ACh-induced relaxation (2). Also, in other rabbit arteries and in arteries from other species, inhibition of cyclooxygenase did not interfere with endothelium-dependent relaxation by ACh (3, 10, 11, 13, 15, 18).

Characteristics of Relaxation by Acetylcholine

The receptor on endothelial cells whose activation by ACh leads to relaxation of arterial smooth muscle is a muscarinic receptor. In arteries from all species tested, ACh-induced relaxation is very sensitive to blockade by atropine (2, 3, 7, 8, 9, 10). In the rabbit aorta, the estimated equilibrium constant (K_B) of atropine acting as a competitive antagonist was 0.35 nM, and the relative potencies of three muscarinic agonists acting in the presence of physostigmine were ACh > methacholine > carbamylcholine (3). Contractions elicited by higher concentrations of muscarinic agonists acting on rabbit aorta and some other arterial preparations are also mediated by muscarinic receptors, but these receptors are located on the smooth muscle cells (2, 5). In rabbit aorta, the degree of contraction with ACh (best studied after removal of endothelium) varies markedly among different preparations. It is not yet established whether the greater sensitivity of the ACh-induced relaxation in comparison to the ACh-induced contraction indicates different subtypes of the muscarinic receptor in the endothelial cells and in the smooth muscle cells respectively.

It is worth noting at this point that muscarinic receptors located on prejunctional adrenergic nerve terminals have also been implicated in the vasodilating effect of ACh. If isolated vessels or perfused vascular beds are vasoconstricted by stimulation of their adrenergic nerves, then ACh acting on the prejunctional receptors can inhibit the stimulation-evoked release of norepinephrine from the nerve terminals and thus inhibit the stimulation-evoked vasoconstriction. [For reviews, see (19, 20).] In the isolated, perfused central ear artery of the rabbit [which generally has its endothelial lining sloughed off during the initial stages of perfusion (O. Steinsland, personal communication)], the prejunctional muscarinic receptor on the adrenergic nerve terminals has pharmacological characteristics similar to the receptor on the endothelial cells (e.g. similar potency ratios for ACh, methacholine, and carbachol, and sensitivity to blockade by atropine (21)). It should be emphasized, however, that the prejunctional muscarinic mechanism for vasodilation is limited to situations where vasoconstriction is the result of adrenergic nerve stimulation, whereas the endothelium-dependent muscarinic mechanism is effective whether or not the vasoconstriction is produced by nerve stimulation.

On rings of rabbit aorta precontracted to moderate tone with norepinephrine, half-maximal relaxation by ACh usually occurs between 0.01 and 0.1 μM (2, 3) and maximal relaxation at 1 μM. The degree of relaxation in percent of the initial contractile tone tends to decrease as the level of initial tone is increased. Rings of rabbit ear artery, celiac artery, renal artery, and superior mesenteric artery are somewhat more sensitive to the relaxing action of ACh than are those of aorta (J. Zawadzki & R. Furchgott, unpublished observations). Preparations of various dog arteries (3, 4, 7, 8, 22, 23), cat arteries (3, 9), rat aorta (10), and pig aorta (11) also exhibit high sensitivity to the relaxing action of ACh. On the other hand, the few human arteries that we have so far tested (branches of mesenteric arteries and an ovarian artery) have shown considerably less sensitivity to the action of ACh than have arteries from experimental animals (R. Furchgott, unpublished observations).

Equal, moderate contractions of rabbit aorta produced by norepinephrine, histamine, serotonin, angiotensin II, or $PGF_{2\alpha}$ have essentially the same sensitivity to the relaxing action of ACh (3). On the other hand, contractions produced by increasing K^+ in the Krebs solution are less sensitive to relaxation by ACh than are equivalent contractions produced by norepinephrine in the case of both rabbit aorta (2, 5) and canine arteries (6, 8, 23, 24). When rabbit aorta is contracted by replacing all Na^+ in the Krebs solution by K^+ and all Cl^- by SO_4^{2-}, maximal relaxation by ACh is about 20% of that obtained in the presence of an equivalent norepinephrine-induced contraction in regular Krebs solution (2, 3, 6). The fact that there is still significant relaxation in the completely depolarizing solution indicates that hyperpolarization of the smooth muscle cells is not required for the endothelium-dependent relaxation by ACh.

Release of an Endothelium-Derived Relaxing Factor (EDRF)

One hypothesis to explain the obligatory role of endothelial cells in the relaxation of arteries by ACh is that activation of the muscarinic receptor in these cells stimulates them to release a factor (or factors) that, on diffusing to the subjacent smooth muscle cells, activates a mechanism for relaxation in the latter cells. First tests of this hypothesis involved superfusion experiments in which an endothelium-free transverse strip of rabbit aorta was superfused with fluid that was first passed over the endothelium-containing intimal surface of a segment of aorta. Occasionally such experiments clearly showed that ACh caused release of an endothelium-derived relaxing factor (EDRF) but results were not consistent (P. Cherry and R. Furchgott, unpublished observations). A second procedure was therefore developed that consistently gave direct evidence for an EDRF (2, 3).

In this procedure, a transverse strip of rabbit aorta freed of endothelial cells (the recipient strip) was tested when mounted separately and also when mounted, intimal surface against intimal surface, with a longitudinal strip with endothelial cells present (the donor strip) in a so-called sandwich mount. The right-angle orientation of the muscle cells of the donor strip prevented them from exerting significant tension changes on the strain gauge during contraction. ACh, which failed to relax contraction of the recipient strip when it was mounted separately, always gave good relaxation of contraction of the same strip when it was mounted as a sandwich with the donor strip. Thus, release of an EDRF by ACh from the endothelial cells of rabbit aorta was demonstrated.

The sandwich procedure has also been used successfully to demonstrate release of an EDRF by the ionophore A23187 in rabbit aorta and by ACh in the dog renal artery (R. Furchgott et al, unpublished observations). Modifications of the procedure have also been used to demonstrate release of an EDRF by ACh and by histamine in rat aorta (10), by ACh in dog femoral artery (J. De Mey, personal communication), and by ACh and bradykinin in dog intrapulmonary arteries (6). In the modification used with the intrapulmonary arteries, the donor strip with endothelium, like the recipient strip without endothelium, was cut transversely, but it was pretreated with the "irreversible" α-adrenergic receptor blocking agent dibenamine prior to being placed in the sandwich mount with the recipient strip. Because of the pretreatment, only the recipient strip was able to contract when norepinephrine was added to produce tone prior to testing ACh or bradykinin for relaxing effects (6).

OTHER AGENTS THAT PRODUCE ENDOTHELIUM-DEPENDENT RELAXATION OF ARTERIES

A number of agents in addition to ACh have now been found to require endothelial cells for producing all or part of their relaxing effects on isolated arteries. It is noteworthy that in most cases to be discussed here, just as in the case of muscarinic agonists, prostaglandins do not appear to have any significant role as mediators of these relaxing effects. It should also be noted that with some of these agents the non-prostaglandin, endothelium-dependent relaxation of isolated arteries is not found in the case of all species tested but may be limited to specific species; in some cases, it may even be limited to specific arteries in specific species.

The Calcium Ionophore A23187

Relaxation of isolated arteries by the ionophore A23187 has been shown to be completely endothelium-dependent in the case of all mammalian species so far tested, including rabbit (4, 25, 26), dog (13), rat (14), pig (11), and man (13). In rabbit aorta, A23187 is 10–30 times more potent than ACh as a relaxing agent (6, 13). It is also more powerful than ACh, so that against high levels of contraction the maximal relaxation by A23187 (0.1 μM) is always greater than that by ACh (1–3 μM). Relaxation by A23187, like that by ACh, is not inhibited by cyclooxygenase inhibitors (13, 25, 26). When A23187 is added to a ring or strip of rabbit aorta at a concentration giving maximal relaxation, and tone is then restored by increasing the concentration of norepinephrine present, additions of ACh now fail to produce any relaxation (6, 13). We have proposed that this interference by A23187 with relaxation by ACh is the result of A23187 activating the production and release of EDRF so fully that any additional activation by ACh is precluded. When a high dose of A23187 (1 μM) is added to a preparation of rabbit aorta for several minutes and then is washed out, its relaxing action persists for long periods after the washout (6, 18). Ionomycin, another calcium ionophore, has about the same potency as A23187 in producing endothelium-dependent relaxation of rabbit aorta (P. Cherry, unpublished observations). On the other hand, monensin, a monovalent cation ionophore selective for Na^+, produces no relaxation (W. Martin, unpublished observations).

ATP and ADP

In isolated preparations of rabbit aorta (4, 13, 16), dog femoral artery (7), and pig aorta (11), the graded, concentration-dependent relaxations by ATP or ADP (1–100 μM) are markedly reduced after removal of endothelial cells. Thus, in all of these species, ATP and ADP exert most of their relaxant effects through an action on endothelial cells. Cyclooxygenase inhibitors such as indomethacin do not inhibit these effects. In the case of rabbit aorta and dog femoral artery, concentration-dependent relaxations by AMP and adenosine (10–3000 µM) are not affected by removal of endothelial cells (7, 13, 16). It is probable that in these arteries the residual relaxation produced by ATP and ADP after removal of endothelial cells is due to the formation of their metabolic products, AMP and/or adenosine, which then act directly on the vascular smooth muscle (6). In pig aorta, a significant part of the relaxation by AMP and adenosine is reported to be endothelium-dependent (11).

Substance P and Some Related Peptides

Relaxation of isolated arteries from rabbits, dogs, and cats by substance P is strictly dependent on the presence of endothelial cells (13, 27). This peptide is the most potent endothelium-dependent relaxing agent studied in our laboratory, with threshold concentrations ranging from about 30 pM in rabbit aorta to 1 pM in dog celiac and superior mesenteric arteries. Desensitization to substance P occurs in all arteries on which it has been tested. Depending on the artery used, desensitization to a maximally effective dose (about 100–1000× threshold) is usually complete within 3–10 minutes. After full development of desensitization to substance P, there is no loss of sensitivity to the relaxing actions of ACh, A23187, and bradykinin. Thus, desensitization appears to be at the level of the receptor for substance P. Full sensitivity to substance P returns readily after washout of a desensitizing dose. Cyclooxygenase inhibitors do not interfere with relaxation by substance P. Recently, we have found that kassanin, physalaemin, and eledoisin also require endothelial cells to produce relaxations of isolated rabbit and dog arteries (28; R. Furchgott, unpublished observations) and that desensitization also develops to these agents. These peptides, which have some structural similarities to substance P near the C-terminal, fail to produce relaxation in the presence of a desensitizing dose of substance P and vice versa. This cross-desensitization strongly suggests that they cause relaxation by acting on the same set of receptors as substance P. Physalaemin is about the same potency as substance P, whereas kassanin and eledoisin are about 1/10th–1/30th as potent. Another peptide, octacholecystokinin, also requires endothelial cells to produce relaxation of rabbit and dog arteries. It is about 1/30000th as potent as substance P (28), and even though its structure has little in common with that of substance P, relaxation to it is lost in preparations desensitized to substance P.

Bradykinin

Bradykinin is a vasodilator that relaxes isolated arteries by one of two different indirect mechanisms depending on the species in question. We found that in rings of superior mesenteric and celiac arteries from rabbit and cat, mechanical removal of endothelial cells did not usually lead to a loss of sensitivity to the relaxing effects of bradykinin (15, 29). However, in these preparations relaxation by bradykinin was completely blocked by cyclooxygenase inhibitors such as indomethacin and flurbiprofen. Thus, in these arteries from rabbit and cat, relaxation by bradykinin appears to be mediated by prostaglandins whose synthesis is stimulated by the peptide, probably in both endothelial and other types of cells. This finding with rabbit arteries was not unexpected in view of the previous results of others indicating that relaxation of certain vascular beds and isolated arteries of the rabbit by bradykinin is mediated by released prostaglandins (30–32). It should be noted that neither bradykinin nor prostaglandins, including PGI_2, relax isolated preparations of rabit aorta and renal artery. On the other hand, PGI_2 is a potent relaxant of rabbit superior mesenteric and celiac arteries and is the prostaglandin that mediates bradykinin-induced relaxation of these arteries (J. W. Aiken, personal communication).

In contrast to arteries from the cat and rabbit, all arteries that we have tested from the dog (splenic, gastric, celiac, femoral, renal, coronary, intrapulmonary, and superior mesenteric) have shown a strict requirement for endothelial cells in the relaxation by bradykinin, and, in addition, their relaxing response to bradykinin has not been interfered with by cyclooxygenase inhibition by either indomethacin or flurbiprofen (15, 29). In dog arteries, bradykinin was usually about ten times more potent than ACh, with a threshold concentration ranging from 0.1–1.0 nM. Similar results with dog intrapulmonary and renal arteries have been reported by others (8, 22). Our results on dog coronary arteries differ somewhat from those of Toda (33), who found that indomethacin reduced to a small extent the relaxation of these arteries by bradykinin. We found that treatment of canine arteries with inhibitors of cyclooxygenase almost always gave considerable potentiation of the contracting activity of the agents used to produce initial tone (usually NE or $PGF_{2\alpha}$). This potentiation presumably occurred because prior to treatment with the inhibitor the isolated arteries were synthesizing prostaglandins with relaxing activity (e.g. PGI_2 and PGE_2) that opposes the contracting activity of added NE or $PGF_{2\alpha}$ (15). Our studies do not exclude the possibility that bradykinin stimulates the release of some prostaglandins (as well as EDRF) in canine arteries, but they do suggest that prostaglandins make little or no contribution to the relaxing effect of bradykinin. In a few experiments on rings of isolated human arteries (branches of mesenteric arteries and ovarian artery), relaxation by bradykinin was found to be dependent on the presence of endothelial cells and was not reduced by inhibition of cyclooxygenase (13, 15). Recently, Gordon & Martin (11) have reported that relaxation of the pig aorta by bradykinin is also endothelium dependent and prostaglandin independent.

Histamine on Rat Aorta

Recently, Van de Voorde & Leusen (10) reported that rings of rat thoracic aorta precontracted with NE exhibit dose-dependent relaxation to histamine (10–

1000 μM). According to them, this relaxation, like that produced by ACh (0.01–10 μM) in rat aorta, is dependent on the presence of endothelial cells and is not blocked by indomethacin. The relaxation by histamine was inhibited by mepyramine but not by cimetidine, indicating that histamine acts on an H_1 receptor of the endothelial cells. Rapoport & Murad (14) have also reported similar results with histamine on rat aorta. Endothelium-dependent relaxation by histamine has not yet been clearly demonstrated in any artery other than the rat aorta.

Serotonin on Canine Coronary Artery

Cohen et al (34) recently made the interesting finding that aggregating human platelets produce relaxation of rings of canine coronary arteries precontracted with $PGF_{2\alpha}$ if endothelial cells are present but produce only contraction if these cells have been previously removed. They propose that part of the relaxation response is the result of serotonin, released from the platelets on aggregation, acting on endothelial cells to produce a signal for relaxation of the coronary smooth muscle cells. Consistent with this proposal is their further finding that serotonin itself causes relaxation of precontracted rings of canine coronary arteries only if endothelial cells are present (35). In these arteries, as in many others, the direct effect of serotonin on the smooth muscle is contraction. The endothelium-dependent relaxing effect of serotonin was not inhibited by indomethacin, was not significantly inhibited by the serotonin antagonist ketanserin, but was largely inhibited by methysergide. Endothelium-dependent relaxation by serotonin has not yet been reported for any arteries other than canine coronary arteries.

Thrombin

De Mey and co-workers (18, 23) demonstrated that bovine thrombin (0.1–10 μ/ml) elicits dose-dependent relaxation of precontracted rings of dog arteries (femoral, splenic, pulmonary, spahenous). Relaxation, like that by ACh, was lost when the rings had been denuded of endothelial cells. Relaxation was not inhibited by inhibitors of cyclooxygenase and prostacyclin synthetase but was inhibited by heparin. Similar findings have been made on thrombin-induced endothelium-dependent relaxation of isolated canine coronary arteries (36). In these arteries, the relaxation response to each addition of thrombin was transient, giving way in time to a contractile response.

Arachidonic Acid

On the basis of our early findings on some conditions and agents that inhibit endothelium-dependent relaxation by ACh, we proposed that ACh acting on the endothelial cells "activates a reaction sequence in which arachidonic (or some other unsaturated fatty acid) is liberated and then oxidized by lipoxygenase to a product that is responsible for the relaxation of the smooth muscle cells" (2). In view of this proposal, a number of laboratories have investigated whether arachidonic acid itself can produce an endothelium-dependent relaxation of isolated arteries. Recently, Singer & Peach (38) reported that this agent, in the concentration range of 10–100 μM, produced transient endothelium-dependent relaxation of rings of rabbit aorta. Indomethacin, which inhibited the acute contractions produced by arachidonic acid in aortic rings freed of endothelium, potentiated both the degree and duration of relaxation produced by this agent in intact rings. After indomethacin pretreatment, these rings, when precontracted to modrate tone by phenylephrine, exhibited a maximum relaxation of about 40% in response to 100 μM arachidonic acid (38). Very similar results have been obtained in our laboratory in experiments with arachidonic acid on rabbit aortic strips precontracted with norepinephrine (6, 39).

De Mey and co-workers (18, 23), using rings of various canine arteries (femoral, saphenous, pulmonary, and splenic), found that arachidonic acid produced graded relaxation over a range extending from about 0.1–10 μM, and that the relaxation was either eliminated or markedly reduced in preparations denuded of endothelial cells. These workers also found that pretreatment of the femoral artery with idomethacin completely inhibited relaxation by arachidonic acid at all concentrations up to 30 μM (18). Using ^{14}C-arachidonic acid as a tracer, they found that a major product formed from the fatty acid was 6-keto-PGF$_{1\alpha}$, the prostaglandin to which prostacyclin (PGI$_2$) is spontaneously converted. Since this product was almost completely eliminated by either removing the endothelial cells or by pretreatment with indomethacin, they concluded that relaxation of dog arteries by arachidonic acid is mainly mediated by PGI$_2$ produced by endothelial cells from the fatty acid. In my laboratory, results with arachidonic acid on isolated canine coronary and superior mesenteric arteries (6, 39) have differed somewhat from those of De Mey et al (18) on femoral arteries: although relaxation produced by low concentrations of arachidonic acid (0.1–1 μM) was blocked by either indomethacin or flurbiprofen, endothelium-dependent relaxation produced by higher concentrations (10–100 μM) still persisted, even after pretreatment with these cyclooxygenase inhibitors.

Recently, Cherry and co-workers (39) reported that other unsaturated fatty acids besides arachidonic (e.g. cis-4, 7, 10, 13, 16, 19-docosohexaenoic, oleic, elaidic, and cis-vaccenic) produce endothelium-dependent relaxations that are not inhibited by cyclooxygenase inhibitors in both rabbit aorta and dog arteries. Since there is some possibility that these fatty acids may facilitate enzymatic reactions in the endothelial cell membranes by increasing "fluidity" of the membranes, Cherry (unpublished results) has recently tested the "membrane mobility agent" A$_2$C on isolated arteries. This agent, which is an ester of an 18-carbon fatty acid with a cyclopropane ring rather than a double bond in the carbon chain (structure: $CH_3(CH_2)_7CH\underset{CH_2}{\overbrace{\qquad}}CH(CH_2)_7COOCH_2$-$CH_2OCH_2CH_2OCH_3$), was developed by Kosower and colleagues as an agent to increase the fluidity of cell membranes (40). Cherry has found that A_2C, like arachidonic acid, produces endothelium-dependent relaxations in concentrations around 100 μM in both rabbit aorta and dog superior mesenteric artery and that the relaxations are not blocked by cyclooxygenase inhibitors.

Other Agents

Recently, Spokas et al (41) reported that the antihypertensive drug hydralazine, particularly at lower concentrations (0.1–1 μM), produced the greater part of its relaxant effect on isolated rings of rabbit aorta by an indirect action mediated by endothelial cells. In contrast, the relaxant effects of nitroglycerin, nitroprusside, minoxidil, and diazoxide were reported to be independent of endothelial cells.

Another agent found to give moderate, transient, endothelium-dependent relaxation of rabbit aorta is nordihydroguiaretic acid. Paradoxically, this agent is a potent inhibitor of endothelium-dependent relaxations by ACh and A23187 (13, 42). It will be further discussed in a later section.

AGENTS AND CONDITIONS THAT INHIBIT ENDOTHELIUM-DEPENDENT RELAXATIONS

Before considering the agents and conditions that inhibit endothelium-dependent relaxations, it should again be emphasized that such relaxations, except in the case of those produced by arachidonic acid in canine arteries (18) and occasionally by bradykinin in certain arteries of rabbits and cats (15), are not inhibited by inhibitors of cyclooxygenase (i.e. by blockade of prostaglandin synthesis). Also, the agents and conditions discussed in this section are for the most part selective inhibitors of endothelium-dependent relaxations, and unless otherwise indicated they have not been found to inhibit endothelium-independent relaxations evoked by direct actions of relaxing agents on vascular smooth muscle.

Anoxia

Without being aware of the role of endothelial cells in the relaxation of arteries by ACh, De Mey & Vanhoutte (24) found that anoxia inhibited this relaxation in rings of canine femoral artery. We subsequently found that anoxia inhibits endothelium-dependent relaxation of rabbit aorta by ACh (2) and by A23187 (25), and of dog arteries (intrapulmonary and renal) by ACh and bradykinin (6). To achieve complete inhibition, special precautions had to be taken to minimize traces of O_2 in the muscle chambers.

5, 8, 11, 14-Eicosatetraynoic Acid (ETYA)

Inhibition of endothelium-dependent ACh-induced relaxation following pretreatment with ETYA, which is an inhibitor of lipoxygenase as well as of cyclooxygenase (43), was first reported for rabbit aorta (2, 3) and later for dog arteries (15, 18) and rat aorta (10). In rabbit aorta, the inhibition by ETYA was found to be irreversible if the pretreatment used 100 μM ETYA (added in an ethanol solution) for 30–60 minutes (2). Inhibition by pretreatment with ETYA has also been reported for the following endothelium-dependent relaxations: those by A23187, ATP, and substance P in rabbit aorta (16, 25, 27); by histamine and A23187 in rat aorta (10, 14); by bradykinin in dog arteries (13, 15); and by arachidonic acid in rabbit aorta (38). Also, ETYA pretreatment completely blocked relaxation by arachidonic acid in the dog femoral artery (18), but in this case its effectiveness was attributable to its inhibition of cyclooxygenase rather than of lipoxygenase. In the dog femoral artery, De Mey et al (18) found no inhibition by ETYA of endothelium-dependent relaxations by either ATP or thrombin.

If ETYA (100 μM) was added during the course of relaxation of rabbit aorta by ACh, the pre-relaxation level of contractile tone was restored almost completely within one minute (2, 3, 6). This type of acute inhibition or antagonism of relaxation by ETYA has also been found in the case of relaxation of rabbit aorta by other endothelium-dependent relaxing agents, such as A23187, ATP, and substance P (4, 6, 16, 25, 27). Acute inhibition, but with only partial restoration of contractile tone, was also found when ETYA was added to canine superior mesenteric artery during relaxation by ACh or bradykinin (15).

Quinacrine

Quinacrine (mepacrine), which is known to be an inhibitor of phospholipase A_2 (43a), effectively inhibits relaxation of rabbit aorta by ACh or methacholine (2, 3, 44). Inhibition develops quickly and is essentially complete at concentrations of 10–30 μM. Quinacrine has also been found to inhibit the following relaxations: that by ACh in dog arteries (3, 18) and rat aorta (14), by substance P in rabbit aorta (27), by bradykinin in dog arteries (15), and by histamine in rat aorta (14). Although quinacrine does inhibit ATP-induced relaxation in rabbit aorta (4), it is reported not to do so in dog femoral artery (18). Relaxation by A23187, unlike that by ACh, is not inhibited by quinacrine in either rabbit aorta or dog arteries (4, 25, 44). It has been proposed that this difference may be accounted for if the inhibition of ACh-induced relaxation is the result of some block by quinacrine of an ion channel coupled to activation of the muscarinic receptor (3, 44).

Nordihydroguiaretic Acid (NDGA)

NDGA, which is an inhibitor of lipoxygenases as well as an anti-oxidant, is a very effective inhibitor of ACh-induced relaxation in rabbit aorta (13, 42, 44), dog renal artery (45), and human mesenteric artery (13). In rabbit aorta, complete inhibition of ACh- or methacholine-induced relaxation is achieved at NDGA concentrations of 30–100 μM (42, 44). The onset of inhibition is rapid and is reversible if the aorta is not exposed to too much NDGA for too long a time (13, 42). NDGA has also been shown to inhibit endothelium-dependent relaxation by A23187 in rabbit aorta (13, 44) and human mesenteric arteries (13), by bradykinin in dog arteries (42, 45), and by arachidonic acid in rabbit aorta (38).

NDGA itself (30 μM), when added to precontracted rings of rabbit aorta, produces moderate relaxation, usually transient, which is strictly dependent on the presence of endothelial cells (13). This endothelium-dependent relaxation by NDGA is more pronounced in some other vessels, such as rabbit superior mesenteric artery and especially cat celiac and superior mesenteric arteries. In the latter vessels, the marked relaxing effects of NDGA itself (both endothelium-dependent and independent) make it difficult to demonstrate the inhibitory action of NDGA against the relaxing effects of ACh or A23187 (R. Furchgott, unpublished observations).

p-Bromophenacylbromide (BPB)

BPB, an alkylating agent that has been shown to be a potent irreversible inhibitor of phospholipase A_2 in cell-free systems (46), is a potent inhibitor of ACh-induced relaxations in arteries of rabbit, dog, cat, and man (13, 42). In rabbit aorta and in other vessels, exposure to 3 μM for 20 minutes or 10 μM for 5 minutes usually sufficed to inhibit relaxation by ACh completely and irreversibly. Such an exposure also inhibited irreversibly the endothelium-dependent relaxations by other agents, such as A23187, substance P, and bradykinin (canine and human arteries) (13). It should be noted that we have recently found that exposure of rings of rabbit aorta to BPB always caused a significant, and sometimes almost total, loss of endothelial cells (6). Although in some experiments complete loss of relaxing response to ACh and A23187 occurred when only about half of the endothelial cells were lost, the possibility of general damage to endothelial cells by BPB must be considered in evaluating its inhibitory action.

Alterations of Extracellular Cations

Partly because of the potent endothelium-dependent relaxing action of A23187, we hypothesized that an increase of calcium ions in the region of some key Ca^{2+}-activated enzyme (perhaps a phospholipase) may be a primary step in the reaction sequence leading to formation and release of an endothelium-derived relaxing substance (now called EDRF) by ACh, A23187, and other agents (3). The results of Singer & Peach (26) on rings of rabbit aorta have provided strong support for a critical role for Ca^{2+}. They found that eliminating Ca^{2+} from the incubation medium inhibited maximum relaxation by A23187 by 92%, and by methacholine (used instead of ACh) by 67%. They proposed that the lesser degree of inhibition of the methacholine-induced relaxations occurred because the muscarinic agonist, but not the ionophore, was able to have access to a separate intracellular pool of Ca^{2+} in the endothelial cells. They also found that the calcium-channel blockers verapamil and nifedipine partially inhibited relaxation by both methacholine and A23187 (26).

De Mey & Vanhoutte (24) found in the case of dog femoral artery that the degree of relaxation by ACh decreased markedly when they replaced most of the Na^+ in Krebs solution with Li^+ or sucrose and was completely inhibited after one hour of exposure of the artery to a K^+-free solution. Since they also obtained inhibition of relaxation on exposure of the artery to ouabain (2–10 μM) or to cooling (22°C), they felt that their results suggested a role for Na^+-K^+-ATPase in ACh-induced relaxation (24). Since their results were obtained before the endothelium-dependency of this relaxation was recognized, it would be well to repeat their experiments giving attention to the possibility that the ionic changes and high ouabain concentrations used may have damaged or even caused a loss of endothelial cells.

Hydroquinone

We tested hydroquinone, a potential free radical scavenger, soon after our early speculation that EDRF released by ACh may be a free radical (3). When hydroquinone (100–300 μM) was added during the course of relaxation of rings of rabbit aorta by ACh or A23187, it very rapidly antagonized the relaxation (4). This inhibitory action was reversible if the exposure to hydroquinone was limited to a few minutes, but prolonged exposure (20 minutes) resulted in complete and irreversible loss of relaxing responses to ACh and A23187 (13). This irreversible loss was accompanied by a severe loss of endothelial cells during the exposure to hydroquinone (R. Furchgott, unpublished observations). Recently, Van de Voorde & Leusen (10) reported that pretreatment with hydroquinone (100 μM, time unspecified) also significantly inhibits relaxation by ACh and histamine in rat aorta.

Methylene Blue

Several studies (47–50) have shown that methylene blue can inhibit significantly the endothelium-independent relaxations of isolated preparations of bovine coronary arteries evoked by $NaNO_2$, glyceryl trinitrate, and nitroprusside, so-called nitrovasodilators that give rise to nitric oxide as the active principle that acts on the smooth muscle (49). Recently, Holtzmann (12) has reported that methylene blue is also a potent inhibitor of the endothelium-dependent relaxation of bovine coronary arteries by ACh. Methylene blue has now been shown to rapidly and completely inhibit relaxation by ACh and by A23187 in rings of rabbit aorta (R. Furchgott, unpublished observations). At a concentration of 10 μM, its inhibition of relaxation by ACh (1 μM) or A23187 (.01 μM) is very much faster in onset and greater in degree than is its inhibition of comparable relaxation by glyceryl trinitrate. This difference probably indicates that inhibition by methylene blue of ACh- and A23187-induced relaxation is the result of an action of the redox dye either in the endothelial cells or on the released EDRF itself.

Hemoglobin

According to Bowman & Gillespie (51), hemolysates of erythrocytes exerted an antagonistic action against relaxation of the bovine retractor penis muscle elicited by an unidentified inhibitory factor extracted from the muscle or by nitroprusside. They obtained similar effects using rabbit aorta. They considered that hemoglobin might be the active antagonistic principle of the hemolysates. We have recently tested hemoglobin on rings of rabbit aorta and have found that at concentrations of 1–10 μM it is an effective inhibitor of ACh- and A23187-induced relaxation (W. Martin & R. Furchgott, unpublished observations). By contrast, methemoglobin is ineffective or only slightly effective as an inhibitor of these endothelium-dependent relaxations.

ENDOTHELIAL CELLS IN THE RELAXATION OF RESISTANCE VESSELS AND VEINS

Resistance Vessels

In our first paper on the endothelium-dependent relaxation of isolated arteries by ACh, we proposed that this mechanism is also responsible for the vasodilation of resistance vessels (arterioles) by ACh (2). Although the validity of this proposal still remains to be proven, preliminary studies are in accord with it. In my laboratory, Carvalho (52) used the isolated arterial vascular bed of the rabbit mesentery perfused at constant flow rate and vasoconstricted with norepinephrine and found that vasodilation produced by ACh was eliminated after perfusing the vascular bed with collagenase to remove endothelial cells. Unfortunately, few experiments with collagenase could be completed successfully because treatment with this enzyme preparation tended to produce marked increases in resistance to flow, probably because of developing edema formation.

Another finding in support of the proposal that vasodilation of resistance vessels by ACh is endothelium-dependent comes from recent work by M.

Owen (personal communication). She has been able to mount rings of second-ary branches of the rabbit ear artery as small as 150 μ O. D. for tension recording and has shown that these branches, like the central ear artery itself, require endothelial cells for ACh-induced relaxation.

Veins

De Mey & Vanhoutte (23) have investigated the responses of rings of several canine veins (femoral, saphenous, splenic, pulmonary) to ACh and other agents that require endothelial cells for relaxing arteries. Results varied some-what, depending on the specific vein, but in general the veins gave much less relaxation in response to ACh than did corresponding arteries. For example, in the saphenous and femoral veins, where relaxation was endothelium-dependent, ACh gave only a small degree of relaxation (20–25% maximum) over the range of 30–300 nM and caused contractions at higher concentrations. Similar results have been obtained in our laboratory with the rabbit portal vein (3, 5). De Mey & Vanhoutte (23) also found that ATP, thrombin, and arachi-donic acid, all of which elicited good-to-excellent endothelium-dependent relaxations in canine femoral, saphenous, splenic, and pulmonary arteries, elicited either no relaxations or transient relaxations of small degree in the corresponding veins. In experiments in our laboratory on the canine femoral vein, bradykinin and A23187, like ACh, gave only very small endothelium-dependent relaxations (R. Furchgott, unpublished observations). The reason for the much smaller relaxations by these vasodilators in veins compared to arteries is not yet clear.

THE ENDOTHELIUM-DERIVED RELAXING FACTOR(S) (EDRF)

The chemical identity of EDRF is not yet known. Early work on the relaxation of rabbit aorta by ACh ruled out adenosine, AMP, or any prostaglandin (2). The finding that the calcium ionophore A23187 was a potent endothelium-dependent relaxing agent and that relaxation by ACh could be inhibited by anoxia, ETYA (a potential lipoxygenase inhibitor), quinacrine (a potential inhibitor or arachidonic-acid release from phosphatides), and hydroquinone (a potential free-radical scavenger) led to the following speculation: (*a*) activation of the endothelial cell muscarinic receptor leads to mobilization of Ca^{++} in the region of a Ca^{++}-activated lipase(s) that releases arachidonic acid from phos-phatides; (*b*) oxidation of the liberated arachidonic acid (or some other unsatu-rated fatty acid) by a lipoxygenase leads to the formation and release of an active, short-lived intermediate, possibly a free radical, which is the relaxing factor (3). As discussed in the next section, one reason for favoring the idea of a free radical as the ACh-evoked EDRF was that certain free radicals were already known to stimulate guanylate cyclase and to cause relaxation of certain smooth muscle preparations (49). Consistent with the speculation that the EDRF released by ACh is a labile product of a lipase-lipoxygenase pathway were the later findings that NDGA (a potential lipoxygenase inhibitor) and BPB (a potential phospholipase A_2 inhibitor) inhibited ACh-induced relaxation. Also, our recent results on rapid acute inhibition of ACh-induced relaxation by methylene blue and by hemoglobin could conceivably indicate reactions of these agents with an EDRF that is a free radical. (For details and references related to the inhibitory agents, see earlier section.)

Because the inhibitory agents cited above may well lack the desired specificity, the results obtained with them are not sufficient for a firm conclusion about the source and nature of EDRF. Indeed, there are other findings that appear inconsistent with the speculative scheme. For example, the lipoxygenase inhibitor BW755C (53) does not inhibit ACh-induced relaxation of rabbit aorta. This lack of inhibition by BW755C could possibly be accounted for in a modified scheme recently proposed by Singer & Peach (35, 44). These workers did find that the endothelium-dependent relaxation of rabbit aorta by arachidonic acid during cyclooxygenase inhibition could be prevented by preincubation with ETYA or NDGA (38), but they proposed that these agents may be inhibiting the oxidation of the fatty acid by cytochrome P450 rather than by a lipoxygenase. If arachidonic acid is actually the precursor of EDRF no matter what oxidizing enzyme system is involved, ETYA or NDGA added during the course of relaxation of cyclooxygenase-inhibited rabbit aorta by arachidonic acid could be expected to acutely antagonize this relaxation just as it does relaxation by ACh and A23187 (13, 42). But neither ETYA nor NDGA acutely antagonizes arachidonic acid-induced relaxation (6). The meaning of this discrepancy is not clear, but a possibility is that the non-prostaglandin EDRF released by arachidonic acid is different from that released by ACh.

The speculation that EDRF released by ACh is a labile oxidation product of arachidonic acid is also difficult to reconcile with the recent findings that endothelium-dependent relaxations in rabbit and dog arteries can be evoked by other unsaturated fatty acids (e.g. cis-4, 7, 10, 13, 16, 19-docosohexaenoic, oleic, elaidic, and cis-vaccenic) and even by a saturated membrane mobility agent, A_2C (39; also see above). Since these agents would be expected to increase membrane fluidity, it has been proposed that such an increase may be a primary step in a reaction sequence in endothelial cells leading to formation of an EDRF (P. Cherry, personal communication). It is conceivable that not only these agents, acting to increase membrane fluidity, but also ACh, stimulating membrane changes via its receptor, alter the membrane to allow the activation of some common ordinarily restrained reaction sequence that gives rise to an EDRF not itself an oxidation product of an unsaturated fatty acid (6).

Regardless of its chemical nature, the EDRF released by A23187 and substance P in rabbit, canine, and feline arteries, and by bradykinin in canine and human arteries, is most likely the same substance (or substances) as the EDRF released by ACh in these arteries. This conclusion is based on the common susceptibilities to inhibitory agents (e.g. anoxia, ETYA, NDGA, BPB) of the relaxation produced by each of these agents and that produced by ACh in any given artery (13; also see above). On the same basis, it seems likely that EDRF released by ATP and ADP in rabbit aorta is similar to that released by ACh (13). However, De Mey et al (18) concluded that in the canine femoral artery relaxation by ATP is mediated by a different "signal" (EDRF?) than is relaxation by ACh, since relaxation by ATP, unlike that by ACh, was not inhibited by pretreatment with ETYA or quinacrine. They also found no inhibition by ETYA or quinacrine of the endothelium-dependent relaxation by thrombin.

STUDIES ON THE MECHANISM OF RELAXATION BY EDRF

Prior to our findings on endothelium-dependent relaxation by ACh, a number of reports indicated that in certain smooth muscles there was a positive relationship between an increase in cyclic GMP and relaxation (49, 54–56), and that guanylate cyclase was markedly stimulated by hydroperoxides of arachidonic acid (57, 58) and by free radicals, particularly nitric oxide and the hydroxyl radical (49). Murad and his colleagues proposed that many potent vasodilators, such as nitroprusside, organic nitrates, azide, and inorganic nitrite, activate guanylate cyclase indirectly via nitric oxide, which they release as a reaction product (49). These findings of others were partly responsible for our speculation that EDRF may be a short-lived hydroperoxide or free radical resulting from the oxidation of arachidonic acid by a lipoxygenase pathway, and that it stimulates the guanylate cyclase of the arterial smooth muscle, causing an increase in cyclic GMP that then somehow activates relaxation (3). Although a causal relationship between increases in cyclic GMP levels and relaxation in vascular smooth muscle has not yet been proven, evidence consistent with such a relationship in the case of relaxation of isolated bovine coronary arteries by nitric oxide and nitric oxide-yielding vasodilators (nitroglycerin, nitroprusside, inorganic nitrite) has recently been presented in several reports (48, 50, 59).

Our speculation that EDRF would stimulate an increase in cyclic GMP of the arterial muscle has been proven correct in recent experiments on rat aorta by Rapoport & Murad (14), and on rabbit aorta by Jothianandan and myself (60). In the former experiments, strips of rat aorta with and without endothelium were exposed to norepinephrine, followed by ACh (10 μM), histamine (100 μM), or A23187 (3 μM), all at concentrations optimal for endothelium-dependent relaxation, for varying times prior to freezing in liquid N_2 (14). Each of these agents produced a marked increase (20- to 40-fold) in cyclic GMP above the control level (about 1 pmol/mg protein) in intact strips. Peak increases occurred in about 30 seconds, followed by a considerable decline over the next 2 minutes. None of the agents produced increases in cyclic GMP in endothelium-free strips. In contrast to these three relaxing agents, nitroprusside (1 μM), which does not depend on endothelium for its relaxant action, produced marked increases in cyclic GMP in both endothelium-free and intact strips. In our laboratory, rings of rabbit aorta were mounted to allow both recording of tension and rapid freezing at any desired stage of contraction or relaxation (60). Norepinephrine produced no change in cyclic GMP from the basal level (about 0.2 and 0.06 pmol/mg protein in intact and endothelium-free rings respectively). Relaxations of norepinephrine-induced contraction by ACh (1 μM) and by A23187 (0.1 μM) in intact rings were accompanied by 5-fold and 7-fold increases in cyclic GMP respectively. The cyclic GMP level peaked between 15 and 30 seconds after ACh addition and then remained at essentially the peak level out to 3 minutes. In endothelium-free rings, ACh and A23187 produced neither relaxation nor any change in cyclic GMP. Glyceryl trinitrate, which relaxed endothelium-free rings and intact rings equally well, produced marked increases in cyclic GMP in both types. In the case of ACh, histamine, and A23187 on rat aorta (14), as well as ACh on rabbit aorta (60), the onset of rise in cyclic GMP occurred before the onset of relaxation. Also, in aortas of both species, relaxation by ACh was not associated with any change in cyclic AMP (14, 60). Evidence that the observed increase of cyclic GMP produced by ACh in strips of aortas of both species was in the vascular smooth muscle rather than in the endothelial cells was obtained in experiments in which rapid removal of endothelial cells in a short interval between incubation with ACh and freezing still left elevated levels of cyclic GMP in the tissue. Removal of the cells was accomplished in rat aorta in 5 seconds by scraping the intimal surface with a scalpel (37), and in rabbit aorta in 3 seconds by dragging that surface over filter paper (R. Furchgott, unpublished observations). Very recently, Holzmann (12) has reported that endothelium-dependent relaxation of bovine coronary arteries by ACh is also accompanied by an increase in cyclic GMP.

Recently, Rapoport and co-workers (61) have reported that the endothelium-dependent increase in cyclic GMP in rat aorta produced by ACh is accompanied by a change in the pattern of phosphorylated proteins. They determined this pattern using two-dimensional gel electrophoresis and autoradiography to ascertain incorporation of ^{32}P-phosphate into tissue proteins. They found that the phosphorylation of nine proteins was increased and that of two proteins (probably myosin light chains) was decreased. This finding is particularly exciting because this change of pattern of phosphorylated proteins is the same as they had previously found in rat aorta after exposure to the endothelium-independent vasodilator sodium nitroprusside and to 8-bromo cyclic GMP (62). They hypothesize that endothelium-dependent relaxation by ACh, as well as endothelium-independent relaxation by nitrovasodilators, is mediated through cyclic GMP-dependent protein phosphorylation and dephosphorylation of myosin light chains.

CONCLUDING REMARKS

It is now well established that a major mechanism for the relaxation of certain isolated arteries by ACh and a number of other potent endogenous vasoactive agents (including ATP and ADP, substance P, bradykinin, histamine, serotonin, and thrombin) is an indirect one in which the agent first acts on endothelial cells to stimulate the production and release of a non-prostaglandin relaxing factor (EDRF), which then in turn acts on the smooth muscle cells of the artery. The chemical identity of EDRF—or perhaps EDRF's, since there is some evidence for more than one factor—is still not known. The original proposal that EDRF is an intermediate product of the oxidation of arachidonic (or some other unsaturated fatty acid) via a lipoxygenase pathway (2, 3) is supported by some but not all recent findings. Regardless of its chemical identity, EDRF does appear to be very labile, and the possibility that it is a free radical is still attractive. The speculation that EDRF would stimulate an increase in cyclic GMP in the arterial smooth muscle (3), just as nitrovasodilators do, has now been proven correct (14, 60). Recent findings suggest that cyclic GMP-dependent protein phosphorylation and dephosphorylation of myosin light chains in arterial muscle may mediate relaxation by ACh and certain other endothelium-dependent relaxing agents (61, 62). The role of endothelial cells in mediating relaxation of blood vessels by a number of endogenous agents must now be a factor in our consideration of the physiological control and pharmacological modifications of regional circulation and probably of certain pathological disorders of circulation.

ACKNOWLEDGMENTS

The research of the author and his collaborators cited in this review was supported by USPHS grant HL21860.

Literature Cited

1. Furchgott, R. F., Zawadzki, J. V. 1980. Acetylcholine relaxes arterial smooth muscle by releasing a relaxing substance from endothelial cells. *Fed. Proc.* 39:581 (Abstr.)
2. Furchgott, R. F., Zawadzki, J. V. 1980. The obligatory role of endothelial cells in the relaxation of arterial smooth muscle by acetylcholine. *Nature* 288:373–76
3. Furchgott, R. F., Zawadzki, J. V., Cherry, P. D. 1981. Role of endothelium in the vasodilator response to acetylcholine. In *Vasodilation*, ed. P. Vanhoutte, I. Leusen, pp. 49–66. New York: Raven. 536 pp.
4. Furchgott, R. F. 1981. The requirement for endothelial cells in the relaxation of arteries by acetylcholine and some other vasodilators. *Trends Pharmacol. Sci.* 2:173–76
5. Furchgott, R. F. 1982. Acetylcholine and blood vessel relaxation: complications and clarifications. In *Trends in Autonomic Pharmacology,* ed. S. Kalsner, 2:497–510. Baltimore: Urban & Schwarzenberg. 363 pp.
6. Furchgott, R. F. 1983. Role of endothelium in responses of vascular smooth muscle. *Circ. Res.* 53:557–73
7. De Mey, J. G., Vanhoutte, P. M. 1981. Role of the intima in cholinergic and purinergic relaxation of isolated canine femoral arteries. *J. Physiol.* 316:347–55
8. Chand, N., Altura, B. M. 1981. Acetylcholine and bradykinin relax intrapulmonary arteries by acting on endothelial cells: Role in lung vascular diseases. *Science* 213:1376–79
9. Lee, T. J. -F. 1982. Cholinergic mechanism in the large cat cerebral artery. *Circ. Res.* 50:870–79
10. Van de Voorde, J., Leusen, I. 1983. Role of endothelium in the vasodilator response of rat thoracic aorta to histamine. *Eur. J. Pharmacol.* 87:113–20
11. Gordon, J. L., Martin, W. 1983. Endothelium-dependent relaxation of the pig aorta: Relationship to stimulation of Rb efflux from isolated endothelial cells. *Br. J. Pharmacol.* 79:531–41
12. Holzmann, S. 1982. Endothelium-induced relaxation by acetylcholine associated with larger rises in cyclic GMP in coronary arterial strips. *J. Cyclic Nucleotide Res.* 8:409–19
13. Furchgott, R. F., Cherry, P. D., Zawadzki, J. V. 1983. Endothelium dependent relaxation of arteries by acetylcholine, bradykinin and other agents. In *Vascular Neuroeffector Mechanisms: 4th International Symposium,* ed. J. Bevan, et al, pp. 37–43. New York: Raven
14. Rapoport, R. M., Murad, F. 1983. Agonist-induced endothelium-dependent relaxation in rat thoracic aorta may be mediated through cGMP. *Circ. Res.* 52:352–57
15. Cherry, P. D., Furchgott, R. F., Zawadzki, J. V., Jothianandan, D. 1982. The role of endothelial cells in the relaxation of isolated arteries by bradykinin. *Proc. Natl. Acad. Sci. USA* 79:2106–10
16. Furchgott, R. F., Zawadzki, J. V. 1980. ATP relaxes rabbit aortic smooth muscle by both an indirect action via endothelial cells and a direct action. *Pharmacologist* 22:271 (Abstr.)
17. Furchgott, R. F., Erreich, S. J. Greenblatt, E. 1961. The photoactivated relaxation of smooth muscle of rabbit aorta. *J. Gen. Physiol.* 44:499–519
18. De Mey, J. G., Claeys, M., Vanhoutte, P. M. 1982. Endothelial-dependent inhibitory effects of acetylcholine, adenosine triphosphate, thrombin and arachidonic acid in the canine femoral artery. *J. Pharmacol. Exp. Ther.* 222:166–73
19. Vanhoutte, P. M. 1977. Cholinergic inhibition of adrenergic transmission. *Fed. Proc.* 36:2444–49
20. Fozard, J. 1979. Cholinergic mechanisms in adrenergic function. See Ref. 5, 1:145–95
21. Steinsland, O. S., Furchgott, R. F., Kirpekar, S. M. 1973. Inhibition of adrenergic neurotransmission by parasympathomimetics in the rabbit ear artery. *J. Pharmacol. Exp. Ther.* 184: 346–56
22. Altura, B. M., Chand, N. 1981. Bradykinin-induced relaxation of renal and pulmonary arteries is dependent upon intact endothelial cells. *Br. J. Pharmacol.* 74:10–11
23. De Mey, J. G., Vanhoutte, P. M. 1982. Heterogeneous behavior of the canine arterial and venous wall. *Circ. Res.* 51:439–47
24. De Mey, J. G., Vanhoutte, P. M. 1980. Interaction between Na$^+$, K$^+$ exchanges and the direct inhibitory effect of acetylcholine on canine femoral arteries. *Circ. Res.* 46:826–36
25. Zawadzki, J. V., Cherry, P. D., Furchgott, R. F. 1980. Comparison of endothelium-dependent relaxation of rabbit aorta by A23187 and by acetylcholine. *Pharmacologist* 22:271 (Abstr.)
26. Singer, H. A., Peach, M. H. 1982. Calcium-and endothelial-mediated vascular

smooth muscle relaxation in rabbit aorta. *Hypertension* 4 (Suppl. 2): III9–25

27. Zawadzki, J. V., Furchgott, R. F., Cherry, P. D. 1981. The obligatory role of endothelial cells in the relaxation of arterial smooth muscle by substance P. *Fed. Proc.* 40:689 (Abstr.)

28. Zawadzki, J. V., Furchgott, R. F., Cherry, P. D. 1983. Endothelium-dependent relaxation of arteries by octasubstance P, kassinin and octacholecystokinin. *Fed. Proc.* 42:619 (Abstr.)

29. Cherry, P. D., Furchgott, R. F., Zawadzki, J. V. 1981. The indirect nature of bradykinin relaxation of isolated arteries: Endothelial dependent and independent components. *Fed. Proc.* 40:689 (Abstr.)

30. Aiken, J. W. 1974. Inhibitors of prostaglandin synthesis specifically antagonize bradykinin- and angiotensin-induced relaxations of the isolated celiac artery from rabbit. *Pharmacologist* 1:295 (Abstr.)

31. Blumberg, A. L., Denny, S. E., Marshall, G. R., Needleman, P. A. 1977. Blood vessel-hormone interactions: Angiotensin, bradykinin and prostaglandin. *Am. J. Physiol.* 232:H305–10

32. Needleman, P., Marshall, G., Sobel, B. E. 1975. Hormone interactions in the isolated rabbit heart: Synthesis and coronary vasomotor effects of prostaglandins, angiotensin, and bradykinin. *Circ. Res.* 37:802–8

33. Toda, N. 1977. Actions of bradykinin on isolated cerebral and peripheral arteries. *Am. J. Physiol.* 232:H267–74

34. Cohen, R. A., Shepherd, J. T., Vanhoutte, P. M. 1983. Inhibitory role of the endothelium in the response of isolated coronary arteries to platelets. *Science* 221:273–74

35. Cohen, R. A., Shepherd, J. T., Vanhoutte, P. M., 1983. 5-hydroxytryptamine released from aggregating platelets can mediate endothelium-dependent inhibition of coronary smooth muscle. *Am. J. Physiol.* In press

36. Ku, D. 1982. Coronary vascular reactivity after acute myocardial ischemia. *Science* 218:576–78

37. Deleted in proof

38. Singer, H. A., Peach, M. J. 1983. Endothelium-dependent relaxation of rabbit aorta. I. Relaxation stimulated by arachidonic acid (AA). *J. Pharmacol. Exp. Ther.* 227:790–95

39. Cherry, P. D., Furchgott, R. F., Zawadzki, J. V. 1983. The endothelium-dependent relaxation of vascular smooth muscle by unsaturated fatty acids. *Fed. Proc.* 42:619 (Abstr.)

40. Kosower, E. M., Kosower, N. S., Faltin, Z., Diver, A., Saltoun, G., Frensdorff, A. 1974. Membrane mobility agents: A new class of biologically active molecules. *Biochim. Biophys. Acta* 363:261–66

41. Spokas, E. G., Folco, G., Quilley, J., Chandler, P., McGiff, J. C. 1983. Endothelial mechanism in the vascular action of hydralazine. *Hypertension* 5 (Suppl. 1): I104–11

42. Furchgott, R. F., Zawadzki, J. V., Jothianandan, D., Cherry, P. D. 1982. Nordihydroguiaretic acid (NDGA) and α,p-dibromoacetophenone (BPB) inhibit endothelium-dependent relaxation of arteries by acetylcholine, bradykinin and A23187. *Fed. Proc.* (Abstr.)

43. Flower, R. J. 1974. Drugs which inhibit prostaglandin biosynthesis. *Pharmacol. Rev.* 26:33–67

43a. Flower, R. J., Blackwell, G. J. 1975. The importance of phospholipase-A_2 in prostaglandin biosynthesis. *Biochem. Pharmacol.* 25:285–91

44. Singer, H. A., Peach, M. J. 1983. Endothelium-dependent relaxation of rabbit aorta. II. Inhibition of relaxation stimulated by methacholine and A23187 with antagonists of arachidonic acid metabolism. *J. Pharmacol. Exp. Ther.* 227:796–801

45. Chand, N., Altura, B. M. 1981. Inhibition of endothelial cell-dependent relaxations to acetylcholine and bradykinin by lipoxygenase inhibitors in canine isolated renal arteries. *Microcirculation* 1:211–23

46. Roberts, M. F., Deems, R. A., Mincey, T. C., Dennis, E. A. 1977. Chemical modification of the histidine residue in phospholipase A_2 (Naja naja naja). *J. Biol. Chem.* 252:2405–11

47. Gruetter, C. A., Kadowitz, P. J., Ignarro, L. F. 1981. Methylene blue inhibits coronary arterial relaxation and guanylate cyclase activation by nitroglycerin, sodium nitrite and amyl nitrite. *Can. J. Physiol. Pharmacol.* 59:150–56

48. Gruetter, C. A., Gruetter, D. Y., Lyon, J. E., Kadowitz, P. J., Ignarro, L. F. 1981. Relationship between cyclic guanosine 3':5'-monophosphate formation and relaxation of coronary arterial smooth muscle by glyceryl trinitrate, nitroprusside, nitrite and nitric oxide: Effects of methylene blue and methemoglobin. *J. Pharmacol. Exp. Ther.* 219:181–86

49. Murad, F., Arnold, W. P., Mittal, C. K., Braughler, J. M. 1979. Properties and regulation of guanylate cyclase and some

proposed functions for cyclic GMP. *Adv. Cyclic Nucleotide Res.* 11:175–204

50. Kukovetz, W. R., Pöch, G., Holzmann, S. 1981. Cyclic nucleotides and relaxation of vascular smooth muscle. See Ref. 3, pp. 339–53

51. Bowman, A., Gillespie, J. S. 1981. An erythrocyte-associated antagonist of inhibitory mechanisms in the bovine retractor penis muscle. *Br. J. Pharmacol.* 74: P181–P82

52. Carvalho, M. H., Furchgott, R. F. 1981. Vasodilation of the rabbit mesenteric vascular bed by acetylcholine and A23187. *Pharmacologist* 23:223 (Abstr.)

53. Higgs, G. A., Copp, F. C., Denyer, C. V., Flower, R. J., Tateson, J. E., Walker, J. M. G. 1978. Reduction of leukocyte migration by a cycleoxygenase inhibitor. *Abstr. 7th Int. Congr. Pharmacol.*, p. 374. Oxford: Pergamon (Abstr.)

54. Katsuki, S., Murad, F. 1977. Regulation of adenosine cyclic 3',5'-monophosphate levels and contractility in bovine tracheal smooth muscle. *Mol. Pharmacol.* 13:330–41

55. Böhme, E., Graf, H., Schultz, G. 1978. Effects of sodium nitroprusside and other smooth muscle relaxants on cyclic GMP formation in smooth muscle and platelets. *Adv. Cyclic Nucleotide Res.* 9:131–43

56. Schultz, K. D., Bohme, E., Kreye, V. W., Schultz, G. 1979. Relaxation of hormonally stimulated smooth muscular tissues by the 8-bromo derivative of cyclic GMP. *Naunyn-Schmiedeberg's Arch. Pharmacol.* 301:1–9

57. Hidaka, H., Asano, T. 1977. Stimulation of platelet guanylate cyclase by unsaturated fatty acid peroxides. *Proc. Natl. Acad. Sci. USA* 74:3657–61

58. Goldberg, N. D., Graff, G., Haddox, M. K., Stephenson, J. H., Glass, D. B., Moser, M. E. 1978. Redox modulation of splenic cell soluble guanylate cyclase activity: Activation by hydrophilic and hydrophobic antioxidants represented by ascorbic and dehydroascorbic acids, fatty acid hydroperoxides, and prostaglandin endoperoxides. *Adv. Cyclic Nucleotide Res.* 9:101–30

59. Ignarro, L. J., Lippton, H., Edwards, J. C., Baricos, W. H., Hyman, A. L., Kadowitz, P. J., Gruetter, C. A. 1981. Mechanism of vascular smooth muscle relaxation by organic nitrates, nitrites, nitroprusside and nitric oxide: Evidence for the involvement of s-nitrosothiols as active intermediates. *J. Pharmacol. Exp. Ther.* 218:739–49

60. Furchgott, R. F., Jothianandan, D. 1983. Relation of cyclic GMP levels to endothelium-dependent relaxation by acetylcholine in rabbit aorta. *Fed. Proc.* 42:619 (Abstr.)

61. Rapoport, R. M., Draznin, M. B., Murad, F. 1983. Endothelium-dependent vascular relaxation may be mediated through cyclic GMP-dependent protein phosphorylation. *Clin. Res.* 31:526A (Abstr.)

62. Rapoport, R. M., Draznin, M. B., Murad, F. 1982. Sodium nitroprusside-induced protein phosphorylation in intact rat aorta is mimicked by 8-bromo cyclic GMP. *Proc. Natl. Acad. Sci. USA* 79:6470–74

Ann. Rev. Pharmacol. Toxicol. 24:199–236
Copyright © 1984 by Annual Reviews Inc. All rights reserved

RATE-CONTROLLED DELIVERY SYSTEMS IN DRUG AND HORMONE RESEARCH

John Urquhart, John W. Fara, and Kay L. Willis

ALZA Research, Palo Alto, California 94304

INTRODUCTION

The advent of implantable devices that give long-duration control over the rate of drug or hormone administration in laboratory animals has opened up both novel and previously impractical experimental methods, protocols, and models for delivering these substances. This review brings together these new methods, protocols, and models for examination from the general perspectives of experimental pharmacology, toxicology, and physiology. They have originated in various specialized fields that infrequently cross-communicate, yet they have a common theme in the controlled deployment of bioactive agents in experimental animals. The novelty in this theme stems both from recent technological advances in drug delivery systems and from the ingenious ways in which individual researchers have put them to use. The focus here is on uses of delivery systems rather than on their technical aspects, which have been well-reviewed elsewhere (1, 2). Some history of the development of these delivery systems is pertinent, however.

Only during the past two decades have practical means existed for multiday, rate-controlled administration of drugs or hormones to both experimental animals and man. Most of the technical advances in delivery systems for clinical use, including infusion pumps, have come since 1974. Among systems for research use, little progress was made with external pumps because of the intricacies of maintaining a leak- and kink-proof flow path from a stationary pump to an uncooperatively revolving animal. An early development was the Rose-Nelson osmotic pump (3)—too bulky for rodents but small enough to be worn externally by dogs—allowing the first multiday infusions of angiotensin

199

II (4, 5). Another stage of miniaturization was needed to make implantable systems suitable for use in rats, mice, and other small laboratory animals.

The first such implants were demonstrated by Folkman & Long in 1964 (6), who showed that drug- or hormone-filled polysiloxane (SILASTIC®) capsules could provide extended-duration, rate-controlled administration of the contained substance by the process of solution diffusion (7). However, these capsules' uses are limited to substances, principally steroids, whose combination of high molar potency and solubility in polysiloxane gives them usefully high rates of release; peptides, as a rule, and many drugs lack the requisite solubility in polysiloxane, and most drugs lack the requisite molar potency.

The development of miniature implantable osmotic pumps in the mid-1970s (8) greatly expanded the range of drugs and hormones, including peptides, for which multiday constant or programmed-rate administration was possible in mice, rats, and larger animals. Osmotic pumps provide a convective stream of drug solution that can be directed through suitable catheter connections to sites in the animal remote from the pump itself, a feature that researchers have ingeniously exploited in many ways. Also in the mid-1970s Folkman & Langer reported a method of loading various agents, including peptides, in ethylene vinyl acetate copolymer pellets to achieve extended-duration release after the pellets are implanted subcutaneously or directly in various tissues, for example the cornea (9); these pellets have played an important role in studies on the biology of new vessel growth into tumors (10).

Although this review concerns drug delivery systems in animal experimentation, it is useful to note briefly recent developments in human pharmaceuticals based on drug delivery systems (11). A number of rate-controlled topical and systemic pharmaceuticals have been registered for human use. Topical products are pilocarpine in a seven-day ocular delivery system (12) and progesterone in a one-year uterine delivery system (13, 14); systemic products are oral forms of theophylline (15) and indomethacin (16, 17) and several transdermal products including three-day scopolamine (18) and one-day nitroglycerin (19, 20); a seven-day transdermal form of clonidine is in advanced clinical trials (21). Concomitantly, there has been a big increase in use of the infusion mode of intravenous drug therapy and the development of many kinds of infusion pumps and controllers for in-hospital use. Drugs that require rate-controlled intravenous (iv) infusion have begun to come into use: dopamine, dobutamine, nitroprusside, and alprostadil. An implantable pump is now in clinical use for chronic infusions (22).

Basic researchers have much more diverse needs for different agents and regimens than do clinicians. Consequently, delivery systems for basic research have been designed to facilitate use with a broad range of agents, minimizing agent-specific formulational issues. Delivery systems for basic research are in effect empty devices that, with due regard for inherent limitations of size, material incompatibilities, and agent solubility, can readily be loaded to infuse whatever agent the researcher chooses. In contrast, delivery systems-based pharmaceuticals are integral units from which it is impossible to remove the drug and substitute another without destroying the system.

This review is organized along the lines of the important new methods, protocols, and models based on delivery system use. It draws on a literature that numbers over 700 publications spanning pharmacology, toxicology, physiology, endocrinology, neural science, environmental studies, experimental psychology, and zoology. It covers literature through mid-1983.

Two Illustrative Studies

Several general principles emerge from analyzing two studies of systemic drug action. Figures 1 and 2, from the work of Smits et al (23), show the hemodynamic responses of the spontaneously hypertensive (SH) rat to propranolol given by constant-rate, five-day infusion (Figure 1) or as a single injection

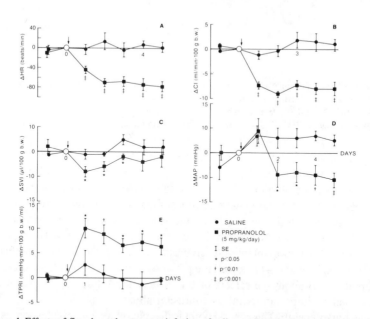

Figure 1 Effects of five-day subcutaneous infusion of saline or 5 mg/kg/day propranolol on (A) heart rate (HR), (B) cardiac index (CI), (C) stroke volume index (SVI), (D) mean arterial pressure (MAP), and (E) total peripheral resistance index (TPRI) in conscious SH rats. Data represent means ± SEM. Redrawn from (23) with permission.

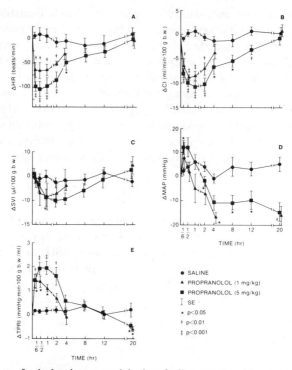

Figure 2 Effects of a single subcutaneous injection of saline, 1 mg/kg or 5 mg/kg propranolol on (A) heart rate (HR), (B) cardiac index (CI), (C) stroke volume index (SVI), (D) mean arterial pressure (MAP), and (E) total peripheral resistance index (TPRI) in conscious SH rats. Data represent means ± SEM. Redrawn from (23) with permission.

(Figure 2). As can be seen from Figure 1, it takes at least two days for the hemodynamic effects of propranolol to become fully developed and to produce the full extent of blood-pressure lowering. The constancy of hemodynamic parameters in the following days establishes that a steady state of response has been achieved after the second day of infusion. By contrast, the responses to a single dose (Figure 2) reveal a rather confusing picture, especially propranolol's clinically important hypotensive action. Using the multiday infusion method, Smits et al (24) resolved the previously conflicting evidence [see, for example, (24)] about the effects of this widely used drug in the SH rat and reconciled an important point of confusion about its validity as a model of human hypertension. The general point is that pharmacodynamic responses are not necessarily expressed completely, or even at all, within the time span of a drug's presence in the body after a single injection; continuing with the infusion until responses stabilize is basic to understanding the full range of a drug's actions.

Figure 3 shows the graded responses of urinary osmolality and volume on the

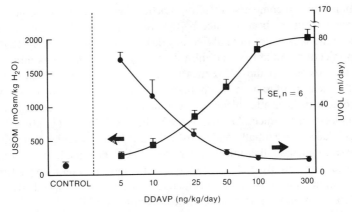

Figure 3 Responses of urine volume (U_{vol}, ●) and osmolality (U_{osm}, ■) to increasing rates of infusion of dDAVP in six rats with congenital diabetes insipidus. Data were collected on the fifth day of infusion. Redrawn from (25) with permission.

fifth day of an infusion of deamino-8-d-arginine vasopressin in rats with hereditary diabetes insipidus (25). The infusion has made the duration of action of this peptide arbitrarily long; the agent's biological activity, in the sense of its bioassay, is defined by the slopes and variances of the two infusion-rate/ response curves. Duration of action is usually regarded as a pharmacokinetic/ pharmacodynamic attribute of the drug substance, but long-duration delivery systems make duration of action a pharmaceutical attribute. Multiday infusions at a series of graded rates, as in Figure 3, appear to provide a more precise way than conventional dose-response testing of defining an agent's pharmacodynamics, a theme that recurs subsequently.

SCHEDULE- OR REGIMEN-DEPENDENCE OF THERAPEUTIC INDEX: THE INJECTION-INFUSION COMPARISON PROTOCOL

Varying the schedule, regimen, or rate of administration has a major influence on the therapeutic index of some drugs; for others, regimen has little such influence. A recently devised protocol to test for this attribute calls for comparative dose-response testing when a drug is administered by a series of injections versus by infusions, each varied over the same range of total doses, given over a fixed time period. Sikic et al devised this protocol for studies of the pharmacodynamics of bleomycin (26); it has subsequently found application with other agents and appears to be a general protocol for basic pharmacodynamic assessment.

The studies by Sikic et al with bleomycin (017) are illustrative of the injection-infusion comparison (IIC) protocol. These researchers administered bleomycin to tumor-bearing mice by three different five-day regimens, each covering the same range of total five-day dose: (*a*) an injection every 12 hours; (*b*) an injection on the first and third days only; (*c*) a continuous infusion by implanted osmotic pumps. The measure of efficacy was reduction in tumor size; the measure of toxicity was pulmonary fibrosis, assessed by hydroxyproline content of lung after bleomycin administration by the three regimens to non-tumor-bearing mice. At each of the higher total doses, the infusion regimen produced substantially and statistically significantly larger reductions in tumor size than did either injection regimen. In contrast, the infusion regimen produced substantially and statistically significantly less pulmonary fibrosis than did either injection regimen at equal total doses. The enhanced efficacy of the bleomycin infusion regimen has been confirmed (27).

The IIC protocol revealed that, in effect, the continuous infusion shifted the dose-response curve for bleomycin toxicity to the right while shifting the dose-response curve for its efficacy to the left. Thus, the therapeutic index of bleomycin in the mouse-tumor model was substantially widened by the use of the infusion regimen relative to that of either injection regimen. Subsequent clinical studies appear to confirm the extrapolation of this conclusion to humans (28, 29).

Recent work by Nau and his colleagues in Berlin (30–32) has added an important dimension to the use of the IIC protocol and the interpretation of its results. They have pointed out that many drugs have large interspecies differences in pharmacokinetics, usually with much shorter half-lives in small animals than in man; when these differences exist, rats or mice will have markedly exaggerated peak-and-trough patterns of drug concentration in plasma when drug is administered to them by once- or twice-daily injections, in contrast to much more modest fluctuations in drug concentrations in humans receiving once- or twice-daily dosing. In this circumstance, not only doses but also *dosing intervals* have to be adjusted in order to have bioequivalence between the regimen for the animal test and the regimen for human use. The work of Nau's group with valproic acid (VPA), described below, illustrates this point and its implications for the design of toxicologic tests; the terminal pharmacokinetic half-life of VPA is 8–16 hours in humans, but only about 0.8 hours in mice.

Nau et al (30) administered VPA by two different regimens in the same range of total doses to pregnant mice from day 7–15 of gestation, by once-daily injections and by constant-rate infusions from implanted osmotic pumps. With infusions, a substantially and statistically significantly higher total dose was required to produce both fetal resorptions and exencephaly than with the once-daily injections; fetal weight was adversely affected by both regimens, but the differences between the two regimens were small. In other words, the dose-response curves for both fetal death and exencephaly were shifted to the right when VPA was given by infusion versus by once-daily injection; the dose-response curve for fetal weight loss was little affected by regimen.

In these studies, VPA concentrations in plasma during the infusions were essentially constant throughout the multiday study. With the injections, drug concentrations in plasma rose and fell quickly, and from about eight hours after each daily injection VPA was undetectable in maternal plasma until the next dose was given; then the cycle repeated itself. In humans, the once-daily therapeutic regimen produces VPA concentrations whose peaks are only about one-tenth as high as those in the mouse, and thereafter decline gradually to a trough level that is not less than about one-fourth that of the peak.

Scaling doses according to body sizes can provide equal time-averaged plasma concentrations in mice and humans, but the hour-to-hour concentration-time profiles differ drastically when VPA is given on the same once-daily basis to mice and to humans: much higher peak concentrations in mice, but much higher trough concentrations in humans. Running the IIC protocol with VPA in pregnant mice amounts to comparing the embryotoxicity of high but briefly maintained peak concentrations versus that of continuously maintained concentrations at far lower levels. Interpretation of the results should consider the fact that an infusion regimen that produces constant VPA concentrations in mouse plasma is much more nearly bioequivalent to the once-daily human therapeutic regimen than is a once-daily dosing regimen in mice.

The virtual absence of VPA during about sixteen hours of each day does not offset embryotoxic effects of injected VPA. With some drugs, such long drug-free intervals—"drug holidays"—may indeed minimize toxicity and show the injection regimen to advantage. With such evidence, it may be useful to study the effects of a combined regimen of daily injections superimposed on a constant infusion, with the infusions serving to maintain certain minimum concentrations at all times. Separate adjustments of the quantities administered by each mode can provide more or less independent control over the peak-and-trough concentrations. Gentamicin is an example of a drug whose toxicity appears to be less by intermittent injections than by constant infusions (33), but there are no animal studies on the effects of a combined regimen. Such a study might help resolve some of the controversy about the appropriate upper and lower limits of gentamicin concentration in human therapeutics.

The large difference in the pharmacokinetic half-life of VPA between mice and humans is not exceptional. The problem of interspecies size- and time-scaling has recently been analyzed by Boxenbaum (34, 35), giving examples of other drugs with large interspecies differences in pharmacokinetic half-life. These are important considerations in the design of pharmacologic and toxicologic studies on small animals, where bioequivalence to the human regimen may be crucial for valid extrapolation of the animal data to humans.

Endocrine Studies with the IIC Protocol

The effects of parathyroid hormone (PTH) on bone formation and resorption have been assessed with the IIC protocol. Tam et al (36) compared the effects of bovine PTH administered by daily injections versus continuous infusions in thyroparathyroidectomized rats. PTH infusion resulted in increased bone apposition and an increase in both bone formation and resorption surfaces, with a net decrease in trabecular bone. Equal doses by injection increased bone apposition rate and bone formation surface but did not increase resorption surfaces; in this case bone volume increased. The authors conclude that the injection regimen provides a way of separating the resorptive effects of PTH from its effects on apposition rate and that intermittent doses of the hormone would be more effective than continuous infusion in promoting anabolic skeletal effects.

Podbesek et al (37, 38) obtained similar results using the IIC protocol to administer PTH to intact greyhounds and found that the injection regimen increased trabecular bone volume while the infusion decreased it. Results with the injections were in agreement with those in patients similarly treated. The authors concluded that an intermittent dosage regimen, even though it only transiently elevates PTH levels, appears more promising than the infusion regimen for the treatment of osteoporosis.

In studies of hormonal feedback in the pituitary-thyroid axis, Connors & Hedge (39) compared injections and infusions of triiodothyronine (T_3) given in graded amounts to thyroidectomized rats. When continuous infusion maintained plasma concentrations of T_3 at slightly below normal levels, thyrotropin (TSH) levels were higher than in intact rats. At higher rates of T_3 infusion plasma concentrations of T_3 were elevated further, though still in the physiological range, and TSH levels were in the normal range. When the same doses of T_3 were given by twice-daily injection, TSH fell to low levels and reduced pituitary responsiveness to thyrotropin-releasing hormone to a greater degree than did the infusion. T_3 was a more potent feedback signal when given by injections, but the more nearly physiological responses were elicited by the infusion regimen.

The growth-promoting effects of human growth hormone (hGH) on hypophysectomized rats were assessed by injections versus infusions; for equal growth responses, injections required about 1.7 times more hGH than did infusions (40).

Conclusion

The IIC protocol appears to be an important new probe in pharmacodynamic testing. As the literature shows, it is not a foregone conclusion which regimen will prove superior for a given agent. The practical significance of the IIC protocol is increased by the variety of new methods for rate-controlled drug administration to humans. If the infusion regimen proves distinctly superior in preclinical studies, there is increasing likelihood that constant-rate administration can be a practical option in therapeutics. Such was not the case a decade ago.

In toxicologic testing, the concept of interspecies bioequivalence in regimen design is new and clearly warrants broader study. A particular value of the IIC protocol may be uncovering toxicity-masking effects of drug holidays that are inescapable when short half-life drugs are given by once- or twice-daily injections. Novel delivery systems allow one to program the concentrations of test agents in plasma and other biophases of experimental animals and thereby equalize disparate pharmacokinetic half-lives. The IIC protocol is only a first step in that direction.

TISSUE MICROPERFUSION

Controlling the flow of drug solutions in the 0.5–1 µl/hour range brings a new way of localizing drug action: tissue microperfusion with drug solution via a fine-gauge cannula inserted directly into a specific tissue site, remote from the osmotic pump. Delivery systems that operate by diffusion do not provide a convective flow of drug solution and so can deliver drug only to their immediate surroundings. Thus, the delivery system and its contained drug has to be inserted into the very tissue that the experimenter seeks to modify. Sometimes that poses limiting problems, which microperfusion avoids.

Because their osmotic driving force is about 300 atm (8), the pumps are capable of delivering drug solutions into solid tissue or against arterial pressures of a few hundred millimeters of mercury without any measurable reduction of flow (41). Also, they can pump solutions directly into tissues through the smallest available cannulae and catheters without flow being impeded by the resulting back pressure. A biologically important point is that flows of 0.5–1 µl/hr appear to be low enough so that hydraulic damage and/or edema is minimal or absent in the microperfused region.

The first use of this method was to test the influence of norepinephrine on cortical neuronal plasticity. Kasamatsu and colleagues tested the hypothesis that norepinephrine regulates plasticity in a variety of ways in feline visual cortex. Microelectrodes measured neuronal firing patterns, allowing assessment of neuronal ability to change ocular dominance as vision was experimentally changed between monocular and binocular. Four important papers (42–45) from Kasamatsu's group established the following: (a) microperfusion of a field of visual cortical neurones with 6-hydroxydopamine (6-OHDA) eliminates the normal plasticity of early postnatal life; (b) microperfusion with norepinephrine of a field previously depleted of catecholamines by 6-OHDA restores the normal plasticity of early postnatal life;

(c) microperfusion with norepinephrine of a region of visual cortex in adult animals partially restores the plasticity of early postnatal life.

The stereotaxically placed cannula was connected to an osmotic pump implanted subcutaneously in the cervical region. The extent of lesion was less than 0.75 mm radius around the 26-ga cannula tip (43), whereas the extent of spread of radiolabelled norepinephrine occurred over a radius of 10 mm from the cannula tip (43, 44); the concentration of microperfused drug was always highest in tissue immediately adjacent to the cannula tip, declined exponentially, and asymptotically approached the background level at distances beyond 10 mm from the cannula tip. Measurements of neuronal electrical activity were routinely made at two mm from the cannula tip, well outside the area of mechanical (or chemical) lesion but near enough to the cannula tip so that the concentration of test agent was about two orders of magnitude higher than that found beyond the microperfused zone.

The 26-ga cannula used by Kasamatsu et al is unnecessarily large; it has an internal diameter (ID) of 254 microns. In microperfusion of rat hypothalamus with labelled amino acids, 30-ga needles (152 microns ID) were used satisfactorily (46), and in rat renal artery infusions plastic tubing with 100 micron ID was satisfactorily used (41). Perhaps a smaller cannula would have lessened the pericannular lesion. Also, Kasamatsu's group used isotonic saline as the perfusion vehicle, which is irritating, as will be apparent to anyone placing a drop of isotonic saline on the surface of the eye, in contrast to Ringer's or other solutions whose ionic compositions approximate that of extracellular or cerebrospinal fluid. Nevertheless, these methodologic fine points cannot detract from the conceptual and technical elegance of the experiments of Kasamatsu and his colleagues. The critical capability that opened up this new line of neurophysiologic/pharmacologic investigation is the nearly atraumatic, direct microperfusion of cortical tissue, allowing direct control over local tissue concentrations of test substances and straightforward within-animal control procedures.

Other laboratories have adopted Kasamatsu's methods, adding further information: Bear et al (47) showed that only microperfused but not systemically administered 6-OHDA is effective in reversing the neuronal plasticity of early postnatal life; Daw et al (48) confirmed Kasamatsu's findings and added the observation that plasticity in directionally sensitive visual cortical cells responds in a qualitatively similar manner to those involved in the monocular/binocular dominance shift; McCall et al (49) showed that chronic intracerebroventricular infusion (icv) of lysergic acid diethylamide influences binocular/monocular shift in the same way as does microperfused norepinephrine.

Mangano & Schwarcz (50) compared the size and nature of local lesions around cannula tips through which solutions of excitatory amino acids were either injected or continuously microinfused. They compared two weeks of 12–hourly 0.5 µl injections with two weeks of continuous infusion of glutamic, aspartic, and cysteine sulfinic acids at 0.5 µl/hour into rat striatum or hippocampus. The injections produced lesions of about 0.5 mm radius around the cannula tip, whereas no lesions occurred with the infusions. The authors concluded that very efficient mechanisms for the cellular uptake of the amino acids exist for protecting neurones against their toxic effects but that the uptake processes appear to have been saturated by the injections, suggesting a model for the neuronal damage in Huntington's disease.

Other CNS microperfusion studies include one-week microperfusion of glucose into basal ventromedial hypothalamus, effecting a 27% reduction in food intake (51); angiotensin II into the olfactory bulb, causing increased nocturnal water intake (52, 53); amphetamine into the caudate-putamen, causing a form of behavioral toxicity that suggests the occurrence of a local lesion, although no demonstrable anatomic lesion could be found at the cannula site (54); dopamine into the nucleus accumbens, producing hyperactive behavior that persisted throughout the fourteen-day microperfusion and for several weeks thereafter (55–57); labelled amino acid precursors into rat hypothalamus (46, 58) and striatonigral tract (59).

Kroin & Penn (60) studied the spatial concentration gradients of cisplatin in brain tissue around a microperfusion cannula. They showed that a platinum concentration of >2 ng/mg can be maintained throughout a 1 cm diameter sphere of tissue. If all the measured platinum were in the form of cisplatin, the observed minimum tissue concentration would lie within the apparent therapeutic concentration range. Kroin & Penn suggested that the microperfusion technique might be used to treat tumors up to 1 cm in size, with multiple cannula-pump units required for larger tumors. Their suggestion warrants further research in animal models of human brain disease in which there are large unmet therapeutic needs, e.g. neoplasms and focal epilepsy, where problems of passage through the blood-brain barrier may be limiting and chemical structural modifications of drugs [see, for example, (61)] to achieve penetration of the blood-brain barrier may not be possible.

Another application of tissue microperfusion has been in the study of trophic influences of nerve activity on skeletal muscle. Drachman et al (62, 63) microperfused rat soleus muscle with α-bungarotoxin in order to effect continuous blockade of acetylcholine at the neuromuscular junction. Microinjection methods had been unsuccessful in getting either the completeness or the continuity of blockade needed to evaluate the role of acetylcholine in neurotrophic regulation of skeletal muscle. Microperfusion established persistent, complete blockade of acetylcholine transmission, evidenced by the complete absence of miniature end-plate potentials and the absence of both electrophysiologic and mechanical response to motor-nerve stimulation. There was no evidence of either histologic or ultrastructural damage to motor-nerve terminals in the microperfused region. This technique allowed Drachman et al to show that blockade of acetylcholine transmission produces changes in resting membrane potential and extrajunctional acetylcholine receptors that are quantitatively equivalent to those of surgical denervation, both in respect to time course of onset and the extent of the fully developed changes. This work supports the conclusion that acetylcholine release, both impulse-related and spontaneous quantal and nonquantal release, is the neurotrophic influence and that loss of postulated other neurotrophic factors is not necessary to account for muscle atrophy after denervation.

Eliason & Maurice (64) described microperfusion of various parts of the rabbit eye, including the corneal stroma. Chappel and colleagues (65) used the microperfusion method to overcome a long-standing point of confusion about whether the site of estradiol feedback action is the anterior pituitary or the hypothalamus.

An important variant of the tissue microperfusion method is the implantation of drug-releasing ethylene vinyl acetate (EVA) copolymer pellets directly in tissue to be studied. The preparation of such pellets has been described by Langer & Folkman (9); they have been used by Folkman and his colleagues in studies of the biology of angiogenesis, the new blood-vessel growth essential to supporting the growth of tumors beyond the few millimeters through which their metabolic needs can be met by diffusion alone. Heparin delivered by EVA pellets is a promoter of angiogenesis and protamine is an inhibitor (66), but heparin or heparin fragments plus cortisone are profound inhibitors of angiogenesis, both locally and, in sufficient doses, systemically (10).

Another variant of the microperfusion method is to infuse blocking or anesthetic agents into special perineural cuffs that bring the drug solution into close contact with the nerve surface. In this manner, Lorkovic (67) obtained motor-nerve transmission blockade with lidocaine and marcaine for 3–7 days, with denervation-like supersensitivity to acetylcholine in muscle innervated by the blocked nerve. Betz and colleagues (68) used this technique with tetrodotoxin to block nerve conduction for 5–13 days without evidence of nerve damage in a study of the factors that can lead to the sprouting of active nerve terminals in muscle.

Another variant of the tissue microperfusion method is an arrangement for the local delivery of substances to the experimentally injured or transected spinal cord in rats (69). A PE10 catheter was positioned over a gelatin sponge pledget that in turn overlay the damaged region of spinal cord; the catheter was supplied by a subcutaneously implanted osmotic pump so that the infusate entered the gelatin sponge and thus had some manner of access to the injury site.

TOLERANCE AND DEPENDENCE

It is well known that repeated administration of many agents can produce tolerance, subsensitivity, or tachyphylaxis to the test agent; if the agent is withheld or if an antagonist is given, a withdrawal syndrome may ensue. It is widely assumed that continuous presence of the test substance will favor development of tolerance, subsensitivity, or tachyphylaxis. Hence, implantable drug delivery systems have found considerable use with a variety of agents in studies on the development or modulation of tolerance and dependence. Whether or not the assumption is valid that constant-rate infusion is always the surest path to tolerance is another question, one that might be advantageously tested with the IIC protocol.

A multiday infusion of sodium barbital in mice produced tolerance, as shown by a significant decrease in sleep time following a challenge dose of barbital 24 hours after cessation of the infusion; physical dependence was demonstrated either by responses to pentylenetetrazol or by convulsions elicited by handling (70). Tabakoff et al (71) infused phenobarbital icv in rats for 72 hours and then removed the pumps; 24 hours later a challenge dose of pentobarbital was given to demonstrate tolerance. Selective destruction of noradrenergic neurons by icv 6-OHDA or by specific lesions of the dorsal or ventral noradrenergic bundles prevented the development of barbiturate tolerance without altering the animal's response to acute barbiturate.

Wei & Loh first demonstrated that physical dependence is a concomitant of centrally acting opiate-like peptides (72). Using multiday infusions of the agents into periaqueductal grey, they resolved the previous confusion about the central actions of these agents that had arisen from contradictory studies with single central injections. Similarly, physical dependence to a whole series of opiate-like peptides has been demonstrated by Wei (73).

A chronically infused, ACTH-related peptide inhibited the formation of tolerance to infused morphine (74). Chronic spinal infusions have been used to demonstrate partial cross-tolerance between an enkephalin and morphine at the spinal level (75, 76).

Another variation in the use of implantable delivery systems in opiate receptor studies is the chronic exposure of animals to a test agent and the subsequent removal of organs from those animals to study mechanisms of tolerance and dependence. This is illustrated by studies from the Max Planck-Munich group of Schulz, Wuster, Herz, and others in which guinea pigs were continuously infused with specific opiates by seven-day delivery from implanted osmotic pumps; subsequently, the animals were sacrificed and the ileum of each was removed for in vitro organ bath studies of cross-tolerance (77, 78). Similar methods have been employed by the same group to study the development of differential tolerance and cross-tolerance in opiate receptors in other tissues (79–87).

Hetta & Terenius (88) demonstrated that multiday maternal infusion of naloxone significantly increased neonatal mortality. Moreover, the young exposed to naloxone in utero showed no significant analgesic response to morphine until 40 days of age.

Implanted pellets of morphine have long been used to maintain the continuous presence of morphine in experimental animals, but the uniformity of morphine-release kinetics has been an unknown since the pellets are made on a small scale in many laboratories. Also, the field of opiate receptor pharmacology now involves many agents besides morphine, not all of which are readily formed into slow-release pellets by simple methods. Thus, it is likely that kinetically validated delivery system implants will gradually replace drug pellets in quantitative studies of opiate receptors and their regulation, as has largely happened in the study of hormone-receptor regulation.

In studies of ethanol dependency, using delivery systems to maintain chronic icv infusions has permitted several new approaches. Volicer et al (89) studied the comparative effects of chronic icv infusion of calcium and a chelator on alcohol dependence and tolerance. Rigter et al (90) demonstrated that vasopressin fragments were capable of enhancing both ethanol dependence and its withdrawal syndrome. Tuomisto et al (91) showed that fourteen-day icv infusions of tetrahydro-β-carbolines in rats substantially increased voluntary alcohol intake, an effect that took more than a week to develop.

Finally, the development of tolerance to chronic treatment with many other agents, including dermorphins (92), d-amphetamine (93), phencyclidine (94), and α- and β-agonists (95) has been studied using periods of chronic infusion of the test agent.

Studies on Receptor Regulation

In this field, delivery systems have been employed to ensure the continuous presence of many different drugs, hormones, and humoral substances at various pre-selected levels. This approach has been used particularly to study receptors for angiotensin II and gonadotropin-releasing hormone (GnRH) as well as for other agents, as is summarized in Table 1.

RATE-CONTROLLED MODULATION OF HORMONE LEVELS

Two major uses of both polysiloxane capsules and osmotic pumps have been to provide a constant background of hormone replacement after removal of the endogenous source of hormone and to maintain continuously high hormone levels. The capsules have been mainly used with estradiol and other steroids for reasons stated earlier.

Knobil and associates (117) mapped the effect of different rates of estradiol

Table 1 Receptor regulation studies done by chronically exposing animals and tissues to test agents delivered via implanted delivery systems

Receptors	Agents delivered	References
Response is to increase receptor population (up-regulation):		
Adrenal angiotensin II	Angiotensin II	96–98
Uterine myometrium angiotensin II	Angiotensin II	99
Pituitary GnRH	GnRH (low dose)	100
Brain opiate	Naltrexone	101
Brain cholecystokinin	Haloperidol	102
Brain dopamine	Prolactin	103
Liver estrogen	Growth hormone	104
Testicular LH	Luteinizing hormone	105
Testicular prolactin	Luteinizing hormone	105
Hepatic prolactin	Growth hormone	106
Lymphocytes-adrenergic	Propranolol	107
Cardiac-adrenergic	Propranolol	107
Lung-adrenergic	Propranolol	107
Hepatic growth hormone and prolactin	Growth hormone	108
Response is to decrease receptor population (down-regulation):		
Pituitary GnRH	GnRH (high dose)	100, 109
	Buserelin	110
Ovarian GnRH	GnRH	111
Testicular LH/hCG	GnRH	112
Cardiac β-adrenoceptors	Isoproterenol and norepinephrine	113
	Isoproterenol	114
Brain α_2-adrenoceptors	Clorgyline	115–116

administration on this hormone's feedback control of gonadotropin secretion, revealing the essential quantitative features of how estradiol can act at times to inhibit gonadotropin secretion but at other times to stimulate it. This work laid the foundation for the subsequent discovery of the integrative mechanisms that control ovulation and the menstrual cycle in man and other primates (118). Having control over the rate, as well as the quantity, of estradiol administration, was essential in resolving the confusion inherent in the sometimes-negative, sometimes-positive feedback actions of estradiol.

Another artful use of steroid-releasing polysiloxane capsule implants is the work of Ewing et al, who showed how graded rates of testosterone release could progressively inhibit spermatogenesis in rabbits (119) and monkeys (120) via dose-rate dependent inhibition of pituitary secretion of luteinizing hormone (LH). In the rabbit, but not in the monkey, it was possible to define a rate of testosterone release that totally suppressed spermatogenesis; however, still higher rates of testosterone release produced dose-rate dependent stimulation of spermatogenesis via a direct testicular effect of the steroid (119–120).

Inability to achieve complete suppression of spermatogenesis in the monkey appears to result because the direct stimulatory effect of testosterone on spermatogenesis occurs at a testosterone dose-rate insufficient to give complete suppression of pituitary LH secretion (120), thereby thwarting the hope that rate-controlled testosterone administration might provide a basis for hormonal contraception in males. Subsequent work has focused on the combined effects of testosterone and estradiol on the inhibition of spermatogenesis (121–122). The paradoxical effects of testosterone only became definable and understandable when the hormone was administered in a rate-controlled manner.

In the absence of endogenous hormone, multiday, rate-controlled replacement at varying rates allows one to probe the adequacy of regimens of hormone replacement. Considerable work has been done with the peptide hormones, whose generally very short half-lives virtually mandate either continuous infusions or very frequent injections in order to achieve chronicity of action, and in some instances any action at all.

The infusion mode has been used to assess effective replacement rates of aldosterone in the rat (123); angiotensin II during captopril blockade in the rat (124–125); insulin in the mouse (126), rat (127), and hamster (128–129); and vasopressin in the Brattleboro rat (130–133). The euglycemic replacement rate of insulin normalized the uterine growth response to estradiol (134), ameliorated proteinuria (135), and normalized gut sterol synthesis (136) in diabetic rats. Hyperinsulinemia has been maintained for as long as eight months by successive osmotic pump implants in a study of sucrose- versus starch-fed rats (137); other metabolic studies (138–140) have used shorter-duration maintenance of hyperinsulinemia. Multiday infusions of aldosterone for 1–4 weeks produced supraphysiologic levels of this steroid and demonstrated its hypertensive effect (141–143) and associated changes of ion transport in arterial walls (141–142). Multiday infusions of glucagon in rats mimicked the effects on hepatic urea cycle enzymes of high-protein intake (144). Multiday infusions of growth hormone induced feminization of hepatic steroid metabolism in an infusion-rate–related manner in the rat (145–148) but to elicit this action by injections required three- or six-hourly injections, whereas twelve-hourly injections were ineffective (148).

Certain assumptions underlie the use of constant-rate parenteral infusion of a single hormone to substitute for an intact gland. With insulin, for example, none of the published studies utilize intraportal infusion to mimic the intraportal secretion of insulin. Intraperitoneal (ip) placement of the delivery system is an uncertain method of approximating intraportal infusion, for some of the released agent may be absorbed across parietal peritoneum into the systemic circulation or across visceral peritoneum into the portal; the ceaseless motions of the viscera invalidate any assumption of constant fractions of ip-administered agent being absorbed by the two routes.

Another assumption is the use of constant-rate replacement to approximate the function of those glands whose secretions have clearly established rhythmic patterns—infradian, circadian, supradian. Fortunately, the constant-rate osmotic pumps can be adapted to deliver test agents in a preprogrammed rhythmic pattern, as Lynch et al (149–150) have elegantly demonstrated with circadian variations in the rate of melatonin infusions (see below). However, evaluation of the significance of rhythmic patterns of hormone secretion/replacement remains an underdeveloped area of research with the notable exception of GnRH, whose physiologic actions depend so clearly on a pulsatile pattern of secretion/replacement (118). As noted earlier, Connors & Hedge (39, 151–152) compared the effectiveness of periodic versus continuous replacement of thyroid hormones as feedback inhibitors of TSH secretion.

Multiday infusions introduce a new type of hormone bioassay; the hormone's actions are assessed in a broader context and over a longer period of time than in the conventional single-dose hormone bioassay. For example, Patel's study (127) of insulin replacement regimens in streptozotocin-diabetic rats spanned 60–80 days, with repeated replacement of two-week duration osmotic pumps. Such experiments call for careful attention to detail, as illustrated by contrasting the design of Patel's study with that of Lopaschuk and colleagues (153), whose work virtually catalogs the technical problems that can confuse the assessment of continuous administration of a peptide hormone for even as short a time as seven days.

Technical Considerations

Important technical considerations in the rate-controlled modulation of hormone levels are: (*a*) to avoid infection at the implantation sites, a special problem in diabetic animals though rarely one in normals. Infected implantation sites may not be purulent and may only show serous or serosanguinous fluid between the implant and a surrounding capsule; (*b*) to formulate the vehicle so as to insure its physical and chemical stability within the delivery system throughout the infusion period; (*c*) to monitor physiologic responses to the infusions at reasonable intervals and to establish with objective evidence, rather than casual surmise, the basis for time-varying responses during a supposedly constant infusion.

With respect to the last point, there are now many proven examples of receptor down-regulation or fade during constant infusions (see above); however, an initially high response that subsequently fades during a presumed constant infusion may be due to: (*a*) decline in infusion rate due to changes in delivery system performance, instability of the agent within the reservoir of the delivery system, or binding of the agent to the delivery system reservoir or infusion tubing; (*b*) changes in pharmacokinetic clearance of the infused agent; (*c*) pharmacodynamic changes, such as receptor "fade." Documentation of the plasma concentration of the infused agent is a logical first step in understanding which of these various mechanisms may be operating. Any peptide solution prepared for chronic infusion has to be regarded as an excellent microbiological growth medium and so should be formulated and handled with strict aseptic technique, with careful consideration given to including an established preservative or other anti-microbial agent in the formulation.

A special problem with insulin is the tendency for solutions of the hormone to aggregate within the reservoir of delivery systems; Grodsky and his colleagues have reported that the inclusion of dicarboxylic acids in the vehicle can prevent aggregation (154). A special problem with parathyroid hormone is its propensity to bind to polymeric surfaces, including those within the osmotic pumps. This problem can be prevented by siliconizing the pumps and any catheters used with them (155).

Use of Delivery Systems to Assess Biological Activities of Hormones and Hormonal Metabolites or Analogs

The use of continuous delivery as the basis for bioassay of estrogenic activities has been explored by Martucci & Fishman (156–157), who assessed the comparative uterotropic activities of 2- , 4- , and 16-hydroxylated metabolites of estradiol in the rat. In prior work, paraffin pellet implants had been used to provide multiday delivery, but Martucci & Fishman had found too much uncertainty in the kinetics of release from the pellets. Using implanted osmotic pumps, these workers showed a sustained uterotropic action of the 4- and 16-hydroxylated metabolites, a short-lived uterotropic activity of 2-hydroxyestradiol, and the ability of 2-hydroxyestrone to increase plasma LH concentrations. These results were confirmed by Ball et al (158–159). A noteworthy point about these multiday infusions of catecholestrogens was their ability to discriminate short-lived versus sustained uterotropic activity.

Naish & Ball (160) examined the effects of estradiol and of 2- and 4-hydroxyestradiol on lordosis behavior in ovariectomized rats, comparing a 2-bolus intravenous injection regimen versus a seven-day subcutaneous infusion from implanted osmotic pumps. For equivalent lordotic responses, it required about one-fiftieth or less the amount of estradiol with the infusion regimen compared to the 2-bolus regimen. For 4-hydroxyestradiol, which also had lordosis-inducing activity, the infusion dose required was about one-tenth that of the bolus regimen. The 2-hydroxy metabolite was without lordosis-inducing activity and did not manifest any inhibitory effect on the activities of either estradiol or 4-hydroxyestradiol. Jellinck et al (161–162) showed the infusion-rate dependent series of biochemical, hormonal, and behavioral effects of estradiol in comparison to those of the 2- and 4-hydroxy metabolites and their differential minimum effective rates for the same biochemical effects in different tissues.

Multiday infusion appears to be a more sensitive method to detect biological activity than the conventional one- or two-injection approach. Another example of this principle is the several hundred-fold greater sensitivity in the response of striatal dopamine receptors to prolactin given by 7–8 day infusion versus 4–6 days of daily injections (163).

The infusion mode may be an important means of testing peptide factors of cellular origin, whose often rapid inactivation makes almost mandatory the use of continuous methods of administration to give the fullest opportunity for expression of biological effects. Some such work has already been reported (164–166).

FETAL DRUG DELIVERY

Fetal hyperinsulinism has been induced in the monkey (167–168) and in the pig (140) by direct implantation of osmotic pumps in the respective fetuses. In both species, fetal growth was normal. Hyperthyroidism has been induced in fetal lambs by chronic infusion of T_3 from fetally implanted osmotic pumps (169–170).

LABELLING STUDIES

^{3}H-thymidine, bromodeoxyuridine, and other radiolabelled metabolic substrates are well-established tools for assessing various aspects of cell turnover. When such substances are administered by single injection, however, the extent of their ensuing incorporation into cellular constituents depends on the turnover of the structure of interest. When turnover is slow, a single injection may not suffice to give adequate labelling and so a schedule of chronic administration of the labelling agent is needed. Repeated injections are an obvious possibility, but the stress of frequent handling can have major effects (171). For these reasons, a number of workers have adopted the use of the continuous infusion technique, using implanted osmotic pumps.

Table 2 indicates the range of applications of labelling studies with ^{3}H-thymidine. The majority of the tissues studied showed low rates of cell turnover, but with the continuing presence of the labelled nucleotide extensive labelling was eventually obtained. In the multiweek studies, animals were reimplanted with fresh one- or two-week duration osmotic pumps.

Bromodeoxyuridine infusions for 1–3 weeks have been reported (179–180), but to date no one has undertaken a formal comparison of the osmotic pump implant with the compressed tablet implant, whose kinetics of release may be capricious and subject to minor variations in formulation and tabletting parameters, as has been observed with compressed tablets in pharmaceutical manufacturing.

Table 2 Tissue labelling after multiday infusions of ^{3}H-thymidine

Species tissue	Duration of infusion	Route	Greatest incorporation	Reference
Hamster/periodontal ligament	6 weeks	IP	47	172
Rat/9L brain tumor	34 hours	SC	43	173
Rat/mammary gland	5 days	IP	80 (young rats); 0 (old rats)	174
liver			53	
intestine			95	
Mouse/lung parenchyma	12 days	IP	40	175
Rat/kidney	7 days	SC	?	176
Mouse/corpus callosum	7 days	SC	40 (subependymal cells) 2 (glia)	177
Mouse/vomeronasal organ	12 days	IP	17	178

Direct-tissue microperfusions with labelled amino acids have demonstrated in vivo synthesis of gonadotropin-releasing hormone from the preoptic area of rat hypothalamus (46) opiomelanocortin from the periarcuate region of rat hypothalamus (58), substance P from rat striatonigral tract (59) and melanotropins from pars intermedia of the amphibian *Xenopus laevis* (181).

Direct-tissue microperfusion with labelled precursors is a powerful and potentially widely applicable method for demonstrating the in vivo synthetic activity of a tissue and, of course, circumstances of activated synthesis. The ability of the microperfusion method to maintain a localized pool of radiolabelled precursor/substrate within a few millimeters of the cannula tip (see above) suggests novel experimental approaches, especially in brain biochemistry.

DO DELIVERY SYSTEMS INCREASE OR DECREASE THE STRESS OF DOSING?

Parenteral administration of bioactive agents to experimental animals requires that the animals be handled, except when the agent can be given by inhalation of ambient air. Unless the animal is domesticated or has received prior training, handling induces tachycardia, acute release of several pituitary hormones—including growth hormone, ACTH, and vasopressin—and usually either aggressive or escape-directed behavior. Adding agents to food or drinking water are ways to avoid repetitive gavage and are used when it is technically possible to do so, and when the imprecision inherent in coupling dosing to appetitive behavior is judged less important than the problems posed by frequent handling.

Delivery systems can reduce handling to once every one, two, or four weeks but they add the need for anesthesia and surgery. Subcutaneous implantation is a minor procedure in an animal that is large relative to the implant, but has to be considered more of a major procedure when the creation of a subcutaneous pocket for the implant involves a tenth or more of the animal's surface area, as it may in the smallest animals. Intraperitoneal implantation can be done through a keyhole incision, avoiding handling of the viscera, but if the peritoneal cavity is opened widely and the viscera handled, there will usually be one or more post-operative days of diminished food intake and deviation from the normal growth curve. Additional procedures, such as leading catheters from the implant to veins, arteries, cerebral ventricles, or the gut lumen, may lengthen the time until food intake is normal and body weight resumes its expected time course. The focus on food intake and body weight as integrated measures of surgical stress reflects clinical judgment above the close interrelations among well-being, appetitive behavior, nutrition, and growth.

Not all stress is surgical nor does all stress manifest itself in diminished food intake and impaired growth. Nontraumatic stress has unfortunately to be described in anecdotal rather than analytical terms. Handling of animals, subjecting them to frequent injections, or restraining them during infusions can all introduce stress into experimental protocols. The usual means of controlling the experiment is to administer only a vehicle to animals selected from the same group as those receiving the test agent, using the same regimen and procedures in both groups. This procedure reveals the effects of the test agent in stressed animals but does not eliminate stress. Therefore, stress is an unintended variable in many studies and is sometimes a confounding one also.

An illustrative and cautionary example is the work of Riley (171), who showed that the appearance of mammary tumors in female mice of the C3H He strain carrying an oncogenic virus was markedly accelerated by a variety of stressful factors, including frequent handling. Embryotoxicity can be enhanced by extra handling of pregnant mice (H. Nau, unpublished observations). A less obvious factor is the possible interaction between stress-related hormonal changes and the agent being administered.

Reported experiences with delivery systems in relation to stress are numerous, mostly anecdotal, but uniform in concluding that neither implantation nor other procedures accompanying implant use appeared stressful (46, 60, 69, 110, 132, 172, 182–183). Most of these studies lasted for 1–2 weeks, but several longer studies, with successive reimplantations, have been performed and assessed from the point of view of the stress involved. De la Torre & Gonzalez-Carvajal (69) have infused several agents to the spinal cord of rats via osmotic pumps for as long as sixteen weeks, reporting that there were no evident adverse effects on the rats. Akhtar et al (110) reported normal body weight and no adverse effects in monkeys over a 20–week period during which these delivery devices were replaced weekly.

The most searching probe of the possible stress associated with implant use has been done by DeLuca and his colleagues in connection with their studies (183) on 20–week infusions of vitamin D metabolites in D-deficient female rats from weaning through a complete reproductive cycle and lactation. The animals were ether-anesthetized every two weeks for osmotic pump replacement. Some of the animals in the study received vitamin D metabolites orally on a thrice-weekly schedule. The maternal growth rates, pregnancy rates, birth rates, litter sizes, litter weights, pup survivorships, and pup weight gains during lactation were comparable between the orally treated and implant-treated animals and compare favorably with normal rats. The only observed difference was that half the animals receiving 25-hydroxyvitamin D_3 by implant had irregular estrous cycles versus one-fourth among those receiving the same agent orally; however, only one-fourth the group receiving the 1,25-dihydroxyvitamin D_3 by implant had irregular estrous cycles, so it is not evident that repetitive implantation alone had an adverse effect on estrous cycling. The authors concluded from the evident normality of growth, reproductive, and nurturing parameters that the removal and reimplantation of the osmotic pumps every other week "did not place a significant stress on the animals" (183).

It appears that delivery system implants can be used on a long-term basis with little or no adverse impact on the experimental animal from the presence of the implant or the procedures for placing it, provided the procedures are done with reasonable skill. It seems that delivery systems add little to the stress of dosing and may be a lower-stress alternative to frequent injections or gavage.

INTRA-ARTERIAL INFUSION

Smits and his colleagues in Maastricht have developed a method for chronic infusion into the rat renal artery (41). Despite the technical obstacles posed by the small size of this vessel and its branches, the rat offers the advantage of uniform pathophysiologic parameters within various strains, plus use of the SH rat model of human hypertension.

Obstruction of renal blood flow was avoided by cannulating the right suprarenal artery and passing the cannula retrogradely so its tip lay at the entrance to the right suprarenal from the right renal artery; the opposite end of the cannula was attached via a larger-bore catheter to an osmotic pump subcutaneously implanted in the neck. Clearance studies (41) showed that the procedures had no adverse effect on right renal function in chronically leftnephrectomized animals during infusion with isotonic saline; the 1 μl/hour infusion rate contrasted with renal plasma flows of about 400 ml/hour.

The first published experimental work with this new method showed the hemodynamic consequences of renal arterial infusion of norepinephrine in normotensive rats: mild hypertension, elevated total peripheral resistance, and slightly diminished cardiac output—all dose-rate dependent—plus a dose-rate–independent, relative bradycardia (184). Many intriguing studies of nephrogenic reflex and humoral mechanisms in normal and SH rats are now possible, and one can anticipate many publications from both the Maastricht group and other laboratories that have adopted their method.

CIRCADIAN RHYTHMS AND OTHER PATTERNED DRUG REGIMENS

Either constancy or gradual decline of rate are characteristic of the four mechanisms used to date in implanted delivery systems: solution diffusion, osmosis, thermally generated vapor pressure, and dissolution. Hence, an additional mechanism is required in order to generate on-off or otherwise oscillatory patterns of release of active agent.

One ingenious solution to the problem of converting constant flow from an implanted pump into a circadian on-off pattern of drug delivery has been provided by Lynch et al (149–150) at MIT. To implanted osmotic pumps they attached a long, narrow-bore polyethylene catheter, carefully filled with an alternating sequence of vehicle and drug solution; the long catheter was formed in a tight coil so that when implanted it occupied about the same amount of space as the osmotic pump to which it was attached. The constant flow from the osmotic pump into the coil displaced the coil's contents from its opposite end, thus putting an alternating sequence of drug solution and vehicle into the animal. The MIT group have used this method to infuse melatonin according to a circadian pattern and have validated it by measuring the temporal patterns of urinary excretion of melatonin and a dye added to one of the two solutions sequenced in the infusion coil. Ewing et al (185) have used this method to produce 0.5 hour pulses of LH and other pituitary hormones every two hours, in order to mimic the pulsatile pattern of LH secretion in the rat (186).

Patterned administration of certain hormones has only recently been recognized to be fundamental to expression of their physiological activities. The work by Knobil and colleagues (118) with GnRH has introduced an entirely new concept to the dynamics of hormone action: using an on-off pattern of delivery, they demonstrated that the physiologic actions of GnRH, and attempts to mimic those actions in therapy, depend on the frequency and amplitude of its administration. Neither dose nor fixed rate provides a basis for expressing this hormone's actions. Such results should stimulate the explorations of time-varied patterns in the administration of many other biological substances to determine the extent to which their actions depend on frequency or amplitude of administration.

In a somewhat different experimental approach to circadian rhythms, other investigators have employed constant-rate infusions to influence the characteristics of physiologic rhythms. For example, Nakagawa (187) infused insulin continuously into various regions of the brain to investigate the role of this substance and that of carbohydrate metabolism in the generation of the circadian feeding rhythm in rats. Other investigators have continuously infused anti-depressant drugs to study their influence on the rest-activity cycle of female hamsters (188–189); for example, multiday infusion of clorgyline lengthens the circadian rest activity cycle (189). Additionally, infusion of clorgyline or imipramine for two weeks was found to induce dissociation of many of the components of the circadian activity rhythm (189), suggesting that chronic use of agents of this nature can modify circadian frequency and/or coupling between circadian rhythms.

Thus, novel delivery systems bring new capabilities to the study of biorhythms. In addition to the programmed coil method of the MIT group, it is useful to recall that the combination of injections and infusions can in principle give quite varied patterns, though if injections have to be very frequent handling stress may be a problem. Future technical advances in delivery-system design may bring versatile rate-programming capability in implantable delivery systems—and indeed some intriguing research indicates that external magnetic fields may be one means of programming rate (190)—but complex rate programs are thus far a very minor theme in pharmacology, though a growing one in endocrinology.

ENVIRONMENTAL STUDIES

Doherty, Ferm, & Smith (191) have called attention to the utility of chronic infusions as a model for environmental exposures. They studied the toxicity of chronically infused sodium cyanide to mimic the metabolism of nitriles or other cyanogenic agents. They found a narrow, steep relation between infusion rate and the appearance of teratogenic effects in pregnant hamsters; the evident minimum effective rate for teratogenicity is 95% of the rate that produces uniform fetal death and significant signs of maternal toxicity. It is doubtful that an injection regimen could have revealed this narrow range in which cyanide is teratogenic but not lethal. This is not an academic point because of the relative constancy of cyanide release from some aliphatic nitriles and amygdalin [see, for example, (191)]. For analogous reasons, Johnson & Foulkes used cadmium infusions instead of bolus injections to approximate better the time course of cadmium ingestion via the diet (192).

DELIVERY SYSTEMS IN PHARMACOKINETIC STUDIES

The measurement of the total clearance of drug is simplified when measurements can be made in the steady state attained when constant-rate infusion of drug has been maintained for longer than 4–5 times the drug's terminal half-life (193). This is a useful approach when studies on small animals preclude the multiple blood samples required for pharmacokinetic characterization of drugs administered by injection or other bolus mode, as illustrated by the studies of Betlach & Tozer on genetic variations in theophylline biodisposition in mice (194–195) and the study of the steady-state tissue distribution of propranolol and its metabolites in the rat (196–197). The infusion mode is also useful to detect and characterize relatively slowly occurring changes in drug metabolism, e.g. those due to diurnal variations (198), those due to autoinduction as seen during continuous administration of phenobarbital in the rat (199), or those due to autoinhibition, as occurs during continuous administration of haloperidol in the rat (200) or p-chloroamphetamine in the mouse (201). The infusion mode also simplifies the study of spatial gradients in drug concentration within the body (193), as illustrated by work in rats on propranolol in various tissues (196–197) and on gentamicin in perilymph and endolymph (202–203).

REBOUND PHENOMENA AFTER WITHDRAWAL OF ANTIHYPERTENSIVE DRUGS

Thoolen et al have developed an animal model for the study of the withdrawal syndrome that occurs upon ceasing chronic administration of clonidine and other centrally acting α-agonist drugs. In a series of papers (204–209) they have established that the abrupt cessation of a 12–day infusion of clonidine leads to a several-day period of tachycardia and to a peculiar cyclic variation of arterial blood pressure: 3–6 minute episodes of 30–50 mm Hg elevations in arterial pressure, 7–8 times per hour, for 24–36 hours after cessation of the drug infusion. These findings have been confirmed (210). The infusion rate used by Thoolen and colleagues reduced blood pressure in the SH rat but had no effect on blood pressure in normal rats, yet the heart rate and blood pressure responses after cessation of the infusion were similar in the two kinds of animal. Centrally administered morphine prevented the tachycardia but not the cyclic upswings in blood pressure; these were blocked by centrally administered oxymetazoline.

  Azepexole had a withdrawal syndrome similar to clonidine (207); neither guanfacine (208–209) nor α-methyldopa (209) given in infusion regimens that were equihypotensive to that of clonidine showed a significant withdrawal syndrome (208–209). The intraperitoneal administration of yohimbine on the twelfth day of infusion of clonidine or guanfacine produced tachycardia and cyclic upswings in blood pressure, along with diarrhea, shivering, jumping, and ptosis (209); only slight shivering and minimal changes in blood pressure occurred when yohimbine was administered on the twelfth day of α-methyldopa infusion (209). It took at least five days of clonidine infusion before yohimbine injection precipitated this withdrawal syndrome (209).

These studies provide a useful animal model for the human cardiovascular sequellae of abrupt withdrawal from chronic drug administration. It is another example of an important drug response that takes days to develop.

NEW ANIMAL MODELS

A frequent limitation in preclinical drug studies is the unavailability of suitable animal models of human disease. Chronic duodenal ulcers, for example, do not naturally occur in the common laboratory species, and while injected histamine has been widely used to stimulate the secretion of gastric acid, it is not a very effective ulcerogenic. Recently, however, Hosoda et al (211) demonstrated that a continuous subcutaneous infusion of histamine in an African rodent, *Praomys (Mastomys) natalensis,* successfully produced multiple ulcers. Responses were dose-related and at higher delivery rates some perforations occurred. In contrast, histamine given as a single subcutaneous injection was not ulcerogenic. The authors suggest that the histamine-infused *Mastomys* may be a useful new animal model for the study of peptic ulcer disease. In addition, a rat model of peptic ulcer disease is suggested by the work of Szabo (212), who induced ulcers by chronic infusion of cysteamine.

To discriminate between central and peripheral actions of β-blockers, Smits et al (213) infused propranolol into an intracerebral ventricle or subcutaneously in the unrestrained SH rat. A five-day icv infusion achieved brain concentrations that were approximately 100-fold higher than those achieved by a subcutaneous infusion at equal rates, whereas plasma concentrations were approximately the same; both regimens lowered blood pressure to about the same extent. When the icv infusion rate was reduced so as to produce brain concentrations equal to those produced by subcutaneous infusion, the plasma levels of propranolol were very low and blood pressure remained elevated. These results support the conclusion that the antihypertensive action of propranolol in SH rats is a peripheral, not a central effect. As discussed in the introduction, Smits et al also demonstrated unequivocally the antihypertensive action of propranolol in the SH rat, which is an important piece of evidence supporting the SH rat as a model of human hypertension.

Comparative studies with antihypertensive drugs in models of hypertensive cardiac hypertrophy show a puzzling dissociation between cardiac hypertrophy and hypertension. Greenberg & Wilborn compared the effects of three-week infusions of clonidine versus propranolol on the cardiac hypertrophy (214) of the SH rat: clonidine normalized myocardial mass but propranolol had no effect, even though the rates of infusion of the two drugs gave equal reductions in blood pressure. The propranolol-infused rats showed focal areas of myocardial necrosis whereas no such changes were seen in the clonidine-infused rats, a finding that clearly warrants further investigation. The cardiac hypertrophy that accompanies hypertension induced by continuous iv infusion of norepinephrine in rats is prevented by concomitant β-blocker treatment but not by concomitant α-blocker treatment, despite the fact that blood pressure in the norepinephrine-plus phentolamine-infused rats was lower than normal (215). Perhaps these puzzling differences are relatable to the striking and paradoxical changes in myocardial adrenergic receptors that the FDA group (95) has observed with osmotic-pump infusion of α- versus β-agonists.

In another hypertensive model, continuous-delivery captopril was used to study the role of angiotensin II as a renal component in the maintenance of blood pressure and fluid volume in sodium-depleted rats (216). The complex role of the renin-angiotensin system in the genesis of hypertension after renal-artery constriction has been analyzed with continuously infused captopril in one- and two-kidney rats: hypertension is prevented by captopril infusion in two-kidney rats but not in one-kidney rats (217). Fluid restriction as well as continuous blockade of the converting enzyme is necessary to prevent hypertension when the renal artery is constricted in one-kidney rats (218).

Experimental hypertension has been induced by multiday infusions of norepinephrine, infused intravenously (215, 219–221) or at much lower rates into the renal artery (184).

Mills et al (222) developed a hypoprolactinemic rat model, suppressing endogenous prolactin secretion by the continuous intraperitoneal infusion of lergotrile mesylate.

The X-linked hypophosphatemic mouse is a model of human vitamin D-resistant rickets. Normalization of the bone defect was possible with four-week infusions of 1,25-dihydroxyvitamin D_3 [1,25(OH)$_2D_3$] provided the regimen was commenced in young animals (223); the vitamin D metabolite acts on intestinal absorption of inorganic phosphorus but the genetic defect in renal phosphorus excretion is unaffected (224). By comparing the effects of injections versus infusions of 1,25(OH)$_2D_3$, Hefti et al (225) concluded that this vitamin D metabolite plays an important role in calcium metabolism but is not involved in its hour-to-hour regulation. The physiologic role of 1,25(OH)$_2D_3$ has been assessed in two important studies by DeLuca and his colleagues (183, 226), who infused this metabolite and several of its analogues as the sole forms of vitamin D for 20 weeks through a complete cycle of reproduction and lactation from the time of weaning in vitamin D-deficient rats. The results indicate that 1- but not 24-hydroxylation is required for growth, reproduction, and skeletal mineralization. This work resolves prior confusion about the physiologic role of $24,25(OH)_2D_3$ that arose from experiments in which the short half-lives of the vitamin D metabolites were not taken into account but which use of the delivery system in the most recent studies has obviated. A model for fetal-growth retardation in utero in the rat was developed by Gruppuso et al (227) utilizing subcutaneously implanted osmotic pumps to produce maternal hyperinsulinemia. Previous models had relied on maternal dietary restriction, uterine vessel ligations, or other surgical interventions. Chronic maternal hyperinsulinemia was achieved by continuous infusion of insulin, thereby decreasing the supply of glucose to the fetus in a regulated manner and reducing fetal growth.

Finally, as pointed out in other sections of this review, the use of implanted delivery systems has simplified greatly the chronic infusion of bioactive agents into the central nervous system, either icv or by direct microperfusion of specific brain regions. Implanted delivery systems obviate the need for special restraints that, together with chronicity of drug delivery, greatly facilitate studies of drug and hormonal effects on appetitive (228–235) and other behavior (91, 236).

CONCLUSION

Multiday constant-rate drug administration has considerable research utility as both a pharmacodynamic probe and as a pharmacokinetic equalizer of disparate half-lives. This mode of administering bioactive agents was impractical for so long that its utility has been largely ignored in both drug and hormone research. The advent of novel drug delivery systems at both the research and clinical levels has removed that obstacle and has opened the way to research on programmed-rate administration of bioactive agents. With multiple regimens made practical, identifying the one most nearly optimal for research or therapeutic uses of each agent is both an opportunity and a challenge.

Literature Cited

1. Chandrasekaran, S. K., Benson, H., Urquhart, J. 1978. Methods to achieve controlled drug delivery—The biomedical engineering approach. In *Sustained and Controlled Release Drug Delivery Systems*, ed. J. R. Robinson, 6: 557–93. New York: Marcel Dekker. 773 pp.
2. Urquhart, J. 1982. Rate-controlled drug dosage. *Drugs* 23:207–26
3. Rose, S., Nelson, J. 1955. A continuous long-term injector. *Aust. J. Exp. Biol.* 33:415–19

4. Urquhart, J., Davis, J. O., Higgins, J. T. Jr. 1963. Effects of prolonged infusion of angiotensin II in normal dogs. *Am. J. Physiol.* 205:1241–46
5. Urquhart, J., Davis, J. O., Higgins, J. T. Jr. 1964. Simulation of spontaneous secondary hyperaldosteronism by intravenous infusion of angiotensin II in dogs with an arteriovenous fistula. *J. Clin. Invest.* 43:1355–66
6. Folkman, J., Long, D. M. 1964. The use of silicone rubber as a carrier for pro-

longed drug therapy. *J. Surg. Res.* 4: 139–42

7. Shell, J. W., Baker, R. W. 1974. Diffusional systems for controlled release of drugs to the eye. *Ann. Ophthalmol.* 6: 1037–45

8. Theeuwes, F., Yum, S. I. 1976. Principles of the design and operation of generic osmotic pumps for the delivery of semisolid or liquid drug formulations. *Ann. Biomed. Eng.* 4:343–53

9. Langer, R., Folkman, J. 1976. Polymers for the sustained release of proteins and other macromolecules. *Nature* 263:797–800

10. Folkman, J., Langer, R., Linhardt, R. J., Haudenschild, C., Taylor, S. 1983. Angiogenesis inhibition and tumor regression caused by heparin or a heparin fragment in the presence of cortisone. *Science* 221:719–25

11. Goldman, P. 1982. Rate-controlled drug delivery. *N. Engl. J. Med.* 307:286–90

12. Richardson, K. T. 1975. Ocular microtherapy: Membrane-controlled drug delivery. *Arch. Ophthalmol.* 93:74–86

13. Pharriss, B. B. 1978. Clinical experience with the intrauterine progesterone contraceptive system. *J. Reprod. Med.* 20: 155–65

14. Newton, J., Szontagh, F., Lebech, P., Rowe, P. J. 1979. A collaborative study of the progesterone intrauterine device (PROGESTASERT). *Contraception* 19: 575–89

15. Spangler, D. L., Kalof, D. D., Bloom, F. L., Wittig, H. J. 1978. Theophylline bioavailability following oral administration of six sustained-release preparations. *Ann. Allergy* 40:6–11

16. Theeuwes, F. 1983. Evolution and design of "rate controlled" osmotic forms. *Curr. Med. Res. Opin.* 8(Suppl. 2):20–27

17. Rhymer, A. R., Sromovsky, J. A., Dicenta, C., Hart, C. B. 1983. "Osmosin": A multi-centre evaluation of a technological advance in the treatment of osteoarthritis. *Curr. Med. Res. Opin.* 8(Suppl. 2):62–71

18. Shaw, J., Urquhart, J. 1980. Programmed, systemic drug delivery by the transdermal route. *Trends Pharmacol. Sci.* 1:208–11

19. Müller, P., Imhof, P. R., Burkart, F., Chu, L.-C., Gérardin, A. 1982. Human pharmacological studies of a new transdermal system containing nitroglycerin. *Eur. J. Clin. Pharmacol.* 22:473–80

20. Chien, Y. W. 1982. Transdermal controlled-release drug administration. In *Drugs and the Pharmaceutical Sciences.* Vol. 14, *Novel Drug Deliverys Systems:*

Fundamentals, Developmental Concepts, Biomedical Assessments, ed. J. Swarbrick, pp. 149–217. New York: Marcel Dekker. 584 pp.

21. Mroczek, W. J., Ulrych, M., Yoder, S. 1982. Weekly transdermal clonidine administration in hypertensive patients. *Clin. Pharmacol. Ther.* 31:252 (Abstr.)

22. Blackshear, P. J., Rohde, T. D., Prosl, F., Buchwald, H. 1979. The implantable infusion pump: A new concept in drug delivery. *Med. Prog. Technol.* 6:149–61

23. Smits, J. F. M., Coleman, T. G., Smith, T. L., Kasbergen, C. M., van Essen, H., Struyker-Boudier, H. A. J. 1982. Antihypertensive effect of propranolol in conscious spontaneously hypertensive rats: Central hemodynamics, plasma volume, and renal function during β-blockade with propranolol. *J. Cardiovasc. Pharmacol.* 4:903–14

24. Smits, J. F. M., van Essen, H., Struyker-Boudier, H. A. J. 1980. Cardiovascular effects of chronic infusion of propranolol in the conscious spontaneously hypertensive rat. *J. Pharm. Pharmacol.* 32:139–40

25. Walker, L. A., Frolich, J. C. 1981. Dose-dependent stimulation of renal prostaglandin synthesis by deamino-8-d-arginine vasopressin in rats with hereditary diabetes insipidus. *J. Pharmacol. Exp. Ther.* 217:87–91

26. Sikic, B. I., Collins, J. M., Mimnaugh, E. G., Gram, T. E. 1978. Improved therapeutic index of bleomycin when administered by continuous infusion in mice. *Cancer Treat. Rep.* 62:2011–17

27. Peng, Y.-M., Alberts, D. S., Chen, H. S., Mason, N., Moon, T. E. 1980. Antitumour activity and plasma kinetics of bleomycin by continuous and intermittent administration. *Br. J. Cancer* 41:644–47

28. Coonley, G., Vugrin, D., LaMonte, C., Lacher, M. J. 1981. Bleomycin infusion: Pulmonary toxicity. *Proc. Am. Assoc. Cancer Res.* 22:369

29. Cooper, K. R., Hong, W. K. 1981. Prospective study of the pulmonary toxicity of continuously infused bleomycin. *Cancer Treat. Rep.* 65:419–25

30. Nau, H., Zierer, R., Spielmann, H., Neubert, D., Gansau, C. 1981. A new model for embryotoxicity testing: Teratogenicity and pharmacokinetics of valproic acid following constant-rate administration in the mouse using human therapeutic drug and metabolite concentrations. *Life Sci.* 29:2803–13

31. Nau, H., Zierer, R. 1982. Pharmacokinetics of valproic acid and metabolites in mouse plasma and brain following

228 URQUHART ET AL

constant-rate application of the drug and its unsaturated metabolite with an osmotic delivery system. *Biopharm. Drug Disp.* 3:317–28

32. Nau, H., Spielmann, H. 1983. Embryotoxicity testing of valproic acid. *Lancet* 1:763–64

33. Reiner, N. E., Bloxham, D. D., Thompson, W. L. 1978. Nephrotoxicity of gentamicin and tobramycin given once daily or continuously in dogs. *J. Antimicrob. Chemother.* 4(Suppl. A):85–101

34. Boxenbaum, H. 1980. Interspecies variation in linear weight, hepatic blood flow, and antipyrine intrinsic clearance: Extrapolation of data to benzodiazepines and phenytoin. *J. Pharmacokin. Biopharm.* 8:165–76

35. Boxenbaum, H. 1982. Intraspecies scaling, allometry, physiological time, and the ground time of pharmacokinetics. *J. Pharmacokin. Biopharm.* 10:201–27

36. Tam, C. S., Heersche, J. N. M., Murray, T. M., Parsons, J. A. 1982. Parathyroid hormone stimulates the bone apposition rate independently of its resorptive action: Differential effects of intermittent and continuous administration. *Endocrinology* 110:506-12

37. Podbesek, R. D., Stevenson, R., Zanelli, G. D., Edouard, C., Meunier, P. J., Reeve, J., Parsons, J. A. 1981. Treatment with human parathyroid hormone fragment (hPTH 1–34) stimulates bone formation and intestinal calcium absorption in the greyhound: comparison with data from the osteoporosis trial. In *Hormonal Control of Calcium Metabolism*, ed. D. V. Cohn, R. V. Talmage, pp. 118–23. Amsterdam: Excerpta Med. 506 pp.

38. Podbesek, R., Edouard, C., Meunier, P. J., Parsons, J. A., Reeve, J., Stevenson, R. W., Zanelli, J. M. 1983. Effects of two treatment regimes with synthetic human parathyroid hormone fragment on bone formation and the tissue balance of trabecular bone in greyhounds. *Endocrinology* 112:1000–6

39. Connors, J. M., Hedge, G. A. 1980. Feedback effectiveness of periodic versus constant triiodothyronine replacement. *Endocrinology* 106:911–17

40. Cotes, P. M., Bartlett, W. A., Das, R. E. G., Flecknell, P., Termeer, R. 1980. Dose regimens of human growth hormone: Effects of continuous infusion and of a gelatin vehicle on growth in rats and rate of absorption in rabbits. *J. Endocrinol.* 87:303–12

41. Smits, J. F. M., Kasbergen, C. M., van Essen, H., Kleinjans, J. C., Struyker-Boudier, H. A. J. 1983. Chronic local

infusion into the renal artery of unrestrained rats. *Am. J. Physiol.* 244:H304–7

42. Pettigrew, J. D., Kasamatsu, T. 1978. Local perfusion of noradrenaline maintains visual cortical plasticity. *Nature* 271:761–63

43. Kasamatsu, T., Pettigrew, J. D., Ary, M. 1979. Restoration of visual cortical plasticity by local microperfusion of norepinephrine. *J. Comp. Neurol.* 185: 163–81

44. Kasamatsu, T., Itakura, T., Jonsson, G. 1981. Intracortical spread of exogenous catecholamines: Effective concentration for modifying cortical plasticity. *J. Pharmacol. Exp. Ther.* 217:841–50

45. Kasamatsu, T., Pettigrew, J. D., Ary, M. 1981. Cortical recovery from effects of monocular deprivation: Acceleration with norepinephrine and suppression with 6-hydroxydopamine. *J. Neurophysiol.* 45:254–66

46. Krause, J. E., Advis, J. P., McKelvy, J. F. 1982. In vivo biosynthesis of hypothalamic luteinizing hormone releasing hormone in individual free-running female rats. *Endocrinology* 111:344–46

47. Bear, M. F., Paradiso, M. A., Schwartz, M., Nelson, S. B., Carnes, K. M., Daniels, J. D. 1983. Two methods of catecholamine depletion in kitten visual cortex yield different effects on plasticity. *Nature* 302:245–47

48. Daw, N. W., Rader, R. K., Robertson, T. W., Ariel, M. 1983. Effects of 6-hydroxydopamine on visual deprivation in the kitten striate cortex. *J. Neurosci.* 3:907–14

49. McCall, M. A., Tieman, D. G., Hirsch, H. V. B. 1982. Chronic intraventricular administration of lysergic acid diethylamide (LSD) affects the sensitivity of cortical cells to monocular deprivation. *Brain Res.* 250:301–08

50. Mangano, R. M., Schwarcz, R. 1983. Chronic infusion of endogenous excitatory amino acids into rat striatum and hippocampus. *Brain Res. Bull.* 10:47–51

51. Panksepp, J., Rossi, J. III. 1981. d-Glucose infusions into the basal ventromedial hypothalamus and feeding. *Behav. Brain Res.* 3:381–92

52. Chen, F.-C. M., Healy, D. P., Hawkins, R., Printz, M. P. 1983. Chronic infusion of angiotensin II into the olfactory bulb elicits an increase in water intake. *Brain Res.* 259:335–39

53. Chen, F.-C. M., Healy, D., Hawkins, R., Printz, M. P. 1982. Studies of the functional significance of angiotensin II receptors in the rat olfactory bulb: Evi-

dence for alterations in normal fluid intake. *Clin. Exp. Hyperten. A* 4:623–37
54. Dougherty, G. G. Jr., Ellinwood, E. H. Jr. 1981. Amphetamine behavioral toxicity: Rotational behavior after chronic intrastriatal infusion. *Biol. Psychiatry* 16: 479–88
55. Costall, B., Domeney, A. M., Naylor, R. J. 1981. Behavioural consequences of discrete, chronic infusion of dopamine into the nucleus accumbens of rat. *Br. J. Pharmacol.* 74:899P–900P (Abstr.)
56. Costall, B., Domeney, A. M., Naylor, R. J. 1982. Chronic intra-accumbens dopamine: Behavioural consequences of continuous infusion or single daily injections. *Br. J. Pharmacol. (Suppl.)* 75:37P (Abstr.)
57. Costall, B., Domeney, A. M., Naylor, R. J. 1982. Numbers of striatal (3H) NPA binding sites change to compensate for consequences of chronic mesolimbic dopamine infusion. *Br. J. Pharmacol. (Suppl.)* 76:296P (Abstr.)
58. Advis, J. P., Krause, J. E., McKelvy, J. F. 1982. In vivo biosynthesis and processing of opiomelanocortin-derived peptides in rat brain. *Endocrine Soc. (Abstr) 64th Ann. Meet.* June 16–18, San Francisco. 230 pp.
59. Krause, J. E., Advis, J. P., McKelvy, J. F. 1982. In vivo biosynthesis and transport of the peptide neurotransmitter candidate substance P in the striatonigral trace of individual free-running rats. *Soc. Neurosci. Abstr., 12th Ann. Meet.,* Oct. 31–Nov. 5, Minneapolis, 8:4 (Abstr.)
60. Kroin, J. S., Penn, R. D. 1982. Intracerebral chemotherapy: Chronic microinfusion of cisplatin. *Neurosurgery* 10:349–54
61. Bodor, N., Brewster, M. E. 1983. Problems of delivery of drugs to the brain. *Pharmacol. Ther.* 19:337–86
62. Pestronk, A., Drachman, D. B., Stanley, E. F., Price, D. L., Griffin, J. W. 1980. Cholinergic transmission regulates extrajunctional acetylcholine receptors. *Exp. Neurol.* 70:690–96
63. Drachman, D. B., Stanley, E. F., Pestronk, A., Griffin, J. W., Price, D. L. 1982. Neurotrophic regulation of two properties of skeletal muscle by impulse-dependent and spontaneous acetylcholine transmission. *J. Neurosci.* 2:232–43
64. Eliason, J. A., Maurice, D. M. 1980. An ocular perfusion system. *Invest. Opthalmol. Visual Sci.* 19:102–05
65. Chappel, S. C., Resko, J. A., Norman, R. L., Spies, H. G. 1981. Studies in rhesus monkeys on the site where estrogen inhibits gonadotropins: Delivery of 17β-estradiol to the hypothalamus

and pituitary gland. *J. Clin. Endocrinol. Metab.* 52:1–8
66. Taylor, S., Folkman, J. 1982. Protamine is an inhibitor of angiogenesis. *Nature* 297:307–12
67. Lorkovic, H. 1979. Effects of motor nerve anesthesia and tenotomy on muscle membrane properties. *Pflugers Arch. Eur. J. Physiol.* 379:89–93
68. Betz, W. J., Caldwell, J. H., Ribchester, R. R. 1980. Sprouting of active nerve terminals in partially inactive muscles of the rat. *J. Physiol.* 303:281–97
69. de la Torre, J. C., Gonzalez-Carvajal, M. 1981. Steady state drug or fluid delivery to injured or transected spinal cord of rats. *Lab. Anim. Sci.* 31:701–03
70. Siew, C., Goldstein, D. B. 1978. Osmotic minipumps for administration of barbital to mice: Demonstration of functional tolerance and physical dependence. *J. Pharmacol. Exp. Ther.* 204:541–46
71. Tabakoff, B., Ritzmann, R. F., Oltmans, G. A. 1979. The effect of selective lesions of brain noradrenergic systems on the development of barbiturate tolerance in rats. *Brain Res.* 176:327–36
72. Wei, E., Loh, H. 1976. Physical dependence on opiate-like peptides. *Science* 193:1262–63
73. Wei, E. 1978. Enkephalin analogs: Correlation of potencies for analgesia and physical dependence. In *Characteristics and Function of Opioids,* ed. J. M. Van Ree, L. Terenius, pp. 445–46. Amsterdam: Elsevier/North Holland. 520 pp.
74. Stewart, J. M., Chipkin, R. E., Channabasavaiah, K., Gay, M. L., Krivoy, W. A. 1980. Inhibition of development of tolerance to morphine by a peptide related to ACTH. In *Neural Peptides and Neuronal Communication,* ed. E. Costa, M. Trabucchi, pp. 305–12. New York: Raven. 670 pp.
75. Tseng, L.-F. 1982. Tolerance and cross tolerance to morphine after chronic spinal d-Ala²-d-Leu⁵-enkephalin infusion. *Life Sci.* 31:987–92
76. Tseng, L.-F. 1983. Partial cross tolerance to d-Ala²-d-Leu⁵-enkephalin after chronic spinal morphine infusion. *Life Sci.* 32:2545–50
77. Schulz, R., Seidl, E., Wuster, M., Herz, A. 1982. Opioid dependence and cross-dependence in the isolated guinea-pig ileum. *Eur. J. Pharmacol.* 84:33–40
78. Wuster, M., Schulz, R., Herz, A. 1982. The development of opiate tolerance may dissociate from dependence. *Life Sci.* 31:1695–98
79. Schulz, R., Wuster, M., Krenss, H.,

Herz, A. 1980. Selective development of tolerance without dependence in multiple opiate receptors of mouse vas deferens. *Nature* 285:242–43

80. Wuster, M., Schulz, R., Herz, A. 1980. Highly specific opiate receptors for dynorphin-(1–13) in the mouse vas deferens. *Eur. J. Pharmacol.* 62:235–36

81. Schulz, R., Wuster, M., Krenss, H., Herz, A. 1980. Lack of cross-tolerance on multiple opiate receptors in the mouse vas deferens. *Mol. Pharmacol.* 18:395–401

82. Schulz, R., Wuster, M., Herz, A. 1981. Pharmacological characterization of the ε-opiate receptor. *J. Pharmacol. Exp. Ther.* 216:604–06

83. Wuster, M., Schulz, R., Herz, A. 1980. The direction of opiod agonists towards μ-, δ- and ε-receptors in the vas deferens of the mouse and rat. *Life Sci.* 27:163–70

84. Schulz, R., Wuster, M., Herz, A. 1981. Differentiation of opiate receptors in the brain by the selective development of tolerance. *Pharmacol. Biochem. Behav.* 14:75–79

85. Schulz, R., Wuster, M., Rubini, P., Herz, A. 1981. Functional opiate receptors in the guinea-pig ileum: Their differentiation by means of selective tolerance development. *J. Pharmacol. Exp. Ther.* 219:547–50

86. Schulz, R., Wuster, M. 1981. Are there sybtypes (isoreceptors) of multiple opiate receptors in the mouse vas deferens. *Eur. J. Pharmacol.* 76:61–66

87. Rubini, P., Schulz, R., Wuster, M., Herz, A. 1982. Opiate receptor binding studies in the mouse vas deferens exhibiting tolerance without dependence. *Arch. Pharmacol.* 319:142–46

88. Hetta, J., Terenius, L. 1980. Prenatal naloxone affects survival and morphine sensitivity of rat offspring. *Neurosci. Lett.* 16:323–27

89. Volicer, L., Schmidt, W. K., Hartz, T. P., Klosowicz, B. A., Meichner, R. 1979. Cyclic nucleotides and ethanol tolerance and dependence. *Drug Alcohol Depend.* 4:295–305

90. Rigter, H., Rijk, H., Crabbe, J. C. 1980. Tolerance to ethanol and severity of withdrawal in mice are enhanced by a vasopressin fragment. *Eur. J. Pharmacol.* 64:53–68

91. Tuomisto, L., Airaksinen, M. M., Peura, P., Eriksson, C. J. P. 1982. Alcohol drinking in the rat: Increases following intracerebroventricular treatment with tetrahydro-β-carbolines. *Pharmacol. Biochem. Behav.* 17:831–36

92. Broccardo, M., Erspamer, V., Falco-nierierspamer, G., Improta, G., Linari, G., Melchiorri, P., Montecucchi, P. C. 1981. Pharmacological data on dermorphins: A new class of potent opioid peptides from amphibian skin. *Br. J. Pharmacol.* 73:625–31

93. Nielsen, E. B. 1981. Rapid decline of stereotyped behavior in rats during constant one week administration of amphetamine via implanted ALZET osmotic minipumps. *Pharmacol. Biochem. Behav.* 15:161–65

94. Nabeshima, T., Sivam, S. P., Tai, C. Y., Ho, I. K. 1982. Development of dispositional tolerance to phencyclidine by osmotic minipump in the mouse. *J. Pharm. Meth.* 7:239–53

95. Sun, C.-L. J., Hanig, J. P. 1983. Alteration of sensitivity of adrenergic vascular responses after prolonged exposure to agonists via osmotic minipump (41584). *Proc. Soc. Exp. Biol. Med.* 172:440–44

96. Hauger, R. L., Aguilera, G., Catt, K. J. 1978. Angiotensin II regulates its receptor sites in the adrenal glomerulosa zone. *Nature* 271:176–77

97. Douglas, J. G. 1980. Potassium ion as a regulator of adrenal angiotensin II receptors. *Am. J. Physiol.* 239:E317–21

98. Aguilera, G., Menard, R. H., Catt, K. J. 1980. Regulatory actions of angiotensin II on receptors and steroidogenic enzymes in adrenal glomerulosa cells. *Endocrinology* 107:55–60

99. Douglas, J. G., Brown, G. P. 1982. Effect of prolonged low dose infusion of angiotensin II and aldosterone on rat smooth muscle and adrenal angiotensin II receptors. *Endocrinology* 111:988–92

100. Clayton, R. N. 1982. Gonadotropin-releasing hormone modulation of its own pituitary receptors: Evidence for biphasic regulation. *Endocrinology* 111:152–61

101. Zukin, R. S., Sugarman, J. R., Fitz-Syage, M. L., Gardner, E. L., Zukin, S. R., Gintzler, A. R. 1982. Naltrexone-induced opiate receptor supersensitivity. *Brain Res.* 245:285–92

102. Chang, R. S. L., Lotti, V. J., Martin, G. E., Chen, T. B. 1983. Increase in brain 125I-cholecystokinin (CCK) receptor binding following chronic haloperidol treatment, intracisternal 6-hydroxydopamine or ventral tegmental lesions. *Life Sci.* 32:871–78

103. Levin, P., Haji, M., Joseph, J. A., Roth, G. S. 1983. Effect of aging on prolactin regulation of rat striatal dopamine receptor concentrations. *Life Sci.* 32:1743–49

104. Norstedt, G., Wrange, O., Gustafsson, J.-A. 1981. Multihormonal regulation of

the estrogen receptor in rat liver. *Endocrinology* 108:1190–96

105. Chan, V., Katikineni, M., Davies, T. F., Catt, K. J. 1981. Hormonal regulation of testicular luteinizing hormone and prolactin receptors. *Endocrinology* 108:1607–12

106. Norstedt, G., Mode, A., Eneroth, P., Gustafsson, J.-A. 1981. Induction of prolactin receptors in rat liver after the administration of growth hormone. *Endocrinology* 108:1855–61

107. Aarons, R. D., Molinoff, P. B. 1982. Changes in the density of beta adrenergic receptors in rat lymphocytes, heart and lung after chronic treatment with propranolol. *J. Pharmacol. Exp. Ther.* 221:439–44

108. Norstedt, G. 1982. A comparison between the effects of growth hormone on prolactin receptors and estrogen receptors in rat liver. *Endocrinology* 110:2107–12

109. Hagino, N., Nakamoto, O., Kunz, Y., Arimura, A., Coy, D. H., Schally, A. V. 1979. Effect of d-Trp^6-LH-RH on the pituitary-gonadal axis during the luteal phase in the baboon. *Acta Endocrinol.* 91:217–23

110. Akhtar, F. B., Marshall, G. R., Wickings, E. J., Nieschlag, E. 1983. Reversible induction of azoospermia in rhesus monkeys by constant infusion of a gonadotropin-releasing hormone agonist using osmotic minipumps. *J. Clin. Endocrinol. Metab.* 56:534–40

111. Harwood, J. P., Clayton, R. N., Chen, T. T., Knox, G., Catt, K. J. 1980. Ovarian gonadotropin-releasing hormone receptors. II. Regulation and effects on ovarian development. *Endocrinology* 107:414–21

112. Huhtaniemi, I., Martikainen, H. 1978. Rat testis LH/HCG receptors and testosterone production after treatment with GnRH. *Mol. Cell. Endocrinol.* 11:199–204

113. Chang, H. Y., Klein, R. M., Kunos, G. 1982. Selective desensitization of cardiac beta adrenoceptors by prolonged in vivo infusion of catecholamines in rats. *J. Pharmacol. Exp. Ther.* 221:784–89

114. Kenakin, T. P., Ferris, R. M. 1983. Effects of in vivo β-adrenoceptor downregulation on cardiac responses to prenalterol and pirbuterol. *J. Cardiovasc. Pharmacol.* 5:90–97

115. Cohen, R. M., Aulakh, C. S., Campbell, I. C., Murphy, D. L. 1982. Functional subsensitivity of α$_2$-adrenoceptors accompanies reductions in yohimbine binding after clorgyline treatment. *Eur. J. Pharmacol.* 81:145–48

116. Cohen, R. M., Ebstein, R. P., Daly, J. W., Murphy, D. L. 1982. Chronic effects of a monoamine oxidase-inhibiting antidepressant: Decreases in functional α-adrenergic autoreceptors precede the decrease in norepinephrine-stimulated cyclic adenosine 3':5' monophosphate systems in rat brain. *J. Neurosci.* 2:1588–95

117. Knobil, E. 1974. The Gregory Pincus Memorial Lecture: On the control of gonadotropin secretion in the Rhesus monkey. *Rec. Prog. Horm. Res.* 30:1–46

118. Knobil, E. 1980. The neuroendocrine control of the menstrual cycle. *Rec. Prog. Horm. Res.* 36:53–88

119. Ewing, L. L., Desjardins, C., Stratton, L. G. 1973. Testosterone polydimethylsiloxane implants and contraception in male rabbits. In *Temporal Aspects of Therapeutics*, ed. J. Urquhart, F. E. Yates, pp. 165–80. New York: Plenum. 213 pp.

120. Ewing, L. L., Schanbacher, B., Desjardins, C., Chaffee, V. 1976. The effect of subdermal testosterone filled polydimethylsiloxane implants on spermatogenesis in Rhesus monkeys (Macaca mulata). *Contraception* 13:583–96

121. Ewing, L. L., Desjardins, C., Irby, D. C., Robaire, B. 1977. Synergistic interaction of testosterone and oestradiol inhibits spermatogenesis in rats. *Nature* 269:409–11

122. Lobl, T. J., Kirton, K. T., Forbes, A. D., Ewing, L. L., Kemp, P. L., Desjardins, C. 1983. Contraceptive efficacy of testosterone-estradiol implants in male Rhesus monkeys. *Contraception* 27:383–89

123. Bia, M. J., Tyler, K. A., DeFronzo, R. A. 1982. Regulation of extrarenal potassium homeostasis by adrenal hormones in rats. *Am. J. Physiol.* 242:F641–44

124. Schiffrin, E. L., Gutkowska, J., Genest, J. 1981. Mechanism of captopril-induced renin release in conscious rats (41173). *Proc. Soc. Exp. Biol. Med.* 167:327–32

125. Muller, J., Lund, E.-G., Hofstetter, L., Brunner, D. B., Haldy, P. 1982. Stimulation of aldosterone biosynthesis by sodium sequestration: Role of angiotensin II. *Am. J. Physiol.* 243:E450–57

126. Busby, B. E., Rodman, H. M. 1983. Impairment of T-cell regulation of the humoral immune response to type III pneumococcal polysaccharide in diabetic mice. *Diabetes* 32:156–64

127. Patel, D. G. 1983. Rate of insulin infu-

sion with a minipump required to maintain a normoglycemia in diabetic rats (41529). *Proc. Soc. Exp. Bio. Med.* 172:74–78

128. Frankel, B. J., Schmid, F. G., Grodsky, G. M. 1979. Effect of continuous insulin infusion with an implantable 7-day "minipump" in the diabetic Chinese hamster. *Endocrinology* 104:1532–39

129. Frankel, B. J., Grodsky, G. M. 1979. Effect of continuous low-dose insulin treatment on subsequent incidence of diabetes in genetically pre-diabetic Chinese hamsters. *Diabetes* 28:544–47

130. Kinter, L. B., Beeuwkes, R. III. 1982. Oral antidiuretic therapy: Studies in the diabetes insipidus rat. *Am. J. Physiol.* 243:R491–99

131. Kinter, L. B. 1982. Water balance in the Brattleboro rat: Considerations for hormone replacement therapy. *Ann. NY Acad. Sci.* 394:448–63

132. Cheng, S. W. T., North, W. G., Gellai, M. 1982. Replacement therapy with arginine vasopressin in homozygous Brattleboro rats. *Ann. NY Acad. Sci.* 394:473–80

133. Gash, D. M., Warren, P. H., Dick, L. B., Sladek, J. R., Ison, J. R. 1982. Behavioral modification in Brattleboro rats due to vasopressin administration and neural transplantation. *Ann. NY Acad. Sci.* 394:672–88

134. Kirkland, J. L., Barrett, G. N., Stancel, G. M. 1981. Decreased cell division of the uterine luminal epithelium of diabetic rats in response to 17β-estradiol. *Endocrinology* 109:316–18

135. Pennell, J. P., Millard, M. M., Ashby, M. H. 1981. Proteinuria in the acutely diabetic rat and its response to insulin treatment. *Diabetologia* 21:54–57

136. Feingold, K. R., Wiley, M. H., MacRae, G., Moser, A. H., Lear, S. R., Siperstein, M. D. 1982. The effect of diabetes mellitus on sterol synthesis in the intact rat. *Diabetes* 31:388–95

137. Reiser, S., Hallfrisch, J., Lyon, R., Michaelis, O. E. IV. 1983. Effect of chronic hyperinsulinism on metabolic parameters and histopathology in rats fed sucrose or starch. *J. Nutr.* 113:1073–80

138. McCormick, K. L., Widness, J. A., Susa, J. B., Schwartz, R. 1978. Effects of chronic hyperinsulinaemia on hepatic enzymes involved in lipogenesis and carbohydrate metabolism in the young rat. *Biochem. J.* 172:327–31

139. Severson, D. L., Fletcher, T. 1982. Effect of hyperinsulinemia on acid cholesterol ester hydrolase activity in liver, heart and epididymal fat pad preparations from rats and mice. *Biochim. Biophys. Acta* 718:144–50

140. Spencer, G. S. G., Hill, D. J., Garssen, G. J., Macdonald, A. A., Colenbrander, B. 1983. Somatomedin activity and growth hormone levels in body fluids of the fetal pig: Effect of chronic hyperinsulinaemia. *J. Endocrinol.* 96:107–14

141. Garwitz, E. T., Jones, A. W. 1982. Aldosterone infusion into the rat and dose-dependent changes in blood pressure and arterial ionic transport. *Hypertension* 4:374–81

142. Garwitz, E. T., Jones, A. W. 1982. Altered arterial ion transport and its reversal in aldosterone hypertensive rat. *Am. J. Physiol.* 243:H927–33

143. Morris, D. J., Kenyon, C. J. 1982. Aldosterone and its metabolism in spontaneously hypertensive rats (SHR). *Clin. Exp. Hyperten.* A4:1613–26

144. Snodgrass, P. J., Lin, R. C., Muller, W. A., Hoki, T. T. 1978. Induction of urea cycle enzymes of rat liver by glucagon. *J. Biol. Chem.* 253:2748–53

145. Mode, A., Norstedt, G., Simic, B., Eneroth, P., Gustafsson, J.-A. 1981. Continuous infusion of growth hormone feminizes hepatic steroid metabolism in the rat. *Endocrinology* 108:2103–08

146. Gustafsson, J.-A., Eneroth, P., Hokfelt, T., Mode, A., Norstedt, G., Skett, P. 1981. Role of the hypothalamo-pituitary-liver axis in sex differences in susceptibility of the liver to toxic agents. *Environ. Health Perspect.* 38:129–41

147. Skett, P., Young, C. 1982. The effects of pituitary hormones on hepatic drug metabolism in the rat. *Acta Endocrinol.* 100:421–26

148. Mode, A., Gustafsson, J.-A., Jansson, J.-O., Eden, S., Isaksson, O. 1982. Association between plasma level of growth hormone and sex differentiation of hepatic steroid metabolism in the rat. *Endocrinology* 111:1692–97

149. Lynch, H. J., Rivest, R. W., Wurtman, R. J. 1980. Artificial induction of melatonin rhythms by programmed microinfusion. *Neuroendocrinology* 31:106–11

150. Lynch, H. J., Wurtman, R. J. 1979. Control of rhythms in the secretion of pineal hormones in humans and experimental animals. In *Biological Rhythms & Their Central Mechanism,* ed. M. Suda, O. Hayaishi, H. Nakagawa, pp. 117–31. Amsterdam: Elsevier/North Holland. 453 pp.

151. Connors, J. M., Hedge, G. A. 1981. Feedback regulation of thyrotropin by

thyroxine under physiological conditions. *Am. J. Physiol.* 240:E308–13

152. Connors, J. M., Hedge, G. A. 1981. Effect of continuous thyroxine administration on thyrotropin secretion in thyroidectomized rats. *Endocrinology* 108:2098–02

153. Lopaschuk, G. D., Tahiliani, A. G., McNeill, J. H. 1983. Continuous longterm insulin delivery in diabetic rats utilizing implanted osmotic minipumps. *J. Pharmacol. Methods* 9:71–75

154. Bringer, J., Heldt, A., Grodsky, G. M. 1981. Prevention of insulin aggregation by dicarboxylic amino acids during prolonged infusion. *Diabetes* 30:83–85

155. Hock, J. M., Simmons, H. A., Schiess, M. C., Raisz, L. G. 1982. Use of osmotic minipumps for delivery of parathyroid hormone. *Calcif. Tissue Int.* 34:270–72

156. Martucci, C. P., Fishman, J. 1979. Impact of continuously administered catechol estrogens on uterine growth and luteinizing hormone secretion. *Endocrinology* 105:1288–92

157. Fishman, J., Martucci, C. 1980. Biological properties of 16alpha-hydroxyestrone: Implications in estrogen physiology and pathophysiology. *J. Clin. Endocrinol. Metab.* 51:611–15

158. Ball, P., Emons, G., Gethmann, U. 1981. Effect of low doses of continuously administered catecholoestrogens on peripheral and central target organs. *Acta Endocrinol.* 96:470–74

159. Emons, G., Knuppen, R., Ball, P. 1981. 4-hydroxyestradiol-17β and 4-hydroxyestriol-17α: Comparative studies on central and peripheral effects of two epimeric catecholestrogens. *Endocrinology* 109:1799–801

160. Naish, S. J., Ball, P. 1981. Catecholestrogens and induction of sexual behavior in the ovariectomized rat. *Neuroendocrinology* 32:225–28

161. Jellinck, P. H., Krey, L., Davis, P. G., Kamel, F., Luine, V., Parsons, B., Roy, E. J., McEwen, B. S. 1981. Central and peripheral action of estradiol and catecholestrogens administered at low concentration by constant infusion. *Endocrinology* 108:1848–54

162. Jellinck, P. H., Luine, V., McEwen, B. S. 1982. Differential effects of catechol estrogens, progestins and CI-628 administered by constant infusion on the central and peripheral action of estradiol. *Neuroendocrinology* 35:73–78

163. Hruska, R. E., Pitman, K. T., Silbergeld, E. K., Ludmer, L. M. 1982. Prolactin increases the density of striatal dopamine receptors in normal and hypophysectomized male rats. *Life Sci.* 30:547–53

164. Holmes, S. J. K., Jaspan, J. B., Moossa, A. R. 1982. The effect of somatostatin on postresectional ileal hyperplasia. *Endocrinology* 111:1397–99

165. Schoenle, E., Zapf, J., Froesch, E. R. 1983. Regulation of rat adipocyte glucose transport by growth hormone: No mediation by insulin-like growth factors. *Endocrinology* 112:384–86

166. Lamote, J., Putz, P., Willems, G. 1982. Effect of cholecystokinin-octapeptide, caerulein, and pentagastrin on epithelial cell proliferation in the murine gallbladder. *Gastroenterology* 83:371–77

167. Susa, J. B., McCormick, K. L., Widness, J. A., Singer, D. B., Oh, W., Admsons, K., Schwartz, R. 1979. Chronic hyperinsulinemia in the fetal rhesus monkey. *Diabetes* 28:1058–63

168. Elliott, M., Sehgal, P. K., Susa, J. B., Zeller, W. P., Widness, J. A., Schwartz, R. 1981. Experimentally-induced hyperinsulinemia in a fetus and newborn rhesus monkey (Macaca mulatta). *Lab. Anim. Sci.* 31:286–88

169. Lorijn, R. H. W., Longo, L. D. 1980. Clinical and physiologic implications of increased fetal oxygen consumption. *Am. J. Obstet. Gynecol.* 136:451–57

170. Lorijn, R. H. W., Nelson, J. C., Longo, L. D. 1980. Induced fetal hyperthyroidism: Cardiac output and oxygen consumption. *Am. J. Physiol.* 239:H302–07

171. Riley, V. 1975. Mouse mammary tumors: Alteration of incidence as an apparent function of stress. *Science* 189:465–67

172. Gould, T. R. L., Brunette, D. M., Dorey, J. 1982. Cell turnover in the periodontal ligament determined by continuous infusion of H³-thymidine using osmotic minipumps. *J. Periodontal Res.* 17:662–68

173. Ogashiwa, M., Hoshino, T., Muraoka, I., Hervatin, S. 1980. Variability of radioactive thymidine labeling in the rat brain tumor model. *Neurol. Med. Chir.* 20:395–404 (In Japanese)

174. Russo, J., Russo, I. H. 1980. Influence of differentiation and cell kinetics on the susceptibility of the rat mammary gland to carcinogenesis. *Cancer Res.* 40:2677–87

175. Haschek, W. M., Reiser, K. M., Klein-Szanto, A. J. P., Kehrer, J. P., Smith, L. H., Last, J. A., Witschi, H. P. 1983. Potentiation of butylated hydroxytoluene-induced acute lung damage by oxygen. *Am. Rev. Respir. Dis.* 127:28–34

176. Stott, W. T., Quast, J. F., Watanabe, P.

G. 1981. Differentiation of the mechanisms of oncogenicity of 1,4-dioxane and 1,3-hexachlorobutadiene in the rat. *Tox. Appl. Pharmacol.* 60:287–300

177. Paterson, J. A. 1983. Dividing and newly produced cells in the corpus callosum of adult mouse cerebrum as detected by light microscopic radioautography. *Anat. Anz.* 153:149–68

178. Wilson, K. C. P., Raisman, G. 1980. Age-related changes in the neurosensory epithelium of the mouse vomeronasal organ: Extended period of post-natal growth in size and evidence for rapid cell turnover in the adult. *Brain Res.* 185:103–13

179. Hagan, M. P., MacVittie, T. J. 1981. CFUs kinetics observed in vivo by bromodeoxyuridine and near-uv light treatment. *Exp. Hematol.* 9:123–28

180. Patt, H. M., Maloney, M. A., Lamela, R. A. 1980. Hematopoietic stem cell proliferative behavior as revealed by bromodeoxyuridine labeling. *Exp. Hematol.* 8:1075–79

181. Martens, G. J. M., Soeterik, F., Jenks, B. G., van Overbeeke, A. P. 1983. In vivo biosynthesis of melanotropins and related peptides in the pars intermedia of xenopus laevis. *Gen. Comparative Endocrinol.* 49:73–80

182. Beyler, S. A., Zaneveld, L. J. D. 1982. Antifertility activity of systemically administered proteinase (acrosin) inhibitors. *Contraception* 26:137–46

183. Jarnagin, K., Brommage, R., DeLuca, H. F., Yamada, S., Takayama, H. 1983. 1- but not 24-hydroxylation of vitamin D is required for growth and reproduction in rats. *Am. J. Physiol.* 244:E290–97

184. Kleinjans, J. C. S., Smits, J. F. M., Kasbergen, H. T. M., Vervoort-Peters, H. T. M., Struyker-Boudier, H. A. J. 1983. Blood pressure response to chronic low-dose intrarenal noradrenaline infusion in conscious rats. *Clin. Sci.* 65:111–16

185. Ewing, L. L., Wing, T.-Y., Cochran, R. C., Kromann, N., Zirkin, B. R. 1983. Effect of luteinizing hormone on Leydig cell structure and testosterone secretion. *Endocrinology* 112:1763–69

186. Desjardins, C. 1981. Endocrine signalling and male reproduction. *Biol. Reprod.* 24:1–21

187. Nakagawa, H., Nagai, K., Kida, K., Nishio, T. 1979. Control mechanism of circadian rhythms of feeding behavior and metabolism influenced by food intake. In *Biological Rhythms and their Central Mechanism*, ed. M. Suda, O. Hayaishi, H. Nakagawa, pp. 283–94. Amsterdam:Elsevier/North Holland

188. Morgan, N. T., Vaughn, W. J., Rasband, W. S., Wehr, T. A., Wirz-Justice, A. 1982. A computer-based system for collection and analysis of circadian rest-activity data. *Experientia* 38:1296–301

189. Wirz-Justice, A., Campbell, I. C. 1982. Antidepressant drugs can slow or dissociate circadian rhythms. *Experientia* 38:1301–09

190. Hsieh, D. S., Langer, R., Folkman, J. 1981. Magnetic modulation of release of macromolecules from polymers. *Proc. Natl. Acad. Sci. USA* 78:1863–67

191. Doherty, P. A., Ferm, V. H., Smith, R. P. 1982. Congenital malformations induced by infusion of sodium cyanide in the golden hamster. *Toxicol. Appl. Pharmacol.* 64:456–64

192. Johnson, D. R., Foulkes, E. C. 1980. On the proposed role of metallothionein in the transport of cadmium. *Environ. Res.* 21:360–65

193. Urquhart, J. 1980. Pharmacokinetics—One user's perspective. *Fed. Proc.* 39:2460–64

194. Betlach, C. J., Tozer, T. N. 1980. Biodisposition of theophylline: I. Genetic variation in inbred mice. *Drug Metab. Disp.* 8:268–70

195. Betlach, C. J., Tozer, T. N. 1980. Biodisposition of theophylline: II. Effect of aromatic hydrocarbon treatment in mice. *Drug Metab. Disp.* 8:271–73

196. Struyker-Boudier, H. A. J., Smits, J. F. 1978. The osmotic minipump: A new tool in the study of steady-state kinetics of drug distribution and metabolism. *J. Pharm. Pharmacol.* 30:576–78

197. Smits, J. F. M., Struyker-Boudier, H. A. J. 1979. Steady-state disposition of propranolol and its total metabolites in the spontaneously hyperactive rat: Chronic subcutaneous versus intracerebroventricular infusion with osmotic minipump. *J. Pharmacol. Exp. Ther.* 209:317–22

198. Shen, S. K., Williams, S., Onkelinx, C., Sunderman, F. W. Jr. 1979. Use of implanted minipumps to study the effects of chelating drugs on renal [63]Ni clearance in rats. *Toxicol. Appl. Pharmacol.* 51:209–17

199. Kapetanovic, I. M., Sweeney, D. J., Rapoport, S. I. 1982. Phenobarbital pharmacokinetics in rat as a function of age. *Drug Metab. Disp.* 10:586–89

200. Kapetanovic, I. M., Sweeney, D. J., Rapoport, S. I. 1982. Age effects on haloperidol pharmacokinetics in male, Fischer-344 rats. *J. Pharmacol. Exp. Ther.* 221:434–38

201. Steranka, L. R., Sanders-Bush, E. 1978. Long-term effects of continuous expo-

sure to p-chloroamphetamine on central serotogenic mechanisms in mice. *Biochem. Pharmacol.* 27:2033–37

202. Tran Ba Huy, P., Manuel, C., Meulemans, A., Sterkers, O., Amiel, C. 1981. Pharmacokinetics of gentamicin in perilymph and endolymph of the rat as determined by radioimmunoassay. *J. Infect. Dis.* 143:476–86

203. Tran Ba Huy, P., Meulemans, A., Wassef, M., Manuel, C., Sterkers, O., Amiel, C. 1983. Gentamicin persistence in rat endolymph and perilymph after a two-day constant infusion. *Antimicrob. Agents Chemother.* 23:344–46

204. Thoolen, M. J. M. C., Timmermans, P. B. M. W. M., van Zwieten, P. A. 1981. Withdrawal syndrome after continuous infusion of clonidine in the normotensive rat. *J. Pharm. Pharmacol.* 33:232–35

205. Thoolen, M. J. M. C., Timmermans, P. B. M. W. M., van Zwieten, P. A. 1981. Morphine suppresses the blood pressure responses to clonidine withdrawal in the spontaneously hypertensive rat. *Eur. J. Pharmacol.* 71:351–53

206. Thoolen, M. J. M. C., Timmermans, P. B. M. W. M., van Zwieten, P. A. 1981. Discontinuation syndrome after continuous infusion of clonidine in the spontaneously hypertensive rat. *Life Sci.* 28:2103–09

207. Thoolen, M. J. M. C., Timmermans, P. B. M. W. M., van Zwieten, P. A. 1981. The influence of continuous infusion and sudden withdrawl of Azepexole (B-HT 933) on blood pressure and heart rate in the spontaneously hypertensive and normotensive rat. Suppression of the withdrawal responses by morphine. *J. Pharmacol. Exp. Ther.* 219:786–91

208. Thoolen, M. J. M. C., Timmermans, P. B. M. W. M., van Zwieten, P. A. 1982. Guanfacine and clonidine: Antihypertensive and withdrawal characteristics after continuous infusion and its interruption in the spontaneously hypertensive and normotensive rat. *Naunyn Schmiedebergs Arch. Pharmacol.* 319:82–86

209. Thoolen, M. J. M. C., Timmermans, P. B. M. W. M., van Zwieten, P. A. 1983. Cardiovascular effects of withdrawal of some centrally acting antihypertensive drugs in the rat. *Br. J. Clin. Pharmacol.* 15:491S–505S

210. Conway, E. L., Jarrott, B. 1982. Effects of clonidine infusion and withdrawal on blood pressure and behaviour in the rat. A preliminary study. *Clin. Exp. Hyper. A* 4:1323–34

211. Hosoda, S., Ikedo, H., Saito, T. 1981. Praomys (Mastomys) Natalensis: animal

model for study of histamine-induced duodenal ulcers. *Gastroenterology* 80: 16–21

212. Szabo, S. 1978. Animal model: Cysteamine-induced acute and chronic duodenal ulcer in the rat. *Am. J. Pathol.* 93:273–76

213. Smits, J. F. M., Van Essen, H., Struyker-Boudier, H. A. J. 1980. Is the antihypertensive effect of propranolol caused by an action within the central nervous system? *J. Pharmacol. Exp. Ther.* 215: 221–25

214. Greenberg, S., Wilborn, W. M. 1982. Effect of chronic administration of clonidine and propranolol on the myocardium of spontaneously hypertensive rats. *Arch. Int. Pharmacodyn.* 255:141–61

215. Yamori, Y., Tarazi, R. C., Ooshima, A. 1980. Effect of β-receptor-blocking agents on cardiovascular structural changes in spontaneous and noradrenaline-induced hypertension in rats. *Clin. Sci.* 59:457s–60s

216. Seymour, A. A., Davis, J. O., Freeman, R. H., DeForrest, J. M., Rowe, B. P., Stephens, G. A., Williams, G. M. 1980. Hypertension produced by sodium depletion and unilateral nephrectomy: A new experimental model. *Hypertension* 2: 125–29

217. Freeman, R. H., Davis, J. O., Watkins, B. E., Stephens, G. A., DeForrest, J. M. 1979. Effects of continuous converting enzyme blockade on renovascular hypertension in the rat. *Am. J. Physiol.* 236:F21–F24

218. Seymour, A. A., Davis, J. O., Freeman, R. H., DeForrest, J. M., Rowe, B. P., Stephens, G. A., Williams, G. M. 1981. Sodium and angiotensin in the pathogenesis of experimental renovascular hypertension. *Am. J. Physiol.* 240: H788–92

219. Yamori, Y., Tarazi, R. C., Ooshima, A. 1980. Differential effects of various antihypertensive agents on cardiac hypertrophy in stroke-prone SHR (SHRSP). *Jpn. Heart J.* 21:567

220. Kleinjans, J., Kasbergen, C., Vervoort-Peters, L., Smits, J., Struyker-Boudier, H. A. J. 1981. Chronic intravenous infusion of noradrenaline produces labile hypertension in conscious rats. *Life Sci.* 29:509–14

221. Diz, D. I., Baer, P. G., Nasjletti, A. 1981. Effect of norepinephrine and renal denervation on renal PGE2 and kallikrein in rats. *Am. J. Physiol.* 241:F477–81

222. Mills, D. E., Buckman, M. T., Peake, G. T. 1981. A chronically hypoprolactinemic rat model: Administration of lergotrile mesylate by osmotic minipump

(41087). *Proc. Soc. Exp. Biol. Med.* 166:438–41

223. Marie, P. J., Travers, R., Glorieux, F. H. 1982. Healing of bone lesions with 1,25-dihydroxyvitamin D₃ in the young X-linked hypophosphatemic male mouse. *Endocrinology* 111:904–11

224. Tenenhouse, H. S., Scriver, C. R. 1981. Effect of 1,25-dihydroxyvitamin D₃ on phosphate homeostasis in the X-linked hypophosphatemic (Hyp) mouse. *Endocrinology* 109:658–60

225. Hefti, E., Trechsel, U., Fleisch, H., Bonjour, J.-P. 1983. Nature of calcemic effect of 1,25-dihydroxyvitamin D₃ in experimental hypoparathyroidism. *Am. J. Physiol.* 244:E313–16

226. Brommage, R., Jarnagin, K., DeLuca, H. F., Yamada, S., Takayama, H. 1983. 1- but not 24-hydroxylation of vitamin D is required for skeletal mineralization in rats. *Am. J. Physiol.* 244:E298–304

227. Gruppuso, P. A., Migliori, R., Susa, J. B., Schwartz, R. 1981. Chronic maternal hyperinsulinemia and hypoglycemia. A model for experimental intrauterine growth retardation. *Bio. Neonate* 40:113–20

228. Gronan, R. J., York, D. H. 1979. Effects of chronic intraventricular administration of angiotensin II on drinking behavior and blood pressure. *Pharmacol. Biochem. Behav.* 10:121–26

229. Hsiao, S., Wang, C. H., Schallert, T. 1979. Cholecystokinin, meal pattern, and the intermeal interval: Can eating be stopped before it starts? *Physiol. Behav.* 23:909–14

230. Avrith, D. B., Fitzsimons, J. T. 1980. Increased sodium appetite in the rat induced by intracranial administration of components of the renin-angiotensin system. *J. Physiol.* 301:349–64

231. Halperin, E. S., Summy-Long, J. Y., Keil, L. C., Severs, W. B. 1981. Aspects of salt/water balance after cerebroventricular infusion of angiotensin II. *Brain Res.* 205:219–21

232. Davis, J. D., Wirtshafter, D., Asin, K. E., Brief, D. 1981. Sustained intracerebroventricular infusion of brain fuels reduces body weight and food intake in rats. *Science* 212:81–82

233. Jalowiec, J. E., Panksepp, J., Zolovick, A. J., Najam, N., Herman, B. H. 1981. Opioid modulation of ingestive behavior. *Pharmacol. Biochem. Behav.* 15:477–84

234. Fink, G. D., Bryan, W. J., Mann, M. E. 1983. Effect of forebrain lesions on response to chronic intraventricular angiotensin II. *Am. J. Physiol.* 244:R45–R50

235. Jerome, M. L., Barbella, Y. R., Wurpel, J., Keil, L. C., Severs, W. B. 1983. Eating, drinking and urine output after prolonged cerebroventricular vasopressin infusions in rats. *Pharmacology* 26: 79–84

236. Gmerek, D. E., Cowan, A. 1983. ACTH(1–24) and RX 336-M induce excessive grooming in rats through different mechanisms. *Eur. J. Pharmacol.* 88:339–46

Ann. Rev. Pharmacol. Toxicol. 1984. 24:237–74
Copyright © 1984 by Annual Reviews Inc. All rights reserved

NON-EQUILIBRIUM BEHAVIOR
OF SOME BRAIN ENZYME
AND RECEPTOR SYSTEMS

Arnold J. Mandell

Department of Psychiatry, University of California at San Diego, La Jolla, California
92093

The previous article in this review dealing with the regulatory properties of
brain tyrosine (TOH) and tryptophan hydroxylase (TPOH) systems (1) emphasized (*a*) *multidimensionality:* almost all the components present under physiological and assay conditions, ranging from electromagnetic fields through
hydrophobic ligands to reducing equivalents, influence in one way or another
the rate functions representing catalytic activities; (*b*) *nonlinearity:* critical
zones of ligand concentration, curvilinear, even intermittent amount-effect
functions, and inconsistencies among results depending on small differences in
parameter values are consonant with the prominent role of cooperative interactions among the many stated and unstated dimensions (coordinates) regulating
catalytic systems; (*c*) *conformational instability:* in the protein macromolecular
components of TOH and TPOH, conformational instabilities are evidenced by
20 years of failure to purify the enzyme proteins in amounts useful for systematic extensive kinetic characterization, by their extreme friability under conditions of storage, by their multiplicity of reported molecular weights and kinetic
constants, and by their markedly increased ease of denaturation and precipitation after the removal of components from their normal milieu by dialysis and
enrichment procedures. That article expressed hope that a multivariate
approach to studies of TOH and TPOH regulation could be developed to allow
data reduction through pattern analysis in place of one- or two-variable kinetic
experiments and quantification by Michaelis or Hill constants (1).

This review updates the 1978 one with respect to research on the regulatory
properties of TOH and TPOH as reported in the literature through early 1983
with the exception of the cyclic nucleotide-protein phosphorylation schemata
(recently involving calmodulin), the current status of which is reviewed else-

237

0362-1642/84/415-0237$02.00

where (2–8). The emphasis here will be on a quantitative approach to qualitative patterns in behavior of complex nonlinear systems like these, ones with which the molecular psychopharmacologist must continually deal. The principles derived will be extended to nonlinear phenomena seen in the currently popular ligand-binding systems with a few examples. The relevance of a new approach to cross-disciplinary pharmacological studies of brain function will also be demonstrated. A conjecture concerning a new structure-function approach to brain polypeptides emphasizing solvent-mediated dynamic macromolecular stability will serve to integrate these concepts.

The mathematical formalisms of this approach are properly derived from modern approaches to stochastic differential equations, including phase transition theory (8a–13) as enriched by current advances in nonlinear dynamics (14–20). This difficult and esoteric theoretical route is not practically useful to those of us working in laboratories of biochemical pharmacology. The emphasis therefore will be on geometric intuition (the behavior of functions in the phase plane), physical mechanistic images, quantitative indices derivable from ones familiar to those who have used elementary statistics, and a metaphorically representative equation that, despite the complexity of its behavior, is both easily understood and numerically solvable on a hand calculator. Elementary representations of solvent entropy, the hydrophobic effect, and macromolecular dynamics from current research in the physics of globular proteins in solution will be used to explain the *solvent-mediated allosteric principle* treated here as the prepotent influence of substrates, ligands, and drugs on the nonlinear kinematic behavior of brain enzymes and membrane receptors via alterations in their *dynamical stability*.

THE ALLOSTERIC PRINCIPLE: SOLVENT ENTROPY, THE HYDROPHOBIC EFFECT, AND MACROMOLECULAR STABILITY

Restraint of autonomous motion among 37° heat-perturbed water molecules, decrease in water degrees of freedom, can be caused by the reorganization of the previously random hydrogen-bond-preserving network of water around non-polar solutes (21, 22). This has been called the hydrophobic effect, bond, or interaction (23–25). The energetically significant negative entropy created by hydrogen-bonded water straddling hydrophobic moieties drives them together, configuring the behavior of biopolymers in solution (26, 27) and, along with the finer adjustments of internal and external hydrogen bonding, plays the major role in globular and membrane protein structural and dynamical stability (28–31). Charged hydrophobic solutes in aqueous solution, e.g. biogenic amine or polypeptide salts, reduce the heat capacity and entropy of the system due to both electrostatic influences and those related to hydrophobicity

(32). The intrinsically dynamically unstable viscoelastic globular protein in solution (33) is perturbed by heated solvent molecules into large, rare, autonomous "breathing" motions with time constants in minutes (34–38). The functional implications of this fluctuating protein admittance have been established by studies such as those demonstrating the need for macromolecular motion to make room for the trajectory of CO-to-protoheme and myoglobin internal binding domains (39–41). If the temporal-spatial randomness of the more frequent, small, fast, solvent molecule-driven macromolecular conformational fluctuations is reduced by charged hydrophobic ligands competing for solvent entropy and the protein's motions gather to become large and coherent, heat capacity calculations show that the molecules contain more than enough intrinsic energy (38 kcal mol^{-1} for a protein of molecular weight 25,000) to be driven through a trajectory of progressively less stable, more active states (folding intermediates) (42, 43), ending in denaturation (44). Long-known examples of such ligand-induced processes involve denaturation of protein via the reconfiguration of solvent dynamical structure by urea and guanidine salts (see Figure 12; 45, 46).

When a charged hydrophobic ligand is itself the concentration-dependent participant in the pattern of reaction rates used to characterize the regulation of brain enzymes (e.g. an aromatic amino acid, tetrahydrobiopterin cofactor [BH_4]) or membrane receptor binding (by a drug or polypeptide), the protein stability-dependent catalytic or binding behavior (41, 47) becomes an intrinsically complex nonlinear function of the changing reactant or ligand concentration [R-L]$_i$. We call this dual action of [R-L] the solvent-mediated allosteric principle; as is implicit in the case of t, the index i indicates its consideration in discrete steps over changing concentration. In tightly conserved water spaces like a test tube or the brain (48), all molecules influence the solvent-mediated behavior of all others in an almost infinite system of partial differential relations, which we dimensionally reduce in expression via the solvent entropy, a mediating quantity much like currency in a complex economic system. Such an arrangement represents a global dynamic system requiring statistical rather than deterministic characterization of its flow. Contrived experimental conditions can generate small parameter zones of linear behavior, indices called affinities, and an apparently deterministic kinetic system based on reduced sets of ordinary differential equations, but such approaches suppress the expression of most of the influential variables and the nonlinear phenomena that occur when systems are examined within realistic ranges of concentrations and ratios, particularly in aqueous solvent.

We should note that post-Boltzmann notions of entropy as explored in the context of modern mathematical research in ergodic theory with particular relevance to mixing indicate that between the limits of randomness and strict periodic order there are many, perhaps a practical infinity of, invariant measures reflecting informationally metastable states (14, 15, 49–55). This suggests that exquisitely specific, subtle, distributed brain codes can be built from conditions that have previously been regarded as electromagnetic and chemical randomness. For example, entropy as a distributed property of pharmacologically altered solvent structural dynamics might constitute the code for the 15–20 discriminable drug-state-dependencies of behavioral paradigms that influence all neurobiological functions (56). Systematically applied measures of metastable stochasticity may supply a cross-disciplinary language for the pharmacology of brain function as a global dynamical system (57, 58). As James Clerk Maxwell wrote, "The true logic of this world is the calculus of probabilities."

THE PHYSIOLOGICAL CONDITIONS AND BEHAVIOR OF TOH AND TPOH

Despite its 1:1 reaction stoichiometry (59), relative to its tyrosine (TYR) and tryptophan (TRP) cosubstrates BH_4 is in far-from-equilibrium concentrations in several regions of rat brain (60–66a). As low as 3–5 μM in regions active in biogenic amine biosynthesis such as rat caudate, compared with amino acid concentrations in the range of 15–40 μM, the cofactor is below the affinity constants of the mixed function oxygenases for it (67, 68), including the most recent estimates for purified TOH (220–394 μM) and TPOH (119 μM) (69–71). When the physiological catalytic ratios of 3:15 μM BH_4 to TYR are simulated in vitro in a crude caudate nuclear homogenate (72), dihydroxyphenylalanine (DOPA) synthesis rates range from 3–5 pmol/mg protein/minute. At 10:10 μM ratios of BH_4 to TRP, similar levels of 5-hydroxytryptophan product formation are observed in crude rat raphé nuclear homogenates (73). In vivo measures of rat caudate dopamine turnover (74, 75) show a rate of 30 nmol/gram tissue/hour, which converts to 0.5 pmol/mg tissue/minute, and with a rough estimate of brain weight as 10% Lowry protein, a rate very close to the in vitro catalytic velocities under conditions of physiological reactant ratios emerges: 5 pmol/mg protein/minute.

Steady-state kinetic studies of TOH require very high reactant concentrations to generate linear functions with small (gaussian) variances. They characteristically exploit BH_4 to TYR ratios ranging from 100:30–1100:15 (76–81). However, reaction-sequence studies conducted that way have limited physiological significance because of their order-of-magnitude distortions in reactant concentrations and ratios and the absence of control of the oxygen concentration parameter, TOH and TPOH being unsaturated at ambient levels (1). Recent studies have confirmed work (82) indicating that O_2 is a regulatory ligand as well as a cosubstrate, i.e. an $[R-L]_i$ (82a–87). A recent study combining pyrimidine cofactor analogues and heavy oxygen labeling to examine the reaction mechanism also suggests that a cofactor-oxygen adduct may be the first intermediate in the amino-acid hydroxylation process (88, 89), consistent with the earlier speculation that addition is partially ordered with respect to O_2 (1).

In vitro studies using a BH_4 to amino-acid ratio in the range of 2:1–1:1 tend to make more prominent the inverted U-shaped functions in the kinetics of both TOH (70, 79, 90) and TPOH (67, 71, 91), and similar evidence of this nonlinear behavior has been observed in catecholamine biosynthesis rates in vivo in response to graded loads of TYR (92). In vivo stoichiometry of reaction rates, but not the effect of BH_4 as $[R-L]_i$ on macromolecular stability, may be regulated by apparent rate-limiting levels of quinonoid dihydropterin reductase (QDPR) (93). In addition, the interactive TOH (TPOH)-QDPR shuttle along with a diffusive delay creates an opportunity for the biosynthetic oscillations of a metabolic reaction-diffusion system (94). In contrast, without competitive kinetics, inactivation of either TOH or TPOH by abnormal isomers of BH_4 in a concentration- and (of significance for macromolecular stability) temperature-dependent way reflects the hydrophobic ligand role of BH_4 concentration as an $[R-L]_i$, inducing activating-inactivating conformational transitions (95–99). A similar explanation can be invoked to account for the parabolic shape of uncompetitive DOPA-inhibition functions (81). When still farther from equilibrium, i.e. at more nearly physiological ratios of BH_4 to amino acid, 1:5 for TOH and 1:1 in the TPOH system, over small steps in $[R-L]_i$ or time t the kinetic velocity emerges as pharmacological ligand-sensitive, nonlinear, and bifurcating functions [called multiple saturation plateaus in earlier studies of regulatory enzymes (100–102)], integrals demonstrating discontinuous transitions among multiple stable states induced by the progressive increases in the solvent-mediated force term, $[R-L]_i$.

Examined over t, the same far-from-equilibrium, physiological conditions generated periodic, quasi-periodic, and non-periodic ("chaotic") oscillations characteristic of systems with multiple stability and resembling those seen in studies of the glycolytic and peroxidase-oxidase enzyme systems (103–108). This variety of behaviors over $[R-L]_i$ and t has been observed in brain TOH and TPOH systems (58, 72, 73, 94, 109–112). It appears that the high BH_4 levels and abnormal ratios of reactants used in the past in most studies of TOH and TPOH kinetics in vitro served to linearize catalytic dynamics over $[R-L]_i$ and t, suppressing a more complex and subtle chemical coding capacity intrinsic to multidimensional, nonlinear biogenic amine regulation. Patterns of dynamical behavior in TOH and TPOH are exquisitely sensitive to small changes in BH_4, but perhaps not stoichiometrically as much as to its influence as a charged hydrophobic ligand, an $[R-L]_i$ (72, 73), a conjecture supported by the finding that levels of pterin analogues that induce amphetamine-like hyperactivity and stereotypy altered the dynamics but not the mean catalytic velocity of TOH

(113). In this context it is relevant that in experiments using a coupled QDPR-phenylalanine hydroxylase assay for BH_4 at doses inducing behavioral stereotypy but not decreasing striatal dopamine synthesis (74, 75), L-amphetamine was unique among 35 psychotropic drugs examined in decreasing the pterin significantly (72, 114–116). That finding was confirmed recently using more specific high-performance liquid chromatographic (HPLC)-fluorescence detection (62; E. H. Y. Lee & A. J. Mandell, manuscript in preparation). It is perhaps as charged hydrophobic macromolecular stability ligands, $[R-L]_i$, that both amphetamine and amphetamine-induced changes in BH_4 dynamics (75, 117) alter the regulatory properties of TOH and TPOH (58, 118–125).

The physiological relevance of dynamic patterns in biogenic amine synthesis as seen in vitro with physiological reactant ratios is consistent with growing evidence in vivo of metastable statistical patterns of fluctuation in brain biogenic amine synthesis and nonlinear diffusion in baseline and perturbation-induced biogenic amine waves ("flying W's") revealed by electrochemical voltammetry (R. Adams, personal communication, 1983; 126–131). A time frame in minutes characterizes the in vitro biogenic amine catalytic statistical fluctuations (see above), the electrochemical relaxation waves of voltammetry, the $t^{1/2}$ of the early biogenic amine turnover studies (132–135), the relaxations of the largest motions of globular proteins in solution (34–37, 136–140), the average periods of the glycolytic and peroxidase oscillators (141, 142), and the pulsatile motions of brain cells in tissue culture (143). The relatively narrow range of mean mass of the monomers of globular protein enzymes (50,000–60,000) and their common solvent environment suggest a role for the statistical phasing of their instability-generated, time-dependent motions in sculpting the dynamic geometries of biological process. In this context the pharmacology of the regulatory properties of brain TOH and TPOH may implicate more general features of biochemical stability. In vitro, the use of low, physiological levels of reactants in realistic ratios acts as a noisy catalytic scattering system with non-gaussian behavior to statistically amplify these physicochemical instabilities. In vivo, as has been suggested with respect to the weak-field, extracellular electromagnetic wave processes in brain (144), the informational content of brain chemical processes may reside in these patterns of semi-ordered stochasticity (57, 58), a spatially distributed code generated by ion, solvent-macromolecular, and membrane interactions.

Statistical recurrence, a pattern of repeated zeros of a function, is an intrinsic feature of all bounded finite-dimensional stochastic differential systems (145); in Levy processes without finite higher moments, a characteristic equation representing its probability distribution (the Fourier transform into a distribution of wave numbers as in equilibrium systems), $f:P(x,t) \rightarrow dxP(x,t)e^{ikx}$, scales across the absolute dimensions of $[R-L]_i$ or t (11, 12). Thus, enzyme behavior with near-periodic or aperiodic oscillating behavior in minutes, whose phase distribution is gathered by, for example, the regular perturbations of a light-dark cycle (146), can be expected to demonstrate more coarse-grained oscillations phased into diurnal rhythms in what has been called a self-similarity across scale (147). Such rhythms have been observed in brain and pineal TOH and TPOH (148–153). In the same vein, some protein motions manifest time scales of physical relaxation in months (136), and comparable seasonal rhythms in brain biogenic amine levels were the focus of a recent conference on biological rhythms in psychiatry (154).

Although the physical image of a protein fluctuating between metastable states is helpful, bounded multidetermined cooperative systems generate patterns of recurrence without such specific deterministic, cycle-generating mechanisms—all the participating components contribute to the emergent dynamic patterns. A coherent summation of the motions of the microdomains of a protein monomer can be visualized in this way (140, 155). Thus, TOH and TPOH product oscillations in minutes and seasonal variations in brain biogenic amine dynamics may reflect the same aggregate, scaling properties of a complex system.

Perhaps the simplest way to appreciate this phenomenon is in an examination of the wave forms generated by simple partial differential equation sets (156) and the characteristic scaling behavior of turbulent (dissipative) (157) and Hamiltonian (conservative) (52, 158) systems near zones of transition. Modern work in stability theory indicates that whereas small perturbations generate bifurcation (branching of the solutions of nonlinear equations) in fragile periodic dynamics, patterns of aperiodic recurrence are both sensitive and remarkably stable structurally (159, 159a). Temporal and spatial slippage in a cycle gives it the flexibility necessary to survive, although the biologist is often likely to regard this less regular geometry as meaningless noise. In systems similar to these biochemical and physiological systems, inability to predict behavior precisely using specifiable coefficients in differential equations led mathematicians to call such aperiodic oscillation chaos. A probabilistic approach to these chaotic dynamical systems, however, has shown them to contain invariant measure (160, 161).

THE BEHAVIOR OF TOH AND TPOH AS A MULTIDETERMINED [R-L]$_i$ and t-DEPENDENT FLOW OF PROBABILITY

Consistent with the findings of the previous review (1), there is continuing evidence that TOH and TPOH are sensitive to a large array of physiologically relevant influences. The regulatory importance of the dynamical physical state of rat caudate TOH (162), emphasized in this development and studied previously in relation to membrane and membrane-like components (78, 163–166), appears to be supported by recent confirmation of the role of particulate versus soluble subcellular location in determining the affinity of the enzyme for BH_4 but not for TYR (167); by current ultrastructural immunocytochemical studies demonstrating that 82% of TOH is in membrane-specialized punctate varicosities, TOH-relevant microscopic structures reported for the first time (168); by incubation with bacterial phospholipases altering its kinetic constants (169); and by a demonstration of both kinetic activation and inactivation (the characteristic multiphasic influence of an $[R-L]_i$; see below) by phosphatidylinositol (170). Phospholipid-induced, pH-dependent activation of rat brainstem TPOH has also been reported (171). The charged nature of native brain TOH and TPOH has been studied recently using a new mini-column isoelectric-focusing pH-gradient technique (J. H. Jackson & A. J. Mandell, manuscript in preparation) and is consistent with significant macromolecular and membrane interactions, kinetic changes in interaction with charged tubulin molecules (172), and the need to prepare an HPLC column with albumin to allow TOH recovery (173). The recent failure to relate activity state and adherence to membranes of adrenal TOH using histochemical staining is not surprising in that these membrane-depolarization, ion-sensitive phenomena (166, 174) behave like dynamical and not permanent histological changes (175). The sensitivity of both TOH and TPOH to negative electrostatic fields as first demonstrated for TOH in 1972 (78, 163) has been elegantly confirmed using heparin in interactional studies with polypeptides (176). Some of the same effects of chondroitin sulfate polyelectrolytes have been reported for TPOH (177, 178). The field-like sensitivity of TOH and TPOH to the influence of ions (179) and the electromagnetico-chemical environment in which brain TOH and TPOH function suggest that the regulatory effect of anions, including carboxylic acids (172, 180) and electrical field stimulation (181), may not be unrelated. The Gibbs-Donnan counterpoint to electrical-chemical negativity in neuronal membrane dynamics, the cations including H^+, K^+, Na^+, Ca^{++}, Mn^{++}, Mg^{++}, the actions of chelating agents, organic cations, iontophores, K^+ active cardiac glycosides (and other polyhydroxy compounds, including ascorbic acid and glucose) have also been shown to play influential roles in the regulation of these brain enzymes' conformational-kinetic stability (181a–191). Related to the issue of pH is the role of specificity of the reducing conditions of the enzymatic reaction, including sulfhydryl groups, protection against H_2O_2, and the role of iron, which has not yet been irrefutably demonstrated to be at the enzymes' reaction center (71, 82a, 88, 192–197).

Beyond the long history of both the activation and inactivation properties of BH_4, TYR, and TRP (1), of greatest relevance to the $[R-L]_i$-TOH (TPOH)-solvent interaction with respect to the induction of a destabilizing-activating-denaturing trajectory for the physical change in the enzyme protein is the recent and remarkable report of Kaufman & Mason (198) indicating that hydrophobic amino acids like methionine and norleucine activated the hepatic mixed-function oxygenase phenylalanine hydroxylase with respect to its physiological substrate. In addition, and consistent with the activating induction of large coherent unfolding motions by hydrophobically constrained solvent and resulting increased ease of substrate approach to the buried active site (39–41, 47), the structural requirements of amino-acid substrates were relaxed (both methionine and norleucine were hydroxylated) when the enzyme was activated in any of several different ways. The same solvent-mediated dynamical stability factors may account for uncompetitive influences on TOH by other non-specific hydrophobic moieties such as unphysiological pterins (96–98) and the tetrahydroisoquinolines (199). There have been several demonstrations of the anatomical proximity of a variety of biologically active peptides considered here to be charged hydrophobic ligands for TOH and TPOH (200–204), as well as catalytic activation by some (205–207), including chains as large as albumin (208), which also stabilizes (173). In vivo evidence of enzyme inactivation by large loads of tyrosine (92), and even the mysterious antidepressant efficacy of D-phenylalanine, equivalent to that of a combination of the D and L isomers and manifesting a two-week latency as is required for the antidepressant effects of tricyclic drugs, small doses of phenothiazines, or tryptophan loads (209, 210), may be explained by a charge and hydrophobic-effect increase in brain-solvent free energy and the induction of an associated destabilization-activation conformational trajectory of TOH and TPOH associated with an antidepressant effect-correlated increase in brain biogenic amine synthesis (211).

There is rather clear evidence that a multiplicity of ligands influential on TOH and TPOH is always present in vitro, that in the brain these systems manifest multiple quasistable states, and that physiological reactant concentrations and ratios generate non-equilibrium catalytic scattering behavior rather than gaussian linear or curvilinear functions manifesting only up-and-down regulation. These conditions, then, bring to brain chemical processes the potential for expression as subtle and complex as the behavioral output of the brain itself. We will proceed now to describe kinematic processes as changes in sizes and shapes in the geometries of the flows of probability, which can be quantitated and predicted by suitable equations, and portray both individual and phase-dependent molecular mechanisms as statistically defined patterns of global dynamical behavior. In these considerations the primary unit of data will be the A value:

$$A = \frac{\mathrm{E}x - x_i}{\overline{\mathrm{E}x} + \dot{x}} \qquad\qquad \text{[Eq. 1]}$$

the value of catalytic velocity, x_i, at a particular value of $[\text{R-L}]_i$ or t as a difference from expectation, $\mathrm{E}x$, the value of the corresponding point on a statistically determined regression line representing the aggregate of the data as normalized by the sum of the average level, $\overline{Ex}$, and slope $\dot{x}$. This condition allows a function of increasing or decreasing velocity over $[R\text{-}L]_i$ or t, where t refers to $(dA/dt)_{[R\text{-}L]}$, to be treated as a normalized series of values over a zero slope. The dynamical behavior of the system is represented by a first-order equation in A:

$$\frac{dA}{d([R\text{-}L]_i, t)} = V(A; [R\text{-}L]_i, t) \qquad \text{[Eq. 2]}$$

where V is a velocity function of A. We condense this high-dimensional process into a first-order autonomous equation representing the phase velocity of A, eliminating its explicit dependence on $[R\text{-}L]_i$ or t:

$$\frac{dA}{d(H^+, K^+, Na^+, CA^{++}...[R\text{-}L]_i...t)} = V(A) \qquad \text{[Eq. 3]}$$

and

$$\int [R\text{-}L]_0 - [R\text{-}L]_i, \ t_0 - t_i \ = \int_{A_0}^{A_i} \frac{dA}{V(A)} \qquad \text{[Eq. 4]}$$

Thermal inactivation studies of TOH and TPOH systems evidence three interconvertible kinetic conformations and a dynamical trajectory between them (99, 212–215), with normalized velocity levels of approximately $1.0 \rightarrow 2.5 \rightarrow 0.3$, suggesting an exponential relationship among the states. Conditions that facilitate activation also inactivate (1, 99, 169, 216, 217). Kept at room temperature and sampled every minute, rat raphé TPOH activity as a sequence of A values demonstrates this kinetic-conformational trajectory in one continuous experiment (Figure 1; 73, 218). Purified mouse mastocytoma TPOH also manifests an iron-reducing system $(H_2O_2?)$-sensitive set of three discrete states (219); those studies demonstrate normalized activity ratios of $1.0 \rightarrow 5.0 \rightarrow 0.2$, also suggesting three logarithmically (power law) related activity levels. Assuming a greater than root mean square proportionality under far-from-equilibrium conditions between the catalytic velocities and the average amplitude of the variations, RMS_A, we can represent the changes from activated (a), low activity (l), and baseline (b) states as a birth and death trajectory of A in the phase plane portraying the flow of probability as a one-dimensional dynamical system with a random distribution of phase (Figure 2). Described as the nonlinear spring-like folding-unfolding dynamics of globular proteins in solution with intermediate metastable states (42, 43, 220, 221), the viscoelastic protein (33) with reaction component-sensitive stability properties accrues a nonlinear macroscopic response to heated solvent perturbations over time,

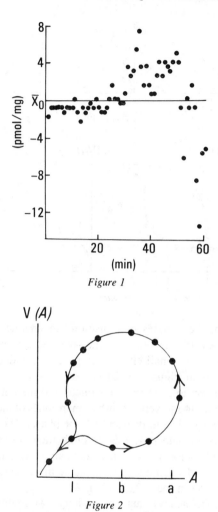

Figure 1

Figure 2

requiring a memory kernel, for example, an exponential instantaneous distribution of states, $G_\tau(b \to a)$ and $G_\tau(a \to l)$. As seen in the substrate activation-inactivation functions below, conditions that facilitate activation also augment the inactivation process rather symmetrically (216, 217), as in Figure 3, so that $G_\tau(b,a,l)$ can be represented by a convolution of exponential processes $(A_0\exp^{kA}, A_{max}\exp^{-kA})$, which reconfigures the phase portrait of $A/V(A)$ into a hysteresis loop with singularities at the $dV(A) = 0$ transitions (Figure 4, left), seen perhaps more clearly in a potential energy graph of $A/U(A)$ (Figure 4, right) representing transitions through metastable states. Synchronization of phase among these globular protein enzymes with nonlinear oscillations of their cosubstrate admittances occurs in the regions of the singularities, $dV(A) = 0$

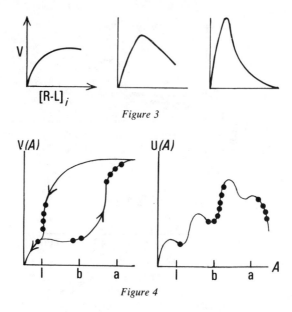

Figure 3

Figure 4

(146). In addition, these zones of transition, degenerate neighborhoods of multivalued inverses, $f:V(A) \rightarrow A$, are the ones showing greatest changes in dynamical behavior with small changes in parameter values. Autonomously emergent changes as in Figure 1 suggest that physiological function and its regulation with respect to changes in chemical information flow require very little energy in addition to solvent perturbation in zones of molecular instability and associated changes in the distributions of phase. The trivial amount of energy required to regulate processes through their instabilities suggests a neurochemical explanation for the thermodynamically paradoxical findings that wild psychosis and sleep manifest the same mean levels of brain glucose and oxygen utilization in man (222, 223).

Periodicity (one frequency), quasi-periodicity (two frequencies), and aperiodicity (three or more distinct frequencies and/or chaos) have been observed in the product concentration fluctuations of TPOH (73, 111) and TOH over t as in Figure 5 (58, 72). Transitions between multiple dynamical regimes (see the protein denaturation curves in Figure 12) have also been observed across $[R\text{-}L]_i$ for TPOH (Ca^{++}) (Figure 6, left) (109) and TOH (TYR) (Figure 6, right) (72).

HOW MACROSCOPIC DYNAMICAL COMPLEXITY CAN EMERGE FROM ACTIVATION-DEACTIVATION PROCESSES IN A POPULATION OF ENZYME PROTEINS

The way in which parabolic manifolds portraying density-dependent processes, like those seen in the substrate kinetics of TOH and TPOH (Figure 3) generate

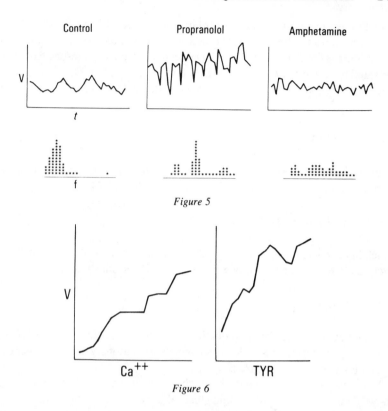

Figure 5

Figure 6

both periodic and aperiodic dynamics across small changes in parameter values is a current focus of interest in statistical physics (17–20). In the interest of a simplification not ordinarily permitted for a far-from-equilibrium system, we linearize $G(\tau)$ so that $d_A(b \rightarrow a)/dt = B(A)$ and $d_A(a \rightarrow l)/dt = D(A)$. The equation of motion for A then becomes:

$$\frac{d(A)}{d([\text{R-L}]_i, t)} = V[B(A) - D(A)] \qquad [\text{Eq. 5}]$$

At low values of $[\text{R-L}]_i$ or t, $B > D$, and beyond some critical transition $D > B$, as in Figure 3. A_0 can be seen as a stable fixed point and the second singularity, a metastable stationary state, is at $A_{\max}$, $d(A) = 0$, $V[B(A)] = V[D(A)]$ as in Figures 3 and 4. It has long been known that increased density of active forms of TOH and TPOH produced by activation, dialysis, or steps toward purification leads to monomeric aggregation, loss of catalytic activity, and precipitation of denatured protein (67, 70, 71, 78, 90, 163, 170, 173, 196, 224–230). The mechanism may involve resonance in large, slow protein motions facilitating coherent, high-amplitude oscillations as in Figure 1 and progression through three metastable states toward irreversible unfolding (44, 231). Thus, two kinds of inactivation are seen: D as a consequence of the trajectory through activation (as in Figures 2–4) and $\tilde{D}$, dependent on the presence of other activated monomers, i.e. $d(A) = A(B - D) - \tilde{D}A^2$. We combine D and $\tilde{D}$ in a single expression representing the density dependence of the inactivation process:

$$d(A) = V(BA - DA^2) \tag{Eq. 6}$$

From the symmetries seen in Figure 3, $B(A) = D(A)$, $B = D = r$, a generalized force term that can represent [R-L], making the manifold:

$$d(A) = V[rA(1 - A)] \tag{Eq. 7}$$

which in the context of the sequence of repeated samplings of TOH and TPOH over discrete steps of $[R\text{-}L]_i$ or t is the classical logistics map (232).

$$A_{t+1} = rA_t(1 - A_t) \tag{Eq. 8}$$

This simple discrete difference equation generates a parabolic curve (Figure 7) whose slope is dependent on $[R\text{-}L]_i$ and whose evolutionary behavior over time resembles that seen in Figure 5.

More detailed development of stoachastic birth and death processes (12) shows them to generate bifurcations that reflect kinematic multistability, seen in Figure 6 and modeled by Equation 8 as in Figure 7. The oxidase-peroxidase system has long been known to display parameter-sensitive bifurcations from equilibrium to single and multiple frequencies and/or chaos (106, 142, 233–236). When periodic versus aperiodic (chaotic) behavior of Equation 8 is plotted as a function of r above values of 3.4 (237, 238), a pattern resembling that in Figure 8 is observed:

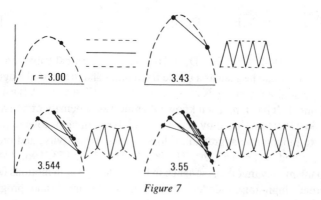

Figure 7

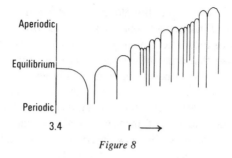

Figure 8

Chaotic regimes and those that are strictly or partially ordered in time are seen closely juxtaposed in parameter space (239). As operative across $[R\text{-}L]_i$, in addition to the feature of sensitivity to differences in initial conditions (161), this principle accounts for the instability manifested by the TOH and TPOH systems when examined under physiological, far-from-equilibrium conditions (72, 73, 111–112). Concentration-dependent stabilization and destabilization by BH_4 (98, 213), activation and inactivation by phospholipids (170), amino-acid substrate activation and inhibition (216, 217), multiphasic effects of increasing levels of in vitro amphetamine (58), and many of the conflicting reports of the influence of various ligands on these systems (1) are examples of these dynamics. The characteristic anomalous and wide clinical dose-response curves of psychotropic drugs, for example the dosage windows for the clinical efficacy of tricyclic antidepressant drugs, are consonant with the nonlinear stability properties of these biogenic amine biosynthetic systems over increasing $[R\text{-}L]_i$ (240, 241).

A STATISTICAL KINEMATICS OF NON-EQUILIBRIUM STEADY STATES: GENERALIZATION ACROSS NEUROPSYCHOBIOLOGICAL LEVELS

Most transform techniques useful in dealing with nonlinear systems (242, 243) are limited by the rather strict requirements of their mathematical assumptions. For example, the stationarity, convergence, and adequate sample length assumed by Fourier transform techniques, displayed qualitatively in Figure 5, are not fulfilled by 100-point studies in triplicate (72) of far-from-equilibrium enzyme system fluctuations (244–246). The third and fourth moments of the probability density distributions reflecting rare, high-amplitude events as seen in computer simulations of protein motion (140)—the critical fluctuations that bifurcate distribution functions (13)—require sample lengths beyond those now possible in brain enzyme kinetic experiments (247). In their place is sought a reliable and meaningful quantitative measure of the pattern of behavior of the A values across $[R\text{-}L]_i$ and t that would reflect the shape of the probability distribution, indicate the frequency content of the A value variations, portray the system's stability along the vertical dimension of Figure 8, reflect the number of independent phases or enzyme forms contributing to the process as its dynamic dimensionality, and scale across a wide range of intervals in time so that drug influences could be compared among several neuropsychobiological data bases. In combination with the RMS_A, the fractional characteristic exponent D_A, the geometric dimensionality of the A value integral (11, 147, 239, 248) serves these purposes quite well (72, 73, 94, 247). This power law dependence of measures made on cooperative biological systems is analogous to the scaling law descriptions of statistical physics (12). Repeated measurements of the catalytic activity of an enzyme homogenate over $[R\text{-}L]_i$ or t, synchronized by continuous rhythmic perturbation in a metabolic shaker (72, 73, 249), are transformed as in Equation 1, $f{:}V_i \rightarrow A_i$, creating the new, normalized series of A values upon which a measure of the texture, D_A, can be made with values ranging from 1 for a smooth line to 2 for an irregular, space-filling (two-dimensional) function.

The relationship between the roughness of the surface of a multidimensional volume representing a dynamic system and its underlying cooperativity as dimensionality (the number of independent coordinates projecting information onto the one-dimensional sequence of A values) can be analogized from the following argument (250). Removing the middle 90% of a line of unit length (dim = 1) leaves 10% at the "surface" of the two ends; removing a circle of diameter 0.9 from the unit disc (dim = 2) leaves about 20% at the surface; in dim = 3 the removal of a concentric ball of diameter 0.9 from the unit sphere leaves about 28% at the surface. In the limit the internal volume of a geometric object of diameter 0.9 and dimension ϕ, $(0.9)^\phi \rightarrow 0$ as $\phi \rightarrow \infty$. In the geometry of multidimensional volumes, the more independent contributors of mechanism or phase, the higher the dimensionality and the greater the arc length of the perimeter relative to its volume. The minimum number of unit balls of diameter ϵ, $N(\epsilon)$, required to cover the function increases with an increase in dimensionality (251), which is seen as an increase in D_A.

D_A is calculated as the slope created when the log of the diameters of a sequence of increasingly larger spheres is plotted on the x-axis against the log of the number of balls of each size required to cover the function projected onto the y-axis. The more irregular the surface, the more crevices are lost by the progressively larger spheres, the steeper the slope, the larger the D_A (72). A microcomputer program for the calculation is available upon request.

With few mathematical assumptions and remarkable statistical stability, the geometric dimension has been applied successfully to electron spin relaxation measurements on myoglobin and ferricytochrome C (252). It can also quantify precisely the elusive behavior of far-from-equilibrium kinematic scattering systems. It serves as the characteristic exponent of non-gaussian distribution functions that are without finite higher moments (11, 253); it describes the shape of the tail of these distributions as an extremal measure that scales as the mean first-passage time (254); it gives a single numerical value to long-range correlations, thus serving as an index of the frequency content of the process (255); it serves as a numerical solution to undifferentiable functions (256); it transforms directly to a measure of the vertical dimension of Figure 8 called the sum of the Lyapounov exponents, quantifying the system's stability (239, 257–259). Since D_A represents the convergence in a relationship between a measure and its measurement, it has symmetry with respect to dilation, i.e. the index is independent of its absolute size. In this way, D_A is self-similar across temporal scales in processes like the internal symmetries of eddies within eddies within eddies in the dissipative dynamics of hydrodynamic turbulence (260, 261), the infinity within conservative Hamiltonian systems in the alternating patterns of invariant curves, and stochasticity seen in the homoclinic regions between attractor domains (14, 15, 52, 158, 262, 263). With the enzymes of the biogenic amine systems omnipresent in brain regions, it is perhaps not surprising that the effects of ligands such as amphetamine, lithium, chlorimipramine, and thyrotropin-releasing hormone (TRH) demonstrate similar alterations in D_A and D_A-like dynamics in TOH and TPOH systems, [3H]-spiroperidol binding, interspike intervals of single units, electroencephalographic dynamics, animal behavior, and clinical response (58, 94, 263a–266). A similarity in the power-law dependence of multiple measures made on a single complex system is consistent with its status as an integrated organization (267), not an unreasonable claim with respect to psychotropic drug-influenced central nervous system function.

The way the D_A to RMS_A relationship as $\delta D_A / \delta RMS_A$ reflects the system's cooperativity as examined over an *ensemble* of experiments under the same conditions can be seen in the two contrasting views of how fluctuations in complex nonlinear systems evolve over time (Figure 9).

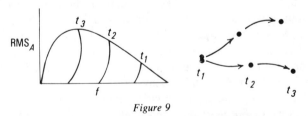

Figure 9

The Eulerian view (Figure 9, left) shows that fluctuations enter the small scales of motion as fast, frequent perturbations by heated solvent molecules and propagate across the 16 time scales of protein motion from 10^{-12} seconds (268) to minutes (136), the total error energy amplitude represented as the RMS_A (269). For globular proteins in solution this process is influenced by changes in solvent ΔG induced by charged and hydrophobic ligands. The Lagrangian view

(Figure 9, right) describes the extent of the maintenance of the neighborhood topology in the evolutionary process, a systems property called mixing reflected in the value of D_A (52, 161); we see a high mixing system in which two points that were together initially become widely separated over time. This effect is regulated by ions, drugs, and other influences on phase that promote or prevent the synchronization of molecular motions. The differential of the D_A to the RMS_A, a dispersion relation shown in Figure 10,

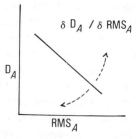

$$\delta D_A \ / \ \delta RMS_A$$

Figure 10

reflects the degree of coupling, the maintenance of the integrity of a neighborhood of values over time, in what can very generally be called a stochastic frequency-amplitude graph. A negative slope reflects a cooperative dynamic that is more subject to bifurcations and phase transitions, whereas a zero to positive slope indicates relative independence among the contributing elements or phases and the greater stability of "noisy periodicity" (94, 159a, 270). The differences between the slopes of the regressions of ensembles from experiments conducted under various psychopharmacological conditions can be tested for statistical significance (73, 230, 247).

Psychotropic drug-induced increases in $-\delta D_A/\delta RMS_A$, as seen at the molecular dynamic level in the TPOH system in the presence of tricyclic antidepressant drugs, are associated with hyperbolic, bifurcating saturation functions and the emergent periodicity and phase transitions characteristic of systems of anharmonic oscillators perturbed by increased coupling (271) in several neurobiological and clinical phenomena (73, 263a, 265, 266, 272). Decreases in $-\delta D_A/\delta RMS_A$ induced by physiological levels of lithium are associated with more sigmoid saturation functions and demonstrate the stability of systems composed of more independent elements (12, 73, 265, 266, 272). Depending upon dose, amphetamine induces both these contrasting conditions in a variety of neuropsychobiological contexts (58, 94, 263a, 273).

NON-EQUILIBRIUM BEHAVIOR AS MULTIPLE RECEPTOR LIGAND-BINDING PROCESSES

The influence of a ligand on the kinetics of its own binding behavior as an $[R-L]_i$, the allosteric principle (274), was invoked long ago to explain the nonlinear behavior of oxygen binding to hemoglobin (275–277). Those classical non-Langmuir, non-Michaelis functions manifested fractional characteristic exponents of about 2.8 (278). Such behavior is easily analogized to more modern views of the nonlinear dynamics of ligand-induced conformational changes in macromolecular and membrane stability via ligand-induced changes in solvent entropy (26–28, 30, 31, 35–37, 279) called the hydrophobic effect (23–25). One recent demonstration of the role of solvent influences on macromolecular motion as reflected in receptor binding kinetics was a direct one exploiting systematic variations in solvent viscosity (41).

Ligand-binding techniques used in current pharmacological studies exploit extremely high concentrations of (cold) hydrophobic ligands, most of which generate multiple discontinuities in the saturation functions (280, 281), not unlike the bifurcational behavior seen in Figure 6 over $[R-L]_i$ and in Figure 5 over t and modeled by Equation 8 and Figure 7 (see also Figure 12). In this context, binding is viewed as adherence to a macromolecular-membrane moiety conformationally altered in a nonlinear manner in the direction of denaturation and precipitation by increasing concentrations of charged and hydrophobic ligands. These dynamics are consistent with a degree of structural-dynamical specificity of the ligand as well as the less specific nonlinear force characteristics of $[R-L]_i$ as seen in Figures 7, 8, and 12. Anomalous behavior in time observed in the early pharmacological ligand-binding studies (282), i.e. the demonstration that the low-affinity system saturated several minutes before the high-affinity one, suggests conformational interconversion as in Figures 1, 2, and 4 rather than the simultaneous presence of multiple receptor membrane proteins. An extensive new literature on specific coding in entropies (see above) makes structural specificity transformable into equal or even more specific solvent-mediated dynamical messages and offers an explanation for the ever growing receptor-system kinetic heterogeneities and inconsistencies in the experimental literature (282a, 282b). Bathing a system of relatively homogeneous nicotinic-cholinergic microsacs from *E. electricus* and *T. marmorata* in high concentrations of cholinergic ligand is the condition under which the depolarization mechanism is desensitized, the time dynamics bifurcate into fast and slow processes (283), and multiple kinetic binding functions can be observed (283–287). Examples of $[R-L]_i$-induced bifurcations in kinetic functions are seen in Figure 11: on the left in [^{3}H]-TRH binding to pituitary cell membrane (288); in the center in [^{3}H]-etorphine binding to liposomes containing cerebrosides (289), a preparation not inconsistent with the orderly and complex kinetics of binding to other non-biological, surface-active materials (290, 291); and on the right in a nonlinear Scatchard plot the use of which is actually inappropriate for nonlinear systems (292), with two high-affinity unstable stationary states in [^{3}H]-spiperone-haloperidol competition binding to an olefactory tubercle crude membrane preparation from the mouse (293).

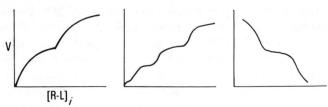

Figure 11

The similarity of these iterative binding functions to classical multiphasic protein denaturation curves over increasing concentrations of solvent-active, charged hydrophobic ligands such as urea or guanidine salts (45) and lithium bromide (294) is rather striking (Figure 12).

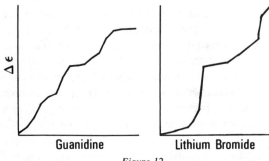

Guanidine   Lithium Bromide

Figure 12

Multiple stable states across increasing concentrations of charged hydrophobic $[R\text{-}L]_i$ as in Figure 11 generate the expected instabilities in the time domain as in Figure 13: [^{3}H]-cAMP binding to purified plasma membranes from *D. discoideum* (295) on the left; cumulative [^{3}H]-spiroperidol binding to crude rat striatal membranes (296) in the center; and a similar preparation with more frequent sampling displayed as differences from mean velocity (264) on the right.

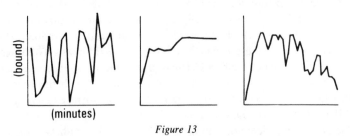

Figure 13

Most of these complex nonlinear behaviors, called surface phenomena in the context of [^{3}H]-spiperone binding to crude striatal membranes (297), were demonstrated several years ago in the context of studies of insulin-receptor interactions (297a, 298) and included the multiphasic, concave upward Eadie-Scatchard plot (299); the same $[R\text{-}L]_i$-induced increases and decreases in binding as seen in Figure 3 and modeled in Equation 8 and Figure 7 (300, 301); and anomalous time-dependent dissociation behavior in the context of the affinities of ligand binding saturation functions (297a, 301, 302). A dynamic (Figure 14, right) in contrast to a structural (Figure 14, left) scheme portraying the interactions between $[R\text{-}L]_i$ and membrane receptors is seen as an exchange of solvent entropies (303) between ligand and receptor polypeptide chains (279), a system with, if anything, more degrees of freedom with respect to the specific encoding of information than that of a static, lock-and-key structure. A successful ligand-membrane receptor interaction may depend upon resonance in the ligand-induced, solvent-mediated receptor response function.

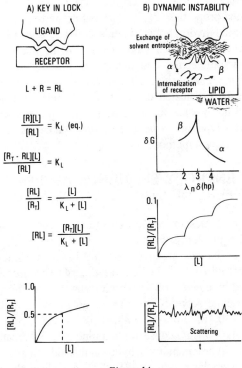

Figure 14

The receptor peptide is portrayed as a transitional β-strand-like form, unstable in water (29, 304–307) and a configuration seen often in binding domains of proteins (308–311). It is perturbed by a [R-L]$_i$-induced change in the neighboring solvent structural dynamics into a volume-reduced, more α-helical form as seen in lysine and leucine copolymer transitions (314), and hydrophobic negative solvent entropy drives it into the lipid bilayer, a process called receptor internalization (312). In this less hydrophobic, lower ΔG environment it can reform. Similar solvent-mediated peptide-peptide dynamics are observed in studies of protein folding (306). It should be noted that there is evidence that the internalization process in non-central nervous system tissue is associated with receptor-mediated endocytosis (313, 314). The membrane perturbation associated with these events could serve as a low-energy, instability-induced trigger for the subsequent transconductional events. Exquisitely solvent structure-sensitive rates of spontaneous depolarization (for example, after small changes in sodium concentration) characterize the behavior of artificial lipid bilayer models of neuronal membranes (315; M. Montal, personal communication, 1981).

Since water structure and dynamics in a closed system are temporally and spatially distributed properties (21, 22), global properties of pharmacological and peptide charged hydrophobic ligands can be rationalized as induced changes in solvent entropy over large regions of the brain and reflected in influences on macromolecular and membrane stability. This suggests that predictions about the relationship between structures and functions of families of [R-L]$_i$'s could be predicated on the basis of their influences on solvent entropies. Due to the precise quantification of this property in kcal for each amino acid, brain polypeptide structure and function can serve as a test of this [R-L]$_i$, solvent entropy hypothesis.

A SOLVENT ENTROPY SEQUENCE APPROACH TO BRAIN POLYPEPTIDE STRUCTURE AND FUNCTION

Recent systematic studies of codon substitution errors and secondary and tertiary structural equivalences in the evolution of polypeptide chains indicate that amino-acid exchanges are made on the basis of similarities in their affinities for water (309, 316, 317). Four families of five amino acids each have been characterized by conversion as energies via their equilibrium kinetics of transport from organic solvents to water as an index of hydrophobicity in kcal/mol: $0.00 \rightarrow 0.10$, $0.66 \rightarrow 0.87$, $1.57 \rightarrow 2.17$, and $2.67 \rightarrow 3.77$ (318–320). In β short spans, consecutive amino acids alternate between low and high values for hydrophobicity; a hydrophobic side chain is surrounded by two hydrophilic or apolar residues (321–323). α-Helical short spans have a two-fold greater wavelength in the hydrophobicity sequence of their residues in which on the average two hydrophobic side chains are followed by two that are hydrophilic or apolar (323–325). The increased adjacency of hydrophobic groups in a longer wavelength, α-helix-like structure leads to more negative solvent entropy-forced self-aggregation between the residues (a critical mass may serve to recruit even more of the chain), a reduced volume of solvent occupancy, and less solvent structural distortion; a sequence varying more frequently between hydrophobic and hydrophilic or apolar residues as in a β-strand occupies a greater solvent volume and induces greater destabilizing ΔG in solvent entropy (307). For example, α-helices become conformationally stable in solution in 10^{-7} seconds (326), whereas the β-conformation requires minutes (327, 328).

On the basis of these findings and the above development involving solvent-mediated macromolecular stability, two members with well-established differences in potency were selected from each of six families of neurobiologically active peptides. The polypeptides were normalized to equivalent lengths; the sequence of deviations from mean hydrophobicity in kcal was determined for each peptide, treated as in Equation 1, and its D_A value calculated (303, 329). As $[R-L]_i$, the faster-frequency, more β-strand-like series, having a higher D_A than the more smoothly varying α-helix sequences, were predicted to generate higher solvent ΔG-mediated macromolecular and membrane instability, with a resulting increase in central nervous system potency (Figure 15).

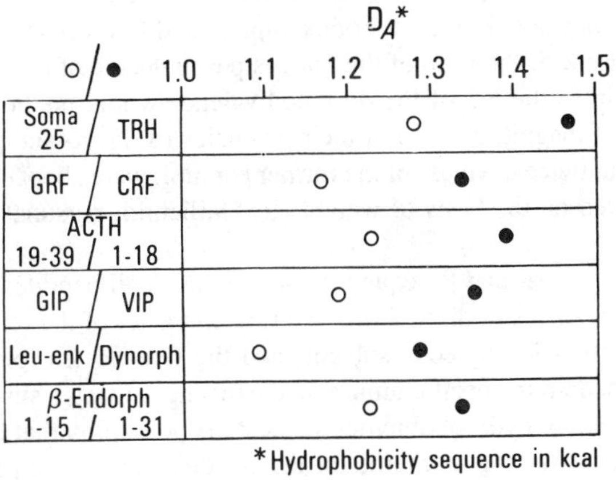

$$D_A{}^*$$

		1.0	1.1	1.2	1.3	1.4	1.5
Soma 25 / TRH					O		●
GRF / CRF				O	●		
ACTH 19-39 / 1-18					O	●	
GIP / VIP				O	●		
Leu-enk / Dynorph			O		●		
β-Endorph 1-15 / 1-31				O	●		

*Hydrophobicity sequence in kcal

Figure 15

The chart demonstrates that a higher D_A (solid dot) is manifested by the more behaviorally activating of each pair of peptides, i.e. by thyrotropin-releasing hormone than by somatostatin-25, by corticotropin-releasing factor than by growth-hormone releasing factor, by the first segment of adrenocorticotrophic hormone than by the second, by vasoactive intestinal peptide than by gastrointestinal peptide, by dynorphin than by leu-enkephalin, and by the entire β-endorphin than by the first half of its sequence (330–336; R. Guillemin, personal communication, 1983; P. Brazeau, personal communication, 1983). The nonlinearity of influences of an $[R-L]_i$ on the activity and stability properties of TOH and TPOH, seen in Figures 3 and 6 as modeled in Equation 8 and Figures 7 and 8, is also observed in the excitatory, inhibitory, and nil effects of the same peptide, depending on neural cell type, anatomical location, and associated neurotransmitter ligands (335, 336). The characteristic partial antagonisms among the participants in a multidetermined system rather than the monotonic ordering of values of the geometric dimension on the hydrophobicity sequence in relation to effect, as in Figure 15, may better predict the actions of related neural peptide pairs. For example, substance P ($D_A = 1.10$), dense in terminals A_{10} mesencephalic dopamine cell bodies, induces an amphetamine-like hyperactivity syndrome when infused into the ventral tegmental region (337); neurotensin ($D_A = 1.34$), located similarly (338), blocks amphetamine-induced hyperactivity and stereotypy when given intracerebrally (339). Perhaps an aggregate of regionally involved brain peptides can be summed logarithmically like Lyapounov exponents of stability (237–239) in order to predict their multiplicatively summed influence on a system (303).

This approach also suggests the possibility that the one ligand molecule-one receptor protein moiety stoichiometry implicit in the use of molarity instead of weight as the meaningful unit in studies of dose-response functions of polypeptides may not be correct. For example, the difference in the exponents, D_A, to the base 2.5, the ratio of the masses per molecule of dynorphin versus leu-enkephalin as the log of the dose equivalence would predict the roughly three orders of magnitude ratio of their potencies (331). α- and β-endorphin, the latter about twice the mass of the former per mol, were about equally potent when compared on the basis of weight (R. Guillemin, personal communication, 1983).

The ubiquity of α- and β-sequence short spans in all peptides and proteins (323), the differences in the stability-altering character of the relationships of the two patterns with aqueous solvent, and the five- to ten-fold increase in degrees of freedom in specific amino-acid exchanges using a simple up-down code of variation in hydrophobicities suggest the possibility that the history of difficulty in constructing a scheme for the custom synthesis of peptides (340) may have been due to a requirement for too much specificity. A macro-code of α and β short span rather than amino-acid sequences is suggested. A recent model with this sort of relaxed structural requirement is explained in terms of an α-helical peptide's asymmetric potential for membrane binding (341). The simplest of all possibilities involves a binary code, a dot versus dash transition probability, each successive residue crossing the mean or not in a mod-2 sequence dynamic of hydrophobicity (303). A perfect β-strand would have a $p(\Delta)$ of 1.0, and an α-helical short span, a $p(\Delta)$ of 0.5. The amino-acid sequences of corticotropin-releasing factor and a polypeptide with very similar actions and potency, urotensin-I (342), differ in 20 of 41 residues. In the binary code of hydrophobicity there are two adjacent transpositions, at 22 and 39, and only two differences, at 27 and 33 (303, 329).

A reflection of the competition for solvent entropy between a macromolecular system (TPOH) and a polypeptide (leu-enkephalin) examined under control conditions and in the presence of the neuropeptide is seen in Figure 16. An $[R-L]_i$-induced change in the kinetic scattering pattern is seen in a more gaussian distribution of A values from multiple simultaneous determinations, although the median velocity remains the same:

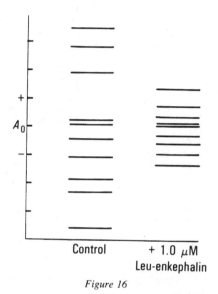

Figure 16

The statistical dynamics of non-equilibrium brain enzyme and receptor systems may offer a new experimental language for studies in molecular psychopharmacology.

ACKNOWLEDGEMENTS

The list of people to whom I feel indebted for stimulating discussions bearing on the issues discussed in this review might be virtually endless, but would certainly include Ralph Abraham, Ralph Adams, Daniel Atkinson, Erol Başar, Floyd Bloom, Paul Boyer, Paul Brazeau, Britton Chance, Jack Cowan, Cindy Ehlers, Marlene DeLuca, Manfred Eigen, Doyne Farmer, George Feher, Hans Frauenfelder, Alan Garfinkel, Albert Goldbeter, Roger Guillemin, Hermann Haken, Stuart Kauffman, Seymour Kaufman, Roy King, Suzanne Knapp, Daniel Koshland, Walter Lovenberg, Benoit Mandelbrot, William McElroy, Maurice Montal, Elliott Montroll, John Ross, David Ruelle, Patrick Russo,

Rob Shaw, Kurt Shuler, René Thom, Kenneth Watson, Norman Weiner, Bruce West, Kent Wilson, and Christopher Zeeman. I am also grateful to Patrick Russo for computer assistance and to Barbara Blomgren for computer, editorial, and production assistance. Our work is supported by grants from the John D. and Catherine T. MacArthur Foundation, the W. M. Keck Foundation, DA–00265–11 and MH16109–04 from the United States Public Health Service, and Contract DAAG20–83-K-0069 from the United States Army Research Office.

Literature Cited

1. Mandell, A. J. 1978. Redundant mechanisms regulating brain tyrosine and tryptophan hydroxylases. *Ann. Rev. Pharmacol. Toxicol.* 18:461–93
2. Joh, T. H., Park, D. H., Reis, D. J. 1978. Direct phosphorylation of brain tyrosine hydroxylase by cyclic AMP-dependent protein kinase: Mechanism of enzyme activation. *Proc. Natl. Acad. Sci. USA* 75:4744–48
3. Weiner, N. 1979. Tyrosine-3-monooxygenase. In *Aromatic Amino Acid Hydroxylases and Mental Disease*, ed. M. B. H. Youdim, pp. 141–90. New York: Wiley. 390 pp.
4. Vulliet, P. R., Langan, T. A., Weiner, N. 1980. Tyrosine hydroxylase: A substrate of cyclic AMP-dependent protein kinase. *Proc. Natl. Acad. Sci. USA* 77:92–96
5. Edelman, A. M., Raese, J. D., Lazar, M. A., Barchas, J. D. 1981. Tyrosine hydroxylase: Studies on the phosphorylation of a purified preparation of the brain enzyme by the cyclic AMP-dependent protein kinase. *J. Pharmacol. Exp. Ther.* 216:647–53
6. Fujisawa, H., Yamauchi, T., Nakata, H., Okuno, S. 1982. Regulation of tryptophan 5-monooxygenase and tyrosine 3-monooxygenase by protein kinases. In *Oxygenases and Oxygen Metabolism,* ed. M. Nazaki, S. Yamamoto, Y. Ishimura, M. J. Coon, L. Ernster, R. W. Estabrook, pp. 281–92. New York: Academic. 664 pp.
7. Kuhn, D. M., Lovenberg, W. 1982. Role of calmodulin in the activation of tryptophan hydroxylase. *Fed. Proc.* 41:2258–64
8. Boadle-Biber, M. C. 1982. Further studies on the role of calcium in the depolarization-induced activation of tryptophan hydroxylase. *Fed. Proc.* 31:2495–503
8a. Haken, H. 1978. *Synergetics.* New York: Springer-Verlag. 355 pp.
9. Ma, S-K. 1976. *Modern Theory of Critical Phenomena.* New York: Benjamin Cummings. 561 pp.
10. Glansdorff, P., Prigogine, I. 1971. *Thermodynamic Theory of Structure, Stability and Fluctuations.* New York: Wiley. 306 pp.
11. Montroll, E. W., West, B. J. 1979. On an enriched collection of stochastic processes. In *Fluctuation Phenomena,* ed. E. W. Montroll, J. L. Lebowitz, pp. 63–175. New York: North-Holland. 350 pp.
12. Reichl, L. E. 1980. *A Modern Course in Statistical Physics,* pp. 307–46. Austin: Univ. Texas Press. 709 pp.
13. Van Kampen, N. G. 1981. *Stochastic Processes in Physics and Chemistry,* pp. 304–38. New York: North-Holland. 419 pp.
14. Moser, J. 1973. Stable and random motions in dynamical systems. *Ann. Math Studies* 77:21–60
15. Bowen, R., Ruelle, D. 1975. The ergodic theory of axiom A flows. *Invent. Math.* 29:181–202
16. Ruelle, D. 1977. *Statistical Mechanics and Dynamical Systems,* pp. 1–108. Durham, NC: Duke Univ. Press. 304 pp.
17. Collet, P., Eckmann, J-P. 1980. *Iterated Maps on the Interval as Dynamical Systems,* pp. 1–62. Boston: Birkhauser. 248 pp.
18. Ott, E. 1981. Strange attractors and chaotic motions of dynamical systems. *Rev. Mod. Phys.* 53:655–71
19. Eckmann, J-P. 1981. Roads to turbulence in dissipative dynamical systems. *Rev. Mod. Phys.* 53:643–54
20. Helleman, R. H. G. 1983. One mechanism for the onsets of large-scale chaos in conservative and dissipative systems. In *Long-Time Prediction in Dynamics,* ed. C. W. Horton, L. E. Reichl, V. G. Szebehely, pp. 95–126. New York: Wiley. 496 pp.
21. Eisenberg, D., Kauzmann, W. 1969. *The Structure and Properties of Water,* pp.

205–27. New York: Oxford Univ. Press. 296 pp.

22. Stillinger, F. H. 1980. Water revisited. *Science* 209:451–57

23. Tanford, C. 1973. *The Hydrophobic Effect*, pp. 24–80. New York: Wiley-Interscience. 233 pp.

24. Tanford, C. 1979. Interfacial free energy and the hydrophobic effect. *Proc. Natl. Acad. Sci. USA* 75:4175–76

25. Ben-Naim, A. 1980. *Hydrophobic Interactions*. New York: Plenum. 311 pp.

26. Cooke, R., Kuntz, I. D. 1974. The properties of water in biological systems. *Ann. Rev. Biophys. Bioeng.* 3:95–126

27. Eagland, D. 1975. Nucleic acids, peptides and proteins. In *Water: A Comprehensive Treatise*, ed. F. Franks, 3:305–18. New York: Plenum. 472 pp.

28. Kauzmann, W. 1959. Some factors in the interpretation of protein denaturation. *Adv. Prot. Chem.* 14:1–68

29. Sturtevant, J. M. 1977. Heat capacity and entropy changes in processes involving proteins. *Proc. Natl. Acad. Sci. USA* 74:2236–40

30. Finney, J. L. 1977. The organization and function of water in protein crystals. *Phil. Trans. R. Soc. London Ser. B* 278:3–32

31. Finney, J. L. 1979. The organization and function of water in protein crystals. In *Water: A Comprehensive Treatise*, ed. F. Franks, 6:47–122. New York: Plenum. 455 pp.

32. Edsall, J. T. 1965. Apparent molal volume, heat capacity, compressibility and surface tension of dipolar ions in solution. In *Proteins, Amino Acids, and Peptides as Ions and DiPolar Ions*, ed. E. J. Cohen, J. T. Edsall, pp. 155–76. New York: Hafner. 686 pp.

33. Yang, J. T. 1961. The viscosity of macromolecules in relation to molecular conformation. *Adv. Prot. Chem.* 16:323–401

34. Careri, G., Fasella, P., Gratton, E. 1975. Statistical time events in enzymes: A physical assessment. *CRC Crit. Rev. Biochem.* 3:141–64

35. Woodward, C. K., Hilton, B. D. 1979. Hydrogen exchange kinetics and internal motions in proteins and nucleic acids. *Ann. Rev. Biophys. Bioeng.* 8:99–127

36. Gurd, F. R. N., Rothgeb, T. M. 1979. Motions in proteins. *Adv. Prot. Chem.* 33:74–165

37. Williams, R. J. P. 1979. The conformational properties of proteins in solution. *Biol. Rev.* 54:389–437

38. McCammon, J. A., Karplus, M. 1980. Simulation of protein dynamics. *Ann. Rev. Phys. Chem.* 31:29–45

39. Austin, R. H., Beeson, K. W., Eisenstein, L., Frauenfelder, H., Gunsalus, I. C. 1975. Dynamics of ligand binding to myoglobin. *Biochemistry* 14:5355–73

40. Alberding, N., Austin, R. H., Chau, S. S., Eisenstein, L., Frauenfelder, H., Gunsalus, I. C., Nordlund, T. M. 1976. Dynamics of carbon monoxide binding to protoheme. *J. Chem. Phys.* 65:4701–11

41. Beece, D., Eisenstein, L., Frauenfelder, H., Good, D., Marden, M. C., Reinisch, L., Reynolds, A. H., Sorensen, L. B., Yue, K. T. 1980. Solvent viscosity and protein dynamics. *Biochemistry* 19:5147–57

42. Karplus, M., Weaver, D. L. 1976. Protein-folding dynamics. *Nature* 260:404–06

43. Baldwin, R. L. 1978. The pathway of protein folding. *Trends Biochem. Sci.* 3:66–68

44. Cooper, A. 1976. Thermodynamic fluctuations in protein molecules. *Proc. Natl. Acad. Sci. USA* 73:2740–41

45. Riddiford, L. M. 1966. Solvent perturbation and ultraviolet optical rotatory dispersion studies of paramyosin. *J. Biol. Chem.* 421:2792–802

46. Hammes, G. G., Swann, J. C. 1967. Influence of denaturing agents on solvent structure. *Biochemistry* 6:1591–96

47. Gavish, B., Werber, M. M. 1979. Viscosity-dependent structural fluctuations in enzyme catalysis. *Biochemistry* 18:1269–75

48. Atkinson, D. E. 1977. *Cellular Energy Metabolism and Its Regulation*, pp. 1–12. New York: Academic. 293 pp.

49. Oxtoby, J. C., Ulam, S. M. 1941. Measure preserving homeomorphisms and metrical transitivity. *Ann. Math.* 42:874–920

50. Kolmogorov, A. N. 1965. Three approaches to the quantitative definition of information. *Prob. Inf. Trans.* 1:1–36

51. Billingsley, P. 1965. *Ergodic Theory and Information*. New York: Wiley. 193 pp.

52. Arnold, V. I., Avez, A. 1968. *Ergodic Problems of Classical Mechanics*, pp. 81–114. New York: Benjamin. 286 pp.

53. Sinai, Y. 1972. Gibbsian measures in ergodic theory. *Russ. Math. Surv.* 27:21–46

54. Yorke, J. A., Yorke, E. D. 1979. Metastable chaos: The transition to sustained chaotic behavior in the Lorenz model. *J. Stat. Phys.* 21:263–74

55. Ford, J. 1983. How random is a coin toss? *Physics Today* 36(4):40–47

56. Overton, D. A. 1974. Experimental

methods for the study of state-dependent learning. *Fed. Proc.* 33:1800–13

57. Mandell, A. J. 1980. Vertical integration of levels of brain function through parametric symmetries within self-similar stochastic fields. In *Information Processing in the Nervous System,* ed. H. M. Pinsker, W. D. Willis, pp. 177–97. New York: Raven. 366 pp.

58. Mandell, A. J., Stewart, K. D., Russo, P. V. 1981. The Sunday syndrome: From kinetics to altered consciousness. *Fed. Proc.* 40:2693–98

59. Kaufman, S. 1958. A new cofactor required for the enzymatic conversion of phenylalanine to tyrosine. *J. Biol. Chem.* 230:931–39

60. Bullard, W. P., Guthrie, P. B., Russo, P. V., Mandell, A. J. 1978. Regional and subcellular distribution and some factors in the regulation of reduced pterins in rat brain. *J. Pharmacol. Exp. Ther.* 206:4–20

61. Levine, R. A., Kuhn, D. M., Lovenberg, W. 1979. The regional distribution of hydroxylase cofactor in rat brain. *J. Neurochem.* 32:1575–78

62. Fukushima, T., Nixon, J. C. 1980. Analysis of reduced forms of biopterin in biological tissues and fluids. *Anal. Biochem.* 102:176–88

63. Nagatsu, T., Yamaguchi, T., Kato, T., Sugimoto, T., Matsuura, S., Akino, M., Tsushima, S., Nakazawa, N., Ogawa, H. 1981. Radioimmunoassay for biopterin in body fluids and tissues. *Anal. Biochem.* 110:182–89

64. Levine, R. A., Miller, L. P., Lovenberg, W. 1981. Tetrahydrobiopterin in striatum: Localization in dopamine terminals and role in catecholamine synthesis. *Science* 214:919–21

65. Lovenberg, W., Levine, R. A., Miller, L. P. 1981. Hydroxylase cofactor and catecholamine synthesis. In *Function and Regulation of Monoamine Enzymes: Basic and Clinical Aspects,* ed. E. Usdin, N. Weiner, M. B. H. Youdim, pp. 225–30. London: Macmillan. 961 pp.

66. Wurtman, R. J., Scally, M. C. 1977. Precursor control of neurotransmitter synthesis. In *Structure and Function of Monoamine Enzymes,* ed. E. Usdin, N. Weiner, M. B. H. Youdim, pp. 231–62. New York: Dekker. 996 pp.

66a. Mandell, A. J., Russo, P. V. 1981. Short-term regulation of hydroxylase cofactor in rat brain. *J. Neurochem.* 37:1573–78

67. Tong, J. H., Kaufman, S. 1975. Tryptophan hydroxylase. Purification and some properties of the enzyme from rabbit hindbrain. *J. Biol. Chem.* 250:4152–58

68. Kaufman, S., Fisher, D. B. 1974. Pterin-requiring aromatic amino acid hydroxylases. In *Molecular Mechanisms of Oxygen Activation,* ed. O. Hayaishi, pp. 285–369. New York: Academic. 678 pp.

69. Oka, K., Ashiba, G., Sugimoto, T., Matsuura, S., Nagatsu, T. 1982. Kinetic properties of tyrosine hydroxylase purified from bovine adrenal medulla and bovine caudate nucleus. *Biochim. Biophys. Acta* 706:188–96

70. Okuno, S., Fujisawa, H. 1982. Purification and some properties of tyrosine-3-monooxygenase from rat adrenal. *Eur. J. Biochem.* 122:49–55

71. Nakata, H., Fujisawa, H. 1982. Purification and properties of tryptophan-5-monooxygenase from rat brain stem. *Eur. J. Biochem.* 122:41–47

72. Mandell, A. J., Russo, P. V. 1981. Striatal tyrosine hydroxylase activity: Multiple conformational kinetic oscillators and product concentration frequencies. *J. Neurosci.* 1:380–89

73. Knapp, S., Mandell, A. J. 1983. Lithium and chlorimipramine differentially alter the stability properties of tryptophan hydroxylase as seen in allosteric and scattering kinetics. *Psychiat. Res.* 8:204–25

74. Kuczenski, R. 1979. Effects of parachlorophenylalanine on amphetamine and haloperidol-induced changes in striatal dopamine turnover. *Brain Res.* 164:217–25

75. Kuczenski, R. 1980. Amphetamine-haloperidol interactions on striatal and mesolimbic tyrosine hydroxylase and dopamine metabolism. *J. Pharmacol. Exp. Ther.* 215:135–42

76. Ikeda, M., Fahien, L. A., Udenfriend, S. 1966. A kinetic study of bovine adrenal tyrosine hydroxylase. *J. Biol. Chem.* 241:4452–56

77. Joh, T. H., Kapit, R., Goldstein, M. 1969. A kinetic study of particulate bovine adrenal tyrosine hydroxylase. *Biochim. Biophys. Acta* 171:378–80

78. Kuczenski, R., Mandell, A. J. 1972. Regulatory properties of soluble and particulate rat brain tyrosine hydroxylase. *J. Biol. Chem.* 247:3114–22

79. Musacchio, J. M., McQueen, C. A., Craviso, G. L. 1973. Tyrosine hydroxylase: Subcellular distribution and molecular and kinetic characteristics of the different enzyme forms. In *New Concepts in Neurotransmitter Regulation,* ed. A. J. Mandell, pp. 69–88. New York: Plenum. 316 pp.

80. Weiner, N., Lee, F-L., Barnes, E.,

Dreyer, E. 1977. Enzymology of tyrosine hydroxylase and the role of cyclic nucleotides in its regulation. See Ref. 66, pp. 109–48

81. Bullard, W. P., Capson, T. L. 1982. Steady-state kinetics of tyrosine hydroxylase. (Privately circulated manuscript)

82. Davis, J. N. 1976. Brain tyrosine hydroxylation: Alteration of oxygen affinity *in vivo* by immobilization of electroshock in the rat. *J. Neurochem.* 27:211–15

82a. Kuhn, D. M., Ruskin, B., Lovenberg, W. 1978. Tryptophan hydroxylase: The role of oxygen, iron, and sulfhydryl groups as determinants of stability and catalytic activity. *J. Biol. Chem.* 255:4137–43

83. Vaccari, A., Brotman, S., Cimino, J., Timiras, P. S. 1978. Adaptive changes induced by high altitude in the development of brain monoamine enzymes. *Neurochem. Res.* 3:295–311

84. Gonzales, C., Kwok, Y., Gibb, J., Fidone, S. 1979. Effects of hypoxia on tyrosine hydroxylase activity in rat carotid artery. *J. Neurochem.* 33:713–19

85. Kuhn, D. M., Ruskin, B., Lovenberg, W. 1979. Studies on the oxygen sensitivity of tryptophan hydroxylase. *Adv. Exp. Med. Biol.* 133:253–63

86. Katz, I. R. 1980. Oxygen affinity of tyrosine and tryptophan hydroxylases in synaptosomes. *J. Neurochem.* 35:760–63

87. Katz, I. R. 1981. Interaction between the oxygen and tryptophan dependence of synaptosomal tryptophan hydroxylase. *J. Neurochem.* 37:447–51

88. Ayling, J. E., Bailey, S. W. 1982. Mechanism of tetrahydrobiopterin-dependent monooxygenases. See Ref. 6, pp. 267–77

89. Benkovic, S. J. 1980. On the mechanism of action of folate and biopterin requiring enzymes. *Ann. Rev. Biochem.* 49:227–51

90. Shiman, R., Akino, M., Kaufman, S. 1971. Solubilization and partial purification of tyrosine hydroxylase from bovine adrenal medulla. *J. Biol. Chem.* 246:1330–40

91. Yamaguchi, T., Sawada, M., Kato, T., Nagatsu, T. 1981. Demonstration of tryptophan-5-monooxygenase activity in human brain by highly sensitive high-performance liquid chromatography with fluorometric detection. *Biochem. Internatl.* 2:295–303

92. Badawy, A. A., Williams, D. L. 1982. Enhancement of rat brain catecholamine synthesis by administration of small doses of tyrosine and evidence for substrate inhibition of tyrosine hydroxylase activity by large doses of the amino acid. *Biochem. J.* 206:165–68

93. Snady, H., Musacchio, J. M. 1978. Quinonoid dihydropterin reductase-II; Regional and subcellular distribution of rat brain enzyme. *Biochem. Pharmacol.* 27:1947–53

94. Mandell, A. J., Russo, P. V., Knapp, S. 1982. Strange stability in hierarchically coupled neuropsychobiological systems. In *Evolution of Chaos and Order in Physics, Chemistry, and Biology*, ed. H. Haken, pp. 270–86. New York: Springer-Verlag. 287 pp.

95. Mann, S. P., Gordon, J. 1979. Inhibition of guinea-pig brain tyrosine hydroxylase by catechols and biopterin. *J. Neurochem.* 33:133–38

96. Kato, T., Yamaguchi, T., Nagatsu, T., Sugimoto, T., Matsuura, S. 1980. Effects of structures of tetrahydropterin cofactors on rat brain tryptophan hydroxylase. *Biochim. Biophys. Acta* 611:241–50

97. Oka, K., Kato, T., Sugimoto, T., Matsuura, S., Nagatsu, T. 1981. Kinetic properties of tyrosine hydroxylase with natural tetrahydrobiopterin as cofactor. *Biochim. Biophys. Acta* 661:45–53

98. Kuhn, D. M. 1983. Deactivation of tyrosine hydroxylase by reduced pterins. *Trans. Am. Soc. Neurochem.* 14:175 (Abstr. 181)

99. Kuhn, D. M. 1984. Further studies on the activation of tryptophan hydroxylase by phosphorylating conditions. *J. Neurochem.* In press

100. Teipel, J., Koshland, D. E. 1969. The significance of intermediary plateau regions in enzyme saturation curves. *Biochemistry* 8:4656–63

101. Levitzki, A., Koshland, D. E. 1969. Negative cooperativity in regulatory enzymes. *Proc. Natl. Acad. Sci. USA* 62:1121–28

102. Walker, E. J., Ralston, G. B., Darvey, I. G. 1975. An allosteric model for ribonuclease. *Biochem. J.* 147:425–33

103. Goldbeter, A., Caplan, S. R. 1976. Oscillatory enzymes. *Ann. Rev. Biophys. Bioeng.* 5:449–75

104. Hess, B., Goldbeter, A., Lefever, R. 1978. Temporal, spatial, and functional order in regulated biochemical and cellular systems. *Adv. Chem. Phys.* 38:363–413

105. Olsen, L. F., Degn, H. 1978. Oscillatory kinetics of the peroxidase-oxidase reaction in an open system. *Biochim. Biophys. Acta* 523:321–34

106. Degn, H., Olsen, L. F., Perram, J. W. 1979. Bistability, oscillation, and chaos in an enzyme reaction. *Ann. NY Acad. Sci.* 316:623–37
107. Boiteux, A., Hess, B., Sel'kov, E. E. 1980. Creative functions of instability and oscillations in metabolic systems. *Curr. Top. Cell Reg.* 17:171–203
108. Decroly, O., Goldbeter, A. 1982. Birhythmicity, chaos, and other patterns of temporal self-organization in a multiply regulated biochemical system. *Proc. Natl. Acad. Sci. USA* 79:6917–21
109. Knapp, S., Mandell, A. J. 1979. Conformational influences on brain tryptophan hydroxylase by submicromolar calcium: Opposite effects of equimolar lithium. *J. Neural Transm.* 415:1–15
110. Deleted in proof
111. Knapp, S., Mandell, A. J., Russo, P. V., Vitto, A., Stewart, K. D. 1981. Strain differences in kinetic and thermal stability of two mouse brain tryptophan hydroxylases. *Brain Res.* 230:317–36
112. Mandell, A. J., Knapp, S. 1982. Regulation of tryptophan hydroxylase: Variational kinetics suggest a neuropharmacology of phase. *Adv. Biochem. Psychopharmacol.* 34:1–15
113. Mandell, A. J., Russo, P. V. 1981. Striatal tyrosine hydroxylase: the role of cofactor concentration in the scaling of enzyme periodicity and behavioral stereotypy. See Ref. 65, pp. 271–80
114. Bullard, W. P., Yellin, J. B., Mandell, A. J. 1979. The pharmacology of striatal pterins and the regulation of dopaminergic function. In *Chemistry and Biology of Pteridines*, ed. R. L. Kisliuk, G. M. Brown, pp. 87–92. Amsterdam: Elsevier/North-Holland. 713 pp.
115. Mandell, A. J., Bullard, W. P., Russo, P. V., Yellin, J. B. 1980. The influence of D-amphetamine on rat brain striatal reduced biopterin concentration. *J. Pharmacol. Exp. Ther.* 213:569–74
116. Lovenberg, W., Alphs, L., Pradham, S., Bruckwick, E., Levine, R. 1980. Longterm haloperidol treatment and factors affecting the activity of striatal tyrosine hydroxylase. *Adv. Biochem. Psychopharmacol.* 24:9–15
117. Kuczenski, R. 1977. Biphasic effects of amphetamine on striatal dopamine dynamics. *Eur. J. Pharmacol.* 46:249–57
118. Hotchkiss, A. J., Morgan, M. E., Gibb, J. W. 1979. The long-term effects of multiple doses of amphetamine on neostriatal tryptophan hydroxylase, tyrosine hydroxylase, choline acetyltransferase, and glutamate decarboxylase activities. *Life Sci.* 25:1373–78
119. Hotchkiss, A. J., Gibb, J. W. 1980. Long-term effects of multiple doses of methamphetamine on tryptophan hydroxylase and tyrosine hydroxylase activity in rat brain. *J. Pharmacol. Exp. Ther.* 214:257–62
120. Trulson, M. E., Jacobs, B. L. 1980. Chronic amphetamine administration decreases brain tryptophan hydroxylase activity in cats. *Life Sci.* 26:329–35
121. Bakhit, C., Kwok, Y. C., Gibb, J. W. 1980. Effects of methamphetamine on kinetic characteristics of neostriatal tyrosine hydroxylase. *Life Sci.* 26:1815–19
122. Bakhit, C., Morgan, M. E., Gibb, J. W. 1981. Propranolol differentially blocks the methamphetamine-induced depression of tryptophan hydroxylase in various rat brain regions. *Neurosci. Lett.* 23:99–103
123. Bordsley, M. E., Bachelard, H. S. 1981. Catecholamine levels and tyrosine hydroxylase activities in rat brain regions after chronic treatment with and withdrawal of methamphetamine. *Biochem. Pharmacol.* 30:1543–49
124. Bakhit, C., Gibb, J. W. 1981. Methamphetamine-induced depression of tryptophan hydroxylase: Recovery following acute treatment. *Eur. J. Pharmacol.* 76:229–33
125. Trulson, M. E., Trulson, V. M. 1982. Effects of chronic methamphetamine administration on tryptophan hydroxylase activity, [^{3}H]serotonin synaptosomal uptake, and serotonin metabolism in rat brain following systematic tryptophan loading. *Neuropharmacology* 21:521–27
126. Wightman, R. M., Strope, E., Plotsky, P., Adams, R. N. 1976. Monitoring of transmitter metabolites by voltammetry in cerebrospinal fluid following neural pathway stimulation. *Nature* 262:145–46
127. Huff, R., Adams, R. N., Rutledge, C. D. 1979. Amphetamine dose-dependent changes of in vivo electrochemical signals in rat caudate. *Brain Res.* 173:369–72
128. Marsden, C. A., Conti, J., Strope, E., Curzon, G., Adams, R. N. 1979. Monitoring 5-hydroxytryptamine release in the brain of the freely moving unanesthetized rat using *in vivo* voltammetry. *Brain Res.* 171:85–99
129. Cespuglio, R., Faradji, H., Ponchou, J. L., Buda, M., Riou, F., Gonon, F., Pujol, J. F., Jouvet, M. 1981. Differential pulse voltammetry in brain tissue. I. Detection of 5-hydroxyindoles in the rat striatum. *Brain Res.* 223:287–98
130. Gonon, F., Buda, M., Cespuglio, R., Jouvet, M., Pujol, J. F. 1981. Voltam-

metry in the striatum of chronic freely moving rats: Detection of catechols and ascorbic acid. *Brain Res.* 223:69–80

131. Plotsky, P. M., DeGreef, W. J., Neill, J. D. 1982. In situ voltammetric microelectrodes: Application to the measurement of median eminence catecholamine release during simulated suckling. *Brain Res.* 250:251–62

132. Costa, E., Gessa, G. L., Kuntzman, R., Brodie, B. B. 1962. The effects of drugs on storage and release of serotonin and catecholamines in brain; pharmacological analysis of central nervous action. In *First International Pharmacology Meeting*, ed. W. D. M. Paton, 8:43–71. New York: Macmillan. 330 pp.

133. Kopin, I. J., Gorden, E. K., Horst, W. D. 1965. Studies of uptake of L-norpinephrine-C^{14}. *Biochem. Pharmacol.* 14:753–68

134. Glowinski, J., Axelrod, J. 1966. Effects of drugs on the disposition of H^3-norepinephrine in the rat brain. *Pharmacol. Rev.* 18:775–85

135. Neff, N. H., Costa, E. 1966. The influence of monoamine oxidase inhibition on catecholamine synthesis. *Life Sci.* 5:951–66

136. Linderstrøm-Lang, K. V. 1958. Deuterium exchange and protein structure. In *Symposium on Protein Structure*, ed. A. Neuberger, pp. 34–51. London: Metheun. 351 pp.

137. Linderstrøm-Lang, K. V., Schellman, J. A. 1959. Protein structure and enzyme activity. In *The Enzymes*, ed. P. D. Boyer, H. Lardy, K. Myrbäck, 1:443–510. New York: Academic.

138. Hvidt, A., Nielsen, S. O. 1966. Hydrogen exchange in proteins. *Adv. Prot. Chem.* 21:287–386

139. Englander, S. W. 1975. Measurement of structural and free energy changes in hemoglobin by hydrogen exchange methods. *Ann. NY Acad. Sci.* 244:10–27

140. McCammon, J. A., Karplus, M. 1979. Dynamics of activated processes in globular proteins. *Proc. Natl. Acad. Sci. USA* 76:3585–90

141. Chance, B., Hess, B., Betz, A. 1964. DPNH oscillations in a cell-free extract of *S. carlsbergensis*. *Biochem. Biophys. Res. Commun.* 16:182–87

142. Degn, H. 1968. Bistability caused by substrate inhibition of peroxidase in an open reaction system. *Nature* 217:1047–50

143. Lumsden, C. E., Pomerat, C. M. 1951. Normal oligodendrocytes in tissue culture. *Exp. Cell Res.* 2:103–14

144. Adey, W. R. 1981. Tissue interactions with nonionizing electromagnetic fields. *Physiol. Rev.* 61:435–74

145. Feller, W. 1968. *An Introduction to Probability Theory and Its Applications*, 1:303–41. New York: Wiley. 509 pp. 3rd ed.

146. Winfree, A. T. 1980. *The Geometry of Biological Time*, pp. 145–75. New York: Springer-Verlag. 530 pp.

147. Mandelbrot, B. B. 1977. *Fractals: Form, Chance, and Dimension*. San Francisco: W. H. Freeman. 365 pp.

148. McLennan, I. S., Lees, G. J. 1978. Diurnal changes in the kinetic properties of tryptophan hydroxylase from rat brain. *J. Neurochem.* 31:557–59

149. Sitaram, B. R., Lees, G. J. 1978. Diurnal rhythm and turnover of tryptophan hydroxylase in the pineal gland of the rat. *J. Neurochem.* 31:1021–26

150. Shibuya, H., Toru, M., Watanabe, S. 1978. A circadian rhythm of tryptophan hydroxylase in rat pineals. *Brain Res.* 138:364–68

151. Natali, J-P., McRae-Degeurce, A., Chouvet, G., Pujol, J-F. 1980. Genetic studies of daily variations of first-step enzymes of monoamine metabolism in the brain of inbred strains of mice and hybrids. I. *Brain Res.* 191:191–203

152. Natali, J-P., McRae-Degeurce, A., Keane, P., Debilly, G., Pujol, J-F. 1980. Genetic studies of daily variations of first-step enzymes of monoamine metabolism in the brain of inbred strains of mice and hybrids. II. *Brain Res.* 191:205–13

153. Cahill, A. L., Ehret, C. F. 1981. Circadian variations in the activity of tyrosine hydroxylase, tyrosine aminotransferase, and tryptophan hydroxylase: Relationship to catecholamine metabolism. *J. Neurochem.* 37:1109–15

154. Wehr, T. A., Goodwin, F. K., eds. 1983. *Circadion Rhythms and Psychiatry*. Los Angeles: Boxwood.

155. Careri, G., Fasella, P., Gratton, E. 1979. Enzyme dynamics: The statistical physics approach. *Ann. Rev. Biophys. Bioeng.* 8:69–97

156. Clauser, F. H. 1956. The behavior of non-linear systems. *J. Aeronaut. Sci.* 23:411–34

157. Swinney, H. L., Gollub, J. P. 1981. *Hydrodynamic Instabilities and the Transition to Turbulence*. New York: Springer-Verlag. 292 pp.

158. Peitgen, H-O. 1982. Phase transitions in the homoclinic regieme of area-preserving diffeomorphisms. See Ref. 94, pp. 197–214

159. Marsden, J. E. 1978. Qualitative

methods in bifurcation theory. *Bull. Am. Math. Soc.* 84:1125–48

159a. Mandell, A. J. 1983. From intermittency to transitivity in neuropsychobiological flows. *Am. J. Physiol.* 245 (Reg. Integ. Comp. Physiol. 14):R484–94

160. Grossmann, S., Thomae, S. 1977. Invariant distributions and stationary correlation functions of one-dimensional discrete processes. *Z. Naturforsch. Teil A* 32:1353–63

161. Ruelle, D. 1979. Sensitive dependence on initial condition and turbulent behavior of dynamical systems. *Ann. NY Acad. Sci.* 316:408–16

162. Mandell, A. J., Knapp, S., Kuczenski, R., Segal, D. S. 1972. Methamphetamine-induced alteration in the physical state of rat caudate tyrosine hydroxylase. *Biochem. Pharmacol.* 21:2737–50

163. Kuczenski, R., Mandell, A. J. 1972. Allosteric activation of hypothalamic tyrosine hydroxylase by ions and sulfated mucopolysaccharides. *J. Neurochem.* 19:131–37

164. Kuczenski, R. 1973. Soluble, membrane-bound, and detergent-solubilized rat striatal tyrosine hydroxylase. *J. Biol. Chem.* 248:5074–80

165. Kuczenski, R. 1974. Effect of sodium dodecyl sulfate on the kinetic properties and molecular weight of rat striatal tyrosine hydroxylase. *Life Sci.* 14:2379–84

166. Kuczenski, R. 1975. Conformational adaptability of tyrosine hydroxylase in the regulation of striatal dopamine biosynthesis. *Adv. Biochem. Psychopharmacol.* 13:109–26

167. Rubio, M. C. 1979. Physical state of tyrosine hydroxylase in the ganglia and nerve endings. *Gen. Pharmacol.* 10:297–302

168. Pickel, V. M., Beckley, S. C., Joh, T. H., Reis, D. J. 1981. Ultrastructural immunocytochemical localization of tyrosine hydroxylase in the neostriatum. *Brain Res.* 225:373–85

169. Kuczenski, R. 1983. Effects of phospholipases on the kinetic properties of rat striatal membrane-bound tyrosine hydroxylase. *J. Neurochem.* 40(3):821–29

170. Lloyd, T. 1979. The effects of phosphatidylinositol on tyrosine hydroxylase: Stimulation and inactivation. *J. Biol. Chem.* 254:7247–54

171. Hamon, M., Bourgoin, S., Hery, F., Simmonet, G. 1978. Phospholipid-induced activation of tryptophan hydroxylase from the rat brainstem. *Biochem. Pharmacol.* 27:915–22

172. Vigny, A., Henry, J-P. 1981. Bovine adrenal tyrosine hydroxylase: Compara-

tive study of native and proteolyzed enzyme and their interaction with anions. *J. Neurochem.* 36:483–89

173. Lloyd, T., Walega, M. A. 1981. Purification of tyrosine hydroxylase by high-pressure liquid chromatography. *Anal. Biochem.* 116:559–63

174. Hamon, M., Bourgoin, S., Artaud, F., Mestikawy, S. E. 1981. The respective roles of tryptophan uptake and tryptophan hydroxylase in the regulation of serotonin synthesis in the central nervous system. *J. Physiol. (Paris)* 77:269–79

175. Stephens, J. K., Masserano, J. M., Vulliet, P. R., Weiner, N., Nakane, P. K. 1981. Immunocytochemical localization of tyrosine hydroxylase in rat adrenal medulla by the peroxidase labeled antibody method: Effects of enzyme activation on ultrastructural distribution of the enzyme. *Brain Res.* 209:339–54

176. Stone, A. L. 1980. Studies on a molecular basis for the heparin-induced regulation of enzymatic activity of mouse striatal tyrosine hydroxylase in vitro. Inhibition of heparin activation and of the enzyme of poly-L-lysyltyrosine and poly-L-lysylphenylalanine and their constituent peptides. *J. Neurochem.* 35:1137–50

177. Kuhn, D. M., Meyer, M. A., Lovenberg, W. 1979. Activation of rat brain tryptophan hydroxylase by polyelectrolytes. *Biochem. Pharmacol.* 28:3255–60

178. Kuhn, D. M., Meyer, M. A., Lovenberg, W. 1980. Comparisons of tryptophan hydroxylase from a malignant murine mast cell tumor and rat mesencephalic tegmentum. *Arch. Biochem. Biophys.* 199:355–61

179. Katz, I. R., Yamauchi, T., Kaufman, S. 1976. Activation of tyrosine hydroxylase by polyanions and salts. *Biochim. Biophys. Acta* 429:84–95

180. Lloyd, T., Ebersole, B. J., Schneider, F. H. 1978. Stimulation of tyrosine hydroxylase activity in cultured mouse neuroblastoma cells by monocarboxylic acids. *J. Neurochem.* 30:1641–43

181. Bustos, G., Roth, R. H., Morgenroth, V. H., Hancke, J. L. 1978. Tyrosine hydroxylase activation and transmitter release from central noradrenergic neurons by electrical field stimulation. *Arch. Pharmacol.* 301:149–56

181a. Kuczenski, R. 1981. Monovalent cations and striatal tyrosine hydroxylase. *J. Neurochem.* 37:681–86

181b. Bustos, G., Roth, R. H. 1979. Tyrosine hydroxylase regulation in rat striatal and olefactory tubercle slices. *Biochem. Pharmacol.* 28:1923–31

182. Chalfie, M., Settipani, L., Perlman, R. L. 1978. Activation of tyrosine 3-monooxygenase in pheochromocytoma cells by lasalocid. *Biochem. Pharmacol.* 27:673–77

183. Mann, S. P. 1978. An improved assay of tyrosine hydroxylase using sodium activation. *J. Neurochem.* 31:747–49

184. Helke, C. J., Yuhaniak, P. A., Keller, K. J., Gillis, R. A. 1978. Effect of deslanoside on brain and spinal cord levels of serotonin and 5-hydroxyindoleacetic acid and tryptophan hydroxylase activity. *Biochem. Pharmacol.* 27:2459–61

185. Hamon, M., Bourgoin, S., Artaud, F., Glowinski, J. 1979. The role of intraneuronal 5-HT and of tryptophan hydroxylase activation in the control of 5-HT synthesis in rat brain slices incubated in K^+-enriched medium. *J. Neurochem.* 33:1031–42

186. Boadle-Biber, M. C. 1979. Decrease in the activity of tryptophan hydroxylase from slices of rat brain stem incubated in a low calcium or a calcium-free manganese-substituted medium. *Biochem. Pharmacol.* 28:3487–90

187. Psychoyos, S., Stanton, B. R., Atkins, C. D. 1979. The influence of glucose, other monosaccharides, and ascorbic acid on tyrosine hydroxylase activity of rat striatal synaptosomes. *Life Sci.* 25:1119–26

188. Bustos, G., Simon, J., Roth, R. H. 1980. Tyrosine hydroxylase regulation: Apparent kinetic alterations following incubation of brain slices in a sodium-free medium. *J. Neurochem.* 35:47–57

189. Kapatos, G., Zigmond, M. J. 1982. Influence of calcium on dopamine synthesis and tyrosine hydroxylase activity in rat striatum. *J. Neurochem.* 39:327–35

190. Yanagisawa, M., Hasegawa, H., Ichiyama, A. 1982. Tryptophan hydroxylase from mouse mastocytoma P-815. Reversible activation by ethylenediamine-tetraacetate. *J. Biochem.* 92:449–56

191. Iuvone, P. M., Marshburn, P. B. 1982. Regulation of tyrosine hydroxylase activity in retinal cell suspensions: Effects of potassium and 8-bromo cyclic AMP. *Life Sci.* 30:85–91

192. Lerner, P., Hartman, P., Ames, M. M., Lovenberg, W. 1977. The role of reductants in the tyrosine hydroxylase reactions. *Arch. Biochem. Biophys.* 182:164–70

193. Lerner, P., Nose, P., Ames, M. M., Lovenberg, W. 1978. Modification of the tyrosine hydroxylase assay. *Neurochem. Res.* 3:641–51

194. Hamon, M., Bourgoin, S., Hery, F., Simmonet, G. 1978. Characteristics of the activation by dithiothreitol and Fe^{++} of tryptophan hydroxylase from the rat brain. *Neurochem. Res.* 3:585–98

195. Hamon, M., Bourgoin, S., Artaud, F., Nelson, D. 1979. Regulatory properties of neuronal tryptophan hydroxylase. *Adv. Exp. Med. Biol.* 133:231–51

196. Kuhn, D. M., Ruskin, B., Lovenberg, W. 1980. Tryptophan hydroxylase. *J. Biol. Chem.* 255:4137–43

197. Okuno, S., Fujisawa, H. 1981. Inactivation of tyrosine-3-monooxygenase by acetone precipitation and its restoration by incubation with a sulfhydryl agent and iron. *Biochim. Biophys. Acta* 658:327–33

198. Kaufman, S., Mason, K. 1982. Novel amino acid substrates and activators for rat liver phenylalanine hydroxylase. See Ref. 6, pp. 305–19

199. Galloway, M. P., Roth, B. L., Coscia, C. J. 1981. The effects of tetrahydroisoquinoline carboxylic acids on tyrosine-3-monooxygenase. *Arch. Biochem. Biophys.* 209:620–27

200. Agnati, L. F., Fuxe, K., Hokfelt, T., Goldstein, M., Jeffcoate, S. L. 1977. A method to measure the distribution pattern of specific nerve terminals in sampled regions. Studies on tyrosine hydroxylase, LHRH, TRH, and GIH immunofluorescence. *J. Histochem. Cytochem.* 25:1222–36

201. Hokfelt, T., Elde, R., Johansson, O., Ljungdahl, A., Schultzberg, M., Fuxe, K., Goldstein, M., Nilsson, G., Pernow, B., Terenius, L., Gauten, D., Jeffcoate, S. L., Rehfeld, J., Said, S. 1978. Distribution of peptide-containing neurons. In *Psychopharmacology: A Generation of Progress*, ed. M. A. Lipton, A. DiMascio, K. F. Killam, pp. 39–66. New York: Raven. 1731 pp.

202. Ajika, K. 1979. Simultaneous localization of LHRH and catecholamines in rat hypothalamus. *J. Anat.* 128:331–47

203. Teitelman, G., Joh, T. H., Reis, D. J. 1981. Linkage of the brain-skin-gut axis: Islet cells originate from dopaminergic precursors. *Peptides* 2:157–68

204. Charnay, Y., Leger, L., Dray, F., Berod, A., Jouvet, M., Pujol, J.-F., Dubois, P. M. 1982. Evidence for the presence of enkephalin in catecholaminergic neurones of cat locus coeruleus. *Neurosci. Lett.* 30:147–51

205. Boadle-Biber, M. C. 1979. Increase in the activity of tryptophan hydroxylase from slices of rat brainstem incubated

with angiotensin-II. *Biochem. Pharma-col.* 28:3243–46

206. Hori, S., Ohtani, S. 1981. Kinetic properties of bovine pineal tryptophan-5-monooxygenase activated by an endogenous activating substance. *J. Neurochem.* 36:551–58

207. Ip, N. Y., Ho, C. K., Zigmond, R. E. 1982. Secretin and vasoactive intestinal peptide acutely increase tyrosine-3-monooxygenase in the rat superior cervical ganglion. *Proc. Natl. Acad. Sci. USA* 79:7566–69

208. Hori, S., Ohtani, S. 1978. Solubilization of tryptophan-5-monooxygenase from the pineal glands and existence of an activating substance in the tissue extract. *J. Neurochem.* 31:663–71

209. Spatz, H., Heller, B., Nachon, M., Fischer, E. 1975. Effects of D-phenylalanine on clinical picture and phenethylaminuria in depression. *Biol. Psychiat.* 10:235–39

210. Beckmann, H., Strauss, M. A., Ludolph, E. 1977. DL-phenylalanine in depressed patients: An open study. *J. Neural Transm.* 41:123–34

211. Schildkraut, J. J. 1978. Current status of the catecholamine hypothesis of affective disorder. See Ref. 201, pp. 1223–34

212. Vitto, A., Mandell, A. J. 1979. Calcium-dependent activation, stabilization, and destabilization of tryptophan hydroxylase from rat midbrain. *Neurosci. Abst.* 5:419

213. Vitto, A., Mandell, A. J. 1981. Stability properties of activated tryptophan hydroxylase from rat midbrain. *J. Neurochem.* 37:601–07

214. Vrana, K. E., Allihiser, C. L., Roskoski, R. 1981. Tyrosine hydroxylase activation and inactivation by protein phosphorylating conditions. *J. Neurochem.* 36:92–100

215. Lazar, M. A., Truscott, R. J. W., Raese, J. D., Barchas, J. D. 1981. Thermal denaturation of native striatal tyrosine hydroxylase: Increased thermolability of the phosphorylated form of the enzyme. *J. Neurochem.* 36:677–82

216. Kaufman, S. 1974. Properties of the pterin-dependent amino acid hydroxylases. In *Aromatic amino acids in the brain. CIBA Symp.* 22:85–107

217. Kaufman, S. 1975. Regulatory properties of tyrosine hydroxylase. In *Neurobiological Mechanisms of Adaptation and Behavior*, ed. A. J. Mandell, pp. 127–36. New York: Raven. 306 pp.

218. Knapp, S., Mandell, A. J. 1983. Scattering kinetics in a complex tryptophan hydroxylase preparation from rat brainstem

raphé nuclei: Statistical evidence that the lithium-induced sigmoid velocity function reflects two states of available catalytic potential. *J. Neural Transm.* In press

219. Hasegawa, H., Yanagisawa, M., Ichiyama, A. 1982. Three discrete activity states of mastocytoma tryptophan-5-monooxygenase. See Ref. 6, pp. 293–304

220. Scheraga, H. A. 1980. Protein folding; application to ribonuclease. In *Protein Folding*, ed. J. Rainer, pp. 261–86. New York: Elsevier/North-Holland

221. Karplus, M. 1981. Aspects of protein dynamics. *Ann. NY Acad. Sci.* 367:407–15

222. Kety, S. S., Woodford, R. B., Harmel, M. H. 1948. Cerebral blood flow and metabolism in schizophrenia. *Am. J. Psychiat.* 104:765–70

223. Sokoloff, L. 1981. Relationships among local functional activity, energy metabolism, and blood flow in the central nervous system. *Fed. Proc.* 40:2311–16

224. Petrack, B., Sheppy, F., Fetzer, V. 1968. Studies on tyrosine hydroxylase from bovine adrenal medulla. *J. Biol. Chem.* 243:743–48

225. Musacchio, J. M., Wurzburger, R. J., D'Angelo, G. L. 1971. Different molecular forms of bovine adrenal tyrosine hydroxylase. *Mol. Pharmacol.* 7:136–46

226. Friedman, P. A., Kappelman, A. H., Kaufman, S. 1972. Partial purification and characterization of tryptophan hydroxylase from rabbit hindbrain. *J. Biol. Chem.* 247:4165–73

227. Knapp, S., Mandell, A. J., Geyer, M. A. 1974. Effects of amphetamines on regional tryptophan hydroxylase activity and synaptosomal conversion of tryptophan to 5-hydroxytryptamine in rat brain. *J. Pharmacol. Exp. Ther.* 189:676–89

228. Knapp, S., Mandell, A. J. 1975. Effects of lithium chloride on parameters of biosynthetic capacity for 5-hydroxytryptamine in rat brain. *J. Pharmacol. Exp. Ther.* 193:812–23

229. Knapp, S., Mandell, A. J. 1976. Coincidence of blockade of synaptosomal 5-hydroxytryptamine uptake and decrease in tryptophan hydroxylase activity: Effects of fenfluramine. *J. Pharmacol. Exp. Ther.* 198:123–35

230. Knapp, S. 1982. Tryptophan hydroxylase: Variational kinetics. *J. Histochem. Cytochem.* 30:847–50

231. Creighton, T. E. 1978. Experimental stud-

ies of protein folding and unfolding. *Prog. Biophys. Mol. Biol.* 33:231–97

232. May, R. M., Oster, G. F. 1976. Bifurcations and dynamic complexity in simple ecological models. *Am. Natur.* 110:573–99

233. Degn, H., Mayer, D. 1969. Theory of oscillations in peroxidase catalyzed oxidation reactions in open system. *Biochim. Biophys. Acta* 180:291–301

234. Seelig, F. F. 1976. Chemical oscillations by substrate inhibition. *Z. Naturforsch. Teil A* 31:731–38

235. Olsen, L. F., Degn, H. 1977. Chaos in an enzyme reaction. *Nature* 267:177–78

236. Kernevez, J-P. 1980. *Enzyme Mathematics*, pp. 57–110, 241–57. New York: North-Holland. 262 pp.

237. Shaw, R. 1981. Strange attractors, chaotic behavior, and information flow. *Z. Naturforsch. Teil A* 36:80–112

238. Geisel, T., Nierwetberg, J., Keller, J. 1981. Critical behavior of the Lyapounov number at the period-doubling onset of chaos. *Phys. Lett.* 86A:75–78

239. Farmer, D. 1982. Chaotic attractors of an infinite-dimensional dynamical system. *Physica* 4D:366–93

240. Kessler, K. A. 1978. Tricyclic antidepressants: mode of action and clinical use. See Ref. 201, pp. 1289–1302

241. Simpson, G. M., Lee, J. H. 1978. A ten-year review of antipsychotics. See Ref. 201, pp. 1131–38

242. Sneddon, I. N. 1972. *The Use of Integral Transforms.* New York: McGraw-Hill. 539 pp.

243. Stakgold, I. 1979. *Green's Functions and Boundary Value Problems.* New York: Wiley. 638 pp.

244. Jenkins, G. M., Watts, D. G. 1968. *Spectral Analysis and Its Applications,* pp. 16–56. San Francisco: Holden-Day. 525 pp.

245. Bendat, J. S. 1978. *Principles and Applications of Random Noise Theory,* pp. 29–77. New York: Krieger. 456 pp. Rev. ed.

246. Bracewell, R. N. 1978. *The Fourier Transform and Its Applications,* pp. 189–214. New York: McGraw-Hill. 444 pp.

247. Mandell, A. J. 1982. Three kinds of enzyme kinetics: Toward a neuropharmacology of phase. *J. Histochem. Cytochem.* 30:841–46

248. Mandelbrot, B. B. 1967. How long is the coast of Britain? Statistical self-similarity and fractional dimension. *Science* 155:636–38

249. Knapp, S., Mandell, A. J. 1981. Calcium, cofactor, and propranolol-induced changes in the kinetic variations of rat

raphé tryptophan hydroxylase activity. See Ref. 65, pp. 215–24.

250. Manin, Y. I. 1981. *Mathematics and Physics,* pp. 35–51. Boston: Birkhäuser. 99 pp.

251. Alexandroff, P. 1961. *Elementary Concepts of Topology.* New York: Dover. 73 pp.

252. Stapleton, H. J., Allen, J. P., Flynn, C. P., Stinson, D. G., Kurtz, S. R. 1980. Fractal form of proteins. *Phys. Rev. Lett.* 45:1456–59

253. Gnedenko, B. V., Kolmogorov, A. N. 1968. *Limit Distributions for Sums of Independent Random Variables,* pp. 162–230. Reading, MA: Addison-Wesley. 293 pp.

254. Seshadri, V., West, B. J. 1982. Fractal dimensionality of Levy processes. *Proc. Natl. Acad. Sci. USA* 79:4501–05

255. Forrest, S. R., Witten, T. A. 1979. Long-range correlations in smoke-particle aggregates. *J. Phys. Math. Gen.* 12:L109–17

256. Berry, M. Y., Lewis, Z. Y. 1980. On the Weierstrass-Mandelbrot fractal function. *Proc. R. Soc. London Ser. A* 370:459–84

257. Kaplan, J., Yorke, J. 1978. The dimension of the strange attractor for a class of difference systems. *Lect. Notes Math.* 730:228–341

258. Mori, H. 1980. Fractal dimensions of chaotic flows of autonomous dissipative systems. *Prog. Theor. Phys.* 63:1044–47

259. Ledrappier, F. 1981. Some relations between dimension and Lyapounov exponents. *Commun. Math. Phys.* 81:229–38

260. Mandelbrot, B. B. 1974. Intermittent turbulence in self-similar cascades: Divergence of high moments and dimension of the carrier. *J. Fluid Mech.* 62:331–58

261. Mandelbrot, B. B. 1977. Fractals and turbulence: Attractors and dispersion. *Lect. Notes Math.* 615:83–93

262. Takens, F. 1972. Homoclinic points in conservative systems. *Invent. Math.* 18:267–92

263. Newhouse, S. 1977. Quasi-elliptic periodic points in conservative dynamical systems. *Am. J. Math.* 99:1061–87

263a. Mandell, A. J. 1981. Statistical stability in random brain systems: Possible implications for polydrug abuse in the borderline syndrome. *Adv. Subst. Abuse* 2:299–341

264. Mandell, A. J. 1982. The influence of a centrally active peptide on receptor macromolecular dynamics: Toward a neuropharmacology of phase. *Ann. NY Acad. Sci.* 398:191–206

265. Knapp, S., Ehlers, C., Russo, P. V., Mandell, A. J. 1981. A cross-

disciplinary approach to the action of lithium: A vertical integration. In *Basic Mechanisms in the Action of Lithium,* ed. H. M. Emrich, J. B. Aldenhoff, H. D. Lux, pp. 102–20. Princeton: Excerpta Medica. 265 pp.

266. Mandell, A. J., Knapp, S., Ehlers, C. L., Russo, P. V. 1983. The stability of constrained randomness: Lithium prophylaxis at several neurobiological levels. In *The Neurobiology of the Mood Disorders,* ed. R. M. Post, J. C. Ballenger. Baltimore: Williams & Wilkins. 967 pp.

267. Apple, M. S., Korostyshevskiy, M. A. 1980. Why many biological parameters are connected by power dependence. *J. Theor. Biol.* 85:569–73

268. Karplus, M., McCammon, J. A. 1979. Protein structural fluctuations during a period of 100 ps. *Nature* 277:578

269. Lorenz, E. N. 1969. The predictability of a flow which possesses many scales of motion. *Tellus* 21:289–307

270. Lorenz, E. N. 1980. Noisy periodicity and reverse bifurcation. *Ann. NY Acad. Sci.* 357:282–91

271. Gollub, J. P. 1980. The onset of turbulence: Convection, surface waves, and oscillators. *Lect. Notes Math.* 132:162–80

272. Ehlers, C. L., Russo, P. V., Mandell, A. J., Bloom, F. E. 1983. Architecture of rat nocturnal locomotion: A predictive descriptor of the effects of antidepressant and antimanic treatments. *Psychopharmacol. Bull.* 19:692–95

273. Wender, P. 1971. *Minimal Brain Dysfunction in Children,* pp. 87–134. New York: Wiley-Interscience. 242 pp.

274. Monod, J., Changeux, J-P., Jacob, F. 1963. Allosteric proteins and cellular control systems. *J. Mol. Biol.* 6:306–29

275. Wyman, J. 1948. Heme proteins. *Adv. Prot. Chem.* 4:407–531

276. Wyman, J., Allen, D. W. 1951. The problem of heme interactions in hemoglobin and the basis of the Bohr effect. *J. Polymer Sci.* 7:499–518

277. Wyman, J. 1963. Allosteric effects in hemoglobin. *Cold Spring Harbor Symp. Quant. Biol.* 28:483–89

278. Levitzki, A. 1978. *Quantitative Aspects of Allosteric Mechanisms,* pp. 11–27. New York: Springer-Verlag. *Molec. Biol. Biochem. Biophys.* 28:11–27

279. Williams, R. J. P. 1977. Flexible drug molecules and dynamic receptors. *Angew. Chem. Int. Ed. Engl.* 16:766–77

280. Lord, J. A. H., Watefield, A. A., Hughes, J., Kosterlitz, H. W. 1977. Endogenous opoid peptides: Multiple agonists and receptors. *Nature* 267:495–99

281. Snyder, S. H., Goodman, R. R. 1980. Multiple neurotransmitter receptors. *J. Neurochem.* 35:5–15

282. Burt, D. R., Snyder, S. H. 1975. Thyrotropin releasing hormone (TRH): apparent receptor binding in rat brain membranes. *Brain Res.* 93:309–28

282a. Taylor, J. E., Richelson, E. 1980. High affinity binding of tricyclic antidepressants to histamine H_1-receptors: Fact and artifact. *Eur. J. Pharmacol.* 67:41–46

282b. Barth, S. 1980. Mass-action model for radioimmunoassays and other saturation assays with atypical performance characteristics. *Math. Biosci.* 51:187–97

283. Colquhoun, D. 1978. The link between drug binding and response: Theories and observations. In *The Receptors,* ed. R. D. O'Brien, 1:93–142. New York: Plenum. 361 pp.

284. Grunhagen, H. H., Changeux, J-P. 1976. Studies on the electrogenic action of acetylcholine with *Torpedo marmorata* electric organ. V. *J. Mol. Biol.* 106:517–35

285. Sakmann, B., Patlak, J., Neher, E. 1980. Single acetylcholine-activated channels show burst kinetics in presence of desensitizing concentrations of agonists. *Nature* 286:71–73

286. Mandell, A. J. 1982. Stochastic markers for an entropic defect. In *Biological Markers in Psychiatry and Neurology,* ed. E. Usdin, I. Hanin, 525–38. New York: Pergamon. 544 pp.

287. Mandell, A. J. 1982. Nonlinear dynamics in brain processes. *Psychopharmacol. Bull.* 18:59–63

288. Grant, G., Vale, W., Guillemin, R. 1973. Characteristics of the pituitary binding sites for thyrotropin-releasing factor. *Endocrinology* 92:1629–33

289. Loh, H. H., Cho, T. M., Wu, Y. C., Harris, R. A., Way, E. L. 1976. Opiate binding to cerebroside sulfate: a model system for opiate-receptor interaction. *Life Sci.* 16:1811–18

290. Cuatrecasas, P., Hollenberg, M. D. 1975. Binding of insulin and other hormones by non-receptor materials: saturability, specificity, and apparent "negative cooperativity." *Biochem. Biophys. Res. Commun.* 62:31–42

291. Hollenberg, M. D., Cuatrecasas, P. 1978. Distinction of receptor from nonreceptor interactions in binding studies. See Ref. 283, pp. 193–214

292. Scatchard, G. 1949. The attractions of proteins for small molecules and ions. *Ann. NY Acad. Sci.* 51:573–672

293. Boehme, R. E., Ciaranello, R. D. 1982. Genetic control of dopamine and seroto-

nin receptors in brain regions of inbred mice. *Brain Res.* 266:51–65

294. Bigelow, C. C. 1960. Difference spectra of ribonuclease and two ribonuclease derivatives. *C. R. Trav. Lab. Carlsberg* 31:305–24

295. King, A. C., Frazier, W. A. 1979. Properties of the oscillatory cAMP binding component of *Dictyostelium discoideum* cells and isolated plasma membrane. *J. Biol. Chem.* 254:7168–76

296. Andorn, A. C., Maguire, M. E. 1980. [³H]Spiroperidol binding in rat striatum: Two high-affinity sites of differing selectivities. *J. Neurochem.* 35:1105–13

297. Leysen, J. E., Gommeren, W. 1981. Optimal conditions for [³H]apomorphine binding and anomalous equilibrium binding of [³H]apomorphine and [³H]spiperone to rat striatal membranes: Involvement of surface phenomena versus multiple binding sites. *J. Neurochem.* 36:201–19

297a. Chang, K. J., Jacobs, S., Cuatrecasas, P. 1975. Quantitative aspects of hormone-receptor interactions of high affinity. Effect of receptor concentration and measurement of dissociation constants of labeled and unlabeled hormones. *Biochim. Biophys. Acta* 406:294–99

298. Jacobs, S., Cuatrecasas, P. 1983. Insulin receptors. *Ann. Rev. Pharmacol. Toxicol.* 23:461–79

299. Cuatrecasas, P. 1974. Membrane receptors. *Ann. Rev. Biochem.* 43:169–214

300. DeMeyts, P. 1976. Cooperative properties of hormone receptors in cell membranes. *J. Supramol. Struct.* 4:241–56

301. Pottet, R. J., Standaert, M. L., Haase, B. A. 1977. Insulin binding to the human lymphocyte receptor. *J. Biol. Chem.* 252:5828–37

302. DeMeyts, P., Roth, J., Neville, D. M., Gavin, J. R., Lesniak, M. A. 1973. Insulin interactions with its receptors: Experimental evidence for negative cooperativity. *Biochem. Biophys. Res. Commun.* 55:154–66

303. Mandell, A. J. 1983. From chemical homology to topological temperature: A notion relating the structure and function of brain polypeptides. In *Synergetics of the Brain*, ed. E. Başar, H. Flohr, H. Haken, A. J. Mandell, pp. 365–76. Berlin: Springer-Verlag. 377 pp.

304. Snell, C. R., Fasman, G. D. 1973. Kinetics and thermodynamics of the α helix ⟷ β transconformation of poly(L-lysine) and L-leucine copolymers. A compensation phenomenon. *Biochemistry* 12:1017–25

305. Lim, V. I. 1978. Polypeptide chain folding through a highly helical intermediate

as a general principle of globular protein structure formation. *FEBS Lett.* 89:10–14

306. Lesk, A. M., Chothia, C. 1980. Solvent accessibility, protein surfaces, and protein folding. *Biophys. J.* 10:35–47

307. Ptitsyn, O. B., Finkelstein, A. V. 1980. Similarities of protein topologies: Evolutionary divergence, functional convergence or principles of folding. *Quart. Rev. Biophys.* 13:339–86

308. Lim, V. I. 1974. Algorithms for prediction of α-helical and β-structural regions in globular proteins. *J. Mol. Biol.* 88:873–94

309. Lesk, A. M., Chothia, C. 1980. How different amino acid sequences determine similar protein structures: The structure and evolutionary dynamics of the globulins. *J. Mol. Biol.* 136:225–70

310. Schiffer, M. 1980. Possible distortion of antibody bonding site of the Mcg Bence-Jones protein by lattice forces. *Biophysical J.* 32:230–32

311. Smillie, L. B., Pato, M. D., Pearlstone, J. R., Mak, A. S. 1980. Periodicity of α-helical potential in tropomyosin sequence correlates with alternating actin binding sites. *J. Mol. Biol.* 136:199–202

312. Gorden, P., Carpentier, J-L., Van Obberghen, E., Barazzone, P., Roth, J., Orci, L. 1979. Insulin-induced receptor loss in the cultured human lymphocyte: Quantitative morphological perturbations in the cell and plasma membrane. *J. Cell Sci.* 39:77–88

313. Carpentier, J-L., Gorden, P., Amheerdt, M., Van Obberghen, E., Kahn, C. R., Orci, L. 1978. ^{125}I-insulin binding to cultured human lymphocytes: Initial localization and fate of hormone determined by quantitative electron microscopic autoradiography. *J. Clin. Invest.* 61:1056–70

314. Hazum, E., Cuatrecasas, P., Marian, J., Conn, P. M. 1980. Receptor-mediated internalization of fluorescent gonadotropin-releasing hormone by pituitary gonadotropes. *Proc. Natl. Acad. Sci. USA* 77:6692–95

315. Nelson, N., Anbolt, R., Lindstrom, J., Montal, M. 1980. Reconstitution of purified acetylcholine receptors with functional ion channels in planar lipid bilayers. *Proc. Natl. Acad. Sci. USA* 77:257–61

316. Wuilmart, C., Urbain, J. 1976. Common origin and evolution of variable and constant regions of immunoglobulins. *J. Immunogenet.* 3:1–14

317. Wolfenden, R., Andersson, L., Cullis, P. M., Southgate, C. C. B. 1981. Affini-

ties of amino acid side chains for solvent water. *Biochemistry* 20:849–55

318. Nozaki, Y., Tanford, C. 1971. The solubility of amino acids and two glycine peptides in aqueous ethanol and dioxane solutions. *J. Biol. Chem.* 246:2211–17

319. Manavalan, P., Ponnuswamy, P. K. 1978. Hydrophobic character of amino acid residues in globular proteins. *Nature* 275:673–74

320. Scheraga, H. A. 1979. Interactions in aqueous solution. *Acc. Chem. Res.* 12:7–13

321. Richardson, J. S. 1977. β-Sheets topology and the relatedness of proteins. *Nature* 268:495–500

322. Sternberg, M. J. E., Thornton, J. M. 1977. On the conformation of proteins: Hydrophobic ordering of strands in β-pleated sheets. *J. Mol. Biol.* 115:1–17

323. Wuilmart, C., Delhaise, P., Urbain, J. 1982. The sharing of amino acid short spans by ancestrally unrelated proteins may be the result of ubiquitous alpha and beta secondary structures. *J. Biosyst.* 15:221–32

324. Schiffer, M., Edmunson, A. B. 1967. Use of helical wheels to represent the structures of protein and to identify segments with helical potential. *Biophys. J.* 7:121–35

325. Delhaise, P., Wuilmart, C., Urbain, J. 1980. Relationships between α and β secondary structures and amino-acid pseudosymmetrical arrangements. *Eur. J. Biochem.* 105:553–64

326. Cummings, A. L., Eyring, E. M. 1975. Helix-coil transition kinetics in aqueous poly(α,L-glutamic acid). *Biopolymers* 14:2107–14

327. Auer, H. E., Patton, E. 1976. Kinetics of the disordered chain-to-β transformation of poly(L-tyrosine) in aqueous solution. *Biophys. Chem.* 4:15–21

328. Arfmann, H. A., Labitzke, R., Wagner, K. F. 1977. Conformational properties of l-leucine, l-isoleucine, and l-norleucine side chains in l-lysine copolymers. *Biopolymers* 16:1815–26

329. Mandell, A. J. 1984. The spectral gap hypothesis and measures on a solvent entropy sequence code for polypeptides influencing neurobiological stability. *Internatl. Rev. Neurobiol.* 25: In press

330. Segal, D. S., Mandell, A. J. 1974. Differential behavioral effects of hypotha-lamic polypeptides. In *The Thyroid Axis, Drugs, and Behavior*, ed. A. J. Prange Jr., pp. 129–34. New York: Raven

331. Goldstein, A., Tachibana, S., Lowney, L. I., Hunkapiller, M., Hood, L. 1979. Dynorphine-(1–13), an extraordinarily potent opiate peptide. *Proc. Natl. Acad. Sci. USA* 76:6666–70

332. Ehlers, C., Henricksen, S. J., Bloom, F. E., Rivier, J., Vale, W. J. 1982. Electroencephalographic and epileptogenic effects of corticotropin releasing factor (CRF) in rats. *Neurosci. Abstr.* 8:1013

333. Lee, E. H. Y., Geyer, M. A., Mandell, A. J. 1983. Effects of corticotropin releasing factor and growth hormone releasing factor on patterns of locomotion and brain monoamines in rats. *Neurosci. Abstr.* 9:385

334. Gispen, W. H., Isaacson, R. L. 1981. ACTH-induced excessive grooming in the rat. *Pharmacol. Ther.* 12:209–46

335. Iversen, L. L. 1983. Nonopioid neuropeptides in mammalian CNS. *Ann. Rev. Pharmacol. Toxicol.* 23:1–27

336. Bloom, F. E. 1983. The endorphins: A growing family of pharmacologically pertinent peptides. *Ann. Rev. Pharmacol. Toxicol.* 23:151–70

337. Kelley, A. E., Stinus, L., Iversen, S. D. 1979. Behavioral activation induced in the rat by substance P infusion into ventral tegmental area: Implication of dopaminergic A_{10} neurones. *Neurosci. Lett.* 11:335–39

338. Palacios, J. M., Kuhar, M. J. 1981. Neurotensin receptors are located on dopamine-containing neurons in rat midbrain. *Nature* 294:587–89

339. Nemeroff, C. B. 1980. Neurotensin: Perchance an endogenous neuroleptic? *Biol. Psychiat.* 15:283–302

340. Guillemin, R. 1978. Peptides in the brain: The new endocrinology of the neuron. *Science* 202:390–402

341. Kaiser, E. T., Kezdy, F. J. 1983. Secondary structures of proteins and peptides in amphiphilic environments. *Proc. Natl. Acad. Sci. USA* 80:1137–43

342. Lederis, K., Letter, A., McMaster, D., Moore, G., Schlesinger, D. 1982. Complete amino acid sequence of urotensin I, a hypotensive and corticotropin-releasing neuropeptide from *Catostomus*. *Science* 218:162–64

Ann. Rev. Pharmacol. Toxicol. 1984. 24:275–328

POSITIVE INOTROPIC AGENTS

A. E. Farah

Sterling Drug, Inc., Rensselaer, New York 12144

A. A. Alousi and R. P. Schwarz, Jr.

Sterling-Winthrop Research Institute, Rensselaer, New York 12144

INTRODUCTION

A large number of naturally occurring and synthetically prepared chemical agents produce a positive inotropic effect on the heart. Analogues of these compounds have been isolated, prepared, and tested, and a number of them also have positive inotropic effects (see Tables 1–6). A number of reviews on inotropic agents and their possible mechanisms have been published (1–7).

Because of space limitations, only compounds that have had extensive pharmacological investigation will be discussed here. Thus, we will consider newer adrenergic agents, new phosphodiesterase inhibitors, some polypeptides, and a number of miscellaneous compounds that have interesting pharmacological properties. The choice of compounds to be discussed was based on the interests of the authors; our readers may disagree with these choices.

THE ADRENERGIC AGENTS

There are three major actions of the effects of adrenergic agents on the heart: the inotropic, chronotropic, and arrhythmogenic effects. Adrenoceptors have been classified into α and β receptors (8) and subgroups of these (α 1, 2, and β 1, 2) have been postulated (9–11). The β-receptor is the one primarily responsible for inotropic and chronotropic effects, with the β-mediated inotropic effects most likely involving adenosine, 3'5'-cyclic phosphate (cyclic AMP) formation (12, 13). However, positive inotropic responses in heart muscle of various species, including man, can also be elicited by the activation of α receptors.

275

0362-1642/84/415-275$02.00

This effect is usually demonstrated in cardiac muscle exposed to β-blocking agents. Here, an α-blocking agent will shift the dose response curve of epinephrine to the right. α-Activators are dopamine, epinephrine, nore-pinephrine, phenylephrine, methoxamine, and related substances (14). In low concentrations (up to 10 μM), the effects of phenylephrine are mostly α effects, while at higher concentrations both β and α effects are involved.

α-Adrenergic effects differ from those of β-mediated effects in having only a weak chronotropic effect and in not increasing cyclic AMP content of the heart. The time to peak tension and relaxation time are not changed by these adrenergic agents and, in contrast to β-adrenergic stimulation, the α activators do not increase cardiac irregularities and may even inhibit arrhythmogenesis (13b).

Although epinephrine (EP), norepinephrine (NE), and isoproterenol (IPN) have powerful positive inotropic effects, their usefulness in the therapy of heart failure has been limited by their poor gastrointestinal absorption and their positive chronotropic and arrhythmogenic properties. These disadvantages have prompted the search for orally effective adrenergic agents whose chrono-tropic, inotropic, and arrhythmogenic effects can be separated.

Separation of Inotropic and Chronotropic Effects

The separation of inotropic and chronotropic effects has been claimed for a number of adrenergic agents, such as dopamine, dobutamine and prenalterol. In general, this separation of effects is most evident in the intact animal. With dopamine, the differential effects are reduced or eliminated after reserpine treatment of the heart, thus suggesting that reflex phenomena contribute to this separation. With dobutamine, the differential effects on contractility and heart rate persist after adrenergic depletion (15, 16, 17). However, when isolated atrial and ventricular tissues are exposed to dobutamine, the heart-rate changes are more sensitive to dobutamine than are the inotropic changes (15, 17). Both pharmacological and ligand binding studies (18–23) show the existence of β-1 and -2 receptors in cardiac muscle. Furthermore, Hedberg et al (24) report that cat- and guinea-pig atria contain 75% β-1 and 25% β-2 receptors, while the ventricles contain mostly the β-2 receptor. These findings have been the basis for explaining the differential effects of an adrenergic agent on heart rate (β-2) and contractile force (β-1). However, Kenakin (25) and Kenakin & Beek (26) have not been able to demonstrate any selectivity for β adrenergic receptors with either dobutamine or prenalterol. Their findings agree with the studies of Bodem et al (15) and Lumley et al (17), which demonstrate no separation of inotropic and chronotropic effects in isolated auricular tissue. Thus, the dif-ferential effects of these agents on heart rate and contractility are very likely characteristics of the heart in situ. Levy & de Oliveira (27) have observed that the blood supply to ventricular muscle is greater than to the atrium, which contains the sinus node. Potter et al (28) have shown that administered catecholamines are retained to the highest degree in those regions of the heart where blood supply is highest. Thus, the retention of H^3 NE per gram of tissue was about 8.4 times greater in the left ventricular, as compared with right atrial, tissue of normal dogs. This is an unexpected finding, since atrial tissue contains larger amounts of adrenergic nerve endings than do the ventricles. The left ventricle received the largest, while the right atrium (and possibly the sinus node) received the smallest amount of NE per unit of weight of cardiac tissue. If one considers that the amounts per gram of tissue thus received are going to be diluted in an equal amount of extracellular space, the concentration of an adrenergic agent would be higher at the ventricular cell surfaces than at the sinus node cells. This would be compatible with the observations that adrenergic agents, when given only in vivo, show this preferential effect on the contractility of the ventricle. The claims purporting preferential effects on contractile force of some of the adrenergic agents are thus best explained by vascular distribution of the injected material and the secondary effects on heart rate resulting from reflex changes caused by these agents. However, in the intact animal, differences in responses between substances with high intrinsic activity (NE) and those with relatively low intrinsic activity (dobutamine, prenalterol) are still apparent. Thus, at doses that produced an equal contractile response, NE and isoproterenol produced a greater increase in heart rate than dopamine, dobutamine, or prenalterol (16, 29, 30). Studies in isolated cat tissue show that equipotent chronotropic doses of NE, EP, IPN, dobutamine, and dopamine produce an equal increase in the contractile response in both auricular and papillary muscle (A. A. Alousi, unpublished data). It is thus likely that the differences between adrenergic agents observed in the intact animal are due to pharmacological differences on vascular smooth muscle, reflex effects, and intrinsic adrenergic blocking actions of a drug (26).

Loss of Cardiac Activity of Adrenergic Agents Following Prolonged Administration

Adrenergic-agonist desensitization of the contractile response and the increase in cyclic AMP content of intact heart muscle has been demonstrated by a large number of investigators (31). All these studies reported that either the chronic administration of an adrenergic agonist or procedures that increase sympathetic activity will cause a reduction in the responsiveness of the heart to an adrenergic β-agonist. Similar findings have been reported in human patients treated with dobutamine (32–35).

In asthmatic patients Galant et al (36) have shown that prolonged therapy with terbutaline, ephedrine, or metaproterenol produces, in polymorphonuclear leukocytes, a reduction in the binding sites of dihydroalprenalol and a reduction in the adenylate cyclase response. However, this reduction probably does not represent desensitization in the bronchial smooth muscle, since Jenne et al (33) could not detect any significant change in the responsiveness of patients to terbutaline in terms of vital capacity and airway resistance. Other parameters, such as decrease in diastolic blood pressure, increase in blood lactate, cyclic AMP, glucose, and lowering in the eosinophil count, show a significant desensitization (37).

Tohmeh et al (38) have shown that short-term infusion of isoproterenol in normal human subjects increased, while a longer infusion time (4–6 hours) decreased, adrenergic binding sites in mononuclear cells of these patients. In all the above situations, prolonged administration of adrenergic agents resulted in a reduction of the effects of the agonist on the heart and circulation but not in bronchial smooth muscle, although the drug concentration in blood seemed to be at a constant level. These data suggest that desensitization of blood constituent must be interpreted with caution, since the appearance of desensitization seems to vary from organ to organ.

Desensitization of tissues to the effects of adrenergic agents is a complex phenomenon that has been recently reviewed by Lefkowitz et al (39), Perkins et al (40), and Harden (31). This seems to involve changes in the coupling mechanism of the receptor to the adenylate cyclase system and a reduction in the number of binding sites, as well as a structural change in a protein moiety of the adrenergic receptor (31).

In some cell types, catecholamine refractoriness can be reduced or prevented by treating the cells with inhibitors of protein synthesis (41, 42), by adrenal cortical hormones, (43, 44, 45), and by quinacrine (46). Both adrenocortical hormones and quinacrine are inhibitors of phospholipase, phosphatidyl choline synthesis has been implicated in receptor affinity (47, 48), and prevention of adrenergic desensitization in rats by quinacrine has been reported by Torda et al (49) and Yamaguchi et al (50).

The appearance of desensitization of adrenoreceptors after prolonged exposure poses a serious practical problem, since both the cardiac inotropic and the vasodilator effects of these substances can be attenuated or lost with chronic administration.

DOPAMINE

Dopamine (see Table 1) is classified as a mixed amine since it produces positive inotropic and chronotropic effects by releasing NE from presynaptic membranes and by acting directly on both α and β receptors in the heart (16, 29).

Thus, dopamine increased the rate of discharge from the sinus node and ectopic foci. It shortened the duration of the action potential and the refractory period of cardiac muscle and increased excitability, automaticity, and contractility of the heart (51, 52).

Table 1 β-Adrenergic compounds that have inotropic effects (only main references are given)

Name	Formula	References
Dopamine		29, 81, 134, 318
Levodopa		134, 319, 320
Ibopamine (SB 7505)		128, 130, 131, 134
Dobutamine		15–17, 77, 82, 92
Butopamine		90, 135a, 135b, 321
Salbutamol		136–138
Pirbuterol		34, 122, 124–126
Prenalterol H 133/22 or H 80/62		19, 113

Table 1 *(Continued)*

Name	Formula	References
RO 363		146, 147
ICI 118587		121
TA 064		142, 144
ASL 7022		322–324

The dopamine-induced inotropic and chronotropic responses are attenuated by the preadministration of cocaine (53), reserpine (54), and desmethylimipramine (16), and potentiated by monoamine oxidase inhibitors (55). β-Adrenergic blockers reduce or eliminate the effects of dopamine on automaticity and increase excitability of the heart (52). They only reduce the inotropic effects in species where both α and β adrenergic receptors have been demonstrated (56a, 56b). Thus, in the dog heart, which does not contain α receptors (57), the positive inotropic and chronotropic effects of dopamine are blocked by a β adrenergic antagonist (58). In frog, rat, guinea pig, rabbit, and human heart muscle, α and β receptors have been demonstrated (59a, 59b). In rabbit hearts, the addition of a β blocker will shift the dose-response curve of dopamine to the right and this curve can be further displaced to the right by the addition of an α adrenergic blocker (60–63). The stimulation of α receptors does not significantly affect heart rate in concentrations that cause positive inotropic effects (59a, 64). It does not influence automaticity or ectopic foci production and may actually inhibit cardiac arrhythmogenesis (52). The α-receptor effects on cardiac contractility are best demonstrated in the presence of a β blocker at low rates of stimulation, at low temperatures, and at low concentrations of the agonist. Under these conditions, an α blocker will further reduce the effects of EP and NE, but not of IPN (60, 65).

It is fairly well established that activation of β-adrenergic receptors in the heart can be correlated with an increase in the cyclic AMP content of myocardial tissue. α-Adrenergic stimulation does not increase the cyclic AMP concentration. Dopamine increased the cyclic AMP content of rat and rabbit cardiac muscle (63, 66, 67); however, this increase was abolished by reserpine pretreatment, although the inotropic effect was reduced. This suggests that NE release is the causative agent of this dopamine effect. However, since dopamine stimulated both α as well as β receptors, one would expect dopamine to increase the cardiac concentration of cyclic AMP; however, no such increase has been observed (62, 68, 69). Huang & Drummond (70) have reported that α adrenoreceptor stimulation reduced the cyclic AMP response produced by isoprenaline. Furthermore, dopamine-induced increases in cardiac cyclic AMP are enhanced by the addition of an α blocking agent (63). The above findings thus suggest that α receptor activation can counteract the increase in cyclic AMP produced by stimulation of the β receptors.

All these findings suggest that dopamine effects on cardiac contractility are predominantly due to β adrenergic stimulation; however, α effects will be observed only under special experimental conditions, especially under those where β receptor activity is reduced. Thus, in hypothyroidism, where sensitivity to β adrenergic stimulation was reduced (71), the response to α receptor stimulation was actually increased (59a). This α adrenergic effect could thus contribute to the effects of dopamine and could be of advantage under hypothyroid shock or arrhythmogenic conditions.

In the intact dog, dopamine effects on cardiac contractility preceded the effects on heart rate. Tuttle & Mills (16) and Lumley et al (17) have shown that this inotropic selectivity is eliminated by pretreatment with adrenergic depleting agents, and in isolated auricular preparation Lumley et al (17) observed that dopamine is actually rate selective. One must conclude that in the intact dog this inotropic selectivity must be related to reflex adjustments, possibly α-adrenergic effects as well as the blood flow distribution effects discussed above. No dopaminergic receptors have been observed in cardiac muscle (72, 73). Thus, presynaptic effects of dopamine on cardiac function are probably not operative.

Dopamine increased the automaticity of the sinus node and ectopic foci and reduced the ventricular fibrillation threshold and the repolarization time of the action potential (52). Under cyclopropane anesthesia, both dopamine and NE produced arrhythmias and ventricular fibrillation, but dopamine had only 1/100 the potency of NE. The arrhythmogenic effects of dopamine were prevented by β-adrenergic blocking agents (52, 74).

Dopamine has been used clinically by the intravenous route for the treatment of shock and acute and chronic heart failure. However, dopamine's propensity to increase heart rate and its arrhythmogenic potential have required careful dose adjustment of this drug. In patients with congestive heart failure, dopamine increased cardiac output, but also increased pulmonary capillary wedge pressure and systemic blood pressure, possibly due to the α-adrenergic effects on vascular smooth muscle; in addition, a vasodilator effect on renal blood vessels has been observed due to its activation of dopaminergic receptors in kidney blood vessels (29).

Dobutamine

Dobutamine has an asymmetric carbon atom attached to the amine group. With the β phenethylamines such as NE, asymmetry occurs in the β-carbon, and the (−)−isomer is about two log units more effective than the (+)−isomer for both the α and β receptors. Maximal effects for both isomers are the same (75). Thus, these isomers have the same "efficacy" but different "affinities" for the receptors. Recently, Kent et al (76) have shown that there are two interconvertible β binding sites for catecholamines on frog red cell membranes, namely, "high" and "low" affinity states. The ability of an agonist to activate the adenylate cyclase system (efficacy) seems to correlate with its ability to form the high affinity state with the receptor.

With dobutamine, the α effects are observed both with the (±)−, (+)− and (−)−isomers and both isomers bind to aortic tissue with equal affinities (77), although only the (−)−isomer is an agonist, while the (+)−isomer is an antagonist to the (−)−isomer of dobutamine as well as to phenylephrine. The β-adrenergic effects of the dobutamine isomers are the same since both produced positive inotropic and chronotropic effects, although, in contrast to the β-phenethylamines, the (+)−isomer of dobutamine has a greater activity (about 1 log unit) than the (−)−isomer. These results indicate that the stereochemical requirements of α- and β-adrenergic receptors are not the same. The asymmetry in the dobutamine molecule governs efficacy rather than affinity as regards the α receptor, while in the β-phenethylamine series, affinity rather than efficacy is governed by the asymmetry in the β carbon atom (77). The effects of the asymmetry in the dobutamine molecule influenced the affinity to the β receptor and had little effect on efficacy. These results indicate that the α- and β-adrenergic receptors have different steric requirements that determine efficacy and affinity of adrenergic agents. The asymmetry observed with dobutamine may be more important in determining efficacy and affinity properties at the β and α receptors than the β carbon asymmetry observed with the phenethylamines (77).

These differing effects of (+)− and (−)−isomers of dobutamine explain the complex actions of the mixed form used clinically.

Dobutamine is active intravenously but is poorly absorbed from the gastrointestinal tract and has a short half-life. It can be classified as an adrenergic agent with β_1-, β_2-, and α-adrenergic actions (25, 78). Its inotropic and chronotropic effects are blocked by β-blocking agents, and here its α effects manifest themselves by increases in blood pressure and peripheral vascular resistance. The β effects are best seen after the administration of an α blocking agent

(15–17, 77, 79, 80–82). Robie et al (80) compared the effects of dobutamine with NE. The dose of dobutamine that reduced femoral blood flow was 15 times the dose that increased femoral blood flow and was about 180 times the equieffective dose of NE. The effects on cardiac contractile force required 40 times the equieffective dose of NE.

In the intact vagotomized dog as well as in the dog treated with syrosingopine, a catecholamine depleter, dobutamine produces a dose-related increase in contractility with minimal increases in heart rate (16, 17, 82). Hinds & Hawthorne (83) administered dobutamine intravenously to instrumented dogs and, with infusion rates of 5–20 μg/kg/min, linear increments of a number of indices of cardiac contractility occurred without a change in left ventricular end diastolic pressure, mean arterial pressure, or heart rate. Similar effects have been observed with infusion rates of 0.1–0.2 μg/kg/min of INE; however, at any level of increased cardiac contractility, heart rate is higher with INE than with dobutamine (83). In dogs with acute myocardial ischemia, Kirlin et al (84), Willerson et al (85), Rude et al (86), and Liang et al (87) observed an increase in heart rate, myocardial contractility, and elevated ST segment of the electrocardiogram, although blood flow to the heart had increased and blood pressure had not changed. Dobutamine administration during coronary occlusion did not increase the area of injury unless doses of dobutamine were administered that substantially increased heart rate (87).

In dogs, Robie & Goldberg (79) and Vatner et al (82) compared dopamine and dobutamine and showed that dopamine increased renal blood flow but did not increase femoral flow; dobutamine, on the other hand, increased femoral blood flow without changing renal flow. In general, dobutamine favors redistribution of blood to muscle and coronary vessels over mesenteric and renal flow.

Bodem et al (15), Lumley et al (17), and Alousi (unpublished data) observed that in isolated preparations heart rate effects were more sensitive to dobutamine than were contractile force changes. Dobutamine increased the cyclic AMP content of the cat (88) and rat hearts (89). The increase in cyclic AMP preceded an increase in phosphorylase-a activity and dobutamine had approximately 1/45 the activity of INE (89).

Clinical studies have been reviewed by Goldberg et al (81), Leier et al (90), Plachetka (91), Sonnenblick et al (92), and Weber & Tuttle (93).

Dobutamine given intravenously to patients with heart failure increased cardiac output linearly with dose, decreased pulmonary capillary wedge pressure, and increased urinary sodium excretion with no significant increase in heart rate or tachyarrhythmias.

Willerson et al (85) and Vasu et al (94) have shown that dobutamine, like a number of other catecholamines, increased the oxygen consumption of the normal heart by augmenting heart rate and increasing ventricular wall tension.

However, in the failing heart, contractility was increased and the left ventricular end diastolic pressure was decreased, the net result being no change in oxygen consumption and an increase in the efficiency of the heart.

When dobutamine was compared with dopamine in low output heart failure, both drugs had approximately equivalent effects on the various indices of positive inotropism and heart rate (91, 95–97). Dopamine increased blood pressure and left ventricular end diastolic pressure, while dobutamine decreased both parameters.

Most of these clinical studies with dobutamine have lasted 24–48 hours. Unverferth et al (32) observed that the cardiac effects of dobutamine in patients were significantly reduced after 96 hours of constant administration. This suggests that with dobutamine desensitization of the heart was occurring, thus limiting the use of this drug to acute situations.

Unverferth et al (32) and Leier et al (98) reported that both symptomatic and hemodynamic improvement persisted for a week in 68% of the patients following discontinuation of three-day therapy with dobutamine. Similar observations have been made with the cardiotonic agent amrinone (99), where the beneficial effects on cardiac function persisted for days or even weeks after drug therapy was stopped and blood concentration of the drug had been dissipated. Very few studies on this aspect of cardiac pharmacology have been published, but the development of an endomyocardial biopsy technique (100, 101) makes it possible to do histological as well as biochemical studies with human heart tissue. Unverferth et al (32) have obtained cardiac tissue from heart failure patients after dobutamine therapy. By means of electron microscope techniques, they made quantitative ultrastructural analysis of these biopsy samples. Simple bed rest had no significant effect on the crista-to-matrix ratio of mitochondria, the size of the mitochondria, or the number of electron-dense particles per mitochondrion. Those patients who had a good clinical response to dobutamine therapy showed a decrease in both the size of the mitochondria and the crista-to-matrix ratio, as well as a decrease in the number of the electron-dense particles in mitochondria. The electron-dense particles are seen in degenerating or ischemic cells (102–104) and cells from failing hearts from hamsters and dogs frequently show the appearance of these dense particles, mitochondrial enlargement, and the change in crista-to-matrix ratio (105, 106). These phenomena indicate an improvement in the physical integrity of mitochondria and possibly mitochondrial function. The mechanism by which dobutamine causes this return toward a normal state of mitochondrial structure is not understood; however, dobutamine and other cardioactive agents produce cardiac blood flow and biochemical changes, which in turn could trigger the repair process in cardiac cells, especially those cells situated at the borderline area of an ischemic zone. This is obviously an important area of cardiac pharmacology and more data should become available in the future.

Prenalterol

Prenalterol (see Table 1) is an orally active β-adrenergic agent (107). In the intact dog, prenalterol produced a positive inotropic effect at dosages that did not increase heart rate, and Carlsson et al (19), Manders et al (30), Strossberg & Montgomery (108), and Williams (109) have attributed this to a selective effect on the β_1 adrenoreceptor. However, binding studies (110, 111) do not support this viewpoint. Studies in isolated cardiac tissue by Kenakin et al (26, 112) have shown that prenalterol does not have positive inotropic selectivity. In coronary arteries and other tissues with β_2 receptors, prenalterol acted as a β blocker (26, 78).

Thus, the in vivo selectivity of prenalterol for inotropic over chronotropic effects cannot be related to receptor binding mechanisms and is most likely due to reflex mechanisms that are initiated when the drug is administered to the intact animal. This is probably due to distribution of the drug in ventricular and auricular tissue and the β-blocking action of this drug. Heart rate and contractility dose-response curves are shifted equally to the right following the administration of a β-blocking agent (113). In intact animals prenalterol produces a greater increase in contractile force than isoprenaline or terbutaline when compared at doses that produce an equal chronotropic effect. Prenalterol doses that produce an inotropic response do not provoke or potentiate cardiac arrhythmias (19).

In man, prenalterol has an elimination half-life of a few minutes, with both fast and slow components. On oral administration, bioavailability was about 25% and elimination half-life was 1.2–1.7 hour. A slow-release form of the drug, which produced effective plasma concentrations for a period of 10 hours, allowed twice daily administration (114).

Prenalterol, when given either intravenously (0.13–0.5 mg) or orally (2.5–10 mg) to humans, increased heart rate, systolic blood pressure, and pulse pressure with either no significant change or a reduction in diastolic pressure (114–116). The above dosages of prenalterol had little effect on renal plasma flow and glomerular filtration rate (117) and had no demonstrable effect on bronchial smooth muscle (118).

A number of clinical studies in post-ischemic heart failure have shown that intravenous and oral administration of prenalterol caused an enhancement of left ventricular function. In some of these studies, increased ectopic activity and ventricular tachycardia were observed (72, 119). The maximum rate of pressure fall (peak negative dp/dt) also increased, suggesting improved relaxation of the stiff ventricle (120).

From the available data, it is not possible to assess the usefulness of this drug following chronic administration. However, experience with other β-adrenergic agents has been disappointing because of the occurrence of the desensitization phenomenon. Kenakin & Beek (26) have shown that in vitro desensitization of guinea pig atria to isoproterenol eliminates the agonist activity of prenalterol. These findings suggest that prolonged therapy with prenalterol could result in desensitization, thus limiting the usefulness of this drug to the treatment of acute heart failure.

ICI 118587

This compound, an analog of prenalterol, is a partial agonist and also has β antagonist properties (121).

Pirbuterol

Pirbuterol is an orally active catecholamine related to salbutamol, which has both β_1 and β_2 effects. It has been studied in both animals and human patients with heart failure. Van Arman et al (122), Moore et al (123), and Constantine et al (124) have described the animal pharmacology of pirbuterol. The data of Gold & Horowitz (125) show that in the unanesthetized instrumented dog, pirbuterol produced equivalent increases in heart rate and cardiac contractile force. Left ventricular end diastolic and systolic volumes were decreased, while left ventricular stroke volume was not changed significantly (0.125–8 µg/kg/min). In those preparations where heart rate was kept constant by pacing, left ventricular end diastolic volume did not change except at the highest rates of pirbuterol infusion, indicating that heart rate changes had contributed to these effects. β blockade shifted the dose-response curve to the right. The heart rate selectivity of pirbuterol in cardiac muscle is not very striking and in this respect the drug resembles isoproterenol.

Clinical findings in heart failure patients have shown that pirbuterol induced both vasodilatation (126) and inotropic effects (127). Due to the symptoms of tremor and nervousness, the dose of pirbuterol was limited to 20 mg three times daily. Exercise tolerance, maximum oxygen uptake, and left ventricular diameters were measured, and after four and seven weeks of therapy, pirbuterol had no demonstrable effects over placebo.

In a similar study, Colucci et al (34) observed a marked attenuation of the hemodynamic effects of pirbuterol in patients. This was correlated with the down regulation of β receptor ligand binding by lymphocytes obtained from these patients. Thus, pirbuterol, like a number of other adrenergic agents, shows evidence of attenuation of its positive inotropic effects, possibly because of reduced binding of the agonist to the β receptors of the heart.

Ibopamine

Ibopamine (see Table 1) is a di-ester of N-methyl dopamine that was synthesized as a renal vasodilator and diuretic. In dogs, oral administration of ibopamine increased renal blood flow with no other observable cardiovascular effect. Large doses also increased femoral blood flow and left ventricular pressure and its rate of increase, dp/dt, as well as systolic and diastolic arterial pressure. These effects are reminiscent of the effects of dopamine, except that ibopamine had much longer-lasting activity and was orally effective. In rats, oral ibopamine increased urinary sodium without affecting potassium excretion. No central nervous system effects were observed (128).

Ibopamine increased the contractility of isolated guinea-pig papillary muscle (129).

In humans, oral ibopamine produced a decrease in systolic time intervals and a diuretic effect (129–134).

In patients with cardiac failure, ibopamine given orally increased cardiac index and stroke volume without significant changes in heart rate or blood pressure. Both pulmonary arterial pressure and systemic vascular resistance were decreased and these effects lasted for 5–7 hours (129). The effects of prolonged administration and its arrhythmogenic potential have not to our knowledge been assessed.

Butopamine

Butopamine (see Table 1) was prepared by Tuttle et al (unpublished data) and has a structure similar to dobutamine. This compound is refractory to the action of catechol-O-methyl transferase and thus it is orally active and has a long-lasting action. Clinical findings in acute heart failure cases have been reported by Thompson et al (135). Intravenous administration produced an increase in the cardiac index and heart rate and shortening of systolic time intervals. A few patients experienced ventricular ectopy, especially with the higher doses used. No data pertaining to oral administration are available.

Salbutamol

Salbutamol (see Table 1) was developed as an oral bronchodilator because of its marked β_2-adrenergic activity on bronchial smooth muscle. The compound has positive inotropic and chronotropic effects on the heart and in heart failure in man it improved all cardiac ventricular parameters and produced only a moderate increase in heart rate (136–138). No data on the chronic use of this drug are available.

Doxaminol (BM 10 1088)

Doxaminol is an orally effective β sympathomimetic agent. In intact animals, it had a positive inotropic selectivity over chronotropic activity, with minimal effects on blood pressure. In combination experiments, the inotropic effects of doxaminol were additive to those of digitoxin without an increase in cardiac arrhythmias (139). Acute clinical studies in normal subjects (140) and heart failure patients (141) have essentially confirmed the animal data. No data for prolonged use of this drug in heart failure patients have been reported, nor are data available to exclude an action by a release mechanism of NE.

TAO64

TAO64 (see Table 1) is an orally effective adrenergic agent. In dogs, Nagao et al (142) and Ikeo et al (143) have shown a separation of inotropic and chronotropic effects. In heart failure patients, Kino et al (144) observed that TAO64, after intravenous and oral administration, produced increases in cardiac output, dp/dt, a reduction in the left ventricular end diastolic pressure, and minimal changes in heart rate. This is another β-adrenergic agent with inotropic selectivity. No chronic use studies in human heart failure patients have come to our attention.

ASL-7022

ASL-7022 (see Table 1) is a tetrahydronaphthalene compound. In dogs it has β-adrenergic properties on cardiac contractility with a slight reduction in heart rate and blood pressure. Experiments in reserpinized dogs have not been reported and it is not clear whether this drug has direct β effects on heart muscle. No clinical data are available to us.

Abbott-47844

Abbott-47844 is a dopamine derivative that has prolonged renal vasodilator and diuretic effects that are not blocked by α- or β-blocking agents.

In larger doses, it had typical β-adrenergic effects on the heart of anesthetized dogs (145).

RO 363

RO 363 (see Table 1), a compound related to prenalterol, was synthesized with the claim that it had β_1 selectivity for adrenoreceptors. Animal studies by Iakovidis et al (146) and Raper et al (147) have shown that RO 363 is about half as active as isoproterenol as an inotropic agent on the heart. No experimental data in intact animals or human patients are available to us.

Bufuralol and Analogs

These benzofuranylethanolamine derivatives have both β-adrenergic activities when tested in anesthetized reserpinized and vagotomized cats. The compounds have no peripheral dilator action and have the expected inotropic and chronotropic effects on the heart (148, 149).

D4975

D4975 is a theophylline dopamine derivative about 100 times more potent than dopamine on heart rate and its effects are difficult to wash out (150). In anesthetized cats, this compound increased cardiac contractile force in a dose of 0.5–1 μg/kg, which had none or only minimal chronotropic effects. It had about five times the activity of dopamine or dobutamine on the heart and had prolonged activity. Propranolol caused a partial antagonism of the cardiac effects of this compound.

The results indicate that D4975's actions on the heart involve both β-adrenoreceptor stimulation and phosphodiesterase inhibition (151). No clinical studies have come to our attention.

Adrenergic Transmitter-Releasing Agents

A large number of substances of varied chemical structure can release NE from sympathetic nerve endings (13, 152). The actions of these substances on the heart are in general similar to those observed with NE. A few of the more recently studied compounds, some of which have mixed actions (inhibition of phosphodiesterase), are listed in Table 2. All these compounds would have limited use in the therapy of heart failure because of their propensity to increase peripheral resistance and because they would be relatively ineffective in the treatment of severe heart failure where the NE content of the heart is reduced.

PHOSPHODIESTERASE (PDE) INHIBITORS

In recent years, interest in phosphodiesterase inhibitors (see Table 3) as inotropic and chronotropic agents has been revived. Much of our information on the action of these agents is based on studies with the methylxanthines, which affect cardiac, skeletal and smooth muscle, as well as the central nervous system and secretory functions.

Three possible mechanisms of action have been considered for the cardiac effects of the methylxanthines: (a) translocation of intracellular calcium; (b) increased concentrations of cyclic AMP resulting from the ability of these compounds to inhibit cyclic AMP phosphodiesterase and concomitant phosphorylation of membrane protein; (c) the ability of the methylxanthines to block adenosine receptors (13b, 153, 154).

As Scholz (13b) and Blinks et al (155) have reported, the methylxanthines in high concentrations produce an array of complex effects on cardiac muscle that defy a simple explanation. In the presence of methylxanthines, the active state is prolonged and intensified. The prolongation of the active state induced by caffeine is antagonized by procaine, while the intensity is not changed. The abbreviation of the contraction produced by catecholamines is blocked by caffeine, although the frequency induced abbreviation is not changed.

From the above findings, Blinks et al (155) postulated that the methylxanthines exert effects on cardiac excitation-contraction coupling by the inhibition of calcium uptake by the sarcoplasmic reticulum and increased calcium influx

Table 2 Compounds that cause the release of norepinephrine in cardiac muscle

Name	Formula	References
Aminotetrahy-drocarba-zole		172, 325
Benzofuranyl-ethanol amine		148
AP10	R = β-D-glucopyranosyl	326
9 Hydroxy-elliptisine		327
Ameziniumetil sulfate (LU1631)		328–331
Dopamine analog (E) and (Z)-2-(3, 4-di-hydroxy-phenyl) cyclopro-pylamine hydro-chlorides		324
Theophylline-dopamine derivative		150, 151
Prolactin	Molecular weight 22,500	332–334

through the sarcolemmal membrane. From recent studies, Blinks et al (156, 157) have concluded that the changes in aequorin light signals obtained from cardiac muscle indicate changes in the amount of intracellular calcium in response to the action potential. The decline of the light signal is probably due

Table 3 Phosphodiesterase inhibitors

Name	Formula	References
MDL 17043 1,3-dihydro-4-methyl-(5-[4-(methyl-thio)benzoyl]-2H-imidazol-2-one		206, 207, 211, 213, 215, 216
Amrinone (Win 40680)		172, 173, 191–192b, 195, 335, 336
Milrinone (Win 47203)		198–200b, 337, 338
Cilostamide OPC 3689		232, 233
USV 2776 6,7-Dimethoxy-1-[3(trifluoro-methyl)phenyl]-3,4, dihydro-isoquino-line HCl		339
Vardax Sulmazole ARL115 BS		220a, 225a, 225b, 340
Buquineran UK 14275		226, 230, 231

Table 3   *(Continued)*

Name	Formula	References
Carbazeran UK 31557		
Phthalazinol		234, 341
Ustimon		342
Visnadin		343
Analogs of Cyclic AMP		310, 311, 344
Trapidil Trapyrin Rocornal		345–347

to the binding of calcium to troponin C, the sarcoplasmic reticulum, and other calcium binding sites. The binding of calcium to the sarcoplasmic reticulum is related to the formation of cyclic AMP and the phosphorylation of phospholamban and sarcolemmal proteins. Rall & West (158) and others (13b) observed that methylxanthines potentiated the effects of a catecholamine in isolated heart muscle, probably due to the inhibition of cyclic AMP phosphodiesterase. The prolonged active state following administration of a methylxanthine was accompanied by a proportional prolongation of the aequorin light signal. The height of the aequorin light signal is not increased by methylxanthines; however, its duration is prolonged and its rate of rise is decreased (157), suggesting that calcium release and uptake are inhibited. Another possible mechanism of methylxanthines has been discussed by Fabiato & Fabiato (159), Guthrie & Naylor (160), and Endoh & Kitazawa (161), who have observed a caffeine-induced increase in calcium sensitivity of skinned muscle. They suggest that sensitization of the contractile mechanism of heart muscle by the methylxanthines is another mechanism of action of phosphodiesterase inhibitors.

Stimulation of the contractility of isolated cardiac papillary muscle requires a concentration of 0.5–1.0 μg of theophylline per ml of bathing fluid (2.5–5.0 μM) (162). Shifting the dose response curve of NE requires about 10^{-4} M (18 γ/ml) theophylline (158). The latter effect may be due to an increased concentration of cyclic AMP. Minimal inhibition of phosphodiesterase requires about 50 μM of theophylline, which is about 50 times the dose that produced a detectable increase in cardiac contractile force in isolated cardiac muscle. This is inconsistent with the concept that the methylxanthines produce a positive inotropic effect in heart muscle by inhibiting cyclic AMP phosphodiesterase (163); however, such inhibition of phosphodiesterase may be of importance when high concentrations of theophylline (above 10^{-4} M) are used (164).

It is well known that adenosine induces a receptor-mediated inhibition of cardiac adenylate cyclase (165, 166). Contraction of cardiac muscle is inhibited by adenosine and partially reversed by a catecholamine or methylxanthines (167, 168). In cardiac muscle, adenosine is bound to the crude microsomal fraction (169). The binding of adenosine to the microsomal fraction satisfies the criteria for membrane binding and this binding was inhibited by ATP, ADP, AMP, and cyclic AMP (166, 170). Guthrie & Nayler (160) reported that caffeine inhibits the adenosine-induced reduction of Ca^{++} uptake by cardiac muscle. It is thus possible that the methylxanthines could act on cardiac contractility by a mechanism related to adenosine regulation of cardiac contractility as well as cardiac cyclic AMP (154, 163).

Specific antagonists to adenosine may have greater organ and tissue selectivity than the methylxanthines and future work in this area of pharmacology may well lead to more specific therapeutic agents than the methylxanthines, as well as to a better understanding of the mechanism of action of the older and newer drugs.

Cardioactive Bipyridines

The cardioactive bipyridines are a new chemical entity with both positive inotropic and vasodilatory activity (171, 172).

Amrinone—Inocor®

EFFECTS ON THE HEART   Amrinone, 5 amino-[3,4'-bipyridine]-6-one (see Table 3), is a positive inotropic agent with vasodilatory properties. A concentration-dependent (3–1000 γ/ml) positive inotropic effect was demonstrated in isolated atrial and/or ventricular tissues of cats, dogs, rabbits, guinea pigs, monkeys, and humans (173–184).

In isolated and failing hearts, amrinone caused significant increases in cardiac contractile force, coronary blood flow, oxygen uptake, and total cardiac work with no significant changes in heart rate and an increase in the efficiency of the heart (175, 185).

The in vivo inotropic activity of amrinone was observed in anesthetized and unanesthetized dogs (173, 185). In intravenous doses of 0.1–1.0 mg/kg or oral doses of 2–10 mg/kg, amrinone caused significant positive inotropic effects, a reduction in peripheral resistance, and no significant effect on heart rate or blood pressure. Higher doses of amrinone further increased contractile force, decreased systolic and diastolic blood pressure, and increased heart rate with no deleterious changes in the ECG (173, 186).

EFFECTS ON BLOOD VESSELS   The vasodilatory properties of amrinone were observed in denervated, isolated, hind-limb preparation (173). Amrinone caused relaxation of untreated or KCl-constricted, isolated, procine coronary arteries (187), norepinephrine- or KCl-constricted, isolated rabbit aorta (168), and phenylephrine-constricted pulmonary arteries (189) and bronchial smooth muscle (190).

Clinical trials with amrinone were conducted in patients with severe congestive heart failure (New York Heart Association Functional Classes III and IV) refractory to conventional therapy. All patients were on digitalis and diuretics; some were on antiarrhythmic and vasodilator agents.

Short-term therapy with intravenous amrinone (bolus injections of 0.50–2.5 mg/kg) showed dose-related improvement in cardiac index with reduction in pulmonary capillary wedge pressure, right atrial pressure (20 to 50%), and no change in heart rate and mean arterial pressure (191, 192a, 192b, 193). Long-term therapy (up to three years) with oral amrinone (100–300 mg, t.i.d.) caused similar improvement in cardiac performance and increased exercise tolerance (194, 195, 196). In patients with ischemic cardiomyopathy, Benotti et al (197) demonstrated beneficial hemodynamic changes, without an increase in myocardial oxygen consumption.

SIDE EFFECTS OF AMRINONE   Of the more than 500 patients treated with amrinone, approximately 15% have demonstrated dose-related, reversible platelet count reduction. A similar number have complained of gastrointestinal disturbances that required dose adjustment or discontinuation of therapy (193, 194, 196). Hepatic enzyme abnormalities and arrhythmias have also been reported.

Milrinone

Milrinone (Win 47203) (see Table 3) is 1,6-dihydro-2-methyl-6-oxo-[3,4-bipyridine]-5-carbonitrile; it is 20–50 times more potent than amrinone (184, 198a, 198b, 199). The pharmacological profile of milrinone is probably similar to amrinone in all test systems, including patients with congestive heart failure. So far, milrinone has been tested in more than 200 subjects and patients using intravenous and oral regimens (200a, 200b, 201). In exploratory efficacy studies in patients with severe congestive heart failure (Classes III and IV), the beneficial effects of milrinone were observed for several months and were not accompanied by any of the side effects observed with amrinone (200b, 201).

Mechanism of Action of the Cardioactive Bipyridines

Both amrinone and milrinone are phosphodiesterase inhibitors; however, it is by no means clear whether this effect is responsible for the inotropic properties of these compounds. Both compounds increase the cyclic AMP content of cardiac muscle; however, here again it is not clear whether this effect is the only mechanism responsible for the inotropic actions of the bipyridines (179, 181, 198a, 198b). The inotropic and chronotropic effects of amrinone are not blocked by α- or β-adrenergic blocking agents, by H_1 or H_2 histamine blocking agents, or by inhibitors of prostaglandin synthesis. The bipyridines do not inhibit cardiac Na^+,K^+-activated ATPase (173, 198a, 198b, 203). A number of investigators have observed that amrinone and milrinone increase calcium uptake in a variety of cells, including heart cells (189, 203, 204). Morgan et al (205) studied the effects of amrinone on the aequorin light signal in cardiac muscle. Amrinone increased the amplitude of both the force of contraction and the light signal, increased the time to peak response, and increased the rate of decline of the light signal. This suggested that amrinone increases both the intracellular Ca^{2+} concentration and the rate of Ca^{++} sequestration to the contractile proteins. Milrinone has a biphasic dose response curve in dog ventricular trabeculae, which suggests the possibility of more than one mechanism of action (A. Farah & P. Canniff, unpublished data), possibly one on Ca^{++} uptake and one due to formation of cyclic AMP and its effects on Ca^{++} uptake and release.

MDL 17043

MDL 17043 (see Table 3) is a phosphodiesterase inhibitor with inotropic, chronotropic, and vasodilator properties (206, 207). Synthesis of this compound was described by Schnettler et al (208). It is active by the intravenous and oral route and, after an oral dose (30 mg/kg) in dogs, its inotropic effect reached a maximum in 30 minutes and lasted about 4–5 hours (207). MDL 17043 is eliminated by biphasic mechanisms and after 3 mg/kg the half-life can be estimated to be about one hour (209). In dogs, it shortened both the QT interval and the atrioventricular conduction time but had no effect on the action potential duration (212).

Similar to other PDE inhibitors, this drug produced positive inotropic effects that are not blocked by α- or β-adrenergic blockers, by H_1 and H_2 blockers, by cardiac denervation, or by reserpine pretreatment (206). MDL 17043 has little effect on cyclic AMP phosphodiesterase I and II activity, but phosphodiesterase III was strongly inhibited by a partially competitive mechanism and 50% inhibition required 1.3 μM, which was only 1/15 the dose required for amrinone (211). However, the in vitro and in vivo effects of MDL and amrinone are about the same, thus suggesting that PDE inhibition may not be the basic mechanism of action of so-called PDE inhibitors. MDL 17043 had minimal effect on dog kidney Na^+K^+ ATPase or on Ca^{++} ATPase obtained from cardiac sarcoplasmic reticulum. Calcium uptake by oxalate-supported cardiac sarcoplasmic reticulum was not changed by MDL 17043 concentrations that produced inotropic effects. In experimental preparations, MDL 17043 had rather similar pharmacological properties to amrinone.

Only limited data on the clinical efficacy of MDL 17043 has so far been published. In normal humans, Belz et al (212) administered the compound either intravenously or orally in a dose of 1–3 mg/kg. These amounts produced cardiac inotropic effects as measured by systolic time intervals and the effects of the drug lasted for more than four hours. Absolute bioavailability was about 60%. In heart failure cases Crawford et al (213), Uretzky et al (214, 215), and Ferry et al (216) have observed with intervenous MDL 17043 (maximum dose 3 mg/kg) an increase in cardiac output and dp/dt, a reduction in the pulmonary capillary wedge pressure, and total peripheral resistance with no arrhythmogenic effects. No data on chronic use of this drug have come to our attention. More recently, Petein et al (217) have published data on the clinical effectiveness of another imidazole derivative (MDL 19205) with results similar to those seen with MDL 17043.

(AR-L115 BS) Vardax, Sulmazole

Vardax (see Table 3) is one of a large series of benzimidazoles synthesized by Amstel & Kutter (218). Following preliminary screening AR-L115 BS was chosen for further development (219).

AR-L115 BS is a phosphodiesterase inhibitor with a K_i of about 315 (K_i of papaverine = 7.9) and at similar concentrations it produced maximal effects on cardiac contractile force in guinea-pig atria. Neither myocardial adenylate cyclase nor cyclic AMP content was changed by this drug. The pharmacology and pharmacokinetics of AR-L115 have been summarized (219) and the data show that AR-L115 is an effective inotropic agent with vasodilator properties. In a dosage that increased cardiac contractility it did not increase heart rate. However, with higher doses, blood pressure was decreased and heart rate was increased.

In the earlier reports, Dahmen & Greeff (220) have claimed that neither pretreatment with reserpine nor β-adrenergic agents reduced the inotropic effect of AR-L115 in guinea-pig auricular muscle. However, Petein et al (221) have shown that AR-L115 increased the release of NE from dog heart. Brutsaert et al (222) have shown that β-adrenergic blocking agents markedly reduced the effects of AR-L115 in rat cardiac tissue and Pouleur et al (223) and Verdouw et al (224) observed a reduction by a β blocker of the inotropic effect of AR-L115 in intact dogs and humans. It is thus likely that this compound, although a phosphodiesterase inhibitor, produced its positive inotropic effect by a second mechanism, namely, release of NE.

The clinical data in man show that AR-L115 has both cardiotonic and vasodilator properties following intravenous and oral administration. However, in cases with severe heart failure, the effects on cardiac output were frequently quite modest, possibly because of the low NE content of the heart observed in severe heart failure. In angina patients AR-L115 improved both hemodynamics and the symptoms of angina (225a, 225b).

No data on prolonged use of AR-L115 in heart failure cases have been reported.

Buquineran (UK 14275)

Buquineran (see Table 3) is a piperidine derivative that inhibits cyclic AMP phosphodiesterase. It also causes the release of NE and its effects on isolated organs and intact animals are reduced by pretreatment with reserpine or a β-adrenergic blocker (210, 226–228).

In animal studies, Buquineran had a positive inotropic and vasodilator effect with minimal effects on heart rate. Studies in normal humans (229, 230) and in patients (103a, 227, 228, 231) all indicated that intravenous infusions of Buquineran (64–256 μg/kg/min) caused a positive inotropic effect in normal subjects and in both acute and chronic heart failure patients. However, many of these positive inotropic effects were abolished by pretreatment with a β-adrenergic blocking agent (227).

Thus, Buquineran is a phosphodiesterase inhibitor with a major effect on NE release that in turn increases the inotropic state of the heart.

Cilostamide

Cilostamide is a cyclic AMP phosphodiesterase inhibitor prepared by Kohri et al (232); its pharmacology was studied by Endoh et al (233).

Cilostamide had one-third the potency of 1-methyl-3-isobutylxanthine (IBMX) in inhibiting a crude amine cyclic AMP phosphodiesterase, but it was 10 times more potent than IBMX in enhancing the isoprenaline-induced increase in cardiac contractility and it potentiated the effects of isoprenaline on cardiac cyclic AMP production (233). Cilostamide increased sinus rate at lower concentrations than those that increased contractile force on isolated auricles, and a β-adrenergic blocker reduced the inotropic effects by about 50%. The results suggest that cilostamide releases NE and is a phosphodiesterase inhibitor with rather modest effects on cardiac contractility.

Phthalazinol (EG626)

Phthalazinol (see Table 3) is a phosphodiesterase inhibitor the cardiac effects of which were studied by Shigenobu et al (234). In comparison with theophylline, it produced greater effects on heart rate and contractile force and showed a separation of inotropic and chronotropic effects in the isolated auricle. All these effects were resistant to β blockade. Phthalazinol potentiated the effects of isoproterenol, which supports the concept that this drug is a phosphodiesterase inhibitor. At lower concentrations, phthalazinol had no effect on the atrial and ventricular action potentials. At high concentrations, the rising phase of the action potential was depressed and it prolonged the action potential. In depolarized muscle, phthalazinol produced the slow response, which was abolished by Mn^{2+}, verapamil, and low Ca^{2+} concentration. It is possible that these effects on inotropism and chronotropism are related to the increase in the slow current, which is induced by the increased concentration of intracellular cyclic AMP.

USV 2776

This compound is one of a series of dihydro- and tetrahydroisoquinolines and is a phosphodiesterase inhibitor, especially of the insoluble fraction obtained from frog and dog heart muscle. It has I_{50} of 4–6 μM on insoluble cyclic AMP and cyclic GMP phosphodiesterase, while papaverine (8–16 μM), theophylline (130–150 μM), and MIX (12–19 μM) were less effective. No data on the cardiac effects of this compound are available.

INHIBITORS OF Na^+K^+-ATPase

This group of substances includes a variety of different chemical entities, including the cardiac glycosides (235) (see Table 4).

A large number of semi-synthetic cardio-active glycosides have been prepared in the hope of improving the therapeutic ratio of the naturally occurring glycosides (4, 5). With few exceptions, the methods used for the determinations of therapeutic efficacy and toxicity ratios are frequently difficult to

Table 4   Substances that inhibit Na^+K^+-ATPase and have positive inotropic effects, excluding cardiac glycosides and related structures

Name	Formula	References
Prednisone bisguanyl hydrazone (PBGH)		348–351
Erythro- phleum- alkaloids cassaine		244, 245, 352–354
Sanguinarine		355, 356
Benzylamino- dihydro- dimethoxy- imidazo- isoquinoline (B11A)		259a, 357–359
Chlorproma- zine and related substances		360–364
p-Chloro- mercuri- benzoate; p-chloro- mercuri benzene sulfonic acid		248, 261, 365, 366
N-ethyl- maleimide		248, 249, 367–369

Table 4 *(Continued)*

Name	Formula	References
Ethacrinic acid		370–373
Vanadate	Na_3VO_4	258, 259, 374
Rubidium	RbCl	235, 254–256b, 375
Thallous ion	$TiNO_3$	235, 255, 376–379
Doxorubicin		380–382

interpret. Methods for determining the minimal therapeutic, toxic, and lethal doses have been described by Farah & Maresh (236) in the isolated heart-lung preparation of the dog and by Walton et al (237) in intact dogs. The general methods have been reviewed by Bahrman & Greeff (238) and Greeff & Hafner (239). With the naturally occurring cardioactive compounds that are slowly inactivated, the constant infusion method of administering the glycosides produced results where the ratio of therapeutic-to-toxic doses was about the same for all compounds studied (236, 240–242). However, with rapidly inactivated and/or rapidly acting substances, such as dihydro cardio-active glycosides, the therapeutic-to-toxic ratio was increased (241). Similar findings have been reported for semi-synthetic cardio-active glycosides by Pastelin & Mendez (199), Mendez et al (242), and Bojorges et al (243). All these substances are rapidly destroyed and have a rapid onset of action, and thus both the therapeutic-to-lethal dose ratio and the toxic-to-lethal dose ratio are greater than the values obtained with ouabain. The rapid onset of action and destruction of these compounds could explain these findings.

Some nonglycosidic Na^+K^+-ATPase inhibitors have a positive inotropic effect in isolated cardiac tissue and only a few will be reviewed here. However, the interested reader is referred to the comprehensive discussion by Akera et al (235).

Erythrophleum Alkaloids

The erythrophleum alkaloids (see Table 4) are diterpenoid acids esterified with β-methylamino ethanol or β-dimethylaminoethanol. The best known of these alkaloids are erythropheleine, cassaine, and cassaidine and all have cardiotonic properties similar to those observed with cardio-active glycosides (244). Krayer et al (245) have shown that erythrophleic acid per se has no positive inotropic effect, although the pertinent amino alcohols, including mono- and di-methylamino ethanol, had positive inotropic effects that were about 1/200 that of cassaine and in high doses produced cardiac irregularities. This suggests that the active moiety is the aminoalcohol and esterification increases the cardiac effects.

Cassaine and related alkaloids like the cardio-active glycosides block the uptake of K^+ in human red blood cells and inhibit Na^+K^+-activated ATPase in homogenates and partially purified enzyme preparations obtained from a variety of tissues and species (235).

Sulfhydryl Inhibitors

Older studies have shown that $HgCl_2$ and organic mercurial diuretics (see Table 4) are negative inotropic and produce severe cardiac irregularities and ventricular fibrillation. On the other hand, p-chloromercuribenzoate was relatively nontoxic to the heart and the end point was a cardiac standstill (246). The diuretic effects of both $HgCl_2$ and organic mercurial diuretics could be inhibited or reversed by p-chloromercuribenzoate (247a, 247b), thus indicating different mechanisms of action of p-chloromercuribenzoate on the heart and kidney. Other sulfhydryl reagents, such as N-ethylmaleimide, inhibit Na^+K^+-ATPase and have a positive inotropic effect in isolated cardiac tissue (235, Table 4), which can sometimes be reduced but not eliminated by reserpine or propranolol pretreatment (248).

However, in a number of instances, the inotropic effect of the sulfhydryl inhibitor does not correlate well with its capacity to block Na^+K^+-ATPase. Thus, Fricke (249) has observed a half-maximal effect on contractile force of guinea-pig papillary muscle at 9 μM concentration of N-methylmaleimide, while 50% inhibition of Na^+K^+-ATPase required 1 mM concentration. Furthermore, the mercurial diuretics and $HgCl_2$ are also powerful inhibitors of the Na^+K^+-ATPase (250, 251) but have predominantly negative inotropic effects on heart tissue (252, 253).

Other Na^+K^+-ATPase inhibitors have a positive inotropic effect, although the correlation between ATPase inhibition and inotropic effect is not always positive. Thus, *rubidium ion* (Rb$^+$), which can replace K^+ in Na^+K^+-ATPase, will inhibit the fully activated ATPase in guinea-pig ventricular tissue and will produce a positive inotropic effect in guinea-pig auricular tissue (254–256a). However, Knight & Nosek (256b) have observed that Rb^+ produced a negative inotropic effect in guinea-pig ventricular tissue, which paralleled a transient shortening of the action potential duration. When active transport of Na^+ was stimulated by a burst of high rate of stimulation (257), Rb^+ produced a block of repolarization in guinea-pig ventricular tissue similar to that observed with cardiac glycosides. These results show that although Rb^+ has inhibitory properties on ATPase and the sodium pump, it does not necessarily follow that this will increase the force of contraction.

Vanadate

Vanadate (see Table 4) is a potent inhibitor of Na^+K^+-ATPase (258) and increases the force of contraction of isolated rat and rabbit auricular and ventricular tissue and ventricular tissue of the cat and guinea pig (235). However, in guinea pig and cat auricular tissue, Vanadate is a negative inotropic agent, although it inhibits the isolated Na^+K^+-ATPase of both these tissues (259a).

Erdman has shown that in rat ventricular muscle Vanadate actually increased Na^+K^+-ATPase activity and Grupp et al (259b) have reported that Vanadate increased cyclic AMP in the presence of propranolol in both ventricular and auricular guinea-pig muscle. Thus, the changes in cyclic AMP produced by Vanadate cannot explain the contractile effects of this ion. With Vanadate, there is a dissociation between inotropic action and inhibition of the Na^+K^+-ATPase; Vanadate inotropic effects may be related to an action on a calcium pool in the glyco-calyx part of the membrane (260) or possibly to prolongation of the sodium current, which manifests itself by a broadening of the action potential in responsive tissue.

Although not all Na^+K^+-ATPase inhibitors produce positive inotropic effects (261), it is rather striking that a number of these, such as p-chloromercuribenzoate, ethacrinic acid, and N-ethylmaleimide, have rather pronounced positive inotropic effects. It should be kept in mind that all these compounds may have effects other than the inhibition of the ATPase and that the inotropic effects could be negated by other effects of this highly reactive group of compounds.

Positive Inotropic Drugs that Prolong the Cardiac Action Potential

To the class of drugs that prolongs the cardiac action potential (see Table 5) belong the veratrum alkaloids, the grayanotoxins, the sea anemone polypeptides, the batrachotoxins, and scorpion poison, all of which prolong the action potential by an action on the sodium current. From studies on the squid

Table 5 Positive inotropic drugs that prolong the cardiac action potential

Name	Formula	References
Veratrum alkaloids Veratridine, Germitrine, Cevadin, Cevine	VERATRIDINE	383–388
Andromedo- toxins Grayanotoxins		262, 263, 389–391
Batrachotoxin		264–266, 392, 393
Anthopleu- rin-A Anthopleura Xantho- grammica	Sequence of amino acids in Anthopleurin-A GLY-VAL-SER-CYS-LEU-CYS-ASP-SER-ASP-GLY-PRO- SER-VAL-ARG-GLY-ASN-THR-LEU-SER-GLY-THR-LEU- TRP-LEU-TYR-PRO-SER-GLY-CYS-PRO-SER-GLY-TRP- HIS-ASN-CYS-LYS-ALA-HIS-GLY-PRO-THR-ILE-GLY- TRP-CYS-CYS-LYS-GLN	271, 277, 283, 286, 394–396
ATXll Anemonia Sulcata	GLY-$^{ILE*}_{VAL}$-PRO-CYS-LEU-CYS-ASP-SER-ASP-GLY-PRO- SER-VAL-ARG-GLY-ASN-THR-LEU-SER-GLY-ILE-ILE- TRP-LEU-ALA-GLY-CYS-PRO-SER-GLY-TRP-HIS-ASN- CYS-LYS-HIS-GLY-PRO-THR-ILE-GLY-TRP-CYS-CYS- LYS-GIN	45, 273, 275
Scorpion poison		397, 398
Tetraethylam- monium ion		399–403
2,4,6,Triamin- opyrimi- dine		267

axon, Purkinje fibers, and cardiac muscle tissue, it has been suggested that these toxins increase sodium influx by increasing the resting sodium permeability (262–265). However, Honerjäger & Reiter (266) suggest that the delay in repolarization produces a prolonged sodium influx that in turn increases Ca^{++} entry. The positive inotropic effects of triaminopyrimidine and tetraethyl ammonium are probably best explained by postulating reduction in potassium conductance by these agents, possibly due to a binding to a calcium site that regulates potassium conductance (267–270).

Anthopleurin-A (AP-A)

Anthopleurin-A (AP-A) (see Table 5) is a polypeptide containing 48 amino acids (molecular weight 5195) that was isolated by Norton et al (271) from the sea anemone *Anthopleura xanthogrammica;* its amino acid sequence was determined by Tanaka et al (272). A closely related single-chain polypeptide, ATX11, was isolated by Beress & Beress (273) from a sea anemone *Anemonia sulcata*. Both these polypeptides seem to have very similar pharmacological effects on cardiac muscle (274–276). Shibata et al (277) determined the effects of AP-A on isolated cardiac tissue and intact cats and dogs. Inotropic effects were observed in rat-, rabbit-, guinea-pig-, and cat-isolated auricular tissue; the toxin was about as effective as isoproterenol (2–5×10^{-9} M) in increasing contractility of the heart but did not increase heart rate significantly. In intact dogs and cats, AP-A (0.5 µg/kg) increased contractile force and dp/dt, decreased heart rate, and produced no change in blood pressure. When large doses (10 µg/kg) were given, cardiac arrhythmias appeared (277–279). In isolated cardiac tissue, the major effects of AP-A were an increased contraction or tension development and an increase in the total duration of contraction, which was mainly due to a prolongation of the rate of relaxation (275).

The effects of AP-A on cardiac contractility were not inhibited by reserpine pretreatment or by a β blocker and no effect on a cardiac Na^+K^+-ATPase preparation could be demonstrated (277). In a calcium-deficient medium AP-A was able to restore contraction, suggesting that external Ca^{++} ion is not required for the inotropic effect of AP-A. However, ryonodine (277) and dantroline (280) inhibited the effects of AP-A on contractile force of the heart. Ryonodine blocked the intracellular translocation of Ca^{++} in cardiac muscle (281) and dantroline reduced calcium release from the sarcoplasmic reticulum of skeletal muscle (282). These data suggest that AP-A action may involve the mobilization of intracellular calcium ion. Electrophysiological studies on heart muscle have shown that the main effect of AP-A is a prolongation of the action potential and an increase in the refractory period. Resting potential and rate of rise of the action potential were not affected; however, the plateau phase was prolonged and repolarization time was increased (275, 277, 283–286). Kodama et al (285) and Beress et al (45) have shown that the anemone toxins prolonged the action potential and this change was greater at lower than at high rates of stimulation. Hashimoto et al (286) have applied voltage clamps to cardiac tissue and have shown that the prolongation of the action potential by AP-A is accompanied by a decreased net outward current. The slow inward current and the potassium outward current were not affected. The prolongation of the action potential by AP-A was reversed by lowering outside Na^+ concentration and by tetrodotoxin (275, 276, 286, 287). The electrophysiological data suggest that AP-A has a major effect on prolonging the sodium current. This would cause an increased Na^+ entry and, indirectly by activating the Na^+-Ca^{++} exchange mechanism, result in increased Ca^{++} concentration and contractile force. However, experiments with ryonodine and dantroline suggest that AP-A may also act by increased translocation of intracellular calcium.

No human data with AP-A have come to our attention. However, because it is a relatively large foreign polypeptide, the formation of antibodies to AP-A may limit its usefulness in therapy.

Miscellaneous Inotropic Agents

FORSKOLIN   Forskolin (see Table 6) is a cardiotonic agent (288) isolated from the Indian herb *Coleus forskohlii* (288, 289). A closely related compound, coleonol, was isolated by Tandon et al (quoted in 290) from *Coleus forskohlii;* it also has inotropic and chronotropic effects on the heart. Forskolin is a diterpene (see Table 6) with an ester bond on Carbon 7. It should be pointed out that the erythrophleum alkaloid cassaine is also a diterpene ester where the alcohol is dimethylamino ethanol.

Lindner et al (288) described the effects of Forskolin on the isolated and in situ heart. This compound is a powerful cardiac stimulant in concentrations as low as 5×10^9 gm/ml. The time to peak tension and relaxation time were not changed by Forskolin. Microelectrode studies have shown that the action potential is shortened, especially with higher concentrations of Forskolin (5 μg/ml); however, the rate of rise of the 0-phase, the overshoot, and the plateau are not significantly changed. In higher concentrations, Forskolin produces spontaneous depolarization (288).

In intact anesthetized cats, Forskolin had positive inotropic and chronotropic effects and reduced blood pressure.

Forskolin does not inhibit either phosphodiesterase or Na^+K^+-ATPase but it depletes K^+ from the heart. In rat heart slices, Metzger & Lindner (291) observed that Forskolin induced a reduction of Na^+K^+-activated ATPase that accompanied the increase in cyclic AMP.

The mechanism of action of Forskolin was studied by Metzger & Lindner (292) and Holzmann et al (293), who observed that in intact cardiac tissue, as well as cardiac slices and membranes from rats, guinea pigs, and rabbits,

Table 6 Miscellaneous compounds

Name	Formula	References
Forskolin		288, 290, 292, 404
Inosine		405, 406
Coenzyme Q$_{10}$ Ubiquinone (10)		299–303, 407
Glucagon	HIS-SER-GEN-GLY-THR-PHE-THR-SER-ASP-TYR-SER-LYS-TYR-LEU-ASP-SER-AVG-AVG-ALA-GLN-ASP-PHE-VAL-GLN-TYR-LEU-HET-ASN-THR	409a, 409b
Secretin	HIS-SER-ASP-GLY-THR-PHE-THR-SER-GLU-LEU-SEV-AVG-LEU-AVG-ASP-SER-ALA-AVG-LEU-GLU-AVG-LEU-LEU-GLU-GLY-LEU-VAL-NH$_2$	410–413
Vasoactive intestinal polypeptide	HIS-SER-ASP-ALA-VAL-PHE-THR-ASP-ASN-TYR-THR-ARG-LEU-ARG-LYS-GLN-MET-ALA-VAL-LYS-LYS-TYR-LEU-ASN-SER-ILE-LEU-ASN	413–415
Allopurinol		416
Ionophore antibiotics Lasalocid (X537A)		417–419
Berberine		420a–423
Aminoethanol	H$_2$N-CH$_2$-CH$_2$OH	245
Na Fluoride	Na	424–429

Table 6   (*Continued*)

Name	Formula	References
Na Fluoro-acetate	FCH_2COOH	426, 430–432
Cholera-toxin	Molecular weight 83,000	309, 433
Imidazole	(imidazole structure)	435
Taurine Frapadil	$HO_3S.\ CH_2CH_2\text{-}NH_2$	435–440
BAYK 8644	(dihydropyridine structure: CF_3, O_2N, $COOCH_3$, H_3C, CH_3, N–H)	441
Histamine	(imidazole structure with $NH_2CH_2\text{-}CH_2$)	442–446

Forskolin increased the cardiac content of cyclic AMP and the activity of protein kinase.

These interesting observations with Forskolin on adenylate cyclase have been extended by Daly and his coworkers and Seamon and Seamon & Daly (290). Daly (294a) has recently reviewed the biochemical aspects of Forskolin action. The data available show that Forskolin increased cyclic AMP by an action on the catalytic unit of the adenylate-cyclase system. Recently, Brooker et al (294b) have observed that the effects of Forskolin on the adenylate-cyclase system of C6–2B rat astrocytoma cells is markedly inhibited by the protein synthesis inhibitors emetine or cycloheximide. These experiments suggest that a protein with a relatively short half-life is essential for the adenylate-cyclase system, which is stimulated by Forskolin. One can surmise that this protein is the site of action of Forskolin and that this protein relates to the activity of the catalytic unit of the adenylate cyclase.

COENZYME Q_{10} Coenzyme Q_{10} (CoQ_{10}) was isolated in 1959 by Crane et al (295) and is concentrated in mitochondria of various organs, including cardiac muscle. The biochemistry and pathophysiology of CoQ_{10} has been recently reviewed (296). The main points of this review are that a 75% depletion of cardiac CoQ_{10} leads to serious impairments of cardiac function and that the concentration of CoQ_{10} was markedly reduced in hearts obtained from heart failure cases (297). Clinical studies, although uncontrolled, have claimed that CoQ_{10} administration causes improvement in patients suffering from congestive heart failure (298).

Recent experimental studies have shown that administration of CoQ_{10} protects the heart from the functional damage produced by ischemia hypoxia or metabolic inhibitors such as adriamycin or dinitrophenol (299–303). All these studies indicate that CoQ_{10} administration reduces the effects of hypoxia and anoxia on both the contractile force and on the slow calcium-dependent action potential observed in depolarized cardiac muscle (303).

The data on CoQ_{10} and cardiac function is quite limited and the usefulness of this compound in the treatment of heart failure will require controlled double-blind clinical evaluation before any judgment can be passed. However, the importance of CoQ_{10} as a redox component between NADH and cytochrome b-c_1 complex makes this coenzyme an essential component for energy production in cardiac muscle and its deficiency will have serious consequences for heart function (304).

CYCLIC NUCLEOTIDE ANALOGS   Earlier studies have shown that exogenously applied cAMP or cyclic AMP analogs (see Table 6) mimic the response to β-adrenergic agonists (159, 305–308). These substances produce a positive inotropic effect, decrease the duration of contraction, suppress potassium contractures, and increase calcium uptake in heart muscle, but are several magnitudes less potent than the adrenergic agonists. These effects are observed after reserpine and β-adrenoreceptor blockade. The findings of Li & Sperelakis (309) that intracellular injection of cyclic AMP increases the slow action potential of cardiac cells depolarized by 22 mM K^+-Tyrode solution is further evidence that cyclic AMP mimics the effects of β-adrenergic agonists.

Since cyclic AMP is rapidly destroyed, more stable analogs have been prepared that have inotropic effects in isolated cardiac preparations (310, 311). It should be kept in mind that these cyclic AMP analogs can act either as activators of protein kinase or as inhibitors of phosphodiesterase, thus mimicking effects of β-adrenergic agonists of phosphodiesterase inhibitors.

CALCIUM IONOPHORES   The ionophores, "ion bearers" (see Table 6), are natural or synthetic products of a molecular weight varying between 200 and 2000. They were discovered serendipitously by Pressman and his colleagues in 1964 through their effect of stimulating energy-linked transport in the mitochondria (312). The ionophores form lipid-soluble complexes with polar cations, such as the monovalent cations Na^+, K^+, Rb^+, Li^+, and Cs^+; the divalent cations Ca^{2+}, Ba^{2+}, Mg^{2+}, Mn^{2+}, and Sr^{2+}; and the biogenic amines epinephrine, norepinephrine, dopamine, and serotonin (313). Most ionophores have some selective affinity and complexing capacity (314).

When ionophores are added to biological membranes, they form lipid-soluble cation complexes capable of rapid diffusion across the membrane. The dynamic reversibility of the complex at the membrane interfaces enables the ionophore to behave as a mobile cation carrier within biological membrane (314).

In rabbit or guinea-pig ventricular strips, the carboxylic calcium ionophore X-537A caused increases in twitch tension and contracture. However, the muscle developed tachyphylaxis to the drug after the first treatment. In addition, no inotropic response was observed after pretreatment of the preparation with propranolol on depletion of cardiac catecholamines with reserpine (315). The catecholamine and Ca^{2+} mobilization effect of the ionophores could be differentiated in cardiac strips treated with propranolol where the inotropic response to small doses of X-537A disappeared while the increase in tension and contracture could still be demonstrated (315).

Studies in anesthetized dogs (316, 317) showed that the intravenous administration of X-537A caused an increase in cardiac contractile force, slight increases in systolic and diastolic blood pressure, and no change in heart rate. The calculated total peripheral resistance was decreased. The translocation of Ca^{2+} and catecholamines was considered the mechanisms for the positive inotropic activity of X-537A.

Literature Cited

1. Taylor, S. H. 1979. Theory and practice in the treatment of heart failure. *European Prazocin Symposium, Vienna*, ed. M. D. Rawlins, pp. 101–31. Excerpta Med. *Intl. Cong. Series 475*
2. Evans, D. B., Weishaar, R. E., Kaplan, H. R. 1982. Strategy for the discovery and development of a positive inotropic agent. *Pharmacol. Ther.* 16:303–30
3. Brittain, R. T., Jack, D., Ritchie, A. C. 1970. Recent β-adrenoreceptor stimulants. *Adv. Drug Res.* 5:197–253
4. Campbell, S. F., Danilewicz, J. C. 1978. Agents for the treatment of heart failure. *Ann. Rep. Med. Chem.* 13:92–102
5. Bristol, J. A., Evans, D. B. 1981. Cardiotonic agents for the treatment of heart failure. *Ann. Rep. Med. Chem.* 16:93–102
6. Mason, D. T., Braunwald, E., Cohn, J. N. 1981. New modalities in the management of heart failure. *Am. Heart J.* 102:485–642
7. Scholz, H. 1983. Pharmacological actions of various inotropic agents. *Eur. Heart J.* 4(Suppl. A.): 161–72
8. Ahlquist, R. P. 1948. A study of the adrenotropic receptors. *Am. J. Physiol.* 153:586–600
9. Lands, A. M., Arnold, A., McAuliff, J. P., Luduena, F. P., Brown, T. G. Jr. 1967. Differentiation of receptor systems activated by sympathomimetic amines. *Nature* 214:597–98
10. Lefkowitz, R. J., Stadel, J. M., Caron, M. G. 1983. Adenylate cyclase-coupled beta-adrenergic receptors. *Ann. Rev. Biochem.* 52:159–86
11. Williams, R. S., Lefkowitz, R. J. 1980. Alpha-adrenergic receptors in rat myocardium. Identification by binding of [^{3}H] dihydroergocryptine. *Circ. Res.* 43:721–27
12. Tsien, R. W. 1977. Cyclic AMP and contractile activity in heart. *Adv. Cyclic Nucleotide Res.* 8:363–420
13a. Kunos, G. 1978. Adrenoreceptors. *Ann. Rev. Pharmacol. Toxicol.* 18:291–311
13b. Scholtz, H. 1980. Effects of beta- and alpha-adrenoceptor activators and adrenergic transmitter releasing agents on the mechanical activity of the heart. In *Handbook of Experimental Pharmacology. Adrenergic Activators and Inhibitors*, ed. L. Szekeres, 54/I; pp. 651–733. Berlin/Heidelberg/New York: Springer-Verlag. 1210 pp.

14. Endoh, M., Schümann, H. J., Krappitz, N., Hillen, B. 1976. α-Adrenoceptors mediating positive inotropic effects on the ventricular myocardium: Some aspects of structure-activity relationship of sympathomimetic amines. *Jpn. J. Pharmacol.* 26:179–90

15. Bodem, R., Skelton, C. L., Sonnenblick, E. H. 1974. Inotropic and chronotropic effects of dobutamine on isolated cardiac muscle. *Eur. J. Cardiol.* 2:181–89

16. Tuttle, R. R., Mills, J. 1975. Dobutamine development of a new catecholamine to selectively increase cardiac contractility. *Circ. Res.* 36:185–96

17. Lumley, P., Broadley, K. J., Levy, G. P. 1977. Analysis of the inotropic:chronotropic selectivity of dobutamine and dopamine in anaesthetised dogs and guinea-pig isolated atria. *Cardiovasc. Res.* 11:17–25

18. Carlsson, E., Åblad, B., Brändström, A., Carlsson, B. 1972. Differentiated blockade of the chronotropic effects of various adrenergic stimuli in the cat heart. *Life Sci.* 11:953–58

19. Carlsson, E., Dahlöf, C.-G., Hedberg, A., Persson, H., Tångstrand, B. 1977. Differentiation of cardiac chronotropic and inotropic effects of β-adrenoreceptor agonists. *Naunyn-Schmiedebergs Arch. Pharmacol.* 300:101–5

20. Dreyer, A. C., Offermeier, J. 1980. *In vitro* assessment of selectivities of various beta-adrenergic blocking agents. *Life Sci.* 27:2087–92

21. O'Donnell, S., Wanstal, J. C. 1980. Pharmacological evidence for differences in the β-adrenoceptor populations influencing atrial rate in guinea pig and cat. *Circ. Res.* 46 (Suppl. 1):55–56

22. Barnett, D. B., Rugg, E. L., Nahorski, S. R. 1978. Direct evidence of two types of β-adrenoceptor binding site in lung tissue. *Nature* 273:166–68

23. Williams, R. S., Bishop, T. 1981. Selectivity of dobutamine for adrenergic receptor subtypes. *J. Clin. Invest.* 67:1703–11

24. Hedberg, A., Matsson, H., Carlsson, E. 1980. Prenalterol, a nonselective β-adrenoceptor ligand with absolute β_1-selective partial agonist activity. *J. Pharm. Pharmacol.* 32:660–61

25. Kenakin, T. P. 1981. An in vitro quantitative analysis of the alpha adrenoreceptor partial agonist activity of dobutamine and its relevance to inotropic selectivity. *J. Pharmacol. Exp. Ther.* 216:210–19

26. Kenakin, T. P., Beek, D. 1982. In vitro studies on the cardiac activity of prenal-

terol with reference to use in congestive heart failure. *J. Pharmacol. Exp. Ther.* 220:77–85

27. Levy, M. N., de Oliveira, J. M. 1961. Regional distribution of myocardial blood flow in dog as determined by Rb[86]. *Circ. Res.* 9:96–98

28. Potter, L. T., Cooper, T., Willman, V. L., Wolfe, D. E. 1965. Synthesis, binding, release, and metabolism of norepinephrine in normal and transplanted dog hearts. *Circ. Res.* 16:468–81

29. Goldberg, L. I. 1972. Cardiovascular and renal actions of dopamine: Potential clinical applications. *Pharmacol. Rev.* 24:1–29

30. Manders, W. T., Vatner, S. F., Braunwald, E. 1980. Cardio-selective beta adrenergic stimulation with prenalterol in conscious dog. *J. Pharmacol. Exp. Ther.* 215:266–70

31. Harden, T. K. 1983. Agonist-induced desensitization of the β-adrenergic receptor-linked adenylate cyclase. *Pharmacol. Rev.* 35:5–32

32. Unverferth, D. V., Leier, C. V., Magorien, R. M., Croskery, R., Svirbely, J. R., et al. 1980. Improvement of human myocardial mitochondria after dobutamine: A quantitative ultrastructural study. *J. Pharmacol. Exp. Ther.* 215:527–32

33. Jenne, J. W., Chick, T. W., Strickland, R. D., Wall, F. J. 1977. Subsensitivity of beta responses during therapy with long-acting beta-2 preparation. *J. Allergy Clin. Immunol.* 59:383–90

34. Colucci, W. S., Alexander, R. W., Williams, G. H., Rude, R. E., Holman, B. L., et al. 1981. Decreased lymphocyte beta-adrenergic-receptor density in patients with heart failure and tolerance to the beta-adrenergic agonist Pirbuterol. *N. Engl. J. Med.* 305:185–90

35. Chang, H. Y., Klein, R. M., Kunos, G. 1982. Selective desensitization of cardiac beta adrenoceptors by prolonged in vivo infusion of catecholamines in rats. *J. Pharmacol. Exp. Ther.* 221:784–89

36. Galant, S. P., Duriseti, L., Underwood, S., Allred, S., Insel, P. A. 1980. Beta adrenergic receptors of polymorphonuclear particulates in bronchial asthma. *J. Clin. Invest.* 65:577–85

37. Plummer, A. L. 1978. Workshop No. 4. Drug tolerance to beta_2 adrenergic agents. *Chest* 73(Suppl. 6):994–1004

38. Tohmeh, J. F., Cryer, P. E. 1980. Biphasic adrenergic modulation β-adrenergic receptors in man. Agonist-induced early increment and late decrement in β-

adrenergic receptor number. *J. Clin. Invest.* 65:836–40

39. Lefkowitz, R. J., Wessels, M. R., Stadel, J. M. 1980. Hormones, receptors, and cyclic AMP: Their role in target cell refractoriness. *Curr. Top. Cell Regul.* 17:205–30

40. Perkins, J. P., Harden, T. K., Harper, J. F. 1982. Acute and chronic modulation of the responsiveness of receptor-associated adenylate cyclases. In *Handbook of Experimental Pharmacology, Cyclic Nucleotides,* ed. J. A. Nathanson, J. W. Kebabian, 58/I:185–224. Berlin/Heidelberg/New York: Springer-Verlag

41. de Vellis, J., Brooker, B. 1974. Reversal of catecholamine refractoriness by inhibitors of RNA and protein synthesis. *Science* 186:1221–23

42. Tarasaki, W. L., Brooker, G., de Vellis, J., Inglish, D., Hsu, C.-Y., et al. 1978. Involvement of cyclic AMP and protein synthesis in catecholamine refractoriness. *Adv. Cyclic Nucleotide Res.* 9:33–52

43. Conolly, M. E., Greenacre, J. K. 1976. The lymphocyte beta-adrenoceptor in normal subjects and patients with bronchial asthma: The effect of different forms of treatment on receptor function. *J. Clin. Invest.* 58:1307–16

44. Stephan, W. C., Chick, T. W., Avner, B. P., Jenne, J. W. 1980. Tachyphylaxis to inhaled isoproterenol and the effect of methylprednisolone in dogs. *Allergy Clin. Immunol.* 65:105–09

45. Beress, L., Ritter, R., Ravens, U. 1982. The influence of the rate of electrical stimulation on the effects of the Anemonia sulcata toxin ATX II in guinea pig papillary muscle. *Eur. J. Pharmacol.* 79:265–72

46. Mallorga, P., Tallman, J. F., Henneberry, R. C., Hirata, F., Strittmatter, W. R., et al. 1980. Mepacrine blocks β-adrenergic agonist-induced desensitization in astrocytoma cells. *Proc. Natl. Acad. Sci. USA* 77:1341–45

47. Hirata, F., Strittmatter, W. J., Axelrod, J. 1979. β-adrenergic receptor agonists increase phospholipid methylation, membrane fluidity, and β-adrenergic receptor-adenylate cyclase coupling. *Proc. Natl. Acad. Sci. USA* 76:368–72

48. Hirata, F., Tallman, J. F. Jr., Henneberry, R. C., Mallorga, P., Strittmatter, W. J., et al. 1980. Regulation of β-adrenergic receptors by phospholipid methylation. In *Receptors for Neurotransmitters and Peptide Hormones: Advances in Biochemical Psychopharmacology,* ed. G. Pepeu, M. J. Kuhar,

S. J. Enna, 21:91–97. New York: Raven

49. Torda, T., Yamaguchi, I., Hirata, F., Kopin, I. J., Axelrod, J. 1981. Quinacrine-blocked desensitization of adrenoceptors after immobilization stress or repeated injection of isoproterenol in rats. *J. Pharmacol. Exp. Ther.* 216:334–38

50. Yamaguchi, I., Torda, T., Hirata, F., Kopin, I. J. 1981. Adrenoceptor desensitization after immobilization, stress, or repeated injection of isoproterenol. *Am. J. Physiol.* 240:H691–96

51. Papp, J. G., Szekeres, L. 1972. The receptor mechanism of some cardioelectrophysiological effects of adrenergic excitants. *Acta Physiol. Acad. Sci. Hung.* 41:339

52. Szekeres, L., Papp, J. G. 1980. Effect of adrenergic activators and inhibitors on the electrical activity of the heart. See Ref. 13b, pp. 597–650

53. Farmer, J. B. 1966. Indirect sympathomimetic actions of dopamine. *J. Pharm. Pharmacol.* 18:261–62

54. Bejrablaya, D., Burn, J. H., Walker, J. M. 1958. The action of sympathomimetic amines on heart rate in relation to the effect of reserpine. *Br. J. Pharmacol.* 13:461–66

55. Goldberg, L. I., Sjoerdsma, A. 1959. Effects of several monoamine oxidase inhibitors on the cardiovascular actions of naturally occurring amines in the dog. *J. Pharmacol. Exp. Ther.* 127:212–18

56. Wagner, J., Rodrigues-Pereira, E., Schümann, H. J. 1975. Alpha-adrenorzeptoren im Ventrikelmyokard der Katze. *Verh. Dtsch. Ges. Kresilaufforsch.* 41:226–29

57. Endoh, M. 1982. Adrenoceptors and the myocardial inotropic response: Do alpha and beta receptor sites functionally coexist? In *Trends in Autonomic Pharmacology,* ed. S. Kalsner, 2:303–22. Baltimore/Munich: Urban & Schwarzenberg. 563 pp.

58. Vatner, S. F., Millard, R. W., Higgins, C. B. 1973. Coronary and myocardial effects of dopamine in the conscious dog: Parasympatholytic augmentation of pressor and inotropic actions. *J. Pharmacol. Exp. Ther.* 187:280–95

59a. Wagner, J., Brodde, O. E. 1978. On the presence and distribution of α-adrenoceptors in the heart of various mammalian species. *Naunyn-Schmiedebergs Arch. Pharmacol.* 302:239–54

59b. Wagner, J., Schümann, H. J., Knorr, A., Rohm, N., Reidemeister, J. C. 1980.

Stimulation by adrenaline and dopamine but not by noradrenaline of myocardial α-adrenoceptors mediating positive inotropic effects in human atrial preparations. *Naunyn-Schmiedebergs Arch. Pharmacol.* 312:99–102

60. Govier, W. C. 1968. Myocardial alpha adrenergic receptors and their role in the production of a positive inotropic effect by sympathomimetic agents. *J. Pharmacol. Exp. Ther.* 159:82–90

61. Schümann, H. J., Motomura, S., Endoh, M., Brodde, O. E. 1977. Comparison of the mechanisms underlying the positive inotropic actions of dopamine, adrenaline and isoprenaline on the isolated rabbit papillary muscle. *Naunyn-Schmiedebergs Arch. Pharmacol.* 297: 257–67

62. Brodde, O. E., Inui, J., Motomura, S., Schümann, H. J. 1980. The mode of direct action of dopamine on the rabbit heart. *J. Cardiovasc. Pharmacol.* 2:567–82

63. Motomura, S., Brodde, O. E., Schümann, H. J. 1978. No evidence for involvement of dopaminergic receptors in the positive inotropic action of dopamine on the isolated rabbit papillary muscle. *Jpn. J. Pharmacol.* 28:145–53

64. Mary-Rabine, L., Hordof, A. J., Bowman, F. O., Maim, J. R., Rosen, M. R. 1978. Alpha and beta adrenergic effects on human atrial specialized conducting fibers. *Circulation* 57:84–90

65. Wenzel, D. G., Su, J. L. 1966. Interactions between sympathomimetic amines and blocking agents on the rat ventricle strip. *Arch. Int. Pharmacodyn. Ther.* 160:379–89

66. Osnes, J.-B., Øye, I. 1976. Adenosine 3′,5′-cyclic monophosphate in perfused rat hearts exposed to isoprenaline and dopamine. *Acta Physiol. Scand.* 96:100–13

67. Osnes, J. B., Christoffersen, T., Øye, T. 1973. Mechanism of the inotropic effect of catecholamines as revealed from experiments in the perfused rat heart. *Acta Physiol. Scand.* (Suppl. 396):6

68. Watanabe, A. M., Hathaway, D. R., Besch, H. R. Jr., Farmer, B. B., Harris, R. A. 1977. α-Adrenergic reduction of cyclic adenosine monophosphate concentration in rat myocardium. *Circ. Res.* 40:596–602

69. Wollemann, M., Borbola, J. Jr., Papp, J. G., Szekeres, L. 1975. Cardiac adenylate cyclase activity in relation to beta-adrenergic responses. *J. Mol. Cell. Cardiol.* 7:523–33

70. Huang, M., Drummond, G. I. 1978.

Interactions between adenosine and catecholamines on cyclic AMP accumulation in guinea pig ventricular myocardium. *Biochem. Pharmacol.* 27:187–91

71. Williams, L. T., Lefkowitz, R. J., Watanabe, A. M., Hathaway, D. R., Besch, H. R. 1977. Thyroid hormone regulation of β-adrenergic receptor number. *J. Biol. Chem.* 252:2787–89

72. Rand, M. J., Story, D. F., McCuloch, M. W. 1975. Inhibitory feedback modulation of adrenergic transmission. *Clin. Exp. Pharmacol. Physiol.* Suppl. 2:21–26

73. Göthert, M., Lox, H. J., Rieckesmann, J. M. 1977. Effects of butyrophenones on sympathetic nerves of the isolated rabbit heart and on postsynaptic α-adrenoceptors of the isolated rabbit aorta. *Naunyn-Schmiedebergs Arch. Pharmacol.* 300:255–65

74. Katz, R. L., Lord, C. O., Eakins, K. E. 1967. Anesthetic-dopamine cardiac arrhythmias and their prevention by beta-adrenergic blockade. *J. Pharmacol. Exp. Ther.* 158:40–45

75. Patil, P. N., Miller, D. D., Trendelenberg, U. 1974. Molecular geometry and adrenergic drug activity. *Pharmacol. Rev.* 26:323–92

76. Kent, R. S., DeLean, A., Lefkowitz, R. J. 1980. A quantitative analysis of beta-adrenergic receptor interactions: Resolution of high and low affinity states of the receptor by computer modeling of ligand binding data. *Mol. Pharmacol.* 17:14–23

77. Ruffolo, R. R. Jr., Spradlin, T. A., Pollock, G. D., Waddell, J. E., Murphy, P. J. 1981. Alpha and beta adrenergic effects of stereoisomers of dobutamine. *J. Pharmacol. Exp. Ther.* 219:447–52

78. Rohm, N., Wagner, J., Schümann, H. J. 1980. The lack of a pronounced preference of prenalterol for the beta-1-adrenoceptor subtype. *Naunyn-Schmiedebergs Pharmacol.* 315:85–88

79. Robie, N. W., Goldberg, L. I. 1975. Comparative systemic and regional hemodynamic effects of dopamine and dobutamine. *Am. Heart J.* 90:340–45

80. Robie, N. W., Nutter, D. O., Moody, C., McNay, J. L. 1974. In vivo analysis of adrenergic receptor activity of dobutamine. *Circ. Res.* 34:663–71

81. Goldberg, L. I., Hsieh, Y. Y., Resnekov, L. 1977. New catecholamines for treatment of heart failure and shock: An update on dopamine and a first look at dobutamine. *Prog. Cardiovasc. Dis.* 19:327–40

82. Vatner, S. F., McRitchie, R. J., Braunwald, E. 1974. Effect of dobutamine on

left ventricular performance, coronary dynamics, and distribution of cardiac output in conscious dogs. *J. Clin. Invest.* 53:1265–73

83. Hinds, J. E., Hawthorne, E. W. 1975. Comparative cardiac dynamic effects of dobutamine and isoproterenol in conscious instrumented dogs. *Am. J. Cardiol.* 36:894–901

84. Kirlin, P. C., Pitt, B., Lucchesi, B. R. 1981. Comparative effects of prenalterol and dobutamine in a canine model of acute ischemic heart failure. *J. Cardiovasc. Pharmacol.* 3:896–905

85. Willerson, J. R., Hutton, I., Watson, J. T., Platt, M. R., Templeton, G. H. 1976. Influence of dobutamine on regional myocardial blood flow and ventricular performance during acute and chronic myocardial ischemia in dogs. *Circulation* 53:828–33

86. Rude, R. E., Izquierdo, C., Buja, M. L., Willerson, J. T. 1982. Effects of inotropic and chronotropic stimuli on acute myocardial ischemic injury. I: Studies with dobutamine in the anesthetized dog. *Circulation* 65:1321–28

87. Liang, C., Yi, J. M., Sherman, L. G., Black, J., Garvas, H., et al. 1981. Dobutamine infusion in conscious dogs with and without acute myocardial infarction. *Circ. Res.* 49:170–80

88. Tuttle, R. R., Hillman, C. C., Tomey, R. E. 1976. Differential β-adrenergic sensitivity of atrial and ventricular tissue assessed by chronotropic, inotropic and cyclic AMP responses to isoprenaline and dobutamine. *Cardiovasc. Res.* 10:452–58

89. McNeill, J. H. 1978. The effect of dobutamine on rat cardiac cyclic AMP, phosphorylase *a* and force of contraction. *Res. Commun. Chem. Pathol. Pharmacol.* 20:597–600

90. Leier, C. V., Heban, P. T., Huss, P., Bush, C. A., Lewis, R. P. 1978. Comparative systemic and regional hemodynamic effects of dopamine and dobutamine in patients with cardiomyopathic heart failure. *Circulation* 58:466–75

91. Plachetka, J. R. 1981. Clinical pharmacology of dobutamine. *J. Cardiovasc. Med.* 6:75–81

92. Sonnenblick, E. H., Frishman, W. H., LeJemtel, T. H. 1979. Dobutamine: A new synthetic cardioactive sympathetic amine. *N. Engl. J. Med.* 300:17–22

93. Weber, R., Tuttle, R. R. 1977. Dobutamine. In *Pharmacological and Biochemical Properties of Drug Substances,* ed.

M. E. Goldberg, 1:109–24. Washington DC: Am. Assoc. Pharm. Sci. 413 pp.

94. Vasu, M. A., O'Keefe, D. D., Kapellakis, G. Z., Daggett, W. M., Powell, W. J. Jr. 1975. Myocardial oxygen consumption and hemodynamic effects of dobutamine, epinephrine and isoproterenol. *Fed. Proc.* 34:435

95. Jewitt, D., Birkhead, J., Mitchell, A., Dollery, C. 1974. Clinical cardiovascular pharmacology of dobutamine, a selective inotropic catecholamine. *Lancet* 2:363–67

96. Loeb, H. S., Khan, M., Sandye, A., Gunnar, R. M. 1976. Acute hemodynamic effects of dobutamine and isoproterenol in patients with low output cardiac failure. *Circ. Shock* 3:55–63

97. Loeb, H. S., Bredakis, J., Gunnar, R. M. 1977. Superiority of dobutamine over dopamine for augmentation of cardiac output in patients with chronic low output cardiac failure. *Circulation* 55:375–81

98. Leier, C. V., Webel, J., Bush, C. A. 1977. The cardiovascular effects of the continuous infusion of dobutamine in patients with severe heart failure. *Circulation* 56:468–72

99. Maskin, C. S., Forman, R., Klein, N. A., Sonnenblick, E. H., LeJemtel, T. H. 1982. Long-term amrinone therapy in patients with severe heart failure: Drug-dependent hemodynamic benefits despite progression of the disease. *Am. J. Med.* 72:113–18

100. Daves, P. K., Stinson, E. B., Graham, A. F., Billingham, M. E., Grehl, T. M., et al. 1973. Percutaneous transvenous endomyocardiol biopsy. *J. Am. Med. Assoc.* 225:288–91

101. Mason, J. W. 1978. Techniques for right and left ventricular endomyocardial biopsy. *Am. J. Cardiol.* 41:887–92

102. Jennings, R. B., Ganote, C. E. 1976. Mitochondrial structure and function in acute myocardial ischemic injury. *Circ. Res.* 38(Suppl. 1):180–89

103a. Jennings, K., Jackson, P. G., Monaghan, M., Jewitt, D. E. 1978. Some aspects of the cardiovascular pharmacology of UK 14,275 in patients with coronary artery disease. *Br. J. Clin. Pharmacol.* 5:13–18

103b. Jennings, R. B., Shen, A. C., Hill, M. L., Ganote, C. E., Herdson, P. B. 1978. Mitochondrial matrix densities in myocardial ischemia and autolysis. *Exp. Mol. Pathol.* 29:55–65

104. Kawamura, K., Cowley, M. J., Karp, R. B., Manta, J. A., Logic, J. R., Rogers, W. J., et al. 1978. Intramitochondrial inclusions in the myocardial cells of hu-

man hearts with coronary disease. *J. Mol. Cell. Cardiol.* 10:797–811

105. Colgan, J. H., Lazarus, M. L., Sachs, H. G. 1978. Post-natal development of the normal and cardiomyopathic Syrian hamster heart: A quantitative electron microscopic study. *J. Mol. Cell. Cardiol.* 10:43–54

106. Prasad, K., Singal, P. K. 1977. Ultrastructure of failing myocardium due to induced chronic mitral insufficiency in dogs. *Br. J. Exp. Pathol.* 58:289–300

107. Åblad, B., Hjalmearson, Å., Johnsson, G. 1982. Pharmacological and clinical effects of prenalterol—a new inotropic β-adrenoceptor stimulant. *Acta Med. Scand.* Suppl. 659:5–8

108. Strossberg, A. M., Montgomery, W. 1981. Cardioselectivity of dobutamine and prenalterol in the pentobarbital anesthetized dog. *Proc. West Pharmacol. Soc.* 24:83–87

109. Williams, R. S. 1983. Selectivity of prenalterol for adrenergic receptor subtypes: A potential mechanism of inotropic selectivity. *J. Cardiovasc. Pharmacol.* 5:266–71

110. Minneman, K. P., Hedberg, A., Molinoff, P. B. 1979. Comparison of beta adrenergic receptor subtypes in mammalian tissue. *J. Pharmacol. Exp. Ther.* 211:502–08

111. Hedberg, A., Minneman, K. P., Molinoff, P. B. 1980. Differential distribution of beta-1 and beta-2 adrenergic receptors in cat and guinea-pig heart. *J. Pharmacol. Exp. Ther.* 212:503–08

112. Kenakin, T. P., Beek, D. 1980. Is prenalterol (H133/80) really a selective beta-1 adrenoceptor agonist? Tissue selectivity resulting from differences in stimulus-response relationships. *J. Pharmacol. Exp. Ther.* 213:406–13

113. Kendall, M. J., Goodfellow, R. M., Westerling, S. 1982. Prenalterol—A new cardioselective inotropic agent. *J. Clin. Hosp. Pharm.* 7:107–18

114. Röhn, O., Fellenius, E., Graffner, C., Johnsson, G., Lundborg, P., et al. 1980. Metabolic and haemodynamic effects and pharmacokinetics of a new selective beta 1-adrenoceptor agonist, Prenalterol, in man. *Eur. J. Clin. Pharmacol.* 17:81–86

115. Rönn, O., Graffner, C., Johnsson, G., Jordö, L., Lundborg, P., et al. 1979. Haemodynamic effects and pharmacokinetics of a new selective beta₁-adrenoceptor agonist, prenalterol, and its interaction with metroprolol in man. *Eur. J. Clin. Pharmacol.* 15:9–13

116. Weiss, A., Pfister, B., Imhof, P., De-

gen, P. H., Burckhardt, D., et al. 1980. Haemodynamic effects, plasma concentrations and tolerance of orally administered prenalterol in man. *Eur. J. Clin. Pharmacol.* 18:383–90

117. Meurer, K. A., Long, R., Hombach, V., Helber, A. 1980. Effect of β₁-selective adrenergic agonist in normal human volunteers. *Klin. Wochenschr.* 53:425–27

118. Löfdahl, C. G., Svedmyr, N. 1981. Prenalterol—A selective β₁-adrenoreceptor agonist in asthmatics. *Eur. J. Respir. Dis.* 62(Suppl. 113):111–12

119. Kirlin, P. C., Pitt, B. 1981. Hemodynamic effects of intravenous prenalterol in severe heart failure. *Am. J. Cardiol.* 47:670–75

120. Erbel, R., Meyer, J., Lambertz, H., Schweitzer, P., Voelker, W., et al. 1982. Hemodynamic effects of prenalterol in patients with ischemic heart disease and congestive cardiomyopathy. *Circulation* 66:361–69

121. Barlow, J. J., Main, B. G., Moors, J. A., Nuttall, A., Snow, H. M. 1979. The cardiovascular activity of ICI 118,587, a novel β-adrenoceptor partial agonist. *Br. J. Pharmacol.* 67:412P

122. Van Arman, C. G., Miller, L. M., O'Malley, M. P. 1961. SC-10049: A catecholamine bronchodilator and hyperglycemic agent. *J. Pharmacol. Exp. Ther.* 133:90–97

123. Moore, P. F., Constantine, J. W., Barth, W. E. 1978. Pirbuterol, a selective beta₂ adrenergic bronchodilator. *J. Pharmacol. Exp. Ther.* 207:410–18

124. Constantine, J. W., McIlhenny, H. M., Moore, P. F. 1979. Pharmacokinetics and cardiopulmonary effects in dogs of sublingual pirbuterol, a new bronchodilator. *J. Pharmacol. Exp. Ther.* 208:371–76

125. Gold, F. L., Horowitz, L. D. 1981. Hemodynamic effects of pirbuterol in conscious dog. *Am. Heart. J.* 102:591–96

126. Awan, N. A., Needham, K. E., Evenson, M. K., Win, A., Mason, D. T. 1980. Hemodynamic actions of prenalterol in severe congestive heart failure due to chronic coronary disease. *Am. Heart J.* 101:158–61

127. Rude, R. E., Turi, Z., Brown, E. J., Orell, B. H., Colucci, W. S., et al. 1981. Acute effects of oral pirbuterol on myocardial oxygen metabolism and systemic hemodynamics in chronic congestive heart failure. *Circulation* 64:139–45

128. Melloni, G. F., Minoja, G. M., Lureti, G. F., Bruni, G. C., Loreti, P., et al.

1979. Effects of SB 7505 on blood pressure, heart rate and diuresis in man. *Curr. Ther. Res.* 25:406–14

129. Dei Cas, L., Bolognesi, R., Cucchini, F., Fappani, A., Riva, S., et al. 1983. Hemodynamic effects of ibopamine in patients with idiopathic congestive cardiomyopathy. *J. Cardiovasc. Pharmacol.* 5:249–53

130. Dei Cas, L., Manca, C., Vasini, G., Mansour, M., Berardini, B., et al. 1980. Non-invasive evaluation of left ventricular function through systolic time intervals following oral administration of SB 7505 in man. *Arzneim. Forsch.* 30:498–500

131. Dei Cas, L., Vasini, G., Manca, C., Bernardini, B., Visioli, O. 1982. Noninvasive evaluation of the effects of oral ibopamine (SB 7505) on cardiac and renal function in patients with congestive heart failure. *J. Cardiovasc. Pharmacol.* 4:436–40

132. Melloni, G. F., Melloni, R., Minoja, G. M., Scarazzati, G., Bruni, G. C., et al. 1981. Clinical tolerability of ibopamine hydrochloride (SB 7505). *Eur. J. Clin. Pharmacol.* 19:409–11

133. Cicchetti, F., Bruni, G. C., Loreti, P., Pamparana, F., Bauer, R., Borghi, C. M. 1980. Behaviour of diuresis, blood arterial pressure and heart rate after SB 7505 (Ibopamine hydrochloride) administration. *Curr. Ther. Res.* 27:741–47

134. Rajfer, S. I., Goldberg, L. I. 1982. Dopamine in the treatment of heart failure. *Eur. Heart J.* 3 (Suppl. D):103–06

135a. Thompson, M. J., Huss, P., Unverferth, D. V., Fasola, A., Leier, C. V. 1980. Hemodynamic effects of intravenous butopamine in congestive heart failure. *Clin. Pharmacol. Ther.* 28:324–54

135b. Nelson, S., Leier, C. V. 1981. Butopamine in normal human subjects. *Curr. Ther. Res.* 30:405–11

136. Gibson, D. G., Coltart, D. J. 1971. Haemodynamic effects of intravenous salbutamol in patients with mitral valve disease: Comparison with isoprenaline and atropine. *Postgrad. Med. J.* 47(Suppl.):40–44

137. Sharma, B., Goodwin, J. F. 1978. Beneficial effect of salbutamol on cardiac function in severe congestive cardiomyopathy. Effect on systolic and diastolic function of the left ventricle. *Circulation* 58:449–60

138. Bourdillon, P. D. V., Dawson, J. R., Foale, R. A., Timmis, A. D., Pool-Wilson, P. A., Sutton, G. D. 1980. Sal-

butamol in treatment of heart failure. *Br. Heart J.* 43:206–10

139. Sponer, G., Dietmann, K., Schaumann, W. 1981. Cardiale Wirkung von Doxaminal Digitoxin und deren Kombination bei Katzen mit akuter Kerz und Kreislauf insuffizienz. *Z. Cardiol.* 70:291

140. Whiting, B., Kelman, A. W., Sumner, D. J., Hillis, W. S., Ledermann, H. 1982. Haemodynamic effects of BM-10,188, a new orally active inotropic agent in healthy volunteers. *Br. J. Pharmacol.* 13:529–32

141. Sauer, E., Sebening, H., Klein, G., Bauer, R., Wirtzfeld, A., Henne, M. 1981. Die Wirkung der positivinotropen Substanz BM 10,188 bei Patienten mit schwerer Herzinsuffizienz. *Hertz/Kreislauf* 6:271–77

142. Nagao, T., Ikeo, T., Sato, M., Nakajima, H., Kyomoto, A. 1981. Positive inotropic effect of (−)-α-(3,4-dimethoxyphenethylaminomethyl)-4-hydroxybenzyl-alcohol (TA-064) in the dog. *Proc. 8th Int. Congr. Pharm., Tokyo,* p. 921

143. Ikeo, T., Nagao, T., Suzuki, T., Yabana, H., Nakajima, H. 1982. Effect of TA-064, a new positive inotropic agent, on left ventricular function in conscious instrumented dogs. *Proc. 55th Gen. Meet. Jpn. Pharmacol. Soc.,* p. 20

144. Kino, M., Hirota, Y., Yamamoto, S., Sawada, K., Moriguchi, M., Kotaka, M., Kubo, S., Kawamura, K. 1983. Cardiovascular effects of a newly synthesized cardiotonic agent (TA-064) on normal and diseased hearts. *Am. J. Cardiol.* 51:802–10

145. Kyncl, J. J., Hollinger, R. E. 1979. Renal and hemodynamic effects of Abbott-47884, L-diacetyl-gamma-glutanyl amide of dopamine, in dogs. *Fed. Proc.* 38:267

146. Iakovidis, D., Malta, E., McPherson, G. A., Raper, C. 1980. In vitro activity of RO 363, a β_1 adreno-receptor selective agonist. *Br. J. Pharmacol.* 68:677–85

147. Raper, C., McPherson, G. A., Iakovidis, D. 1978. A phenoxypropanolamine derivative (RO 363) with selective β_1-receptor stimulant actions. *Eur. J. Pharmacol.* 52:241–42

148. Lövgren, K., Hedberg, A., Nilsson, J. L. 1980. Adrenergic receptor agonists. Benzofuranylethanolamines. *J. Med. Chem.* 23:624–27

149. Fothergill, G. A., Osbond, J. M., Wickens, J. C. 1977. Bufuralol, a new β-adrenoceptor blocking agent. Part 1: Synthesis and structure-activity studies in

a series of benzofuran-2-ethanolamines. *Arzneim. Forsch.* 27:978–81

150. Anttila, P., Dreyer, F.-W., Westermann, E. 1977. Cardiovascular effects of some dopamine derivatives. *Naunyn-Schmiedebergs Arch. Pharmacol.* 297: 128

151. McCaig, D., Parratt, J. R. 1979. The cardiovascular pharmacology of 7-propyl-theophylline-dopamine (DH 975); comparison with dopamine and dobutamine. *Br. J. Pharmacol.* 67:239–45

152. Trendelenburg, U. 1972. Classification of sympathomimetic amines. In *Handbook of Experimental Pharmacology: Catecholamines*, ed. H. Blaschko, E. Muscholl, 33:336–62. Berlin/Heidelberg/New York: Springer-Verlag

153. Eichler, O. 1976. Herz und Kreislauf. In *Kaffee und Coffein*, ed. O. Eichler, pp. 133–170. Berlin/Heidelberg/New York: Springer-Verlag

154. Rall, T. W. 1980. The xanthines: Theophylline, caffeine, and theobromine. In *The Pharmacological Basis of Therapeutics*, ed. L. S. Goodman, A. Gillman, pp. 592–607. New York/Toronto/London: Macmillan. 6th ed.

155. Blinks, J. R., Olson, C. B., Jewell, B. R., Bravany, P. 1972. Influence of caffeine and other methylxanthines on mechanical properties of isolated mammalian heart muscle. *Circ. Res.* 30:367–92

156. Blinks, J. R., Rüdel, R., Taylor, S. R. 1978. Calcium transients in isolated amphibian skeletal muscle fibres: Detection with aequorin. *J. Physiol.* 277:291–323

157. Blinks, J. R., Wier, W. G., Morgan, J. P., Hess, P. 1982. Regulation of intracellular [Ca++] by cardiotonic drugs. In *Advances in Pharmacology and Therapeutics, II/3, Cardiorenal and Cell Pharmacology*, 8th Intl. Congr. Pharmacol., ed. H. Yoshida, Y. Hagihara, S. Ebashi, pp. 205–16. Oxford/New York: Pergamon

158. Rall, T. W., West, T. C. 1963. The potentiation of cardiac inotropic responses to norepinephrine by theophylline. *J. Pharmacol. Exp. Ther.* 139:269–74

159. Fabiato, A., Fabiato, F. 1979. Calcium and cardiac excitation-contraction coupling. *Ann. Rev. Physiol.* 41:473–84

160. Guthrie, J. R., Nayler, W. G. 1967. Interaction between caffeine and adenosine on calcium exchangeability in mammalian atria. *Arch. Int. Pharmacodyn.* 170:249–55

161. Endo, M., Kitazawa, T. 1978. Excitation-contraction coupling in chemically skinned fibers of cardiac muscle, *Proc. 8th World Congr. Cardiol., Tokoyo*, ed. S. Hayase, S. Murao, pp. 800–03. Amsterdam: Excerpta Med. 1163 pp.

162. Marcus, M. L., Skelton, C. L., Grauer, L. E., Epstein, S. E. 1972. Effects of theophylline on myocardial mechanics. *Am. J. Physiol.* 222:1361–65

163. Rall, R. W. 1982. Evolution of the mechanism of action of methyl xanthines: From calcium mobilizers to antagonists of adenosine receptors. *Pharmacologist* 24:277–87

164. Nawrath, H. 1981. Action potential, membrane currents and force of contraction in cat ventricular heart muscle treated with papaverine. *J. Pharmacol. Exp. Ther.* 218:544–49

165. Fain, J. N. 1973. Inhibition of adenosine cyclic 3',5'-monophosphate accumulation in fat cells by adenosine, N^6-(phenylisopropyl)adenosine, and related compounds. *Mol. Pharmacol.* 9:595–604

166. Londos, C., Cooper, D. M. F., Wolff, J. 1980. Subclasses of external adenosine receptors. *Proc. Natl. Acad. Sci. USA* 77:2551–54

167. DeGubareff, T., Sleator, W. Jr. 1965. Effects of caffeine on mammalian atrial muscle, and its interaction with adenosine and calcium. *J. Pharmacol. Exp. Ther.* 148:202–14

168. Urthaler, F., Woods, W. T., James, T. N., Walker, A. A. 1981. Effects of adenosine on mechanical performance and electrical activity in the canine heart. *J. Pharmacol. Exp. Ther.* 216:254–60

169. Dutta, P., Mustafa, J. 1979. Saturable binding of adenosine to the dog heart microsomal fraction: Competitive inhibition of aminophylline. *J. Pharmacol. Exp. Ther.* 211:496–501

170. Bruns, R. F., Daly, J. W., Snyder, S. H. 1980. Adenosine receptors in brain membranes: Binding of N^6-cyclohexyl (^{3}H)adenosine and 1,3-diethyl-8-(^{3}H)phenylxanthine. *Proc. Natl. Acad. Sci. USA* 77:5547–51

171. Alousi, A. A., Farah, A. E., Lesher, G. Y., Opalka, C. J. Jr. 1978. Cardiotonic activity of amrinone (Win 40680): 5-Amino-3,4'-bipyridin-6(1H)-one. *Fed. Proc.* 37:914 (Abstr.)

172. Farah, A. E., Alousi, A. A. 1978. New cardiotonic agents: A search for digitalis substitute. *Life Sci.* 22:1139–48

173. Alousi, A. A., Farah, A. E., Lesher, G. Y., Opalka, C. J. Jr. 1979. Cardiotonic activity of amrinone—Win 40680 [5-

Amino-3,4'-bipyridin-6(1H)-one]. *Circ. Res.* 45:666–77

174. Gaide, M. S., Baker, S. P., Ezrin, A. M., Gelband, H., Bassett, A. L. 1981. Amrinone, isoproterenol and ouabain modification by cardiac K⁺ contracture. *Eur. J. Pharmacol.* 73:253–60

175. Onuaguluchi, G., Tanz, R. D. 1981. Cardiac effects of amrinone on rabbit papillary muscle and guinea pig Langendorff heart preparations. *J. Cardiovasc. Pharmacol.* 3:1342–55

176. Rendig, S. V., Amsterdam, E. A., Mason, D. T. 1981. Elevated Ca^{++} reduces positive inotropic effect of amrinone in cat papillary muscle. *Circulation* 64:IV-70

177. Rosenthal, J. E., Ferrier, G. R. 1982. Inotropic and electrophysiologic effects of amrinone in untreated and digitalised ventricular tissues. *J. Pharmacol. Exp. Ther.* 22:188–96

178. Adams, H. R., Thody, J., Sutko, J. L. 1982. Amrinone activates K^{+}-depolarized atrial and ventricular myocardium of guinea pigs. *Circ. Res.* 51:662–65

179. Honerjaeger, P., Schaefer-Korting, M., Reiter, M. 1981. Involvement of cyclic AMP in the direct inotropic action of amrinone. Biochemical and functional evidence. *Naunyn-Schmiedebergs Arch. Pharm.* 318:112–20

180. Evans, D. B., Potoczak, R. E., Lomas, T. E., Haleen, S. J., Kaplan, H. R. 1980. In vitro and in vivo cardiostimulant actions of amrinone and prenalterol. *Pharmacologist* 22:287 (Abstr.)

181. Endoh, M., Hamashita, S., Taira, N. 1982. Positive inotropic effect of amrinone in relation to cyclic nucleotide metabolism in the canine ventricular muscle. *J. Pharmacol. Exp. Ther.* 221:775–83

182. Komai, H., Rusy, B. F. 1982. Inotropic effect of amrinone in rabbit papillary muscle. *Fed. Proc.* 41:1309 (Abstr.)

183. Binah, O., Rosen, M. R. 1981. Developmental changes in the inotropic effects of amrinone. *Circulation* 64:22

184. Alousi, A. A., Edelson, J. 1981. Amrinone. See Ref. 93, 3:120–47

185. Barcenas, L., Kabela, E. 1979. Acciones de un Neuvo Agente Inotropico Positivo Sobre el Flujo Coronario, el Consumo de Oxigeno y la Contractilidad del Preparado Cardiopulmonar del Perro. *Bol. Estud. Med. Biol.* 30:294 (Abstr.)

186. Grupp, I., Grupp, G., Fowler, N. O., Gabel, M., Alousi, A. A., Millard, R. W. 1980. Hemodynamic and inotropic responses of normal and depressed dog

hearts to amrinone. *Fed. Proc.* 39:976 (Abstr.)

187. Millard, R. W., Dube, G., Grupp, G., Grupp, I., Alousi, A., Schwartz, A. 1980. Direct vasodilator and positive inotropic actions of amrinone. *J. Mol. Cell. Cardiol.* 12:647–52

188. Meisheri, K. D., Hwang, O., Van Breemen, C. 1981. Evidence for two separate Ca^{2+} pathways in smooth muscle plasmalemma. *J. Membr. Biol.* 59:19–25

189. Martorana, M. G., Rodge, I. W., Shahid, M. 1982. Effects of amrinone on tension responses and cyclic nucleotide levels in rabbit depressed papillary muscle. *Br. J. Pharmacol.* 77:385P (Abstr.)

190. Mielens, Z. E., Buck, D. C. 1982. Relaxant effects of amrinone upon pulmonary smooth muscle. *Pharmacology* 25:262–71

191. Benotti, J. R., Grossman, W., Braunwald, E., Davolos, D. D., Alousi, A. A. 1978. Hemodynamic assessment of amrinone. A new inotropic agent. *N. Engl. J. Med.* 299:1373–77

192a. LeJemtel, T. H., Keung, E., Sonnenblick, E. H., Ribner, H. S., Matsumoto, M., Davis, R., Schwartz, W., Alousi, A. A., Davolos, D. D. 1979. Amrinone: A new nonglycosidic nonadrenergic cardiotonic agent effective in the treatment of intractable myocardial infarction in man. *Circulation* 59:1098–04

192b. LeJemtel, T. H., Keung, E. C., Schwartz, W. J., Maskin, C. S., Greenberg, M. A., Davis, R. S., Forman, R., Ribner, H. S., Sonnenblick, E. H. 1979. Hemodynamic effects of intravenous and oral amrinone in patients with severe heart failure: Relationship between intravenous and oral administration. *Trans. Assoc. Am. Physicians* 92:325–33

193. Wynne, J., Malacott, R. F., Benotti, J. R., Curfman, G. D., Grossman, W., Holman, B. L., Smith, T. W., Braunwald, E. 1980. Oral amrinone in refractory congestive heart failure. *Am. J. Cardiol.* 45:1245–49

194. LeJemtel, T. H., Keung, E., Ribner, H. S., Davis, R., Wexler, J., Blaufox, M. D., Sonnenblick, E. H. 1980. Sustained beneficial effects of oral amrinone on cardiac and renal function in severe congestive heart failure in man. *Am. J. Cardiol.* 45:123–29

195. Weber, K. T., Andrews, V., Janicki, J. S., Wilson, J. R., Frishman, A. P. 1981. Amrinone and exercise performance in patients with chronic heart failure. *Am. J. Cardiol.* 48:164–69

196. Maskin, C. S., Forman, R., Klein, N. A., Sonnenblick, E. H., LeJemtel, T. H.

1982. Long-term amrinone therapy in patients with severe heart failure: Drug-dependent hemodynamic benefits despite progression of the disease. *Am. J. Med.* 72:113–18

197. Benotti, J. R., Grossman, W., Braunwald, E., Carabello, B. A. 1980. Effects of amrinone on myocardial energy metabolism and hemodynamics in patients with severe congestive heart failure due to coronary artery disease. *Circulation* 62:28–34

198a. Alousi, A. A., Canter, J. M., Montenaro, M., Fort, D. J., Ferrari, R. A. 1983. Cardiotonic activity of milrinone, a new and potent cardiac bipyridine, on the normal and failing heart of experimental animals. *J. Cardiovasc. Pharmacol.* 5:792–803

198b. Alousi, A. A., Stankus, G. P., Stuart, J. C., Walton, L. H. 1983. Characterization of the cardiotonic effects of milrinone, a new and potent cardiac bipyridine, on isolated tissues from several animal species. *J. Cardiovasc. Pharmacol.* 5:804–11

199. Pastelin, G., Mendez, R., Kabela, E., Farah, A. 1983. The search for a digitalis substitute II milrinone (Win 47203). Its action on the heart-lung preparation of the dog. *Life Sci.* 33:1787–96

200a. Maskin, C. S., Sonnenblick, E. H., LeJemtel, T. H. 1983. Acute and sustained clinical benefits of a new inotropic agent, Win 47203. *J. Am. Coll. Cardiol.* 1:675

200b. Maskin, C. S., Sinoway, L., Chadwick, B., Sonnenblick, E. H., LeJemtel, T. H. 1983. Sustained hemodynamic and clinical effects of a new cardiotonic agent, Win 47203, in patients with severe congestive heart failure. *Circulation* 67:1065–70

201. Baim, D. S., McDowell, A. V., Cherniles, J., Monrad, E. S., Parker, J. A., Edelson, J., Braunwald, E., Grossman, W. 1983. Evaluation of a new bipyridine inotropic agent—Win 47203—in patients with severe congestive heart failure. *N. Engl. J. Med.* 309:748–56

202. Schwartz, A., Grupp, I., Grupp, G., Johnson, C. L., Verner, P., Wallick, E. T., Imai, K. 1979. Amrinone: A new inotropic agent studies organelle systems. *Circulation* 60:II–16

203. Parker, J. C., Harper, J. R. Jr. 1980. Effect of amrinone, a new cardiotonic drug, on calcium movements in red blood cells. *Clin. Res.* 28:472A

204. Frangakis, C. J., Lasher, K. P., Alousi, A. A. 1982. Physiological and biochemical effects of amrinone on cardiac

myocytes. *Circulation* 66:II–57

205. Morgan, J. P., Lee, N. K. M., Blinks, J. R. 1980. Mechanism of inotropic action of amrinone: Unusual pattern of Ca^{++} transients as detected with aequorin. *Fed. Proc.* 39:854

206. Roebel, L. E., Dage, R. C., Cheng, H. C., Woodward, J. K. 1982. Characterization of the cardiovascular activities of a new cardiotonic agent, MDL 17043 (1,3-dihydro-4-methyl-5-[4-methylthio)-benzoyl]-2H-imidazol-2-one). *J. Cardiovasc. Pharmacol.* 4:721–29

207. Dage, R. C., Roebel, L. E., Hsieh, C. P., Weiner, D. L., Woodward, J. K. 1982. Cardiovascular properties of a new cardiotonic agent: MDL 17043 (1,3-dihydro-4-methyl-5-[4-(methylthio)-benzoyl]-2H imidazol-2-one). *J. Cardiovasc. Pharmacol.* 4:500–08

208. Schnettler, R. A., Dage, R. C., Grisar, J. M. 1982. 4-Aroyl-1,3-dihydro-2H-imidazol-2-ones, a new class of cardiotonic agents. *J. Med. Chem.* 25:1477–81

209. Chan, K. Y., Lang, J., Okerholm, R. A. 1983. Quantitative determination of cardiotonic agent MDL 17,043 in plasma by reversed-phase high-performance liquid chromatography. *J. Chromatogr.* 272:396–400

210. Russell, D. C., Smith, H. J., Oliver, M. F. 1979. Electrophysiological and haemodynamic effects of a new inotropic agent (UK 14275) in the dog. *Clin. Exp. Pharmacol. Physiol.* 6:585–89

211. Kariya, T., Wille, L. J., Dage, R. C. 1982. Biochemical studies on the mechanism of cardiotonic activity of MDL 17,043. *J. Cardiovasc. Pharmacol.* 4:509–14

212. Belz, G. G., Alken, R. G., Haegele, K. D., Meinicke, T., Belz, G., Schechter, P. J. 1983. Pharmacodynamic and pharmacokinetic studies on MDL 17,203, a new cardiotonic agent. *Clin. Pharmacol. Ther.* 33:202

213. Crawford, M. H., Sorensen, S. G., Richards, K. L., Sodums, M. 1982. Demonstration of combined vasodilator-inotropic effect of MDL 17043 in patients with reduced left ventricular performance. *Clin. Res.* 30:866A

214. Uretsky, B. F., Generalovich, T., Reddy, P. S., Spangenberg, R. B., Follansbee, W. P. 1982. Acute hemodynamic effects of a new inotropic agent, MDL 17043. *Clin. Res.* 30:762A

215. Uretsky, B. F., Generalovich, T., Reddy, P. S., Spangenberg, R. B., Follansbee, W. P. 1983. The acute hemodynamic effects of a new agent, MDL 17,043,

in the treatment of congestive heart failure. *Circulation* 67:823–28

216. Ferry, D. R., Crawford, M. H., Kennedy, G. T., O'Rourke, R. A. 1982. Effectiveness of a new agent with positive inotropic and vasodilator properties in the treatment of severe congestive heart failure. *Clin. Res.* 31:182A

217. Petein, M., Garberg, V., Carlyle, P., Cohn, J. N., Levine, T. B. 1983. Acute hemodynamic and neurohumoral effects of MDL 19205, a new inotropic agent, in congestive heart failure. *J. Am. Coll. Cardiol.* 1:675

218. Austel, V., Kutter, E. 1981. The theory of sets as a tool in systematic drug design. *Arzneim. Forsch.* 31:130–35

219. Diederen, W., Kadatz, R. 1981. Effects of AR-L 115 BS, a new cardiotonic compound, on cardiac contractility, heart rate and blood pressure in anaesthetized and conscious animals. *Arzneim. Forsch.* 31:146–50

220. Dahmen, M., Greeff, K. 1981. Analysis of the positive-inotropic activity of the benzimidazole derivative AR-L 115 BS in isolated guinea pig atria. *Arzneim. Forsch.* 31:161–65

220a. See papers in *Arzneim. Forsch.* 1981. 31:129–278

221. Petein, M., Pierpont, G. L., Cohn, J. N., From, A. H. L. 1982. In vivo interaction of AR-L 115 BS with the adrenergic nervous system. *Circulation* 66(4, Pt. II):II–138

222. Brutsaert, D. L., De Clerck, N. M., Housmans, P. R., Van Ocken, E. R. 1982. Effects of ARL-115 on contraction and relaxation of isolated mammalian cardiac muscle. *J. Cardiovasc. Pharmacol.* 4:333–43

223. Pouleur, H., Rousseau, M. F., van Mechelen, H., Roncoroni, L., Ries, A., Charlier, A. A. 1982. Cardiovascular effects of AR-L115 in conscious dogs with and without chronic congestive heart failure. *J. Cardiovasc. Pharmacol.* 4:409–18

224. Verdouw, P. D., Hartog, J. M., Rutteman, A. M. 1981. Systemic and regional myocardial responses to AR-L 115 BS, a positive inotropic imidazopyridine in the absence or in the presence of the bradycardic action of alinidine. *Basic Res. Cardiol.* 76:328–43

225a. Thormann, J., Schlepper, M., Kramer, W. 1982. AR-L 115 in coronary artery disease: Positive inotropic effects and increase in left-ventricular pump function without inducing angina. *Clin. Exp. Pharmacol. Physiol.* 9:235–43

225b. Thormann, J., Kramer, W., Schlepper, M. 1982. Hemodynamic and myocardial energetic changes induced by the new cardiotonic agent, AR-L 115, in patients with coronary artery disease. *Am. Heart J.* 104:1294–02

226. Alabaster, C. T., Blackburn, K. J., Joice, J. R., Massingham, R., Scholfield, P. C. UK-14,275, a novel orally-active cardiac stimulant. *Br. J. Pharmacol.* 60:284P–85P

227. Jewitt, D., Jennings, K., Jackson, P. G. 1978. Efficacy of new inotropic drugs in clinical coronary heart failure. *Am. J. Med.* 65:197–202

228. Jackson, P. G., Jackson, G., Kitson, D., Jewitt, D. E. 1978. The inotropic effects of UK 14,275, a phosphodiesterase inhibitor, in man. *Br. J. Clin. Pharmacol.* 5:7–11

229. Follath, F., Kersting, F., Lewis, G. R. J., Dollery, C. T. 1975. Cardiovascular effects of UK 14,275: Evaluation of a new phosphodiesterase inhibitor with inotropic properties in animals and human volunteers. *Br. J. Clin. Pharmacol.* 2:372P–73P

230. Follath, F., Kersting, F., Lewis, G. R. J., Walden, R. J., Woolhouse, N. M., Dollery, C. T. 1976. Cardiovascular effects of a new inotropic drug in dog and normal man. *Clin. Pharmacol. Ther.* 20:24–30

231. Hutton, I., Hillis, W. S., Langhan, C. E., Conely, J. M., Lawrie, T. D. V. 1977. Cardiovascular effects of a new inotropic agent, U. K. 14275, in patients with coronary heart disease. *Br. J. Clin. Pharmacol.* 4:513–17

232. Kohri, H. Y., Kimura, Y., Watanabe, K., Kanbe, T., Wishi, T., Nakagawa, K., Hayashi, H., Hidaki, H. 1978. Selective inhibition of cyclic AMP phosphodiesterase by OPC 3689, an antithrombotic agent. *7th Intl. Congr. Pharmacol., Paris,* p. 125. Oxford/New York: Pergamon

233. Endoh, M., Satoh, K., Yamashita, S. 1980. Inhibition of cyclic AMP phosphodiesterase activity and myocardial contractility: Effects of cilostamide, a novel PDE inhibitor, and methylisobutylxanthine on rabbit and canine ventricular muscle. *Eur. J. Pharmacol.* 66:43–52

234. Shigenobu, K., Iwayama, Y., Sakai, R., Kasuya, Y. 1980. Cardiotonic effect of phthalazinol (EG-626) in the isolated guinea pig myocardium: Mechanical and electrophysiological studies. *J. Pharmacol. Bio-Dyn.* 3:543–52

235. Akera, T., Fox, A. L., Greeff, K. 1981. Substances possessing inotropic properties similar to cardiac glycosides. In

Handbook of Experimental Pharmacology, Cardiac Glycosides, ed. K. Greeff, 56/I:459–86. Berlin/Heidelberg/New York: Springer-Verlag

236. Farah, A., Maresh, G. 1948. Determination of the therapeutic irregularity and lethal doses of cardiac glycosides in the heart-lung preparation of the dog. *J. Pharmacol. Exp. Ther.* 92:32–42

237. Walton, R. P., Leary, J. S., Jones, H. P. 1950. Comparative increase in ventricular contractile force produced by several cardiac glycosides. *J. Pharmacol. Exp. Ther.* 98:346–57

238. Bahrmann, H., Greeff, K. 1981. Evaluation of cardiac glycosides in the intact animal. See Ref. 235, pp. 117–52

239. Greeff, K., Hafner, D. 1981. Evaluation of cardiac glycosides in isolated heart preparations other than papillary muscle. See Ref. 235, pp. 161–84

240. Gruhzit, C. C., Farah, A. E. 1953. Determination of the therapeutic range of gitalin in the heart-lung preparation of the dog. *J. Pharmacol. Exp. Ther.* 108:112–16

241. Vick, R. L., Kahn, J. B. Jr., Acheson, G. H. 1957. Effects of dihydro-ouabain, dihydrodigoxin and dihydrodigitoxin on the heart-lung preparation of the dog. *J. Pharmacol. Exp. Ther.* 121:330–39

242. Mendez, R., Pastelin, G., Kabela, E. 1974. The influence of the position of attachment of the lactone ring to the steroid nucleus on the action of cardiac glycosides. *J. Pharmacol. Exp. Ther.* 188:189–97

243. Bojores, R., Cardenas, M., Pastelin, G., Mendez, R. 1974. Accion de la Actodigina (AY-22241) en pacientes con insuficiencia Cardiaca y fibrilacion o flutter auriculares chonicos. *Arch. Inst. Cardiol. Mex.* 44:615–23

244. Maling, H. M., Krayer, O. 1946. The action of the erythrophleum alkaloids upon the isolated mammalian heart. *J. Pharmacol. Exp. Ther.* 86:66–78

245. Krayer, O., Farah, A., Uhle, F. C. 1946. Pharmacology and chemistry of substances with cardiac activity. IV. Effect of methylaminoethanol, dimethylaminoethanol and related substances on the isolated mammalian heart. *J. Pharmacol. Exp. Ther.* 88:277–86

246. Farah, A., Mook, W., Johnson, R. 1951. Some actions of mercury compounds on the heart. *Proc. Soc. Exp. Biol. Med.* 76:403–06

247a. Miller, T. B., Farah, A. E. 1962. Inhibition of mercurial diuresis by non-diuretic mercurials. *J. Pharmacol. Exp. Ther.* 135:102–11

247b. Miller, T. B., Farah, A. E. 1962. On the mechanism of the inhibition of mercurial diuresis by p-chloromercuribenzoic acid. *J. Pharmacol. Exp. Ther.* 136:10–19

248. Temma, K., Akera, T., Ku, D. D., Brody, T. M. 1978. Sodium pump inhibition by sulfhydryl inhibitors and myocardial contractility. *Naunyn-Schmiedebergs Arch. Pharmacol.* 302:63–71

249. Fricke, U. 1978. Myocardial activity of inhibitors of the Na^+-K^+-ATPase: Differences in the mode of action and subcellular distribution pattern of N-ethylmaleimide and ouabain. *Naunyn-Schmiedebergs Arch. Pharmacol.* 303: 197–204

250. Schwartz, A., Laseter, A. H. 1964. A sodium- and potassium-stimulated triphosphatase from cardiac tissue-II. The effects of ouabain and other agents that modify enzyme activity. *Biochem. Pharmacol.* 13:337–48

251. Taylor, S. R. 1963. The effect of mercurial diuretics on adenosinetriphosphatase of rabbit kidney in vitro. *Biochem. Pharmacol.* 12:539–50

252. Long, W. K., Farah, A. 1946. The influence of certain sulfhydryl compounds on the toxicity of an organic mercurial diuretic. *J. Pharmacol. Exp. Ther.* 88:388–99

253. Halbach, S. 1975. Effect of mercuric chloride on contractility and transmembrane potential of the guinea-pig myocardium. *Naunyn-Schmiedebergs Arch. Pharmacol.* 289:137–48

254. Ku, D., Akera, T., Tobin, T., Brody, T. M. 1974. Effects of Rubidium on cardiac tissue: Inhibition of Na^+,K^+-ATPase and stimulation of contractile force. *Res. Comm. Chem. Path. Pharmacol.* 9:431–40

255. Ku, D., Akera, T., Tobin, T., Brody, T. M. 1975. Effects of monovalent cations on cardiac Na^+,K^+-ATPase activity and on contractile force. *Naunyn-Schmiedebergs Arch. Pharmacol.* 290:113–31

256a. Ku, D. D., Akera, T., Tobin, T., Brody, T. M. 1976. Comparative species studies on the effect of monovalent cations and ouabain on cardiac Na^+K^+-adenosine triphosphatase and contractile force. *J. Pharmacol. Exp. Ther.* 197:458–569

256b. Knight, R. G., Nosek, T. M. 1981. Effects of Rubidium on contractility and sodium pump activity in guinea-pig ventricle. *J. Pharmacol. Exp. Ther.* 219:573–79

257. Vassalle, M. 1970. Electrogenic suppression of automaticity in sheep and

dog Purkinje fibers. *Circ. Res.* 27:361–77

258. Cantley, L. C. Jr., Josephson, L., Warner, R., Yanagisawa, M., Lechene, C., Guidotti, G. 1977. Vanadate is a potent (Na,K)-ATPase inhibitor found in ATP derived from muscle. *J. Biol. Chem.* 252:7421–23

259a. Borchard, U., Fox, A. A. L., Greeff, K., Schlieper, P. 1979. Negative and positive inotropic action of vanadate on atrial and ventricular myocardium. *Nature* 279:339–41

259b. Grupp, G., Grupp, I., Johnson, C. L., Wallick, E. T., Schwartz, A. 1979. Effects of Vanadate on cardiac contraction and adenylate cyclase. *Biochem. Biophys. Res. Commun.* 88:440–47

260. Takeda, K., Temma, K., Akera, T. 1982. Inotropic effects of Vanadate in isolated rat and guinea-pig heart under conditions which modify calcium pools involved in contractile activation. *J. Pharmacol. Exp. Ther.* 222:132–39

261. Schwartz, A., Lindenmayer, G. E., Allen, J. C. 1975. The sodium-potassium adenosine triphosphatase: Pharmacological, physiological and biochemical aspects. *Pharmacol. Rev.* 27:3–134

262. Seyama, I., Narahashi, T. 1973. Increase in sodium permeability of squid axon membranes by α-dihydrograyanotoxin II. *J. Pharmacol. Exp. Ther.* 184:299–307

263. Narahashi, T., Sayama, I. 1974. Mechanism of nerve membrane depolarization caused by grayanotoxin I. *J. Physiol.* 242:471–87

264. Hogan, P. M., Albuquerque, E. X. 1971. The pharmacology of batrachotoxin. III. Effect on the heart Purkinje fibers. *J. Pharmacol. Exp. Ther.* 176:529–37

265. Shotzberger, G. S., Albuquerque, E. X., Daly, J. W. 1976. The effects of betrachotoxin on cat papillary muscle. *J. Pharmacol. Exp. Ther.* 196:433–44

266. Honerjäger, P., Reiter, M. 1977. The cardiotoxic effect of batrachotoxin. *Naunyn Schmiedebergs Arch. Pharmacol.* 299:239–52

267. Frank, M., Flom, L. L., 1978. Effects of 2,4,6-triaminopyrimidine on the electromechanical properties of guinea pig myocardium. *J. Pharmacol. Exp. Ther.* 204:175–82

268. Meves, H., Pichon, Y. 1975. Effects of 4-aminopyridine on the potassium current in internally perfused giant axons of the squid. *J. Physiol.* 251:60–62P

269. Yeh, J. Z., Oxford, G. S., Wu, C. H., Narahashi, T. 1976. Dynamics of aminopyridine block of potassium channels

in squid axon membrane. *J. Gen. Physiol.* 68:519–35

270. Kass, R. S., Malloy, K. J., Scheuer, T. 1981. Iontophoretic injection of quaternary ammonium compounds blocks outward currents in cardiac Purkinje fibers. *Biophys. J.* 33:A71

271. Norton, T. R., Shibata, S., Kashiwagi, M., Bentley, J. 1976. Isolation and characterization of the cardiotonic polypeptide Anthopleurin-A from the sea anemone. *Anthopleura xanthogrammica. J. Pharm. Sci.* 65:1368–74

272. Tanaka, M., Hanin, M., Yasunobu, K. T., Norton, T. R. 1977. Aminoacid sequence of the anthopleura xanthogrammica heart stimulant, Anthopleurin A. *Biochemistry* 16:204–08

273. Beress, L., Beress, R. 1975. Isolation and characterization of three polypeptides with neurotoxic activity from Anemonia Sulcata. *FEBS Lett.* 50: 311–14

274. Alsen, C. 1975. Cardiotoxic effect of two toxins isolated from the sea anemone. *Naunyn Schmiedebergs Arch. Pharmacol.* 287:R105

275. Ravens, U. 1976. Electromechanical studies of an anemonia sulcata toxin in mammalian cardiac muscle. *Naunyn Schmiedebergs Arch. Pharmacol.* 296: 73–78

276. Romey, G., Renaud, J. F., Fosset, M., Lazdunski, M. 1980. Pharmacological properties of the interaction of a sea anemone polypeptide toxin with cardiac cells in culture. *J. Pharmacol. Exp. Ther.* 213:607–15

277. Shibata, S., Norton, T. R., Izumi, T., Matsuo, T., Katsuki, S. 1976. A polypeptide (AP-A) from sea anemone (Anthopleura Xanthogrammica) with potent positive inotropic action. *J. Pharmacol. Exp. Ther.* 199:298–309

278. Blair, R. W., Peterson, D. F., Bishop, V. S. 1978. The effects of Anthopleurin A on cardiac dynamics in conscious dogs. *J. Pharmacol. Exp. Ther.* 207:271–76

279. Scriabine, A., Van Arman, C. G., Morris, A. A., Morgan, G., Bennett, C. D. 1977. Cardiotonic activity of anthopleurin-A (AP-A), a polypeptide from sea anemone (Anthopleura Xanthogrammica), in dogs. *Fed. Proc.* 36:973

280. Bailey, L. E., Shibata, S., Seriguchi, D. G., Dresel, P. E. 1980. Inhibition of the positive inotropic effect of anthopleurin-A (AP-A) by Dantroline. *Life Sci.* 26:1061–68

281. Nayler, W. G., Daile, P., Chipperfield, D., Gan, K. 1970. Effect of Ryanodine

on calcium in cardiac muscle. *Am. J. Physiol.* 219:1620–26

282. Putney, J. W., Bianchi, C. P. 1974. Site of action of Dantrolene in frog sartorius muscle. *J. Pharmacol. Exp. Ther.* 189:202–12

283. Shimizu, T., Iwamura, N., Toyama, J., Yamada, K., Shibata, S. 1979. Effect of cardiotonic polypeptide Anthopleurin-A on canine Purkinje and ventricular muscle fibers. *Eur. J. Pharmacol.* 56:7–13

284. Fujiwara, M., Muramatsu, I., Hidaka, H., Ikushima, S., Ashida, K. 1979. Effect of goniopora toxin, a polypeptide isolated from coral, on electromechanical properties of rabbit myocardium. *J. Pharmacol. Exp. Ther.* 210:153–57

285. Kodama, I., Shibata, S., Toyama, J., Yamada, K. 1981. Electromechanical effects of Anthopleurin A (AP-A) on rabbit ventricular muscle. Influence of driving frequency, calcium antagonists, tetrodotoxin, lidocaine and ryanodine. *Br. J. Pharmacol.* 64:29–37

286. Hashimoto, K., Ochi, R., Hashimoto, K., Inui, J., Miura, J. 1980. The ionic mechanism of prolongation of action potential duration of cardiac ventricular muscle by Anthopleurin-A and its relationship to the inotropic effect. *J. Pharmacol. Exp. Ther.* 215:479–85

287. Low, P. A., Wu, C. H., Narahashi, T. 1979. The effect of Anthopleurin-A on crayfish giant axon. *J. Pharmacol. Exp. Ther.* 210:417–21

288. Lindner, E., Dohadwalla, A. N., Bhattacharya, B. K. 1978. Positive inotropic and blood pressure lowering activity of a dieterpene derivative isolated from coleus forskohli: Forskolin. *Arzneim. Forsch.* 28:284–89

289. Bhat, S. V., Bajwa, B. S., Dornàuer, H., de Souza, N. J. 1977. Structures and stereochemistry of new labdane dieterpenoids from coleus forskohlii briq. *Tetrahedron Lett.* 19:1669–72

290. Seamon, K. B., Daly, J. W. 1981. Forskolin: A unique dieterpene activator of cyclic AMP-generating systems. *J. Cyclic Nucleotide Res.* 7:201–24

291. Metzger, H., Lindner, E. 1982. Forskolin-dependent activation of an adenylate cyclase of rat heart membranes leads to inhibition of membrane-bound Na,K-ATPase. *Hoppe-Seyler's Z. Physiol. Chem.* 363:466–67

292. Metzger, H., Lindner, E. 1981. The positive inotropic acting Forskolin, a potent adenylatecyclase. *Arzneim. Forsch.* 31:1248–50

293. Holzmann, S., Schmidt, K., Dittrich, P., Kukovetz, W. R. 1982. Zum Mechanis-

mus der positiv inotropen und gefäs serweiternden Wirkung von Forskolin aus Coleus forskohlii. *Planta Med.* 45:133

294a. Daly, J. W. 1983. Forskolin, adenylate cyclase and cell physiology: An overview. *Proc. Int. Symp. Cyclic Nucleotides and Protein Phosphorylation, Milan, June.* New York: Raven

294b. Brooker, G., Pedone, C., Barovsky, K. 1983. Selective reduction of Forskolin-stimulated cyclic AMP accumulation by inhibitors of protein synthesis. *Science* 220:1169–70

295. Crane, F. L., Hatefi, Y., Lester, R. L., Widmer, C. 1959. Isolation of a quinone from beef heart mitochondria. *Biochim. Biophys. Acta* 25:220–25

296. Yamamura, Y., Folkers, K., Ito, Y., eds. 1980. *Biomedical and Clinical Aspects of Coenzyme Q*, Vol. 2. Amsterdam: Elsevier/North Holland

297. Folkers, K., Littarru, G. P., Ho, L., Runge, T. M., et al. 1970. Evidence for a deficiency of coenzyme Q_{10} in human heart disease. *Intl. J. Vitam. Nutr. Res.* 40:380–90

298. Yamamura, Y., Folkers, K., Ito, Y., eds. 1980. Clinical status of coenzyme Q and prospects. See Ref. 296, pp. 281–98

299. Yamamura, Y., Folkers, K., Ito, Y., eds. 1980. The use of coenzyme Q_{10} to protect ischemic heart muscle. See Ref. 296, pp. 409–25

300. Yamamura, Y., Folkers, K., Ito, Y., eds. 1980. Effect of coenzyme Q_{10} on action potentials and contractions during metabolic inhibition in isolated guinea pig ventricular muscle. See Ref. 296, pp. 47–64

301. Yamamura, Y., Folkers, K., Ito, Y., eds. 1980. The restorative of coenzyme Q_{10} on the adriamycin induced depression of myocardial contractility. See Ref. 296, pp. 225–50

302. Furuta, T., Kodoma, I., Kondo, N., Toyama, J., Yamada, K. 1982. A protective effect of Coenzyme Q_{10} on isolated rabbit ventricular muscle under hypoxic conditions. *J. Cardiovasc. Pharmacol.* 4:1062–67

303. Arita, M., Kiyosue, T., Imuanishi, S., Aomine, M. 1982. Electrophysiological and inotropic effects of Coenzyme Q_{10} on guinea pig ventricular muscle depolarized by potassium under hypoxia. *Jpn. Heart J.* 23:961–74

304. Folkers, K., Watanabe, T., Kaji, M. 1977. Critique of Coenzyme Q in biochemical and biomedical research and in ten years of clinical research on cardiovascular disease. *J. Mol. Med.* 2:431–39

305. Kukovetz, Von W. R. 1968. Über die Wirkung von Dibutyryl-3',5'-AMP am isolierten Herzen. *Naunyn Schmiedebergs Arch. Pharmacol.* 260:163–64

306. Meinertz, T., Nawrath, H., Scholz, H. 1973. Dibutyryl cyclic AMP and adrenaline increase contractile force and ^{45}Ca uptake in mammalian cardiac muscle. *Naunyn Schmiedebergs Arch. Pharmacol.* 277:107–12

307. Meinertz, T., Nawrath, H., Scholz, H. 1976. Possible role of cyclic AMP in the relaxation process of mammalian heart: Effects of dibutyryl cyclic AMP and theophylline on potassium contractures in cat papillary muscles. *Naunyn Schmiedebergs Arch. Pharmacol.* 293:129–37

308. Tsien, R. W. 1973. Adrenaline-like effects of intracellular iontophoresis of cyclic AMP in cardiac Purkinje fibres. *Nature* 245:120–22

309. Li, T., Sperelakis, N. 1983. Stimulation of slow action potentials in guinea pig papillary muscle cells by intracellular injection of cAMP, Gpp(NH)p and cholera toxin. *Circ. Res.* 52:111–17

310. Miller, J. P., Boxwell, K. H., Meyer, R. B. Jr., Christensen, L. F., Robins, R. K. 1980. Synthesis and enzymatic and inotropic activity of some new 8-substituted and 6,8-disubstituted derivatives of adenosine cyclic 3',5'-monophosphate. *J. Med. Chem.* 23:242–51

311. Revankar, G. R., Robins, R. K. 1982. Chemistry of cyclic nucleotides and cyclic nucleotide analogs. See Ref. 40, pp. 17–151

312. Moore, C., Pressman, B. C. 1964. Mechanism of action of valinomycin on mitochondria. *Biochem. Biophys. Res. Commun.* 15:562–67

313. Pressman, B. C., de Guzman, N. T. 1974. New ionophores for old organelles. *Ann. NY Acad. Sci.* 227:380–91

314. Pressman, B. C. 1976. Biological applications of ionophores. *Ann. Rev. Biochem.* 45:501–30

315. Levy, J. V., Cohen, J. A., Inesi, G. 1973. Contractile effects of a calcium ionophore. *Nature* 242:461–63

316. Schwartz, A., Lewis, R. M., Hanley, H. G., Munson, R. G., Dial, F. D., Ray, M. V. 1974. Hemodynamic and biochemical effects of a new positive inotropic agent. *Circ. Res.* 34:102–11

317. Hanley, H. G., Lewis, R. M., Hartley, C. J., Franklin, D., Schwartz, A. 1975. Effects of an inotropic agent RO 2–2985 (X-537A), on regional blood flow and myocardial function in chronically instrumented conscious dogs and anesthetized dogs. *Circ. Res.* 37:215–25

318. White, D. H., Crawford, M. H., O'Rourke, R. A. 1979. Beneficial effects of prolonged low dose dopamine in hospitalized patients with severe refractory heart failure. *Clin. Cardiol.* 2:135–39

319. Whitsett, R. L., Goldberg, L. I. 1972. Effects of levodopa on presystolic ejection period, blood pressure, and heart rate during acute and chronic treatment of Parkinson's disease. *Circulation* 45:97–106

320. Rajfer, S. I., Anton, A. H., Rowland, J., Goldberg, L. I. 1983. Beneficial hemodynamic effects of oral Levodopa in heart failure: Relationship to the generation of dopamine. *Clin. Res.* 31:526A

321. Thompson, M. J., Leier, C. V. 1980. Butopamine, a new inotropic agent, administered intravenously in patients with congestive heart failure. *Clin. Res.* 28:591A

322. Gorczynski, R. J., Anderson, W. G., Stout, D. V. 1981. N-aralkyl substitution of 2-amino-5,6-6,7-dyhydroxy-1,2,3,4-tetrahydronaphthalenes. 1. Cardiac and pressor/depressor activities. *J. Med. Chem.* 24:835–39

323. Gorczynshi, R. J. 1982. Cardiovascular pharmacology of ASL-7022, a novel catecholamine. 1. Inotropic, chronotropic and pressor actions. *J. Pharmacol. Exp. Ther.* 223:7–11

324. Erhardt, P. W., Gorczynski, R. J., Anderson, W. G. 1979. Conformational analogues of dopamine. Synthesis and pharmacological activity of (E) and (Z)-2 - (3,4 - dihydroxyphenyl)cyclopropylamine hydrochlorides. *J. Med. Chem.* 22:907–11

325. Mooradian, A., Hlavac, A. G., Dupont, P. E., Bell, M., Alousi, A. 1975. Hydroxylated 2,3,4,9-tetrahydro-1H-carbazol-3-amines. A new class of experimental cardiotonic drugs. *J. Med. Chem.* 18:640–41

326. Prigent, A. F., Nemoz, G., Roche, M., Pacheco, H. 1979. In vitro and in vivo myocardial effects of a cyclic AMP phosphodiesterase inhibitor structurally related to natural cardenolides. *Arch. Int. Pharmacodyn. Ther.* 241:131–52

327. Chanh, P. H., Xuong, N. D., LePecq, J. B., Paoletti, C. 1976. Cardiovascular activity of 9-hydoxy-ellipticine. *Pharmacology* 14:490–98

328. Steppeler, A., Starke, K. 1980. Selective inhibition by Amezinium of intraneuronal monoamine oxidase. *Naunyn*

Schmiedebergs Arch. Pharmacol. 314: 13–16

329. Steppeler, A., Pfändler, R., Hedler, L., Starke, K. 1980. An analysis of the effects of Amezinium on post-ganglionic sympathetic neurones. *Naunyn Schmiedebergs Arch. Pharmacol.* 314: 1–11

330. Lehmann, H. D., Schuster, J., Giertz, H. 1979. Haemodynamic effects of a new sympathomimetic: Amezinium metil sulfate (LU 1631). *Naunyn Schmiedebergs Arch. Pharmacol.* 308:R16

331. Lenke, D., Gries, J., Kratzschmar, R. 1979. Pharmacological studies on the mechanism of action of Amezinium metil sulfate (LU 1631). A new compound with sympathomimetic action. *Naunyn Schmiedebergs Arch. Pharmacol.* 308: R12

332. Nassar, B. A., Manku, M. S., Reed, J. D., Tynan, M., Horrobin, D. F. 1974. Actions of prolactin and frusemide on heart rate and rhythm. *Br. Med. J.* 2:27–29

333. Nassar, B. A., Horrobin, D. F., Tynan, M., Manku, M. S., Davies, P. A. 1975. Seasonal and sexual variations in the responsiveness of rabbit hearts to prolactin. *Endocrinology* 97:1008–13

334. Karmazyn, M., Daly, M. J., Moffat, M. P., Dhalla, N. S. 1982. A possible mechanism of inotropic action of prolactin on rat heart. *Am. J. Physiol.* 243:E458–E463

335. Cardenas, L. M., Vidaurri, D. A. 1979. Estudio de los Efectos Hemodinamicos de Diferentes Dosis de un Neuvo Inotropico: La amrinona. *Arch. Inst. Cardiol. Mex.* 49:961–68

336. Chesebro, J. H., Fuster, V., Robertson, J. S., Dewanjee, M. K., Wahner, H. W., Burnett, J. C. 1982. Shortened platelet survival in cardiac failures: predisposition to amrinone-induced platelet reduction. *Circulation* 66:II-382

337. Alousi, A. A., Helstosky, A., Montenaro, M. J., Cicero, F. 1981. Intravenous and oral cardiotonic activity of Win 47203. A potent amrinone analogue in dogs. *Fed. Proc.* 40:663 (Abstr.)

338. McDowell, A., Baim, D., Cherniles, J., Bekele, T., Braunwald, E., Grossman, W. 1983. Hemodynamic effects of a new inotropic agent (Win 47203) in patients with refractory heart failure. *J. Am. Coll. Cardiol.* 1:675

339. Van Inwegen, R. G., Salaman, P., St. Georgiev, V., Weinrye, I. 1979. Dihydro- and tetrahydroisoquinolines as inhibitors of cyclic nucleotide phosphodiesterases from dog heart. *Biochem. Pharmacol.* 28:1307–12

340. Ziskoven, R., Achenbach, C., Wiemer, J., Hauswirth, O. 1982. A voltage clamp study of the effects of AR-L 115 BS on the pacemaker current of cardiac Purkinje fibres. *Basic Res. Cardiol.* 77:536–51

341. Adachi, K., Numano, F. 1977. Phosphodiesterase inhibitors: Their comparative effectiveness in vitro in various organs. *Jpn. J. Pharmacol.* 27:97–103

342. Kraupp, V. O., Heistracher, P., Wolner, E., Tuisl, E. 1964. Die Wirkung von N,N'-Dimethyl-N,N'-bis[3-(3',4',5'-trimethoxybenzoxy) - propyl] - äteylendiamin auf Herz- und Kreislaufdynamik sowie O_2-Versorgung des Herzmuskels und des Gehirnes. *Arzneim. Forsch.* 14:1086–98

343. Erbring, V. H., Uebel, H., Vogel, G. 1967. Zur Chemie Pharmakologie und Toxikologie von Visnadin. *Arzneim. Forsch.* 17:283–87

344. Meyer, R. B. Jr., Uno, H., Robins, R. K., Simon, L. N., Miller, J. P. 1975. 2-Substituted derivatives of adenosine and inosine cyclic 3',5'-phosphates. Synthesis, enzymic activity, and analysis of the structural requirements of the binding locale of the 2-substituent on bovine brain protein kinase. *Biochemistry* 14:3315–21

345. Füller, H., Hauschild, F., Modersohn, D., Thomas, E. 1971. Pharmakologie des 5-Methyl-7-diamino-s-triazolo [1,5-a] pyrimidin (Trapymin, Rocornal), einer Verbindung mit koronargefässerweiternder Wirkung. *Pharmazie* 26:554–62

346. Takenaka, F., Ishihara, T., Hiraki, I., Higuchi, M., Umeda, T., Nozaki, M. 1974. Effects of 5 - methyl - 7 -diethylamino - s - triazolo[1,5 - a] pyrimidine (Trapymin, Rocornal) on the cardiovascular system in the dog. *Pharmacometrics* 8:339–48

347. Azuma, J., Sawamura, A., Harada, H., Tanimoto, T., Morita, Y., Sperelakis, N., Yamamura, Y. 1981. Trapidil stimulation of slow Ca^{2+} current in cardiac muscle. *Eur. J. Pharmacol.* 72:199–208

348. Ehmer, A., Jahr, K., Küschinsky, G., Lüllmann, H., Reuter, H., Wollert, U. 1964. Über die Herz glykosidartige Wirkung von Progesteronbisguanylhydrazon (Progesteronbiguazon). *Naunyn Schmiedebergs Arch. Pharmakol.* 248:521–39

349. Greeff, K., Meng, K., Schwarzmann, D. 1964. Digitalisähnliche Eigenschaften des Prednison- und Prednisolonbisguanylhydrazons: Ihre Wirkung auf die Kaliumbilanz isolierter Herzpräparate und den Na/K-Transport an Erythrocyten. *Naunyn Schmiedebergs Arch. Pharmakol.* 249:416–24

350. Drausfeld, H., Greeff, K. 1964. Der Einfluss des Prednison- und Prednisolon bisguanylhydrazons auf die Na⁺K⁺ stimulierte membrane-ATPase des Meerschweinchen herzens. *Naunyn Schmiedebergs Arch. Pharmakol.* 249:425–31

351. Yamamoto, S., Akera, T., Brody, T. M. 1978. Prednisolone - 3,20 - bisguanylhydrazone: Binding in-vitro to sodium- and potassium-activated adenosine triphosphatase of guinea pig heart ventricular muscle. *Eur. J. Pharmacol.* 51:63–69

352. Kahn, J. B. Jr. 1962. Effects of two Erythrophleum alkaloids on potassium transfer in human erythrocytes. *Proc. Soc. Exp. Biol. Med.* 110:412–14

353. Kahn, J. B. Jr., Van Atta, R. A. Jr., Johnson, G. L. 1963. Some effects of cassaine on cardiovascular dynamics in the dog. *J. Pharmacol. Exp. Ther.* 142:215–22

354. Repke, K., Portius, H. J. 1963. Über die Identität der ionenpumpen-ATPase in der Zellmembran des Herzmuskels mit einem Digitalis-Rezeptorenezym. *Experientia* 19:452–58

355. Seifen, E., Straub, K. D. 1974. Effects of sanguinarine on the isolated mammalian heart. *Pharmacologist* 16:245

356. Pitts, B. J. R., Myerson, L. R. 1978. Inhibition of ouabain binding to NaK-ATPase by sanguinarine: Correlation with the inotropic effect. *Fed. Proc.* 37:240

357. Szekeres, L., Papp, J. G., Udvary, E. 1974. On two isoquinoline derivatives with marked antianginal and antiarrhythmic actions. *Naunyn Schmiedebergs Arch. Pharmacol.* 284:R79

358. Fox, A. A. L., Borchard, U., Greeff, K. 1979. Digitalisähnliche und antiarrhythmische Wirkung des Isoquinolinderivates BIIA. *Z. Kardiol.* 68:244

359. Fox, A. A. L., Greeff, K. 1981. Mechanism of inhibition of sodium- and potassium-dependent adenosine triphosphatase by the isoquinoline derivative BIIA: A specific interaction with sodium activation. *Biochem. Pharmacol.* 30:611–17

360. Borchard, U., Fox, A. A. L., Greeff, K. 1980. The positive inotropic, antiarrhythmic and Na⁺,K⁺-ATPase inhibitory effects of isoquinoline derivative, BIIA. *Naunyn Schmiedebergs Arch. Pharmacol.* 312:187–92

361. Järnefelt, J. 1962. Properties and possible mechanism of action of the Na⁺ and K⁺-stimulated microsomal adenosinetriphosphatase. *Biochim. Biophys. Acta* 59:643–54

362. Davis, P. W., Brody, T. M. 1966. Inhibition of Na⁺K⁺-activated adenosine triphosphatase activity in rat brain by substituted phenothiazines. *Biochem. Pharmacol.* 15:703–10

363. Akera, T., Brody, T. M. 1970. Inhibitory sites on sodium- and potassium-activated adenosine triphosphatase for chlorpromazine free radical and Ouabain. *Mol. Pharmacol.* 6:557–66

364. Akera, T., Ku, D. D., Brody, T. M., Manian, A. A. 1978. Inotropic action of hydroxylated chlorpromazine metabolites and related compounds. *Biochem. Pharmacol.* 27:995–98

365. Temma, K., Akera, T., Brody, T. M. 1977. Hydroxylated chlorpromazine metabolites: Positive inotropic action and release of catecholamines. *Mol. Pharmacol.* 13:1076–85

366. From, A. H. L., Probstfield, J. L. 1971. P-chloromercuribenzene sulfonic acid induced inotropism. *Fed. Proc.* 30:632

367. Glynn, I. M. 1963. Transport adenosinetriphosphatase in electric organ. The relation between ion transport and oxidative phosphorylation. *J. Physiol.* 169:452–65

368. Bennett, D. R., Andersen, K. S., Andersen, M. V. Jr., Robertson, D. N., Chenoweth, M. B. 1958. Structure-activity analysis of the positive inotropic action of conjugated carbonyl compounds on the cat papillary muscle. *J. Pharmacol. Exp. Ther.* 122:489–98

369. Yamamoto, H., Kitano, T., Nishino, H., Murano, T. 1973. Studies on pharmacodynamic action of N-ethylmaleimide (NEM). 1st report: Influence of NEM on synaptic transmission of sympathetic nerves in guinea pigs. *Jpn. J. Pharmacol.* 23:151–60

370. From, A. H. L. 1970. N-ethyl maleimide (NEM) induced inotropism. *Clin. Res.* 18:306

371. Duggan, D. E., Knoll, R. M. 1965. Effects of ethacrynic acid and cardiac glycosides upon a membrane adenosine triphosphatase of renal cortex. *Arch. Biochem. Biophys.* 109:388–96

372. Askari, A., Rao, S. N. 1970. Drugs affecting sodium transport in human erythrocyte ghosts. *J. Pharmacol. Exp. Ther.* 172:211–23

373. From, A. H. L., Probstfield, J. L., Smith, T. R. 1975. Ethacrynic acid induced inotropism. *Proc. Soc. Exp. Biol. Med.* 149:1059–62

374. Law, R. O. 1976. The effects of ouabain and ethacrynic acid on the intracellular sodium and potassium concentrations in renal medullary slices incubated in cold potassium-free Ringer solution and

reincubated at 37°C in the presence of external potassium. *J. Physiol.* 254:743–58

375. Prasad, K., Midha, K. K. 1972. Effect of rubidium on cardiac function. *Jpn. Heart J.* 13:317–24

376. Britten, J. S., Blank, M. 1968. Thallium activation of the (Na^+-K^+)-activated ATPase of rabbit kidney. *Biochim. Biophys. Acta* 159:160–66

377. Skulskii, I. A., Manninen, V., Järnefelt, J. 1975. Thallium inhibition of Ouabain-sensitive sodium transport and of the (Na^+K^+)-ATPase in human erythrocytes. *Biochim. Biophys. Acta* 394:56–76

378. Winter, U., Achenbach, C., Wiemer, J., Ziskoven, R. 1982. The influence of Thallium(1)-ions on myocardial contractility. *Pfluegers Arch.* 392:R2 (Abstr.)

379. Wiemer, J., Ziskoven, R., Achenbach, C., Hauswirth, O. 1982. Effect of Thallium (1)-ions on dV/dt max i_{si} and I_{K2}. *Pfluegers Arch.* 392:R2 (Abstr.)

380. Kobayashi, T., Nakayama, R., Takatani, O., Kimura, Y. 1972. Positive chronotropic and inotropic actions of new antitumor agent adriamycin and its cardiotoxicity—Its special references to myocardial contractile force and the change of the transmembrane action potential. *Jpn. Circ. J.* 36:259–65

381. Van Boxtel, C. J., Olson, R. D., Boerth, R. C., Oates, J. A. 1978. Doxorubicin: Inotropic effects and inhibitory action on Ouabain. *J. Pharmacol. Exp. Ther.* 207:277–83

382. Gosalvez, M., van Rossum, G. D. V., Blanco, M. F. 1979. Inhibition of sodium-potassium-activated adenosine 5'-triphosphate and ion transport by adriamycin. *Cancer Res.* 39:257–61

383. Krayer, O., Acheson, G. H. 1946. The pharmacology of the veratrum alkaloids. *Physiol. Rev.* 26:383–446

384. Benforado, J. M. 1967. The veratrum alkaloids. In *Physiological Pharmacology*, ed. W. S. Root, F. G. Hoffmann, 4:331–98. New York: Academic. 2nd ed.

385. Ohta, M., Narahashi, T., Keeler, R. F. 1973. Effects of veratrum alkaloids on membrane potential and conductance of squid and crayfish giant axons. *J. Pharmacol. Exp. Ther.* 184:143–54

386. Honerjäger, P., Reiter, M. 1975. The relation between the effects of veratridine on action potential and contraction in mammalian ventricular myocardium. *Naunyn Schmiedebergs Arch. Pharmacol.* 289:1–28

387. Honerjäger, P., Reiter, M. 1977. Sarcolemmal sodium permeability and con-

tractile force of guinea pig papillary muscle: Effects of germitrine. *Circ. Res.* 40:90–98

388. Horackova, M., Vassort, G. 1974. Excitation-contraction coupling in frog heart. *Pfluegers Arch.* 352:291–302

389. Ku, D. D., Akera, T., Frank, M., Brody, T. M., Iwasa, J. 1977. The effects of grayanotoxin I and α-dihydrograyanotoxin II on guinea-pig myocardium. *J. Pharmacol. Exp. Ther.* 200:363–72

390. Akera, T., Ku, D. D., Frank, M., Brody, T. M., Iwasa, J. 1976. Effects of grayanotoxin I on cardiac Na^+,K^+-adenosine triphosphate activity, transmembrane potential and myocardial contractile force. *J. Pharmacol. Exp. Ther.* 199:247–54

391. Moran, N. C., Dresel, P. E., Perkins, M. E., Richardson, A. P. 1954. The pharmacological actions of andromedotoxin, an active principle from Rhodedendron Maximum. *J. Pharmacol. Exp. Ther.* 110:415–32

392. Narahashi, T., Albuquerque, E. X., Deguchi, T. 1971. Effects of batrachotoxin on membrane potential and conductance of squid giant axons. *J. Gen. Physiol.* 58:54–70

393. Albuquerque, E. X., Seyama, I., Narahashi, T. 1973. Characterization of batrachotoxin-induced depolarization of the squid giant axons. *J. Pharmacol. Exp. Ther.* 184:308–14

394. Shibata, S., Izumi, T., Seriguchi, D. G., Norton, T. R. 1978. Further studies on the positive inotropic effect of the polypeptide anthopleurin-A from a sea anemone. *J. Pharmacol. Exp. Ther.* 205:683–92

395. Low, P. A., Wu, C. H., Narahashi, T. 1979. The effect of anthopleurin-A on crayfish giant axon. *J. Pharmacol. Exp. Ther.* 210:417–21

396. Romey, G., Abita, J. P., Schweitz, H., Wunderer, G., Lazdunski, M. 1976. Sea anemone toxin: A tool to study molecular mechanisms of nerve conduction and excitation-secretion coupling. *Proc. Natl. Acad. Sci. USA* 73:4055–59

397. Coraboeuf, E., Deroubaix, E., Taxieff-Depierre, F. 1975. Effect of toxin II isolated from scorpion venom on action potential and contraction of mammalian heart. *J. Mol. Cell. Cardiol.* 7:643–53

398. Romey, G., Lazdunski, M. 1975. Scorpion and sea anemone toxin actions on axonal membranes. *Proc. 5th Intl. Biophys. Congr., Copenhagen*, p. 503

399. Acheson, G. H., Moe, G. K. 1945. Some effects of tetraethyl ammonium on the

mammalian heart. *J. Pharmacol. Exp. Ther.* 84:189–95

400. Ochi, R., Nishiye, H. 1974. Effect of intracellular tetraethylammonium ion on action potential in guinea pig's myocardium. *Pfluegers Arch.* 348:305–16

401. Woods, W. T., Urthaler, F., James, T. N. 1978. Chronotropic effects of tetraethylammonium and 4-aminopyridine in canine sinus node pacemaker cells. *Circulation* 57/58 (Suppl.):II–46

402. Kenyon, J. L., Gibbons, W. R. 1979. Influence of chloride, potassium, and tetraethylammonium on the early outward current of sheep cardiac Purkinje fibers. *J. Gen. Physiol.* 73:117–38

403. Kass, R. S., Malloy, K. J., Scheuer, T. 1981. Iontophoretic injection of quaternary ammonium compounds blocks outward currents in cardiac Purkinje fibers. *Biophys. J.* 33:71A (abstr. M-PM-C6)

404. Seamon, K. B., Daly, J. W. 1983. Forskolin, cyclic AMP and cellular physiology. *Trends Pharmacol. Sci.* 4:120–23

405. Juhász-Nagy, A., Aviado, D. M. 1977. Inosine as a cardiotonic agent that reverses adrenergic *beta* blockade. *J. Pharmacol. Exp. Ther.* 202:683–95

406. Faucon, G., Lavarenne, J., Collard, M., Evreux, J. C. 1966. Effets d'un nucleoside, l'hypoxanthine-d-riboside sur l'activite et l'irrigation myocardiques. *Therapie* 21:1239–52

407. Ohhara, M., Kanaida, H., Yoshimura, R., Okada, M., Nakamura, M. 1981. A protective effect of coenzyme Q_{10} on ischemia and reperfusion of the isolated perfused rat heart. *J. Mol. Cell. Cardiol.* 13:65–74

408. Evans, D. B., Parham, C. S., Schenck, M. T., Laffan, R. J. 1976. Stimulation of myocardial contractility by a new cyclic nucleotide analog, 8-(benzylthio)-N^6-n-butyl-adenosine cyclic $3',5'$-phosphate. *J. Cyclic Nucleotide Res.* 2:307–19

409a. Farah, A. 1983. Glucagon and the circulation. *Pharmacol. Rev.* 35:181–217

409b. Farah, A. 1983. Glucagon and the heart. In *Handbook of Experimental Pharmacology, Glucagon*, ed. P. Lefebvre, 66/II, pp. 553-609. Berlin/Heidelberg/New York: Springer-Verlag

410. Jorpes, J. E., Mutt, V. 1973. Secretin and cholecystokinin (CCK). In *Secretin, Cholecystokinin, Pancreozymin and Gastin*, ed. J. E. Jorpes, V. Mutt, 34: 1–179. Berlin / Heidelberg / New York: Springer-Verlag

411. Ross, G. 1970. Cardiovascular effects of secretin. *Am. J. Physiol.* 218:1166–70

412. Chiba, S. 1976. Effect of secretin on pacemaker activity and contractility in

the isolated blood-perfused atrium of the dog. *Clin. Exp. Pharmacol. Physiol.* 3:167–72

413. Chatelain, P., Deschodt-Lanckman, M., De Neef, P., Christophe, J., Robberecht, P. 1979. Effect of secretin, glucagon and vasoactive intestinal peptide hormone-sensitive rat cardiac adenylate cyclase. *Arch. Intl. Physiol. Biochim.* 87:783–84

414. Said, S. I., Bosher, L. P., Spath, J. A., Kontos, H. A. 1972. Positive inotropic action of newly isolated vasoactive intestinal polypeptide (VIP). *Clin. Res.* 20:29

415. Brown, J. C., Otte, S. C. 1978. Gastrointestinal hormones and the control of insulin secretion. *Diabetes* 27:782–89

416. Sheridan, D. J., Terry, G., Tynan, M. J. 1978. Allopurinol—an agent for myocardial protection during hypoxia. *Cardiovasc. Med.* 3:1207–10

417. Pressman, B. C., de Guzman, N. T., Somani, P. 1975. Correlation of inotropic and transport properties of carboxylic ionophores. *Pharmacologist* 17:245

418. Sutko, H. L., Besch, H. R. Jr., Bailey, J. C., Zimmerman, G., Watanabe, A. M. 1977. Direct effects of monovalent cations, ionophores monensin and nigericin on myocardium. *J. Pharmacol. Exp. Ther.* 203:685–700

419. Shlafer, M., Somani, P., Pressman, B. C., Palmer, R. F. 1978. Effects of the carboxylic ionophore monensin on atrial contractility and Ca^{2+} regulation by isolated cardiac microsomes. *J. Mol. Cell. Cardiol.* 10:333–46

420a. Krol, R., Zalewski, A., Maroko, P. R. 1982. Beneficial effects of berberine, a new positive inotropic agent, on digitalis-induced ventricular arrhythmias. *Circulation* 66:II–56

420b. Krol, R., Zalewski, A., Cheung, W., Maroko, P. R. 1982. Additive effects of berberine and ouabain on myocardial contractility. *Clin. Res.* 30:673A

421. Ribeiro, L. G. T., Bowker, B. L., Maroko, P. R. 1982. Beneficial effects of Berberine on early mortality after experimental coronary artery occlusion in rats. *Circulation* 66(Suppl.):II–56

422. Maroko, P. R., Zalewski, A., Krol, R., Cheung, W. 1982. Protoberberine alkaloids—A new family of inotropic agents. *Circulation* 66(Suppl.):II–137

423. Zalewski, A., Krol, R., Maroko, P. R. 1983. Berberine, a new inotropic agent—Distinction between its cardiac and peripheral responses. *Clin. Res.* 31:227A

424. Loewi, O. 1955. On the mechanism of the positive inotropic action of fluoride, oleate, and calcium on the frog's heart. *J. Pharmacol. Exp. Ther.* 114:90–99

425. Katzung, B., Rosin, H., Scheider, F. 1957. Frequency-force relationship in the rabbit auricle and its modification by some metabolic inhibitors. *J. Pharmacol. Exp. Ther.* 120:324–33

426. Covin, J. M., Berman, D. A. 1959. Metabolic aspects of the positive inotropic action of fluoride on rat ventricle. *J. Pharmacol. Exp. Ther.* 125:137–41

427. Reiter, M. 1965. The effect of various anions on the contractility of the guinea-pig papillary muscle. *Experientia* 21:87–89

428. Opit, L. J., Potter, H., Charnock, J. S. 1966. The effect of anions on (Na$^+$ + K$^+$)-activated ATPase. *Biochim. Biophys. Acta* 120:159–61

429. Tobin, T., Akera, T., Dworin, J. Z., Brody, T. M. 1974. Fluoride nephropathy: Lack of involvement of renal ATPase. *Can. J. Physiol. Pharmacol.* 52:589–95

430. Chenoweth, M. B., Pengsritong, K. 1950. Positive inotropic and other actions of fluoracetate. *Fed. Proc.* 9:263

431. Bennett, D., Chenoweth, M. B. 1951. Metabolism associated with positive inotropic action. *Fed. Proc.* 10:280

432. Korth, M., Weger, N., Reiter, M. 1978. The positive inotropic action of sodium fluoroacetate on guinea-pig ventricular myocardium. *Naunyn Schmiedebergs Arch. Pharmacol.* 303:7–14

433. Lai, C. Y. 1980. The chemistry and biology of cholera toxin. *CRC Crit. Rev. Biochem.* 9:171–206

434. Knope, R., Moe, G. K., Saunders, J., Tuttle, R. 1973. Myocardial effects of imidazole. *J. Pharmacol. Exp. Ther.* 185:29–34

435. Dietrich, J., Diacono, J. 1971. Comparison between ouabain and taurine effects on isolated rat and guinea pig hearts in low calcium medium. *Life Sci.* 10:499–507

436. Dolara, P., Ledda, F., Mugelli, A., Mantelli, L., Zilletti, L., et al. 1978. Effect of taurine on calcium, inotropism, and electrical activity of the heart. In *Taurine and Neurological Disorders*, ed.

A. Barbeau, R. J. Huxtable, pp. 151–59. New York: Raven

437. Schaffer, S. W., Chovan, J. P., Werkman, R. F. 1978. Dissociation of cAMP changes and myocardial contractility in taurine perfused rat heart. *Biochem. Biophys. Res. Commun.* 81:248–53

438. Darsee, J. R., Heymsfield, S. B. 1981. Decreased myocardial taurine levels and hypertaurinuria in a kindred with mitral-valve prolapse and congestive cardiomyopathy. *N. Engl. J. Med.* 304:129–35

439. Sawamura, A., Azuma, J., Harada, H. 1982. Positive inotropic action of taurine abstract. *Jpn. Circ. J.* 46:838

440. Azuma, J., Hasegawa, H., Sawamura, A., Awata, N., Ogura, K., et al. 1983. Therapy of congestive heart failure with orally administered taurine. *Clin. Ther.* 5:398–408

441. Schramm, M., Thomas, G., Towart, R., Franckowiak, G. 1983. Novel dihydropyridines with positive inotropic action through activation of Ca^{2+} channels. *Nature* 303:535–37

442. McNeill, J. H. 1979. Cyclic AMP and myocardial contraction. See Ref. 57, 1:421–41

443. Tran, V. T., Chang, R. S. L., Snyder, S. H. 1978. Histamine H$_1$ receptors identified in mammalian brain membranes with [^{3}H]mepyramine. *Proc. Natl. Acad. Sci. USA* 75:6290–94

444. Levi, R., Malm, J. R., Bowman, O., Rosen, M. R. 1981. The arrhythmogenic actions of histamine on human atrial fibers. *Circ. Res.* 49:545–50

445. Trzeciakowski, J. P., Levi, R. 1982. Reduction of ventricular fibrillation threshold by histamine: Resolution into separate H$_1$- and H$_2$-mediated components. *J. Pharmacol. Exp. Ther.* 223:774–83

446. Taylor, J. E., Richelson, E. 1982. High-affinity binding of [^{3}H] doxepin to histamine H$_1$-receptors in rat brain: Possible identification of a subclass of histamine H$_1$-receptors. *Eur. J. Pharmacol.* 78:279–85

Ann. Rev. Pharmacol. Toxicol. 1984. 24:329–60
Copyright © 1984 by Annual Reviews Inc. All rights reserved

GOSSYPOL: A POTENTIAL ANTIFERTILITY AGENT FOR MALES

Shao-Zhen Qian

Department of Basic Medical Research, Jiangsu Family Planning Institute, 123 Tian Fei Xiang, Nanjing 210005, People's Republic of China

Zhen-Gang Wang

Department of Pharmacology, Institute of Basic Medical Sciences, Chinese Academy of Medical Sciences, 5 Dong Dan San Tiao, Beijing, People's Republic of China

INTRODUCTION

Gossypol is a yellowish phenolic compound occurring naturally in certain species of cotton plants of the family Malvaciae, mostly in the seeds and root bark. At one time, gossypol was considered only a toxic waste in the processing of cottonseed products (1). In 1957, however, Liu (2) reported that Wang village in Jiangsu, China, had not had a single childbirth for as long as 10 years, from the 1930s to the 1940s, while before and after this period of collective infertility the villagers had been fecund. It was found that in these unprolific years the villagers had switched for economic reasons from soybean oil to crude cottonseed oil for cooking purposes. In the face of this evidence, Liu suggested that gossypol, the biologically active substance in cottonseed, might cause female infertility, particularly since many of the female villagers suffered menstrual disturbances at the same time. Later, the Hubei Provincial Group (3) documented the antispermatogenic effects of crude cottonseed oil in rats and monkeys, and since then a number of workers have investigated the active principle(s) in cottonseed and cotton root bark. Several groups (4–11) almost simultaneously demonstrated the male antifertility effect of gossypol.

The work on gossypol as an antifertility agent, initiated by Liu (2) and pursued actively by these groups, has stimulated nationwide attention; after the

329

0362-1642/84/415-0329$02.00

publication of a review article by the National Coordinating Group (12), it attracted universal interest. Various aspects of the subject have been reviewed by many authors (13–22). The present paper is a general review of gossypol as a potential male contraceptive, focusing on the pharmacological features not fully discussed in previous review articles.

THE CHEMISTRY OF GOSSYPOL

Gossypol has a molecular weight of 518.54 and a structure of (2,2'-binaphthalene)-8,8'-dicarboxaldehyde-1,1',6,6',7,7'-hexahydroxy-5,5'-diisopropyl-3,3'-dimethyl, as documented by Edwards (23) through total synthesis of the molecule. If gossypol is recrystallized in different solvents three crystalline substances with different melting points can be obtained. These substances have different optical properties and crystalline forms but show no weighty differences in their chemical and spectral behavior, suggesting not much dissimilarity in their chemical structures. However, many reactions of gossypol cannot be explained by this structure.

In an attempt to clarify the multiplicity of reactions of gossypol, Adams & Geissman (24) proposed that gossypol exists in three tautomeric forms: the aldehyde, the ketonoid, and the hemiacetal (Figure 1). Although the presence of the three tautomers of gossypol can be authenticated by the preparation of their respective derivatives, substantial concentrations of the hemiacetal or ketonoid forms have not yet been ascertained. Recently, the use of NMR to

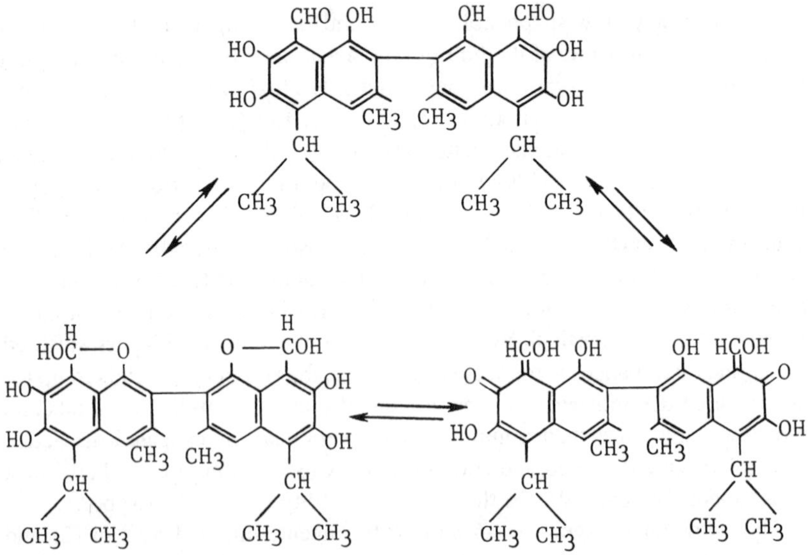

Figure 1   Tautomeric forms of gossypol

study the chemical shifts of gossypol in various solutions has shed further light on its structural changes. In ordinary inert solvents, gossypol exists mainly in aldehyde form, while in polar solvents, such as DMSO, the hemiacetal form occurs in dynamic equilibrium with the aldehyde form (25).

There are two optical isomers of gossypol. Initially, gossypol was only isolated from the Gossypium species as a racemate. Not long ago, the (+)−isomer was isolated first from Thespesia populnea, then from the Gossypium species (26, 27). The spectral characteristics and melting points of the (+)−isomer and the racemate are identical, but the former is more soluble in ordinary organic solvents than the latter. The melting points of the corresponding derivatives of the (+)−isomer and the racemate are different. Resolution of the racemate has recently been achieved (27a). It has been suggested that the optical activity of gossypol is the consequence of atropisomerism, i.e. the restriction of rotation of the two naphthalene units about the interlinking C-C bond.

THE ANTIFERTILITY EFFECT OF GOSSYPOL

Three forms of gossypol, gossypol, gossypol acetic acid, and gossypol formic acid, have been used in laboratory investigations and clinical trials. They are very much the same in their biological activities; therefore, they will be discussed as a whole under the generic name gossypol. Unless specified otherwise, the term refers to the racemate administered orally.

There are pronounced differences among animal species in their sensitivity to the antifertility action of gossypol. Among the laboratory animals tested, hamsters seemed to be the most sensitive, followed by rats, monkeys, and dogs in decreasing order, while rabbits and mice appeared to be insensitive (7, 12, 28–31). The effective dose for hamsters was 5–10 mg/kg per day, given for 6–12 weeks; recovery of fertility occurred 4–14 weeks after withdrawal of the drug (29, 30, 32, 33).

The effective dose for rats ranged from 10 to 30 mg/kg per day, given for 3–10 weeks. Onset of infertility was dose-dependent; the recovery of fertility after treatment ceased was also related to the dose, occurring 3–12 weeks after withdrawal (5, 7, 9, 12, 34–43). Gossypol at a dose of 7.5 mg/kg per day administered for longer period of time could also induce infertility in rats (5, 42, 45), but 3 mg/kg per day given for 16 weeks was without effect (5). With regard to the minimal effective dose, reports are inconsistent. 5 mg/kg per day given for 6 weeks (7) or 4 weeks (46) led to infertility, but 6 mg/kg per day given for 5 weeks was said to be ineffective (39). The sensitivity of rat testes toward gossypol showed marked individual variation; long-term treatment might cause complete atrophy of the seminiferous epithelium in some of the animals, and sterility is the likely consequence (47, 48) of this condition.

In dogs, gossypol appeared to be barely antispermatogenic, although toxic doses of gossypol could more or less inhibit spermatogenesis (28, 49). In rabbits, gossypol did not induce infertility. 10mg/kg per day given for 14 weeks hardly affected the sperm concentration and motility in the ejaculate; the pregnancy rate and the implantation sites of female rabbits inseminated with spermatozoa from the treated males did not differ significantly from the control (29). When rabbits were given gossypol at a dose of 10 mg/kg per day for 77 to 250 days, both the sperm data and fertility were not significantly affected despite severe toxicity resulting in eventual death (31). Gossypol did not inhibit spermatogenesis in mice. An oral dose of 15–30 mg/kg per day did not significantly affect the motility of epididymal and vasal spermatozoa (7, 50); the same was true with toxic doses (7, 30). It is interesting to note that, although gossypol did not affect spermatogenesis in mice, it inhibited pregnancy in female mice during the first two weeks of gestation (30).

Monkeys are moderately sensitive to the antispermatogenic action of gossypol. When rhesus monkeys were given a dose of 4 mg/kg per day for two years, spermatogenesis was completely inhibited in two of the three animals; in the third a few normal spermatids and spermatozoa could still be found in some of the seminiferous tubules (28). In cynomolgus monkeys, gossypol at a dose of 10 mg/kg per day given for as long as 6 months only decreased the sperm count and motility in the ejaculate (51).

It may be worth mentioning that it is gossypol itself and not the impurities present in the crude preparation that is antispermatogenic (32), and that the (+)−isomer isolated from Thespesia populnea is not antispermatogenic in rats (7, 52) and hamsters (52a) at dose levels higher than the effective dose of the racemate. Both the (+)−isomer and the racemate inhibited implantation in female rats, the suggested mechanism being inhibition of histamine release (53) or blocking of the LH effect (54). Gossypol inhibited sperm motility in vitro and in vagino (44, 55–61a), as well as when it was injected into the periepididymal fat (62) or directly into the epididymis (63). The spermicidal effect in vitro of the water-soluble coprecipitate of gossypol-polyvinylpyrolidone was more powerful than that of gossypol (57). Gossypol also reduced the ability of human sperm to penetrate both cervical mucus and zona-free hamster ova (61a).

THE METABOLISM OF GOSSYPOL

Gossypol is absorbed through the intestine as well as through the epithelial lining of the stomach (64). In this connection, it is interesting to note that, in an attempt to mitigate the gastric side effects of gossypol, one group of clinicians adopted enteric-coated tablets for the clinical trial. They found that both the antifertility effect and the systemic side effects of these tablets were much less than those of ordinary tablets (R. A. Zhang, personal communication). Apparently the differing response was due to decreased gastric absorption of gossypol caused by the enteric coat. Fecal excretion was the major route by which gossypol, administered either orally or parenterally, was removed from the animal body. Most of the absorbed gossypol was excreted via the bile, suggesting biliary circulation of gossypol between the liver and the intestine (64–73). High concentrations of gossypol in the bile are in harmony with the tentative conclusion that compounds of high molecular weight containing polar anionic groups and two or more aromatic rings tend to be excreted into the bile.

In rats given a single oral dose of (^{14}C) gossypol (64) in a 13-day experimental period, 77.4% of the ingested radioactivity was recovered from the feces, 12.1% from the expired CO_2, and 3.1% from the urine. The accumulation of radioactivity in the tissues was relatively low, totaling 12.5% of the administered dose one day after administration. Besides the gastrointestinal contents, which contained the highest radioactivity, the tissues examined one day after administration arranged according to their specific activity in decreasing order were as follows: gastrointestinal tract, liver, heart, kidney, spleen, lung, blood, muscle, adipose tissue, testis, and brain. After 24 hours, the activities of all these tissues gradually decreased, with minor fluctuations, and on the 13th day total tissue activity was only 0.28% of the administered dose. The peak of radioactivity in almost all the tissues examined was on the first day after administration. Reabsorption of gossypol from the renal tubule through the mechanism of nonionic absorption might account for the low urinary excretion of radioactivity.

A relatively large quantity of the ingested activity was recovered from the expired CO_2; for this reason, the investigators believed that decarbonylation was a major route of gossypol biodegradation in rats. The biological half-life of radioactivity in the body was 48 hours. Skutches & Smith indicated that the binaphthalene nucleus of the gossypol molecule was not degraded and only the formyl carbon was metabolized to CO_2 (74). More or less similar results were obtained by Xue et al (70, 71), but they showed that after a single oral administration of (^{14}C) gossypol to rats, the bioliogical half-life in the body was 60 hours, and that in many of the tissues examined, including heart, spleen, kidney, adrenal, pituitary, muscle, and testis, the peak of radioactivity occurred in the fourth to ninth days post-administration. They also indicated that the pituitary, adrenal, and thyroid glands exhibited very high specific activity, even outstripping that of the liver on the second, fourth, and ninth days. The results of repeated dosing of (^{14}C) gossypol were very much the same as those of the single-dose experiment (70, 71). Wang et al (72) pointed out that the distribution and excretion of gossypol in rats and monkeys were quite similar, and that in rats the half-life of gossypol in the gastrointestinal tract was 9.6 hours, indicating a low rate of absorption. Tang et al (73) compared the metabolism of (^{14}C) gossypol in mouse, rat, dog, and monkey and found that the pattern of distribution of activity in various tissues following a single dose of gossypol was much alike in the four species. Among them, the specific activity of the heart was the highest in the dog, that of the testis was the highest in the rat; the circulatory half-life was the longest in the dog, and the fecal excretion was higher in monkey and rat than in the other two species. Sang et al (28) indicated the greater excretion and lesser absorption of gossypol in monkey than in dog. These two groups of authors believed that the discrepancies in the metabolism of different species might have important bearing on their differential responses to the antifertility and toxic effects of gossypol. The fact that antifertility doses of gossypol selectively damaged the spermatogenic cells of rats, leaving the vital organs, which contained much higher concentrations of gossypol than did the testes, unaffected (12, 17), speaks strongly in favor of a specific vulnerability of the testicular cells to the action of gossypol. In rats treated orally with gossypol at a dose of 40 mg/kg per day for 8 weeks, the concentrations of free and bound gossypol in the liver, spleen, kidney, lung, and testis were found to increase gradually over the experimental period (75).

In pigs, the metabolism of (^{14}C) gossypol was similar to that of rats, but the tissue deposit of radioactivity was higher and the recovery from the expired CO_2 was lower. The total tissue deposit one day after administration was 32.9% in pigs (12.5% in rat), and the total recovery from expired CO_2 in a 20–day experiment was 2.1% of the dose ingested (12.1% in rats in a 13–day experiment). Low recovery from expired CO_2 indicated that decarbonylation was not an important route of gossypol biodegradation in pigs. The researchers also opined that the higher toxicity of gossypol in pig than in rat might be related to the difference in tissue deposition and decarbonylation of gossypol in these species (69).

Iron and protein form nonabsorbable Fe-gossypol chelate and protein-gossypol complex in the gastrointestinal tract; therefore, they are used to detoxify gossypol present in the cottonseed feed for livestock (1). In rats, the addition of ferrous salts to the feed reduced tissue deposition, accelerated fecal excretion, and shortened the half-life of (^{14}C) activity in the body; it also increased the respiratory elimination of (^{14}C), which might be explained by the postulation that iron catalyzes the decarbonylation process of gossypol (64). Protein supplements to the diet increased fecal excretion and decreased tissue deposition of (^{14}C) gossypol (65). In passing, it may be worth mentioning that Mg-gossypol complex has been shown to be antispermatogenic in rats, with a relatively low toxicity compared with gossypol (76).

THE TOXICITY OF GOSSYPOL

Single-Dose Toxicity

The single-dose oral LD_{50} of gossypol suspended in water is listed for some animal species in Table 1; if the drug is given in oil, the values will be 10% less

Table 1   Single-dose oral LD_{50} of gossypol (mg/kg) in water for several species

Rat	Mouse	Rabbit	Guinea Pig	Pig
2400–3340	500–950	350–600	280–300	550

[see(1)]. In rats, the single-dose oral LD_{50} of gossypol in peanut oil was 2590 ± 310 mg/kg (9).

Repeated-Dose Toxicity

The manifestations of repeated-dose oral toxicity of gossypol in some laboratory animals are outlined in Tables 2, 3, 4, and 5.

After reviewing the prolific literature relevant to the study of the toxicity of gossypol, including those not cited in this article, we have drawn the following conclusions:

1. Tolerance to gossypol varies greatly in different species. Among mice, rabbits, rats, guinea pigs, dogs, pigs, and monkeys, rats and the monkeys seem to be the most tolerant, dogs and rabbits the least. Preliminary results indicate that hamsters are even more tolerant than rats (29); female hamsters appear to be less tolerant to gossypol than males (77).
2. In rats, ordinary antifertility doses of gossypol seem to be nontoxic; only if the total dose is elevated to about 5–9 times the proposed minimal effective dose (7.5 mg/kg per day, given orally for 12 weeks), i.e. 20 mg/kg per day for 39 weeks or 30 mg/kg per day for 16 weeks, do minor lesions occur first in the liver, then in the heart or the kidneys in a few of the treated animals. Rats, as mentioned above, are sensitive to the antispermatogenic action of gossypol.
3. Monkeys tolerate the toxic effect of gossypol but are only moderately sensitive to its antispermatogenic action.
4. Dogs are very sensitive to the toxic effect but barely sensitive to the antispermatogenic effect of gossypol. Almost every dog died at each of the dose levels tested. The organs most seriously damaged are the heart and the liver: low doses seem to damage the heart more, leading to acute cardiac failure and sudden death; high doses seem to damage the liver more, causing cachexia and death. Fatal doses of gossypol induce only slight to moderate inhibition of spermatogenesis.
5. Rabbits are sensitive to the toxic but not the antispermatogenic effects of gossypol. Although the toxic manifestations are very conspicuous after gossypol administration, leading to fatality, the animals are still fertile shortly before death.

Table 2   Repeated-dose oral toxicity of gossypol in rats

Regimen (mg/kg/d)	Weeks	Manifestations	References
7.5	52	SGPT, BUN, ECG normal; histology of heart, liver, kidney normal; bone marrow and blood picture normal. Fertility suppressed, mating normal; germinal epithelium damaged but with no gross degeneration. Leydig cells unaffected.	78
7.5	12	Histology of organs normal; majority infertile, mating normal.	45
10	12	ECG normal; SGPT and gamma globulin slightly increased, but recovered after withdrawal of gossypol; in 1 out of 12 rats, SGPT highly increased with focal necrosis of liver, but histology of kidney and heart normal; for the rest, liver, kidney, heart normal. All infertile, Leydig cell unaffected.	7
10	26	Bone marrow and blood picture normal; histology of vital organs normal; no change in oil red "O" staining, G6Pase, G6PDH, ATPase, AKPase, ACPase, RNA, and DNA of liver; oil red "O" staining, G6PDH, ATPase, AKPase, ACPase of kidney; oil red "O" and Sudan Black staining and 3-OH-steroid dehydrogenase of adrenal gland. Infertile, mating normal.	79
15	10	Histology of heart, lung, kidney, liver, spleen, stomach and small intestine normal; bone marrow picture normal.	5
20	39	MAO, AKPase, PAS and oil red "O" staining of liver normal; individual animal showed slight degenerative changes in liver cell and increased SDH activity.	17
30	10	No effect on body weight and weight of accessory sex glands; hCG binding in testis normal; SDH and ATPase of testis and liver normal. Infertile; germinal epithelium damaged in part of animals.	43
30	16	No effect on body weight and weight of accessory sex glands; histology of heart, liver, lung, kidney and spleen normal; occasional minor focal inflammatory infiltration in different organs. Infertile since fifth week, damage to germinal epithelium began at second week; no effect on Leydig cell seen under electron microscope.	80

THE GENETIC EFFECT OF GOSSYPOL

Offspring Observation

Gossypol-treated rats were mated with untreated females after recovery of fertility. On gross examination, the offspring of the F_1 and F_2 generations were normal (7). Of the 8806 human volunteers taking gossypol, the spouses of 266

Table 3 Repeated-dose oral toxicity of gossypol in rabbits

Regimen (mg/kg/d)	Days	Manifestations	References
16	14–140	SGPT, NPN and blood picture normal; bradycardia and ECG changes in part of animals. 6 out of 10 died 14–140 days after dosing began	81
80	8–17	Loss of weight, loss of appetite, dyspnea, hind limb paralysis, collapse. Died 8–17 days after dosing began. Autopsy: congestion of liver and lungs. Fertility and semen spermatozoa normal shortly before death.	31
40	23–35	Similar to above. Died 23–35 days after dosing began	31
20	35–84	Similar to above. Died 35–84 days after dosing began	31
10	77–250	Similar to above. Died 77–250 days after dosing began	31

subjects conceived after withdrawal of gossypol or during the regimen. 53 gave birth to apparently normal babies; the rest of the fetuses were artificially aborted (18).

Dominant Lethal Mutagenic Effects

Male rats were given 20 mg/kg of gossypol per day for 4 weeks to make them infertile, then the animals were allowed to mate with untreated females for three rounds on days 37–40, 47–50, and 57–60 post-regimen. On the thirteenth day of pregnancy, the researchers sacrificed the females and recorded the numbers of live and dead fetuses and the number of implantation sites. They found that after the first and second rounds of mating, the ratio of dead fetuses to the number of implantation sites was significantly higher in the treated than in the control animals. However, after the third round, the ratio of the treated animals dropped to a level that did not differ significantly from that of the control. Results suggest that gossypol may damage the genetic material but the effect is transient and may decrease with time (87).

Embryotoxicity and Teratogenicity

In Wistar rats and long-haired rabbits, gossypol in dose levels 5- or 30-fold the clinical dose did not show significant embryotoxicity or teratogenicity (88).

Ames Test

De Peyster & Wang (89) indicated that gossypol was not mutagenic to the five standard tester strains of Salmonella typhimurium either with or without the inclusion of a rat-liver metabolic enzyme fraction. Similar results were obtained by many other researchers (90–94). It may be worth mentioning that

Table 4 Repeated-dose oral toxicity of gossypol in dogs

Regimen (mg/kg/d)	Days	Number of animals	Manifestations	References
1.5	60–141	4	Loss of weight, loss of appetite, weakness, caddy stool, dyspnea. All animals died suddenly 60–141 days after dosing began. Autopsy: cardiac dilatation; edema, lysis and atrophy of myocardium; congestion of liver; cloudy swelling and hyaline degeneration of renal tubules; pulmonary congestion and edema. Cause of death: acute cardiac failure. Germinal epithelium: slight to moderate damage.	49
3.0	51–64	4	Similar to above, except liver showed additional slight fatty degeneration; germinal epithelium slightly damaged.	49
30	18–28	4	Severe anorexia, loss of weight, weakness, nausea, vomiting, tarry stool, anaemia, cachexia; died 18–28 days after dosing began. Autopsy: similar to above, except liver showed moderate fatty degeneration and pachy necrosis. Cause of death: cachexia. Germinal epithelium damage: slight to moderate.	49
1.0	129–130	2	Anorexia, loss of weight, weakness, tachycardia. ECG, NPN, SGPT normal. Died suddenly 129 and 130 days after dosing began. Autopsy: myocarditis and endocarditis.	82
5.0	73	2	One dog died on day 73 of dosing, manner of death unnoticed; another sacrificed on the same day. Other manifestations similar to above.	82
1.0–3.0	25–131	12	Anorexia, vomiting, diarrhea, weakness, bradycardia, ECG abnormalities (flattening of T and prominant U). Some dogs died on day 25, 43, 60, 63, and 131 of dosing. Autopsy: cardiac dilatation and hypertrophy, endocarditis, congestion of kidney and spleen, fatty degeneration and necrosis of liver, edema and hemorrhage of lungs. Inhibition of spermatogenesis: not obvious.	17

Table 5 Repeated-dose oral toxicity of gossypol in monkeys

Regimen (mg/kg/d)	Months	Number of animals	Manifestations	References
1–2	14	3	Renal function, histology of heart and kidney, renal LDH and ATPase normal. Liver showed temporary ultrastructural changes (distension of endoplasmic reticulum, increase in lysosomes).	17
4.0	24	3	Serum Na, K, Mg, Cl, creatinine, LDH, NPN and SGOT normal. Urinary Na, K, Mg, Cl, creatinine, LDH, SGOT, AKP normal; urine concentrating ability normal. Cellular K normal, cellular Na increased. Myocardium: slightly congested, LDH-1,2 decreased, LDH-3,4,5 increased, ATPase unchanged, SDH increased or unchanged. Ultrastructure essentially normal. Liver: hepatic sinusoid slightly distended, partial vacuolation in central zone of lobule; temporary changes in ultrastructure (distension and vacuolation of endoplasmic reticulum, lysosomes increased, ribosomes decreased, mitochondrial damage, decrease of cristae); LDH, G6PDH, ATPase and RNA unchanged. Kidney: cloudy swelling of proximal tubules, mitochondrial damage; ATPase and ACPase decreased, G6PDH and juxtaglomerular cell granules unchanged. Histology of spleen, stomach, intestine and adrenal normal. Germinal epithelium markedly damaged in two animals, but in the third a few normal spermatids and spermatozoa still present.	17, 28, 83–86a
8.0	4	2	Myocardial striation obscure with occasional cloudy swelling and acidocytosis. Liver: slight cloudy swelling, fatty infiltration, focal inflammation and acidocytosis. Cloudy swelling of renal tubule.	17
5 or 10	6		No serious clinico-pathological side effects. Sperm count and motility depressed.	51

in mice skin-painting tests, gossypol showed tumor-inducing or promoting activity (95). Lifetime carcinogenicity data so far are unavailable.

Chromosomal Observations

The effect of gossypol on the frequency of occurrence of sister chromatid exchange (SCE), micronuclei, and chromosomal aberrations has been investigated repeatedly by different groups and the results are roughly consistent: low (5-fold clinical dose) or medium (around 10-fold clinical dose) dose levels did not appear to damage the genetic material in vivo, while high doses (more than 30-fold clinical dose) did. The same dose-dependent relationship also seems to hold true with in vitro experiments. In humans, routine clinical dosages did not seem to affect genetic material. The results reported by different workers are listed in Table 6.

THE ENDOCRINE EFFECT OF GOSSYPOL

Gossypol does not demonstrate androgenic, antiandrogenic, estrogenic, or antiestrogenic activity, but it does potentiate the androgenicity of methyl testosterone (30). In regard to the effect of gossypol on the endocrine glands or tissues, three main kinds of investigations have been carried out, including morphological studies, in vitro studies, and studies of the effect on blood hormone levels. The results of these investigations will be discussed separately in the following paragraphs.

Morphological Studies

THE EFFECT ON THE HYPOTHALAMUS   In gossypol-treated rats, the cell size, the volume of cytoplasm, and the number of cytoplasmic granules in the neurons of the paraventriculus nucleus were decreased, while the nuclei of these cells were distended, assuming a vesicular appearance (108).

THE EFFECT ON THE PITUITARY   In rats, gossypol reduced the number of cytoplasmic granules in the gonadotrophs (108), increased the number of active-stage gonadotrophs, decreased the number of quiescent-stage gonado-trophs, and led to the appearance of cells similar to castration cells (109). It may bring about hydropic degeneration of β_1 cells and more or less affect all types of pars distalis cells (110).

THE EFFECT ON THE LEYDIG CELL   A majority of the researchers working on the question reported that gossypol does not affect the morphology of Leydig cells (7, 28, 80, 109, 111, 112). However, in testicular biopsy specimens from sterile men with a history of using crude cottonseed oil, Leydig cells were reduced in number and showed early signs of degeneration (113). Moreover, in rats treated with gossypol, the cell size, the volume of cytoplasm, and the smooth endoplasmic reticulum of Leydig cells were reduced, with increased number of lysosomes and occasional vacuolization (113a).

In Vitro Studies on Testicular Steroidogenesis

Lin et al (114) found that adding 10^{-5}M and 10^{-7}M of gossypol to rat Leydig cell culture reduced LH-stimulated production of testosterone (T) in the culture;

Table 6 Chromosomal observations[a]

Species	Dose (μg/ml in vitro; mg/kg/d per os)	Chromosomal aberration (cell type)	SCE (cell type)	Micronuclei (cell type)	References
Hamster	0.23–2.3 in vitro		Negative (CHO)		96
Hamster	0.2–2.0 in vitro		Negative (CHO)		97
Rat	20, oral 9 days	Negative (SG, SC)		Negative (LP)	98
ICR mice	4, oral 4 days		Negative (BM)		99
ICR mice	1–10, oral 19 days	Negative (SG, SC)	Negative (SG)		100
ICR mice	3 and 8, oral 9 days		Negative (SG)		101
ICR mice	20–50, oral 19 days		Increased (SG, SC)	Increased (SG)	100
ICR mice	20, oral 9 days		Increased (SG)		101
Kunming mice	4, oral 14 days	Negative (SG)	Negative (SG)		102
Man	10 in vitro		Negative (LP)		92
Man	1–9 in vitro	Negative (LP)	Increased (LP)		103
Man	0.2–2.0 in vitro		Negative (LP)		97
Man	0.005–0.1 in vitro	Negative (LP)			104
Man	Routine 2 years		Negative (LP)	Negative (LP)	105
Man	20 mg/day 78–85 days	Negative (LP)			106
Man	Routine 34–50 months	No significant effect on number of nucleolar organizing regions and occurrence of acrocentric chromosome association in peripheral lympocytes.			107

[a]BM = bone marrow cell; CHO = Chinese hamster ovary cell; LP = peripheral lymphocyte; SC = spermatocyte; SG = spermatogonium; routine = 20 mg/day for 60–70 days, followed by a maintenance dose of 40–50 mg/week orally.

they also discovered that LH-stimulated T production by Leydig cells from rats treated with gossypol was significantly lower than that by Leydig cells from control rats. Therefore, these authors concluded that gossypol depressed testicular steroidogenesis. Several other groups obtained similar results in rats (41, 115, 116) and in rabbits (31). However, Zhuang (117) indicated that these concentrations of gossypol did not decrease hCG-induced T production per 10^6 Leydig cells of rat and that T concentration in the culture media was lowered as a consequence of the decreased number of Leydig cells, apparently due to the addition of gossypol. The (^{125}I) hCG binding in testis homogenate of gossypol-treated (25–30 mg/kg/d over 10 weeks) rats was similar to that of untreated animals, suggesting noninterference of gossypol in hormone action at the target level (43).

In connection with these in vitro experiments, it is advisable to note that the actions of gossypol in vitro and in vivo are remotely different in many respects. For example, in isolated rabbit heart, Qian et al (118) found that gossypol 0.5 or 1.0 μg/ml in Locke's solution completely inhibited ventricular contractility, while free gossypol 2.13–2.25 μg/ml in blood (donated by other rabbits fed gossypol at a dose of 30 mg/kg per day for 8–12 days) did not inhibit it at all. It has been reported that most, if not all, gossypol in the body is conjugated with different molecules of the organism and that so-called free gossypol is actually conjugates of gossypol with micromolecules. Their actions will naturally differ from those of gossypol in vitro. Therefore, special care should be taken in the interpretation of in vitro experimental results.

Effect on Blood Hormone Levels

As can be seen from Table 7, the results from various experiments are largely inconsistent, particularly in regard to the effect of gossypol on T level, which may be due to differences in animal species (strains), drug purity and dosage, or other experimental conditions employed.

CLINICAL TRIALS OF GOSSYPOL

The initial clinical trials of gossypol as a male antifertility agent were carried out by Qian et al (11) in 1972. Although customarily undertaking clinical trials so soon after documentation of an antifertility effect in animals would be unseemly, in this case the trial was completely justified. In the first place, humans have used gossypol and gossypol-containing drugs and foods for a long period of time with few adverse consequences (123–127). Second, generally accepted standards have been set for gossypol consumption by humans, being 450 mg/kg in food in the United States and 600 mg/kg as recommended by international groups (128). Moreover, before the discovery of the antifertility action of gossypol, Qian's group had documented gossypol as the active

Table 7 Effect of gossypol on blood hormone levels

Species	Regimen (mg/kg/d)	Weeks	T	LH	FSH	References
Rat			Negative	Negative	Negative	12
Rat	7.5	12	Negative	Negative	Negative	42, 45
Rat	12	6	Negative			7
Rat	15	12	Negative	Negative	Negative	42, 114
Rat	25	10	Negative	Negative		43
Rat	30	5		Negative		119, 120
			Response to LHRH normal			
Rat	30	5 or 6	Lowered	Lowered	Negative	41, 42, 114
Rat	30	5	Lowered	Negative	Negative	40
Rat	20	4	Lowered	Negative		113a
Young rat	20	8	Lowered	Negative		113a
Hamster	10 or 15	5	Negative	Negative		33
Hamster	10 or 15	10, 8	Lowered	Negative		33
Rabbit	20 or 10	12–20	Lowered			31
Monkey	2	13	Negative	Negative	Negative	45
Monkey	4	39–87	Negative			7
Monkey	8	7	Negative	Negative		45
Monkey	8	17	Negative			7
Monkey	10	36	Negative			51
Man	Routine		Negative	Negative	Negative	12, 17, 18
			Response to LHRH normal			143, 145
Man	Routine	36–52	Negative	Negative		121
			Response to LHRH and hCG normal			
Man	Routine		Negative	Negative		146
Man	Routine total dose 3–17 gm		25% increased	Negative	50% increased	122

principle of cotton root bark, a Chinese folk medicine for the treatment of chronic bronchitis and cough, and had carried out clinical trials of gossypol on bronchitic patients.

Qian et al (11) found that gossypol given orally at a dose of 60–70 mg per day for 35–42 days caused a gradual increase in the percentage of nonmotile spermatozoa in the ejaculate, followed by oligospermia, necrospermia, and azoospermia in all 25 volunteers. Interestingly, sperm motility decreased markedly as early as the second week of administration, suggesting that gossypol may act on epididymal or testicular spermatozoa. Recovery occurred around three months after withdrawal. The side effects of this dosage were reversible and generally of mild degree, mainly including decrease or increase in appetite, fatigue, dryness of mouth, diarrhea, inconsiderable elevation of

SGPT, and a tendency to sleepiness; individual cases suffered slight oedema of the eyelid, seemingly decreased libido and potency, and insignificant depression of serum potassium levels. When the dose was decreased to 24–35 mg per day and the duration of treatment appropriately prolonged, the side effects were much reduced and the antifertility effect was retained. In all subjects except three who had trivial complaints, health status was good one year after the gossypol regime ended. The investigators concluded that gossypol was an effective antispermatogenic agent in men, but that the significance of the side effects necessitated further toxicological studies (11).

After a series of toxicological studies, second- and then third-phase trials were carried out in several parts of China. Until 1980, the total number of volunteers had amounted to 8806 (18). Optimal or routine loading and maintenance doses were determined to be 20 mg/day for 60–70 days and 40–50 mg/week respectively. With this dosage level, antifertility efficacy was 99.07%. The common side effects in men taking routine doses were similar to those reported by Qian et al (11); additionally, an infrequent but important side effect, hypokalemic paralysis, was uncovered during the expanded trials, the overall occurrence being 0.75% (18), although in certain districts it was as high as 4.7% (129). Hypokalemic paralysis was always preceded by a prodromal stage characterized by muscular weakness and/or severe fatigue, and the use of potassium salt at this stage could prevent paralysis (129). The problem of hypokalemia will be discussed separately below.

Changes in sperm count and motility in subjects taking the optimal doses of gossypol were similar to those in men taking 60–70 mg/day, although these subjects took longer to show evidence of necrospermia and azoospermia. Recovery ensued in most subjects after cessation of gossypol treatment, but around 10% of the volunteers remained azoospermic six months to 4.5 years post-regimen, indicating the possibility of irreversibility of fertility (18). The recovery rate was much higher in subjects taking gossypol for less than two years than in those taking it for more than two years. Quantitative histological studies of testicular biopsy specimens of infertile men taking gossypol-containing crude cottonseed oil also indicated the possibility of irreversibility of spermatogenesis if large amount of the oil had been used, particularly for a long period of time (113).

The pattern of exfoliated cells in human semen has been studied by several groups (131–134). Zong (131) indicated that in men taking routine doses of gossypol, exfoliated cells, mainly mid- and late-stage spermatids and a few double- or multinucleated cells, could be seen at the end of the first month, followed by gradually increasing numbers of primary spermatocytes and spermatogonia. At the end of fifth month, the semen pictures showed wide individual variations. In general, the following three patterns could be differentiated: (a) no-cell semen, (b) semen with spermatids predominant, (c) semen with primary spermatocytes predominant. Zong believed that the second was the most ideal pattern. In this case both the spermatogonia and the spermatocytes were capable of division, giving rise to an incessant number of new spermatids. In no-cell semen, all cell types were seriously inhibited and sterility would have resulted if treatment had continued. In these cases, suspension of gossypol treatment for some period of time may obviate this possibility.

Shi et al (132) studied changes in the pattern of exfoliated cells in human semen during and after gossypol treatment. They found, in addition to what Zong reported (131), that the peak of exfoliation of spermatids, spermatocytes, and spermatogonia occurred in the sixth, twenty-fourth, and thirty-sixth months of maintenance dosing respectively, and that after withdrawal of gossypol the recovery of fertility seemed to be related to the prominent cell type exfoliated at the time of withdrawal. If the cell type was spermatogonia, the chances for recovery were less. As a result of these discoveries, these researchers also advocated the examination of exfoliated cells in semen as a means of decreasing the occurrence of gossypol-induced sterility. Chen & Li indicated that, in men taking gossypol, the LDH-X activity of spermatozoa decreased dose-dependently, which might serve as another index for the individualization of the dosage (130). Later, several groups documented the inhibitory effect of gossypol on LDH-X activity (135–139a) and considered it to be gossypol's target of action. Gossypol did not induce autoimmune reaction to sperm in men (140).

Investigators in Shandong province recommended the use of gossypol formic acid for clinical trials because, they claimed, the side effects appeared fewer than those associated with gossypol and gossypol acetic acid (36, 141, 142).

There is no clear evidence on whether all the side effects associated with gossypol treatment, such as decreased libido, can be ascribed entirely to the drug. Factors other than gossypol may cause these symptoms as well. For the resolution of this problem, well-controlled double-blind clinical studies have been initiated (143, 144). Coutinho carried out the first clinical trial outside China in 8 men for periods of 6–12 months (121). Treatment consisted of oral administration of 20 mg daily for 4 months, followed by 20 mg every other day. Reduction in sperm count occurred after 45 days and azoospermia at the end of 4 months of treatment. No change in semen volume was detected. None of the subjects reported loss of libido or potency. Blood chemistry, serum potassium, and testosterone levels were normal throughout the treatment. Response to LHRH and hCG was normal. There were no significant changes in blood pressure and body weight. Recovery of semen values was faster in men who took the drug for short periods of time. These results are consistent with those obtained by Chinese scientists.

HYPOKALEMIC PARALYSIS

Hypokalemic paralysis is an infrequent side effect of gossypol, but for the time being it is the most important stumbling block to the general application of the drug as an antifertility agent. Hypokalemic paralysis associated with gossypol administration usually occurs in March, when vegetable food is in short supply, and in September, when people sweat a great deal. Nothing particular has been found in the history of the subjects, no family or past history of paralysis or thyrotoxicosis. The clinical picture is that of hypokalemic syndrome: fatigue, muscular weakness, followed by flaccid paralysis starting from the lower extremity and gradually spreading upward, but usually not affecting the respiratory muscles. The principal laboratory findings are hypokalemia with corresponding ECG changes; 24-hour urinary potassium increased; renal concentrating and diluting ability, renal acidifying power and renogram normal; blood pH, aldosterone level, and thyroid function normal. Recovery is prompt and complete after potassium repletion in most cases, but a few may remain hypokalemic for a long time after cessation of gossypol treatment. These cases require intermittent potassium therapy; otherwise, paralysis may recur.

For several years during the past decade, the problem of whether gossypol can induce hypokalemia had been the subject of dispute. Attempts to produce hypokalemia by administering gossypol to various experimental animals have not been successful. Next, although the clinical and laboratory findings on hypokalemia associated with gossypol are undeniably different from those of the more familiar forms of hypokalemia, such as familial periodic paralysis (thyrotoxic or non-throtoxic), it is difficult to differentiate hypokalemia associated with gossypol from hypokalemia of unknown diagnosis (147). One would naturally think that hypokalemia associated with gossypol administration might simply be hypokalemia of unknown diagnosis.

In 1975, Qian et al (148) showed that gossypol decreased the potassium content of myocardium in isolated rabbit heart. A little later the same group (149) found that gossypol reduced the intracellular potassium ion concentration in low-K–fed rats but not in regularly fed rats. Similar results were obtained in isolated skeletal muscles by Xu & Qian (150). These were the first experimental evidences documenting a definite effect of gossypol on potassium metabolism. Moreover, Qian et al (15, 129) pointed out that the incidence of hypokalemic paralysis was astonishingly higher in subjects taking gossypol than in the control population and that among the gossypol takers hypokalemic paralysis occurred only in those with a relatively low K intake, a phenomenon curiously similar to what happened in rats (149). Putting all these facts together, one may conclude that hypokalemic paralysis in gossypol takers is not a casual coexistent hypokalemia of unknown diagnosis but is related to the administration of gossypol. In regard to the mechanism of development of gossypol-induced hypokalemia, Qian et al (148) suggested that gossypol might inhibit the activity of Na-K-ATPase or some other Mg-dependent enzyme systems associated with energy metabolism. This hypothesis is based on the following facts: (a) the potassium-depleting effect of gossypol on isolated heart can be reversed by Mg ion (148), which is a cofactor for Na-K-ATPase; (b) the effect of gossypol on K metabolism is apparent only in rats and men having a low-K intake (15, 149), and it is well known that Na-K-ATPase is more susceptible to specific inhibitors in a low-potassium environment (152).

The effect of gossypol on Na-K-ATPase activity has been investigated by several groups. Gossypol inhibited renal Na-K-ATPase activity in guinea pigs fed a relatively low K diet and in renal slices cultured in a low K medium; the addition of K to the diet or the medium could mitigate this inhibition (153). In rats, guinea pigs, rabbits, and monkeys fed regular diets, ordinary antifertility doses of gossypol did not significantly affect renal Na-K-ATPase activity (154–156; H. P. Lei, personal communication). When large doses were given to rats and guinea pigs, the enzyme was inhibited (156, 157), however. In guinea pigs, large doses of gossypol also inhibited the Na-K-ATPase activity of the skeletal muscle (157). Na-K-ATPase activity in rat brain synapses (158), in guinea-pig renal cortex (158a), and in spermatozoa of sea urchin (159) was inhibited by gossypol in vitro in a dose-dependent manner. Na-K-ATPase is the principal enzyme system responsible for the maintenance of a high intracellular K ion concentration (152). Inhibition of the activity of this enzyme will inevitably lead to a decrease in intracellular K content, renal K loss, and depletion of body K, all of which happened in hypokalemic patients administered gossypol (129, 145, 160). In gossypol-treated rats, the urinary excretion of (^{42}K) was increased in certain phases after administration of (^{42}K) (161). Recently, it has been shown that gossypol decreases the K ion concentration of spermatozoa (162).

Hypokalemia is a low-incidence side effect of gossypol administration. Most of the subjects taking gossypol do not show hypokalemia and the body K level of these subjects are normal (151). The production in animal models of low-incidence side effects is a very difficult problem in toxicology. As has been mentioned, attempts to produce hypokalemia were not successful in all the experimental animals tested. In rats, gossypol did not significantly affect the urinary and fecal excretion of K (149, 163), or the (^{42}K) distribution in tissues (161, 164), nor did it aggravate hypokalemia produced by deoxycorticosterone acetate (165). Plaa (166) stressed that, in the development of such low-incidence side effects, factors other than the drug may play a contributing role; if these factors are not operational, the effects can not be produced. K deficiency may be one of the contributing factors in gossypol-induced hypokalemia (15, 149). Recently, Wang et al (167) indicated that the in vitro inhibitory effect of gossypol on vas deferens, uterus, and ileum is exaggerated in a low K medium.

In the two cases of gossypol-induced chronic hypokalemia that occurred in Jiangsu, Qian (15) found that the urinary prostaglandin E_2-like substances (PGEL) was greatly increased, reaching 1599 and 2416 ng/24 hours respectively, more than 3- to 5-fold the normal value in his laboratory (168). In the case with higher urinary PGEL, potassium repletion for one month did not elevate the serum K level nor ameliorate the hypokalemic symptoms. Addition of indomethacin brought about a dramatic short-term therapeutic effect, with normalization of serum K and urinary PGEL levels (15). This finding strongly suggests the participation of prostaglandin in the development of chronic hypokalemia induced by gossypol. It has been known that prostaglandin of the E series increases urinary K excretion (169) and that K deficiency could enhance renal PGE and F biosynthesis (170). On the basis of these evidences, Qian postulated an explanation for the mechanism of development of chronic hypokalemia induced by gossypol treatment (15). Gossypol might initiate a sequence of events, including inhibition of Na-K-ATPase, leakage of intracellular K extracellularly, and renal loss of K, resulting in hypokalemia. K deficiency would augment the renal biosynthesis of PGE, which in turn would lead to a greater loss of K from the kidney. A vicious circle is thus formed. In this regard it is interesting to note that both PGE (171) and low extracellular K level (152) are inhibitory to Na-K-ATPase activity, and that gossypol itself may stimulate PG biosynthesis (15, 172). All these relationships may prompt the formation of a hypokalemia-causing cycle, as can be seen in Figure 2. The cycle, once established, seems to continue even after the withdrawal of the

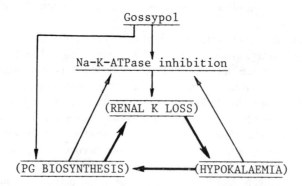

Figure 2   Possible mechanism for the development of chronic hypokalemia

causative factor. The addition of indomethacin to the cycle may block the PG biosynthesis link.

THE SITE AND MECHANISM OF ACTION

Several groups of researchers reported that, in the spermatogenic series, the cell types most sensitive to gossypol are the late spermatids and pachytene spermatocytes (17, 80, 112, 173–175). This view is consistent with the results of epididymal ligation experiments indicating that the target organ of gossypol action is the testis and not the epididymis (34). However, damage to epididymal spermatozoa (5, 176), testicular and epididymal spermatozoa, and epididymal epithelium (177) has been shown to be the earliest finding discernible after gossypol administration. Moreover, in young guinea pigs, gossypol interfered with the formation of the tight junction of Sertoli cells (178); in man and animal, gossypol might cause degenerative changes in Sertoli cells (112, 174, 179, 180). In gossypol-treated rats, one of the earliest signs of gossypol action is Sertoli cell damage, including vacuolization and breakage of tight junctions (177). In vitro studies indicated that gossypol causes marked morphological changes in Sertoli cells with decreased formation of androgen-binding protein (181). Therefore, the initial action of gossypol on these cellular sites should also be considered. In regard to the effect of gossypol on the Sertoli cells, it has been reported that gossypol does not affect the permeability of the blood-testis barrier in adult rats (182) and the protein synthesis of Sertoli cells (183).

Gossypol has long been known as an uncoupler of oxidative phosphorylation (1). It uncouples spermatozoal oxidative phosphorylation (184), first stimulates and then inhibits respiration (59, 185), and reduces ATP production (55, 184, 186, 187). In rats given (^{14}C) gossypol, the mitochondrial fraction of the testis homogenate revealed the highest radioactivity compared with other fractions (188). Among the cellular organelles of the spermatogenic cells, the earliest and most conspicuous damage caused by gossypol occurred in the mitochondria (17, 37, 80, 112, 133, 134, 145, 173, 176, 189–191). Therefore, Xue and his colleagues (17, 192) postulated that the mitochondria of spermatogenic cells may be the subcellular target of gossypol action. As indicated above, gossypol inhibits Na-K-ATPase and LDH-X activity. The former has been suggested as the molecular site of the gossypol effect causing hypokalemia (15, 148, 153) and the latter as the molecular site causing infertility (135, 136). Xue et al (192) noted that both of these enzymes are present in the mitochondria. Another mitochondrial enzyme, pyruvate dehydrogenase, is also inhibited by gossypol (159). However, Tso & Lee (162) indicated that, although gossypol lowers the K content of spermatozoa apparently as a consequence of the inhibition of membrane Na-K-ATPase activity, this inhibition does not seem to be the cause of decreased sperm motility.

Qian (15, 172) proposed that prostaglandins might participate in the antisper-matogenic mechanism of gossypol. This hypothesis is based on the following facts: (*a*) the antispermatogenic but not the toxic effect of gossypol can be reversed by aspirin, a prostaglandin synthetase inhibitor, and augmented by K deficiency (15, 193, 194); (*b*) in rats fed a normo- or low-K diet, gossypol increases the plasma, renal, and testicular PG levels (193; Y. Xu, S. Z. Qian, et al, unpublished data); (*c*) systemic administration of PGE damages similar cell types in rat testes, as does gossypol (195). In another report gossypol was shown to lower the plasma PGF_{2a} level but to leave the PGE level unaffected (196).

In regard to the antagonism of gossypol action, it may be worth mentioning that Smilax reverses the toxicity but not the antifertility effect of gossypol (197). Wang et al (167) suggested that the cyclic nucleotide system might participate in the mechanism of gossypol action. They indicated that gossypol increases the ratio of cAMP/cGMP, which is known to inhibit the motility, respiration, and metabolism of spermatozoa. Yu et al (198) indicated that the Zn content of atrophied testis and epididymis of gossypol-treated rat decreased and suggested that chelation of Zn by gossypol might be related to its antisper-matogenic activity. Kalla & Vasudev pointed out that gossypol does not affect the Zn content of human sperm (199).

Gossypol has been shown to interfere with the transition in the synthesis of nuclear histone from lysine-rich to arginine-rich ones in the late spermatid, as shown by Chen et al (200). These researchers believed that this inhibition of transition might play a role in the antispermatogenic mechanism of gossypol, as it is well known that the transition is indispensable to the fertility of spermato-zoa. Spermatozoal acrosin, proacrosin, LDH-X, NAD-isocitrate dehy-drogenase, succinyl-CoA synthetase, and fumarase are highly sensitive to gossypol; acrosin has the lowest inhibition threshold (201, 202). Gossypol also inhibits testicular ATPase (203) and testis-specific LDH-X (130, 135–139a) activity, inhibits the utilization of fructose by spermatozoa (204), and is cytotoxic in vitro (104). All these factors may participate in the mechanism of gossypol action.

Results are inconsistent concerning the effect of gossypol on DNA synthesis (46, 119, 205–208). Pathways involved in the metabolism of succinate have been shown to be more sensitive to gossypol than those of pyruvate and maleate, and the succinate-to-cytochrome C segment is the most sensitive in the chain. However, as this inhibition threshold is higher than either the uncoupling threshold or the concentration inhibiting sperm motility, the seg-ment might not be the main target of gossypol effect (209). In hamsters, substantial reduction in sperm population occurred before the suppression of serum T level (33), and in rabbits gossypol significantly lowered the serum T level while the animals remained fertile (31). Therefore, it has been suggested that the antifertility effect of gossypol does not seem to be mediated through its suppressive effect on testicular steroidogenesis.

Several miscellaneous effects of gossypol are worth mentioning, including:

1. Lengthening of pentobarbital sleeping time (210) and inhibition of glutathione-S-transferase activity (136), indicating a harmful influence on detoxification mechanisms.
2. Mitochondrial degeneration of the skeletal muscle (211, 211a), depression of catechol-O-methyltransferase activity (212), blocking of neuromuscular transmission, and lowering of the cholinergic responses in vitro (213–215). However, Wang et al (145) indicated that gossypol does not notably affect the vegetative nervous system.
3. Decrease of Ca absorption (216) and lowering of low-density lipoprotein level of blood (51, 217).
4. Interferon induction (218), antitumor, antimicrobial, and antiviral activities (1, 219, 220).

Gossypol does not appear to affect the function and morphology of the adrenal cortex (108, 221, 222). It was shown to inhibit the endometrial cells and has been used clinically for the treatment of functional bleeding, endometriosis, and leiomyoma with promising results (223–227).

CONCLUDING REMARKS

Gossypol is an effective antispermatogenic agent for certain susceptible animals and for humans. The source of the drug, the cotton plant, is abundant and the preparation inexpensive. Prasad & Diczfalusy (20) wrote: "The discovery of gossypol and the demonstration of its antifertility action mark an important milestone in the search for a new male antifertility agent. . . . For the present, gossypol represents the only approach which has a reasonable chance to reach the stage of large scale clinical testing before the end of this decade." These words appropriately reflect the views of most of the researchers in this field. However, quite a lot of work, particularly in regard to its toxicology, must be done before it (or one of its analogues) can be developed into a practical male antifertility drug. The following points appear to indicate the main directions for future research in the scope of pharmacology and toxicology.

1. Hypokalemia: exploration of the contributing factor(s), means to prevent its occurrence, mechanism(s) of development, production of animal model, etc.
2. Irreversibility: exploration of the contributing factor(s), measures to detect impending sterility, etc.
3. General toxicological assessment: effects on the endocrine system, liver, heart, and kidney; lifetime carcinogenicity studies, etc.
4. Studies on the mechanism(s) of action. These studies may also be helpful in the development of gossypol analogue(s) exhibiting satisfactory antifertility and minimal toxic effects.

ACKNOWLEDGMENTS

We are greatly indebted to Mmes. S.Q. Chen, Y. Xu, H. Q. Ying, and Z. R. Zhang, and Drs. J. H. Ding, X. H. Wang, and C. Q. Zhong for their assistance in the preparation of this manuscript.

Literature Cited

1. Abou-Donia, M. B. 1976. Physiological effects and metabolism of gossypol. *Residue Rev.* 61:124–59
2. Liu, B. S. 1957. A tentative idea of the use of cooking cottonseed oil for fertility control. *Shanghai J. Chin. Med.* 6:43–47
3. Hubei Provincial Epidemic Prevention Station. 1967. Prevention and treatment of "Hanchuan Fever" and "Xinzhou Paralysis". Restricted publication
4. Wu, X. R. 1972. *Study on the antifertility effect of cottonseed and gossypol.* Presented at 1st Natl. Conf. Male Antifertil. Agents, Sept., Wuhan
5. Wang, N. G., Lei, H. P. 1972. *Antifertility effect of gossypol acetic acid on male rats.* Presented at 1st Natl. Conf. Male Antifertil. Agents, Sept., Wuhan. Republished 1979 in *Natl. Med. J. China* 59:402–5
6. Dai, R. X., Pang, S. N., Lin, X. K., Ke, Y. B., Liu, Z. L., Dong, R. H. 1972. *A study of antifertility of cottonseed.* Presented at 1st Natl. Conf. Male Antifertil. Agents, Sept., Wuhan. Republished 1978 in *Acta Biol. Exp. Sinica* 11:1–10
7. Wang, Y. E., Luo, Y. D., Tang, X. C. 1972. *Studies on the antifertility action of cottonseed meal and gossypol.* Presented at 1st Natl. Conf. Male Antifertil. Agents, Sept., Wuhan. Republished 1979 in *Acta Pharm. Sinica* 14:662–69
8. Shandong Coord. Group Antifertil. Plants. 1972. *Animal screening of antifertility effective constituents of cottonseed.* Presented at 1st Natl. Conf. Male Antifertil. Agents, Sept., Wuhan
9. Zhang, Y. G., Shi, Q. X. 1972. *Antifertility effect of gossypol on male rats.* Presented at 1st Natl. Conf. Male Antifertil. Agents, Sept., Wuhan. Republished 1980 in *Zhejiang J. Med.* 2:56–57
10. Jiangsu Coord. Group Male Antifertil. Agents. 1972. *Antifertility effect of gossypol on male rats.* Presented at 1st Natl. Conf. Male Antifertil. Agents, Sept., Wuhan
11. Qian, S. Z., Hu, J. H., Ho, L. X., Sun, M. X., Huang, Y. Z., Fang, J. H. 1972. *The first clinical trial of gossypol on male antifertility.* Presented at 1st Natl. Conf. Male Antifertil. Agents, Sept., Wuhan. Republished 1980 in *Clinical Pharma-cology and Therapeutics,* ed. P. Turner, pp. 489–92. London: MacMillan. 576 pp.
12. Natl. Coord. Group Male Antifertil. Agents. 1978. Gossypol—A new male antifertility agent. *Chin. Med. J.* 91:417–28
13. Qian, S. Z. 1972. *The pharmacology and clinical application of gossypol.* Presented at 1st Natl. Conf. Male Antifertil. Agents, Sept., Wuhan
14. Qian, S. Z. 1975. *Effect of gossypol on the energy metabolism.* Presented at 4th Natl. Conf. Male Antifertil. Agents, Oct., Suzhou. Republished 1977 in *Acta Acad. Med. Wuhan* 1:71–74
15. Qian, S. Z. 1981. Effect of gossypol on potassium and prostaglandin metabolism and mechanism of action of gossypol. In *Recent Advances in Fertility Regulation,* ed. C. F. Chang, D. Griffin, A. Woolman, pp. 152–59. Geneva: Atar. 399 pp.
16. Qian, S. Z., Xu, Y. 1981. The effect of gossypol on potassium and prostaglandin metabolism. *Reprod. Contracep. China* 1:6–10
17. Xue, S. P. 1981. Studies on the antifertility effect of gossypol, a new contraceptive for males. See Ref. 15, pp. 122–46
18. Liu, Z. Q., Liu, G. Z., Hei, L. S., Zhang, R. A., Yu, C. Z. 1981. Clinical trial of gossypol as a male antifertility agent. See Ref. 15, pp. 160–63
19. Ying, H. Q. 1981. The isomerism of gossypol. *Reprod. Contracep. China* 4:8–13
20. Prasad, M. R. N., Diczfalusy, E. 1982. Gossypol. *Int. J. Androl. Suppl.* 5:53–70
21. Lei, H. P. 1982. Review and prospect of gossypol research. *Acta Pharm. Sinica* 17:1–4
21a. Lei, H. P. 1983. Prospect of gossypol as a pill for males. *Acta Pharm. Sinica* 18:321–24
22. Gu, Z. P. 1983. A glimpse of studies of gossypol in foreign countries. *Reprod. Contracep. China* 1:8–10
23. Edwards, J. D. Jr. 1958. Total synthesis of gossypol. *J. Am. Chem. Soc.* 80:3798–99
24. Adams, R., Geissman, T. A. 1960. Gossypol, a pigment of cottonseed. *Chem. Rev.* 60:555–74
25. Baram, N. I., Ismailov, A. I., Kamaev,

F. G., Leont'ev, V. B. 1976. NMR spectroscopic study of different samples of gossypol. *Khim. Prir. Soedin.* 2:249–52

26. King, T. J., de Silva, L. B. 1968. Optically active gossypol from Thespesia populnea. *Tetrahedron Lett.* 3:261–63

27. Dechary, J. M., Pradel, P. 1971. The occurrence of (+)−gossypol in Gossypium species. *J. Am. Oil Chem. Soc.* 48:563–64

27a. Si, Y. K., Zhou, J., Huang, L. 1983. Resolution of racemic gossypol. *Bull Sci. China* 28:640

28. Sang, G. W., Zhang, Y. G., Shi, Q. X., Shen, K. Y., Lu, F. Y., Zhao, X. J., Wang, M. Q., Liu, X. L., Yuan, Y. Y. 1980. Chronic toxicity of gossypol and the relationship to its metabolic fate in dogs and monkeys. *Acta Pharmacol. Sinica* 1:39–43

29. Chang, M. C., Gu, Z. P., Saksena, S. K. 1980. Effect of gossypol on the fertility of male rats, hamsters and rabbits. *Contraception* 21:461–69

30. Hahn, D. W., Rusticus, C., Homn, R., Johnson, A. N. 1981. Antifertility and endocrine activities of gossypol in rodents. *Contraception* 24:97–105

31. Saksena, S. K., Salmonsen, R., Lau, I. F., Chang, M. C. 1981. Gossypol: Its toxicological and endocrinological effects in male rabbits. *Contraception* 24:203–14

32. Waller, D. P., Fong, H. H. S., Cordell, G. F., Soejarto, D. D. 1981. Antifertility effects of gossypol and its impurities on male hamsters. *Contraception* 23:653–60

33. Saksena, S. K., Salmonsen, R. A. 1982. Antifertility effects of gossypol in male hamster. *Fertil. Steril.* 37:686–90

34. Dai, R. X., Dong, R. H. 1973. *Studies on the antifertility effect of gossypol. I. An experimental analysis by epididymal ligature.* Presented at 2nd Natl. Conf. Male Antifertil. Agents, Aug., Qingdao. Republished 1978 in *Acta Biol. Exp. Sinica* 11:15–22

35. Shandong Coord. Group Antifertil. Plants. 1973. *Studies on the antifertility effect of gossypol on male rats.* Presented at 2nd Natl. Conf. Male Antifertil. Agents, Aug., Qingdao

36. Yuan, J. Y. 1979. Gossypol formic acid, a male contraceptive. *J. Shandong Med. Drug* 2:36–37

37. Nadakavukaren, M. J., Sorensen, R. H., Tone, J. N. 1979. Effect of gossypol on the ultrastructure of rat spermatozoa. *Cell. Tissue Res.* 204:293–96

38. Weinbauer, G. F., Rovan, E., Frick, J. 1982. Antifertility efficacy of gossypol

acetic acid in male rats. *Andrologia* 14:270–75

39. Shi, Q. X., Zhang, Y. G., Yuan, Y. Y. 1981. Studies on the antifertility effect of gossypol. II. Effect on spermatogenesis in rats. *Acta Zool. Sinica* 27:22–28

40. Hoshiai, H., Uehara, S., Nagaike, F., Momono, K., Mori, R., Suzuki, M., Lin, Y. C. 1981. Action mechanism of gossypol on rats as male contraceptive agent: *In vivo* study. *Jpn. J. Fertil. Steril.* 26:35–39

41. Hadley, M. A., Lin, Y. C., Dym, M. 1981. Effect of gossypol on the reproductive system of male rats. *J. Androl.* 2:190–99

42. Chang, C. C., Gu, Z. P., Tsong, Y. Y. 1982. Studies on gossypol. I. Toxicity, antifertility, and endocrine analysis in male rats. *Intl. J. Fertil.* 27:213–18

43. Kalla, N. R., Foo, T. W. J., Sheth, A. R. 1982. Studies on the male antifertility agent gossypol acetic acid. V. Effect on the fertility of male rats. *Andrologia* 14:492–500

44. Zhejiang Acad. Med. Sci. 1975. *In vitro spermicidal action of gossypol.* Presented at 4th Natl. Conf. Male Antifertil. Agents, Oct., Suzhou

45. Bartin, C. W., Sundaram, K. S., Chang, C. C. 1980. *Toxicology, endocrine and histopathologic studies in small animals and Rhesus monkeys administered gossypol.* Presented at PARFR Workshop on Gossypol, March, Chicago

46. Kalla, N. R., Vasudev, M., Arora, G. 1981. Studies on the male antifertility agent gossypol acetic acid. III. Effect on rat testis. *Andrologia* 13:242–49

47. Zhou, L. F., Lei, H. P. 1981. Recovery of fertility in rats after gossypol treatment. See Ref. 15, pp. 147–51

48. Dai, R. X., Pan, S. Y. 1980. Studies on the antifertility effect of gossypol. VI. Observations of testicular atrophy of rats administered gossypol for long terms. *Acta Exp. Biol. Sinica* 13:192–99

49. Jiangsu Coord. Group Male Antifertil. Agents. 1972. *Studies on the repeated-dose toxicity of gossypol in dogs.* Presented at 1st Natl. Conf. Male Antifertil. Agents, Sept., Wuhan

50. Shi, Q. X., Zhang, Y. G. 1980. Studies on antifertility effect of gossypol. I. Effect of gossypol on androgen-dependent organs. *Acta Zool. Sinica* 26:311–16

51. Shandilya, L. H., Clarkson, T. B., Adams, M. R., Lewis, J. C. 1982. Effect of gossypol on reproductive and endocrine functions of male cynomolgus monkey. *Biol. Reprod.* 27:241–52

52. Yao, X. Y., 1981. Studies on the isola-

tion and the antifertility effect of
(+)−gossypol. *Reprod. Contracep. China* 2:51–52

52a. Waller, D. P., Bunyapraphatsara, N., Martin, A., Vournazos, C. J., Ahmed, M. S., Soejarto, D. D., Cordell, G. A., Fong, H. H. S. 1983. Effect of (+)−gossypol on fertility in male hamsters. *J. Androl.* In press

53. Murthy, R. S. R., Basu, D. K., Murti, V. V. S. 1981. Antifertility effect of (+)−gossypol. *Curr. Sci.* 50:64–66

54. Yuan, Q. X., Gao, D. W., Li, C. Z. 1983. Effects of gossypol on the implantation of female rats and its possible mechanism. *Reprod. Contracep. China* 2:25–30

55. Kalla, N. R., Vasudev, M. 1980. Studies on the male antifertility agent gossypol acetic acid, *in vitro* study on the effect on human spermatozoa. *IRCS Med. Sci.: Libr. Compend.* 8:375–76

56. Burgos, M. H., Chang, C. Y., Nelson, L., Segal, S. J. 1980. Gossypol inhibits motility of Arbacia sperm. *Biol. Bull.* 159:467–68

57. Waller, D. P., Zaneveld, L. J. D., Fong, H. H. S. 1980. In vitro spermicidal activity of gossypol. *Contraception* 22:183–87

58. Ridley, A. J., Blasco, L. 1981. Testosterone and gossypol effects on human sperm motility. *Fertil. Steril. Suppl.* 35:244

59. Tso, W. W., Lee, C. S. 1981. Effect of gossypol on boar spermatozoa in vitro. *Arch. Androl.* 7:85–88

59a. Tso, W. W., Lee, C. S. 1982. Cottonseed oil as a vaginal contraceptive. *Arch. Androl.* 8:11–14

60. Williams, W. L. 1980. New antifertility agents active in rabbit vaginal contraception method. *Contraception* 22:659–72

61. Cameron, S. M., Waller, D. P., Zaneveld, L. J. D. 1982. Vaginal spermicidal activity of gossypol in Macaca arctoides. *Fertil Steril.* 37:273–74

61a. Aitken, R. J., Liu, J., Best, F. S. M., Richardson, D. W. 1983. Analysis of the direct effect of gossypol on human spermatozoa. *Int. J. Androl.* 6:157–67

62. Hadley, M. A., Burgos, M. H. 1981. *Inhibition of rat epididymal sperm by gossypol.* Presented at NY Acad. Sci. Meet. Cell Biol. Testis, April

63. Yu, Z. H. 1982. Spermatocidal action of some fat-soluble chelating agents in pouch of cauda epididymides in rats. *Acta Pharmacol. Sinica* 3:260–63

64. Abou-Donia, M. B., Lyman, C. M., Dieckert, J. W. 1970. Metabolic fate of

gossypol: The metabolism of gossypol-^{14}C in rats. *Lipids* 5:938–46

65. Lyman, C. M., Cronin, J. T., Trant, M. M., Odell, G. V. 1969. Metabolism of gossypol in the chick. *J. Am. Oil Chem. Soc.* 46:100–4

66. Abou-Donia, M. B., Lyman, C. M. 1970. Metabolic fate of gossypol: The metabolism of [^{14}C] gossypol in laying hens. *Toxicol. Appl. Pharmacol.* 17:160–73

67. Albrecht, J. E., Clawson, A. J., Smith, F. H. 1972. Rate of depletion and route of elimination of intravenously injected gossypol in swine. *J. Animal Sci.* 35:941–46

68. Abou-Donia, M. B., Dieckert, J. W. 1974. Urinary and biliary excretion of (^{14}C) gossypol in swine. *J. Nutr.* 104:754–60

69. Abou-Donia, M. B., Dieckert, J. W. 1975. Metabolic fate of gossypol: The metabolism of (^{14}C) gossypol in swine. *Toxicol. Appl. Pharmacol.* 31:32–46

70. Xue, S. P., Zhou, Z. H., Liu, Y., Wu, Y. W., Zong, S. D. 1975. *The pharmacokinetics of (^{14}C) gossypol acetic acid in rats. I. Whole body and microautoradiographic studies on the distribution and fate of (^{14}C) gossypol in rat body.* Presented at 4th Natl. Conf. Male Antifertil. Agents, Oct., Suzhou. Republished 1979 in *Acta Biol. Exp. Sinica* 12:179–94

71. Xue, S. P., Liu, Y., Fei, R. R., Han, S. M., Su, S. Y. 1975. *The pharmacokinetics of (^{14}C) gossypol acetic acid in rats. II. Quantitative studies on the kinetics of distribution, excretion and metabolism of (^{14}C) gossypol acetic acid in rat body.* Presented at 4th Natl. Conf. Male Antifertil. Agents, Oct., Suzhou. Republished 1979 in *Acta Biol. Exp. Sinica* 12:275–87

72. Wang, N. G., Li, G. X., Chen, Q. Q., Lei, H. P. 1973. *The metabolism of gossypol in vivo.* Presented at 2nd Natl. Conf. Male Antifertil. Agents, Aug., Qingdao. Republished 1979 in *Natl. Med. J. China* 59:596–99

73. Tang, X. C., Zhu, M. K., Shi, Q. X. 1980. Comparative study on the absorption, distribution and excretion of (^{14}C) gossypol in four species of animals. *Acta Pharm. Sinica* 15:212–17

74. Skutches, C. L., Smith, F. H. 1974. Metabolism of gossypol, biosynthesized from methyl (^{14}C)- and carbosyl (^{14}C)-labeled sodium acetate in rat. *J. Am. Oil Chem. Soc.* 51:413–15

75. Jensen, D. R., Tone, J. N., Sorensen, R. H., Bozek, S. A. 1982. Deposited pat-

tern of the antifertility agent, gossypol, in selected organs of male rats. *Toxicology* 24:65–72

76. Shi, C. Z., Ding, W. P., Yu, M. Q., Wu, X. R. 1981. Preparation, antifertility effect and toxicity of Mg-gossypol. *Acta Acad. Med. Wuhan* 4:6

77. Wu, Y. M., Chappel, S. C., Flickinger, G. L. 1981. Effect of gossypol on pituitary-ovarian endocrine function, ovulation and fertility in female hamster. *Contraception* 24:259–68

78. Zhou, L. F., Chen, Q. Q., Wang, N. G., Lei, H. P. 1975. *Observation on the effect of prolonged administration of gossypol acetic acid to rats*. Presented at 4th Natl. Conf. Male Antifertil. Agents, Oct., Suzhou. Republished 1980 in *Natl. Med. J. China* 60:343–44

79. Zhou, L. F., Lei, H. P., Gao, Y., Liu, Y., Wang, N. Y., Guo, Y. 1982. Further observation on the effect of prolonged administration of gossypol acetic acid to rats. *Acta Pharm. Sinica* 17:245–52

80. Xue, S. P., Zong, S. D., Su, S. Y., Wu, Y. W., Lin, Y., Zhou, Z. H., Ma, X. X. 1973. *Antifertility effect of gossypol on the germinal epithelium of the rat testis. A cytological, autoradiographical and ultrastructural observation*. Presented at 2nd Natl. Conf. Male Antifertil. Agents, Aug., Qingdao. Republished 1980 in *Sci. Sinica* 23:642–57

81. Shandong Coord. Group Male Antifertil. Plants. 1973. *Repeated-dose toxicity of gossypol in rabbits*. Presented at 2nd Natl. Conf. Male Antifertil. Agents, Aug., Qingdao

82. Inst. Materia Medica, Chinese Acad. Med. Sci. 1973. *Repeated-dose toxicity of gossypol in dogs*. Presented at 2nd Natl. Conf. Male Antifertil. Agents, Aug., Qingdao

83. Shi, Q. X., Zhang, Y. G., Sang, G. Y., Wang, M. Q., Shen, K. Y., Lu, F. Y. 1979. Effect of long-term administration of gossypol on the potassium metabolism and renal function of rhesus monkey. *Bull. Pharm. Sinica* 14:89–90

84. Feng, Z. Q. 1980. *Electronmicroscopic observation on the effect of long-term administration of gossypol on the structure of liver in rhesus monkey*. Presented at Ann. Meet. Chin. Anat. Soc., Chengdu

85. Liu, Y., Su, S. Y., Chen, X. M., Xue, S. P. 1980. Electronmicroscopic observation on the ultrastructure and histochemical changes of LDH and SDH of cardiac muscle in male monkeys. *Acta Anat. Sinica* 11:428–32

85a. Zhuang, Y. Z., Xu, M. Y., Zhao, X. J.,

Liu, Y., Su, S. Y. 1981. Electronmicroscopic observation of the effect of gossypol on the liver and kidney of rhesus monkey. *Zhejiang J. Med.* 1:27

86. Feng, Z. Q. 1982. *Electronmicroscopic observation on the effect of long-term administration of gossypol on the structure of kidney in monkey*. Presented at Ann. Meet. Chin. Anat. Soc., Guilin

87. Zhang, Z. S., Pan, X. X., Wang, M. M., Yao, Y. L. 1979. Dominant lethal mutagenic effect of gossypol in male rat. *Med. Industry* 7:20–22

88. Tan, Y. B., Zheng, H. Z., Zhang, Z. S., Wang, M. M., Yao, Y. L. 1982. Embryotoxicity and teratogenicity of gossypol acetic acid. Restricted publication

89. de Peyster, A., Wang, Y. Y. 1979. Gossypol, proposed contraceptive for men passes the Ames test. *N. Engl. J. Med.* 301:275–76

90. Colman, N., Gardner, A., Herbert, V. 1979. Non-mutagenicity of gossypol in the Salmonella mammalian-microsome plate assay. *Environ. Mutagen* 1:315–20

91. Wuhan Med. College. 1980. Assaying of mutagenicity of gossypol by Ames test. *Acta Acad. Med. Wuhan* 1:87

92. Li, C. B., Ding, F., Ma, Z. R., Zhao, S. Y. 1981. Determination of the genetic safety of gossypol by Ames test and SCE frequency. *Acta Fu Dan Univer.* 20:361–65

93. Zhang, H. J., Wei, Z. W., Zhu, Y. Z. 1982. Determination of the mutagenicity of gossypol by Ames test. Restricted publication

94. Majumdar, S. K., Thatcher, J. D., Dennis, E. H., Cutrone, A., Slockage, M., Hammond, M. 1982. Mutagenic evaluation of two male contraceptives: 5-thio-D-glucose and gossypol acetic acid. *J. Hered.* 73:76–77

95. Haroz, R. K., Thomasson, J. 1980. Tumor initiating and promoting activity of gossypol. *Toxicol. Lett. Suppl.* 6:72

96. Lei, S. P., Xu, S. W., Wang, Y. C. 1980. Effect of gossypol acetic acid on SCE of Chinese hamster ovary K-1 cell. *Acta Biol. Exp. Sinica* 13:426

97. Zhang, Z. S., Zheng, H. Z., Ding, Y. N., Jiang, X. R. 1982. In vitro effect of gossypol acetic acid on human lymphocyte SCE. Restricted publication

98. Zhang, Z. S., Pan, X. X., Wang, M. M., Yao, Y. L. 1981. Genetic studies on gossypol. I. Comparative study of the cytogenetic effects of gossypol acetic acid on male germ cell and lymphocytes in rats. *Reprod. Contracep. China* 1:33–36

356   QIAN & WANG

99. Zhang, Z. S., Wang, M. M., Zheng, H. Z., Tan, Y. B., Lu, Q., Yao, Y. L., Jiang, X. R., Wang, R. L. 1981. Genetic studies on gossypol. II. The effect of gossypol acetic acid on sister chromatid exchange in mouse. *Reprod. Contracep. China* 2:42–44

100. Zhuo, J. M., Lu, Q. J., Jiang, S. H. 1982. Effect of gossypol on germ cell chromosomes in mice. *Reprod. Contracep. China* 3:49–52

101. Wang, R. L., Wang, M. M., Lu, Q., Zheng, H. Z., Yao, Y. L., Jiang, X. R., Zhang, Z. S. 1982. Genetic studies on gossypol. III. Mutagenic effect of gossypol acetic acid on SCE of mice spermatogonia. Restricted publication

102. Yang, Y. H., Shieh, S. P. 1982. Studies on the gossypol effect on chromosome aberration and SCE in mice. *Acta Anat. Sinica* 13:215–20

103. Cai, Y. Y., Liu, Y., Xu, G. L., Shieh, S. P. 1981. Effect of gossypol on frequency of chromosomal aberration and SCE in human peripheral lymphocyte in vitro. *Acta Anat. Sinica* 12:293–98

104. Ye, W. S., Liang, J. C., Hsu, T. C. 1983. Toxicity of a male contraceptive, gossypol, in mammalian tissue. *In Vitro* 19:53–57

105. Zhang, Z. S., Lu, Q., Tan, Y. B., Jiang, X. R., Zheng, H. Z., Wang, M. M., Yao, Y. L. 1983. SCE and micronucleus test in subjects taking gossypol formic acid. *Acta Genet. Sinica* 10:157–60

106. Zhang, Z. S., Lu, Q., Tan, Y. B., Jiang, X. R., Zheng, W. Z., Wang, R. L. 1983. Chromosome aberration studies in gossypol formic acid users. *Reprod. Contracep. China* 1:56–57

107. Huang, T. H., Fan, Y. S., Chen, L. F., Li, P., Miao, Y. S., Li, C. C. 1983. Effect of gossypol acetic acid on function of rRNA and acrocentric chromosome association in human cells. *Natl. Med. J. China* 63:97–100

108. Yuan, D. X., Liu, X. Y., Gao, Y. H., Wang, J. Y., Fu, Z. L. 1980. Histochemical observations on pituitary, adrenal cortex and hypothalamus in rats after gossypol administration. *Acta Anat. Sinica* 11:331–36

109. Ye, S. J., You, M. M., Shieh, S. P. 1982. Ultrastructural observations on the gonadotrophic cells of adenohypophysis and Leydig cell in gossypol treated rats. *Acta Anat. Sinica* 13:206–10

110. Zhou, J. Y., Zhung, Y., Zhang, S. X., Bo, A. H., Han, S. Q. 1981. A histological study on the effect of gossypol on anterior lobe of pituitary of castrated hogs. *Acta Anat. Sinica* 12:101–6

111. Luo, Y., Dong, Z. Q., Feng, Y. Z. 1980. Effect of gossypol acetic acid on histology of human testis. *Chin. J. Urol.* 1:198–99

112. Hoffer, A. P. 1982. Ultrastructural studies of the seminiferous and epididymal epithelium and epididymal sperm in rats treated with gossypol. *Arch. Androl* 9:35

113. Wang, Y. F., Wu, M. Z., Wang, Z. X., Gu, D. Q., Gu, J. Z., Wu, Q. H. 1982. Quantitative histological investigation of testes from normal adults and men infertile after taking raw cottonseed oil. *Reprod. Contracep. China* 24:31–34

113a. Liang, S. X., Pang, S. N., Dong, R. H., Dai, R. X. 1981. Radioimmunoassay of serum T and LH in male rats administered gossypol. *Acta Biol. Exp. Sinica* 14:191–97

114. Lin, Y. C., Hadley, M. A., Llingener, D., Dym, M. 1980. Effect of gossypol on the reproductive system of male rats. *Biol. Reprod.* 22(Suppl. 1):95A

115. Lin, T., Murono, E. P., Osterman, J., Nankin, H. R., Ciulson, P. B. 1981. Gossypol inhibits testicular steroidogenesis. *Fertil. Steril.* 35:563–66

116. Hoshiai, H., Uehara, S., Nagaike, F., Momono, K., Hoshi, K., Suzuki, M. 1982. Action mechanism of gossypol as a male contraceptive agent: In vitro study on Leydig cell of rat. *Jpn. J. Fertil. Steril.* 27:156–60

117. Zhuang, L. Z. 1981. Effect of gossypol on the growth and function of Leydig and Sertoli cells in culture. *Biol. Reprod.* 24(Suppl. 1):229

118. Qian, S. Z., Xu, Y., Zhang, X. L. 1974. *Effect of gossypol on the isolated rabbit heart.* Presented at 3rd Natl. Conf. Male Antifert. Agents, Feb., Beijing

119. Wang, T. G. 1979. *Some pharmacological studies on gossypol.* Presented at the Int. Coop. Contraceptive Res. (ICCR), Population Council, May, New York

120. Wang, H. Y., Xu, Y. S., Jiang, L. G., De, S. L., Shi, Y. Q., Zhou, Z. M. 1979. Effect of sex steroid hormone and gossypol on LH secretion of rat pituitary by RIA. *Acta Physiol. Sinica* 31:337–42

121. Coutinho, E. M. 1982. Clinical studies with gossypol. *Arch. Androl.* 9:37–38

122. Zhang, G. Y., Zhou, X. Y., Gao, S. M., Guo, Z. S., Liu, G. Z., Cao, J. 1983. Comparison of changes of serum gonadotropins and steroid hormones in azoospermic men caused by gossypol and other factors. *Reprod. Contracep. China* 2:31–35

123. Bressani, R., Aguifre, A., Scrimshaw, N. S. 1959. All vegetable protein mixture

for human feeding. *J. Nutr.* 65:351–55

124. Bydagyan, F. E., Vladimirev, B. D., Levitskii, L M., Shchurov, K. A. 1947. Influence of prolonged consumption of small amount of cottonseed meal on the human organism. *Gigiena Sanit.* 7:28–33

125. Cook, E. F., Martin, E. W. 1948. *Reminton's Practice of Pharmacy*, p. 798. Mack

126. Erynimov, L. C. 1966. Treatment of tumor of urinary bladder with gossypol and ionol in combination with surgery. *Vop. Onkol.* 2:29–35

127. Harper, G. A., Smith, K. J. 1968. Status of cottonseed protein. *Econ. Bot.* 22:63–72

128. Beradi, L. C., Goldblatt, L. A. 1969. Gossypol. In *Toxic Constituent of Plant Foodstuff*, ed. I. E. Liener, pp. 211. New York: Academic. 500 pp.

129. Qian, S. Z., Jing, G. W., Wu, X. Y., Xu, Y., Li, Y. Q., Zhou, Z. H. 1977. *Gossypol-related hypokalaemia, clinicopharmacologic studies*. Presented at 5th Natl. Conf. Male Antifertil. Agents, Aug., Qinhuangdao. Republished 1980 in *Chin. Med. J.* 93:477–82

130. Chen, X. M., Li, H. Y. 1978. *Effect of gossypol on LDH-X of human spermatozoa.* Proc. Ann. Meet. Chin. Anat. Soc., Guilin, p. 127

131. Zong, S. D. 1977. *Studies on the exfoliated cells in semen of men taking gossypol.* Presented at 5th Natl. Conf. Male Antifertil. Agents, Aug., Qinhuangdao. Republished 1979 in *Med. Res. Commu.* 2:24

132. Shi, Q. X., Qiu, J. X., Zhang, G. Y. 1981. Analysis on exfoliated cells in human semen after oral administration of gossypol acetic acid. *Acta Pharmacol. Sinica* 2:262–66

133. Tung, S. M., Zhou, X. H., Zhou, Y. X. 1980. Studies on antifertility effect of gossypol: Cytological observation of human semen. *Acta Acad. Med. Prim. Shanghai* 7:19–26

134. Shao, T. S., Zhang, B. C., Ye, W. S., You, M. M. 1982. Cytological, cytochemical and ultrastructural observation on the human sperm following gossypol administration. *Acta Anat. Sinica* 13:201–5

135. Lee, C. Y., Malling, H. V. 1981. Selective inhibition of sperm-specific LDH-X by an antifertility agent, gossypol. *Fed Proc.* 40:718

136. Maugh, T. H. II. 1981. Male "pill" blocks sperm enzyme. *Science* 212:314

137. Tso, W. W., Lee, C. S. 1982. LDH-X: An isoenzyme particularly sensitive to

gossypol inhibition. *Int. J. Androl.* 5:205–9

138. Lee, C. Y. G., Moon, Y. S., Gomel, V. 1982. Inactivation of LDH-X by gossypol. *Arch. Androl.* 9:34–35

138a. Giridharan, N., Bamji, M. S., Sankaram, A. V. B. 1982. Inhibition of rat testis LDH-X by gossypol. *Contraception* 26:607–15

139. Lee, C. Y. G., Moon, Y. S., Yuan, J. H., Chen, A. F. 1982. Enzyme inactivation and inhibition by gossypol. *Mol. Cell. Biochem.* 47:65–70

139a. Eliasson, R., Virji, N. 1983. Effect of gossypol acetic acid on the activity of LDH-C₄ from human and rabbit spermatozoa. *Int. J. Androl.* 6:109–12

140. Xie, W. Y., Ni, Y. X., Jiang, Y., Wang, Y. X., Wu, Y. L. 1981. Observation on sperm immunity to gossypol. *Reprod. Contracep. China* 4:35–37

141. Shandong Coord. Group Antifert. Plants. 1975. *Preliminary report on the experimental study and clinical trial of gossypol formic acid.* Presented at 4th Natl. Conf. Male Antifert. Agents, Oct., Suzhou

142. Shandong Coord. Group Antifert. Plants. 1977. *A concluding report on the clinical trial of gossypol for male fertility control, 1312 cases.* Presented at 5th Natl. Conf. Male Antifert. Agents, Aug., Qinhuangdao

143. Liu, G. Z. 1982. Double-blind study of gossypol: The loading phase. *Arch. Androl.* 9:38–39

144. Lyle, K. C. 1982. Controlled clinical trial of gossypol: Methodological considerations. *Arch. Androl.* 9:38

145. Wang, Z. G., Zhou, Z. M., Shi, Y. Q., Liu, J. S., Li, Y. M. 1975. Preliminary report on the clinical trial of gossypol in peasants. Restricted publication

146. Frick, J., Danner, C., Köhle, R., Kunit, G. 1981. Male fertility regulation. In *Research on Fertility and Sterility*, ed. J. Cotes-Prieto, A. Campos-da-Pas, M. Neves-e-Castro, pp. 291. Lancaster: MTP. 456 pp.

147. Kjerulf-Jensen, K., Krarup, N. B., Warming-Larsen, A. 1951. Persistent hypokalaemia requiring constant K therapy. *Lancet* 260:372–75

148. Qian, S. Z., Xu, Y., Jing, G. W. 1975. *The K-depleting effect of gossypol on isolated rabbit heart and its possible mechanism.* Presented at 4th Natl. Conf. Male Antifert. Agents, Oct., Suzhou. Republished 1979 in *Acta Pharm. Sinica* 14:116–19

149. Qian, S. Z., Xu, Y., Chen, Z. C., Cao, L. M., Sun, S. G., Tang, X. C., Wang,

Y. E., Shen, L. Y., Zhu, M. K. 1977. *Influence of gossypol on the K metabolism of rats and effect of some possible contributing factors (low-K and low-Mg intake)*. Presented at 5th Natl. Conf. Male Antifert. Agents, Aug., Qinhuangdao. Republished 1979 in *Acta Pharm. Sinica* 14:513–20

150. Xu, Y., Qian, S. Z. 1981. The influence of gossypol on the potassium content of isolated skeletal muscle. *Bull. Pharm. Sinica* 16:78

151. Kuming Med. College 1st Hospital. 1981. K balance study on subjects taking gossypol acetic acid. *Chin. J. Urol.* 2:143–44

152. Schwartz, A., Lindenmayer, G. E., Allen, J. C. 1975. Na-K-ATPase, pharmacological, physiological and biochemical aspects. *Pharmacol. Rev.* 27:1–134

153. Bi, X. F., Zheng, Y. J., Yang, H. F., Zhang, Z. Y. 1980. Effect of gossypol on renal Na-K-ATPase activity. *Sci. Sinica* 9:914–19

154. Fu, Y. F., Zhao, R. S., Liu, J. G. 1979. Effect of gossypol acetic acid on renal Na-K-ATPase activity of rabbit and rat. *Nature China* 2:724–25

155. Wu, Y. W., Wang, N. Y., Tong, D. S., Shieh, S. P. 1981. Ultra-cytochemical observations on the effect of gossypol on renal Na-K-ATPase of rat and guinea pig. *Acta Anat. Sinica* 12:289–92

156. Fei, R. R., Liang, D. C., Gao, Y., Liu, Y., Guo, X. Y., Zhou, Z. H., Xue, S. P. 1982. Gossypol effect on the activity of renal cell membrane Na-K-ATPase of rats and guinea pigs. *Reprod. Contracep. China* 1:42–45

157. Su, S. Y., Liu, Y., Zhou, Z. H., Shieh, S. P., Zhao, X. J., Xu, M. Y., Zhuang, Y. Z. 1982. Relationship between gossypol administration and activity of Na-K-ATPase in animal. *Acta Anat. Sinica* 13:85–91

158. Feng, B. Y., Xu, M. Y. 1982. Effect of gossypol on the ATPase activity of the brain synapses. *Bull. Sci. Sinica* 17:1072–75

158a. Ye, Y. X., Zheng, Y. J., Yang, H. F. 1983. Effect of gossypol on ATPase activity and (³H)-ouabain binding in kidney cortex membranes. *Chin. J. Nucl. Med.* 3:38–41

159. Adeyemo, O., Chang, Y. C., Segal, S. J., Koide, S. S. 1982. Gossypol action on the production and utilization of ATP in sea urchin spermatozoa. *Arch. Androl.* 9:343–49

160. Bi, X. F., Ye, Y. X., Yang, H. F., Zhang, Z. R. 1981. Preliminary study on

gossypol in causing hypokalaemia. *Acta Acad. Med. Sinica* 3:175–78

161. Xue, S. P., Liang, D. C., Shao, T. S., Wu, Y. W., Liu, Y., Zhou, Z. H., Wang, N. Y. 1979. Studies on the effect of gossypol on (⁴²K) metabolism of rat. *Acta Anat. Sinica* 10:78–87

162. Tso, W. W., Lee, C. S. 1982. K leakage: Not the cause of gossypol induced antimotility in spermatozoa. *Int. J. Androl. Suppl.* 5:53–70

163. Sun, Y. B., Chen, Q. Q., Wang, Y., Su, M. 1982. Effect of gossypol on K excretion of male rat. *Acta Acad. Med. Sinica* 4:126–27

164. Wang, Z. G., Zhou, Z. M., Shi, Y. Q., Liu, J. S., Li, Y. M. 1975. Effect of gossypol on the distribution of [⁴²K] in rats. Restricted publication

165. Yu, T. H., Zhang, X. D., Wang, Z. H. 1981. Gossypol did not affect the hypokalaemia by DOCA in rat. *Reprod. Contracep. China* 2:39–41

166. Plaa, G. L. 1978. The problem of low-incidence response. In *Proc. 1st Int. Congr. Toxicol*, ed. G. L. Plaa, W. A. M. Duncan, pp. 207–19. New York: Academic. 670 pp.

167. Wang, Z. G., Gao, H. Q., Hu, A. Z., Wu, T., Zhang, Z. R., Li, Y. M., Shen, R. G. 1983. Studies on the mechanism of gossypol action. *Bull. Sci. China*. In press

168. Cheng, D. D., Li, Y. Q., Ye, G. C., Qian, S. Z. 1981. A simplified method for solvent extraction of PGE₂-like substances from human urine. *Reprod. Contracep. China* 2:57–59

169. Shea-Donohni, P. T., Bolger, P. M., Eisner, G. M., Slotkoff, L. M. 1979. Effect of PGE₂ on electrolyte and fluid excretion: Evidence of direct tubular effect. *Can. J. Physiol. Pharmacol.* 57:1448–52

170. Düsing, R., Attallah, A. A., Presyna, A. P., Lee, J. B. 1978. Renal biosynthesis of PGE₂ and F₂ₐ, dependence on extracellular potassium. *J. Lab. Clin. Med.* 92:669–72

171. Mozsik, G., Kutas, J., Nagy, L., Nemeth, G. 1974. Inhibition of Na-K-ATPase system from human gastric mucosa by PGE₁ and PGE₂. *Eur. J. Pharmacol.* 29:133–37

172. Qian, S. Z. 1982. Participation of prostaglandin in the mechanism of action of gossypol. *Arch. Androl.* 9:36–37

173. Dai, R. X., Pan, S. N., Liu, Z. L. 1975. *Studies on the antifertility effect of gossypol. II. A morphological analysis of the antifertility effect of gossypol.* Presented at 4th Natl. Conf. Male Antifert. Agents,

Oct., Suzhou. Republished 1978 in *Acta Biol. Exp. Sinica* 11:27–30

174. Hei, L. S., Cai, G. Z., Ying, G. H., Lei, J. Z. 1981. Electronmicroscopic observation of the effect of gossypol on spermatogenesis in cancer patients. *Natl. Med. J. China* 61:527–29

175. Ye, W. S., Lin, T. S., Liu, Z. H., You, M. M., Guo, Y. 1982. Effect of gossypol on protein and nucleic acid synthesis in spermatogenic cells of rat in vivo and in vitro. *Acta Anat. Sinica* 13:92–96

176. Hoffer, A. P. 1982. Ultrastructural studies of spermatozoa and the epithelial lining of the epididymis and vas deferens in rats treated with gossypol. *Arch. Androl.* 8:233–46

177. Gu, Z. P., Zong, S. D., Chang, C. C. 1983. Morphological changes in testes and epididymides of rat after gossypol. *Acta Pharmacol. Sinica* 4:40–45

178. Pelletier, R. M., Friend, D. S. 1981. Effect of gossypol on the postnatal seminiferous epithelium and Sertoli cell junction of guinea pig. *Biol. Reprod.* 24(Suppl. 1):25

179. Wang, D. X., You, M. M., Xue, S. P. 1982. Ultrastructural observation of gossypol effect on the Sertoli cells in rat. *Acta Anat. Sinica* 13:211–14

180. Oko, R., Hrudka, F. 1982. Effect of gossypol on spermatozoa. *Arch. Androl.* 9:39–43

181. Zhuang, L. Z., Phillips, D. M., Gunsalus, G., Bardin, C. W., Mather, J. P. 1983. Effect of gossypol on rat Sertoli and Leydig cells in primary culture. In press

182. Yang, Y. Z., Wu, D., Wang, N. Y., Chen, X. M. 1982. Studies on the effect of gossypol on blood-testis barrier in rat. *Reprod. Contracep. China* 22:52–55

183. Zhou, X. M. 1982. Gossypol effect on protein synthesis in Sertoli cells in rats. *Reprod. Contracep. China* 1:39–41

184. Tso, W. W., Lee, C. S., Tso, M. Y. W. 1982. Effect of gossypol on boar spermatozoal ATP metabolism. *Arch. Androl.* 9:319–32

185. Tso, W. W., Lee, C. S. 1982. Gossypol uncoupling of respiratory chain and oxidative phosphorylation in ejaculated boar spermatozoa. *Contraception* 25:649–56

186. Ke, Y. B. 1982. Studies on the mechanism of antifertility effect of gossypol. *Jiangsu J. Med. Pharm.* 8:23–24

187. Ke, Y. B., Tso, W. W. 1982. Variations of gossypol susceptibility in rat spermatozoa during spermatogenesis. *Int. J. Fertil.* 27:42–46

188. Liang, D. C., Fei, R. R., Liu, Y., Yang, S. L., Su, S. Y., Guo, X. Y., Liu, Z. H., Zhou, Z. H., Xue, S. P. 1981. Studies on the distribution of (^{14}C) gossypol in subcellular fractions of rat testis and site of gossypol action. *Acta Acad. Med. Sinica* 3:153–57

189. Feng, Z. Q. 1975. Effect of gossypol on human sperm, a electronmicroscopic study. Presented at 4th Natl. Conf. Male Antifert. Agents, Oct., Suzhou

190. Hang, Z. B., Wang, Y. P., Gan, D. Q., Liu, Y., Zong, S. D. 1980. Electronmicroscopic observation of the effect of gossypol on human spermatozoa. *Acta Anat. Sinica* 11:299–302

191. Oko, R., Hrudka, F. 1982. Segmental aplasia of the mitochondrial sheath and sequelae induced by gossypol in rat spermatozoa. *Biol. Reprod.* 26:183–86

192. Xue, S. P., Liang, D. C., Fei, R. R., Chen, X. M., Ye, S. J., Wu, Y. W., You, M. M., Guo, X. Y. 1982. Subcellular target site of antifertility effect of gossypol and its hypothetical action mechanism. *Sci. Sinica B* 12:1095–108

193. Xu, Y., Wang, W. H., Qian, S. Z. 1983. Antagonism of antifertility effect of gossypol by aspirin. *Acta Pharmacol. Sinica* 4:122–24

194. Qian, S. Z., Xu, Y., Wu, S. Y. 1983. The antispermatogenic effect of gossypol in K-deficient rats. *Acta Pharmacol. Sinica.* 4:183–85

195. Ye, G. C., Xu, Y., Qian, S. Q., Jiang, X. J., Sun, W. K., Tang, X. C. 1983. Effect of large dose of PGE on spermatogenesis and tissue PG levels in rats. *Acta Pharm. Sinica* 18:406–10

196. Wang, Z. G., Cheng, J. X., Yang, W. 1980. Effect of gossypol on plasma PG levels in rats. *Bull. Sci. China* 25:720

197. Wang, W. H., Yu, J. H., Zhou, Z. R., Chen, Z. W., Zhao, N. J., Li, Y. Q. 1982. Antagonism of gossypol toxicity by Smilax. *Bull. Chin. Materia Med.* 7:32–34

198. Yu, T. H., Chang, H. T., Hsieh, P. L. 1981. The in vivo effect of gossypol on Zn, Fe, and Mn concentration in rats. *Acta Physiol. Sinica* 33:17–23

199. Kalla, N. R., Vasudev, M. 1981. Studies on the male antifertility agent gossypol acetic acid. II. Effect on motility and ATPase activity of human spermatozoa. *Andrologia* 13:95–98

200. Chen, X. M., Zhou, W. Y., Ma, X. X., Feng, J. B., Xue, S. P. 1982. Gossypol effect on synthesis and turnover of basic nucleoprotein in spermatids of rat. *Acta Anat. Sinica* 13:193–200

201. Tso, W. W., Lee, C. S. 1982. Gossypol:

360   QIAN & WANG

An effective acrosin blocker. *Arch.
Androl.* 8:143–47
202. Tso, W. W., Lee, C. S., Tso, Y. W.
1982. Sensitivity of various spermatozoal enzymes to gossypol inhibitor.
Arch. Androl. 9:31–32
203. Kalla, N. R., Wei, J. F. T. 1981. Effect
of gossypol acetic acid on respiratory enzymes in vitro. *IRCS Med. Sci: Biochem.*
9:792
204. Pösö, H., Wichmann, K., Jänne, J.,
Luukkainen, T. 1980. Gossypol, a
powerful inhibitor of human spermatozoal metabolism. *Lancet* 1:885–86
205. Shandong Coord. Group Antifert. Plants.
1976. *DNA content of human sperm in
subjects taking gossypol.* Presented at 5th
Natl. Conf. Male Antifert. Agents, Aug.,
Qinhuangdao
206. Wu, K., Liu, H. M., Zhang, X. L.,
Zhou, W. Y. 1980. Effect of gossypol on
DNA content of human sperm. *Acta
Sichuan Med. College* 11:127–29
207. Zhou, W. Y., Xue, S. P. 1981. Effect of
gossypol acetic acid on DNA content of
primary spermatocytes of rat. *Reprod.
Contracep. China* 3:26–29
208. Ye, Y. X., Liang, D., Gao, H. Y., Ye,
G. Y. 1982. Effect of gossypol on the
incorporation of (^{3}H) thymidine in liver,
testis and small intestine of experimental
animals. *Acta Pharm. Sinica* 16:390–93
209. Tso, W. W., Lee, C. S. 1981. Variation
of gossypol sensitivity in boar spermatozoal electron transport chain segment.
Contraception 24:569–76
210. Lei, H. P., Li, G. X., Wang, N. G.,
Chen, Q. Q., Guan, M. Z. 1979. Effect
of gossypol acetic acid on the liver. *Natl.
Med. J. China* 59:330–32
211. Yu, M. Q., Chen, W. J., Wu, X. R.
1979. Histochemical study on the effect
of gossypol acetic acid on some enzymic
activity of neuro-muscular junction,
skeletal and cardiac muscles. *Acta Acad.
Med. Wuhan* 2:93
211a. Su, S. Y., Liu, Y., Zou, Y. H. 1983.
Electronmicroscopic observation of gossypol effects on gastronemius muscle in
laboratory animals. *Acta Anat. Sinica*
14:98–103
212. Tang, F., Tsang, A. Y. F., Lee, C.,
Wong, Y. P. D. 1982. Inhibition of
catechol-O-methyltransferase by gossypol: The effect of plasma (serum) protein.
Contraception 26:515–19
213. Ma, R. H., Yu, D. Q., Wu, X. R. 1979.
Inhibitory effect of gossypol acetic acid
on neuro-muscular system. *Acta Acad.
Med. Wuhan* 3:71–72
214. Shu, H. D., Yang, Q. Z., Xu, K. 1982.

Effect of gossypol acetic acid on neuro-
muscular transmission. *Acta Pharmacol.
Sinica* 3:17–21
215. Ma, R. H., Jiang, C. S., Li, F., Wu, X.
R. 1980. Effect of gossypol on some
functions of autonomic nervous system.
Acta Acad. Med. Wuhan 1:65–67
216. Liu, X. M., Zhao, Q. R., Lin, H. 1982.
Radiotracer study on the effect of gossypol acetic acid on Ca metabolism of rat.
Chin. J. Nucl. Med. 2:175–77
217. Clarkson, T. B. 1982. Hypolipidemic
effect of gossypol in cynomolgus monkey (Macaca fascicularis). *Lipids*
17:285–90
218. Khadzhibaeva, G. S., Pogodina, V. V.,
Laterpova, R. V., Bil'ner, L. M. 1978.
Interferonogenic activity of low-molec-
ular weight gossypol. *Antibiotiki* 23:
365–68
219. Aizikov, M. I., Kurmukov, A. G., Isa-
mukhamedov, I. 1977. Antimicrobial
and wound-healing effect of gossypol.
Dokl. Akad. Nauk Uzb SSR 6:41–42
220. Wichman, K., Valteri, A., Luukkainen,
T. 1982. Inhibiting herpes simplex virus
type 2 infection in human epithelial cells
by gossypol, a potent spermicidal and
contraceptive agent. *Am. J. Obstet.
Gynecol.* 142:593–94
221. Zhang, N. Z., Fu, Y. F., Dou, S. Y.
1981. The effect of gossypol acetic acid
on adrenocortical function. *Natl. Med. J.
China* 61:412
222. Ye, S. J., You, M. M., Xue, S. P. 1982.
Ultrastructural effect of gossypol on
adrenal cortex of rats. *Acta Anat. Sinica*
13:324–27
223. Han, M. L. 1980. Gossypol treatment for
menopausal functional bleeding, leiomyoma and endometriosis, a preliminary
report. *Acta Acad. Med. Sinica* 2:167–
70
224. Cheng, K. F., Wu, W. Y., Tang, M. Y.,
Chu, P. T. 1980. Endometrial changes
after administration of gossypol for
menorrhagia. *Am. J. Obstet. Gynecol.*
138:1227–29
225. Liu, Y. X., Jia, X. Z., Zou, A. M.,
Zhao, M. 1981. Effect of gossypol on the
amount of receptors of sex steroid hormone in human endometrium. *Chin. J.
Obstet. Gynecol.* 16:129–31
226. Wuhan Med. College. 1981. Clinical
observation on the use of gossypol in
gynecology. *Chin. J. Obstet. Gynecol.*
16:132–36
227. Zhou, S. W. 1981. A concluding report
on the use of gossypol in gynecology
clinic. *Chin. J. Obstet. Gynecol.* 16:137–
41

Ann. Rev. Pharmacol. Toxicol. 1984. 24:361–86

NEUROLEPTIC CONCENTRATIONS AND CLINICAL RESPONSE

Leonor Rivera-Calimlim

Department of Pharmacology, University of Rochester Medical Center,
Rochester, New York 14642

Linda Hershey

Department of Neurology, Case Western Reserve University School of Medicine,
Cleveland, Ohio 44106

INTRODUCTION

The clinical effectiveness of antipsychotic chemotherapy has been proven
worldwide, yet a multitude of problems remain concerning that significant
percent of the target population who do not benefit from such chemotherapy.
Since the introduction of chlorpromazine in the early 1950s, other phenothiazines, the butyrophenones, the thioxanthenes, the dihydroindolones, and
the dibenzoxazepines have been introduced and have proven therapeutically
effective with varying degrees of potency and side effects(1). Non-responders
to chlorpromazine have responded to some of the newer drugs, but the parameters of safe and effective dosage remain to be set. In the many uncontrolled and
controlled clinical trials and anecdotal case reports, drug dosing has been
mainly empirical, based on pushing doses to toxic levels or on a trial-and-error
titration of dose and clinical effect. The lack of therapeutic guidelines in the
clinical use of the antipsychotic drugs has moved interested groups to attack the
problem of wide variability in drug dosage and clinical response among
psychiatric patients.

The introduction of sensitive antipsychotic drug assays in biologic fluids (2)
revolutionized pharmacokinetic and pharmacodynamic knowledge about the
various antipsychotic drugs used in different types of clinical disorders. It

361

0362-1642/84/415-0361$02.00

became evident that the pharmacokinetics of antipsychotics vary considerably with age, duration of illness, duration of previous drug therapy, and interactions with drugs prescribed with the antipsychotics (3). These facts, together with indistinct and nonspecific clinical end points, rating scales of varying sensitivity, and technical problems in the chemical assay of antipsychotic drugs, have contributed to the failure of studies in different laboratories to establish a correlation between the plasma concentration of antipsychotic drugs and clinical improvement or side effects (4–12).

This review will summarize recent studies on therapeutic monitoring of plasma concentration of neuroleptics in psychiatric patients and emphasize data that are of significance in establishing guidelines in the clinical use of these drugs.

CHLORPROMAZINE

Correlation of Biologic Fluid Concentrations and Clinical Effect

The value of plasma chlorpromazine (CPZ) monitoring in the therapeutic management of psychiatric patients depends on the existence of a positive correlation between plasma CPZ concentration and clinical response. Several studies using sophisticated assay techniques have measured CPZ and its metabolites in various biologic fluids other than plasma, such as RBC (13), CSF (9, 14), urine (15), saliva (16), and whole blood (17), in an attempt to establish a therapeutic concentration range. Whereas data from a number of studies (18–21) suggest that plasma concentrations of CPZ greater than 30 ng/ml are required for clinical effectiveness and that concentrations higher than 200–300 ng/ml may be associated with signs of toxicity, there is much disagreement about a "therapeutic window" based on these studies. Several critical reviews in the last decade (22–25) have expressed concern about the validity of the conclusions claimed by the various studies aimed at establishing a correlation between plasma concentration and clinical response. Deficiencies involving assay methodology, study design, study population, and statistical data analysis were pointed out in both positive and negative studies. Studying the correlation of plasma concentration with clinical responses requires a specific, sensitive, and accurate assay method for the compound, a controlled randomized double-blind design, and a sensitive and reliable clinical assessment scale for specific target clinical signs or symptoms.

Unfortunately, strictly randomized controlled studies are often unachievable for several reasons. First, population homogeneity may be compromised by (a) "good-prognosis" patients with self-limited types of schizophrenia who do well with or without drugs; (b) "treatment-resistant" patients with "organic-type" schizophrenia who do not or will never respond to any dose of any antipsychotic drug; (c) the use of the word *acute* to describe either a de novo acute episode, a relapse in a first episode, or a chronic relapsing schizophrenia; and (d) the use of the word *chronic* to include patients, previously treated or untreated, who are either drug responsive or drug resistant. Second, fixed doses, which are highly desirable in most controlled trials, may be inappropriate for antipsychotic drugs, where plasma concentrations are consistently shown not to correlate with dose. Since antipsychotic therapeutic trials often run for 6–8 weeks, it is ethically inappropriate to fix a dose that obviously does not work or that induces significant toxicity in a particular patient. Third, placebo use involves ethical and legal risks in the acute schizophrenic, who needs treatment and whose drug response is readily measured compared to the chronic population. And, finally, a wide spectrum of target manifestations in different types of schizophrenia, including delusions, withdrawal, retardation, depression, and thought disorders, respond differentially to neuroleptics.

In the cited studies on plasma CPZ and clinical response, Wode-Helgodt (21) was the first investigator to support the earlier claims of Rivera-Calimlim et al (18–20) of a positive correlation between plasma concentration of CPZ and clinical response by doing a randomized, placebo-controlled, double-blind clinical trial in 48 acute schizophrenics. This study attempted to obtain a fairly homogenous group of patients with acute schizophrenic psychosis, focusing on thought disorders, delusions, and hallucinations as inclusion criteria. By *random assignment* patients received one of the three doses tested (200, 400, and 600 mg daily) after a placebo period. Plasma and cerebrospinal fluid (CSF) CPZ concentrations were measured by a mass fragmentographic method. Clinical improvement and side effects were rated according to the comprehensive psychopathological rating scale (CPRS) of Asberg et al (26) and side effects by a scale introduced by Simpson & Agnus (27). They showed a positive correlation between CPZ concentrations in CSF and plasma, and both CSF and plasma concentrations were correlated with clinical response, with CSF concentrations showing a better correlation. There was more interindividual variation in plasma CPZ concentrations than in CSF concentrations; this may be explained by individual variations in plasma protein binding. Rank correlation coefficients with clinical measures for psychotic morbidity were highest for CPZ concentration in CSF, followed by CPZ concentration in plasma, dose per kg body weight, and total dose.

Wode-Helgodt's study suggested that for the achievement of a more than 50% reduction in the morbidity score, CSF concentrations of CPZ should be above 1 ng/ml and plasma concentrations of CPZ above 40 ng/ml. These findings are in agreement with previous studies (9, 19, 20) that showed a correlation of CSF and plasma concentrations of CPZ with clinical effects. Data from our prospective studies of acute psychiatric inpatients treated with

CPZ in a naturalistic design suggested that the various symptoms of schizophrenia respond differentially to CPZ (19–20). Stratification of symptoms to form the major categories of thought disorder, paranoid delusions, withdrawal retardation, and depression facilitated assessment of the correlation of plasma CPZ with clinical improvement. Our study suggested that the correlation was best with thought disorder, less good with the total brief psychiatric rating scale (BPRS) score and paranoid delusion, and least good with depression and withdrawal retardation. In 1978 (20), data from 46 acute psychiatric patients studied following the protocol utilized in 1976 (19) were analyzed by multiple-regression analysis to correlate CPZ plasma concentration with clinical improvement. Scores for the total BPRS, thought disorder, paranoid delusion, depression, and withdrawal and retardation, corrected for initial clinical status, were examined as dependent variables at the end of the third week of treatment with CPZ. The mean CPZ plasma concentration, hospital, year of illness, CPZ dose, and preadmission BPRS were used as independent variables. The analysis supported the early suggestions that thought disorder, paranoid delusion, and total BPRS scores correlated significantly ($p=0.007$, 0.04, and 0.02 respectively) with plasma CPZ levels. As in the Wode-Helgodt study, the percent variation explained (r^2) by the plasma concentration was about 26–53%.

Garver et al (13) suggested that erythrocyte (RBC) concentration is a better predictor of brain concentrations and reported that dystonic patients have higher RBC levels of butaperazine than do non-dystonic patients. Whether butaperazine and chlorpromazine kinetics are similar is not known. Others have suggested that saliva is a more logical fluid to measure, as it would reflect the free neuroleptic, which is the form that distributes to the brain (16), but methodological problems in saliva assays have been reported (28). CSF concentration unquestionably should relate best to brain concentration, as has recently been shown (9, 14), but for routine clinical application such measurements are impractical. Since both Axelsson (9) and Wode-Helgodt (21) have established a positive correlation between CSF and plasma concentrations of CPZ in psychiatric patients, studies using plasma concentrations measured by reliable, specific, accurate, and sensitive methods should be acceptable.

The availability of several sophisticated assays for neuroleptic drugs in different biologic fluids and tissues has been comprehensively and critically reviewed by Usdin (2) and Curry (29). The development of sophisticated methods for neuroleptic assay, from thin-layer chromatography, spectrometry, fluorometry, gas-liquid chromatography with electron-capture detector, mass fragmentography, and radioimmunoassay to the most recent radioreceptor assay, has outstripped the development of specific, critical, and structured clinical design and assessment of drug response in psychiatry. While drug assay is objective, clinical assessment and scoring for drug response are subjective. Despite the availability of numerous validated diagnostic and clinical assessment scales (4–12), the users of these scales are so heterogeneous in skills and experience for subjective assessment of patients that reasonable concerns for the validity of clinical assessment of drug response are inevitable. This may be the foremost reason for the conflicting reports on the correlation of plasma neuroleptic concentration and clinical effects.

Radioreceptor Assay

The introduction of the radioreceptor assay for plasma levels of neuroleptics was claimed to be a solution to the question of whether the parent compound or a metabolite is the clinically therapeutic moiety (30). If both parent compound and its metabolites are suspected to be therapeutic agents, then an assay measuring "neuroleptic activity" in plasma or other biologic fluids based on dopamine receptor binding would be a logical approach.

Radioreceptor assay of neuroleptics is based on the hypothesis that effective antischizophrenic drugs act by selectively blocking the brain dopamine receptors. The principle of the assay is the in vitro competitive binding of plasma neuroleptics with radio-labelled butyrophenones (^{3}H-haloperidol or ^{3}H-spiroperidol) that bind selectively and with high affinity to striatal dopamine receptor sites in mammalian brain (30).

Possible pitfalls of the assay lie in the many assumptions that need to be met to insure accuracy and reliability of the method. Some of the assumptions that have not been documented are (a) that neuroleptic binding affinity to striatal or caudate dopamine receptors is identical to the binding to mesolimbic dopamine receptors; (b) that receptor binding affinity of the neuroleptic and all metabolites is at least equal to or higher than the binding affinity of spiroperidol or haloperidol and that the neuroleptic concentration in the plasma should be high enough to achieve displacement of the ligand; (c) that the active metabolites are proven to be dopamine antagonists and not partial agonists.

Some investigators have found that levels of active metabolites correlate better with clinical response than do the parent compound (8, 31–35). This evidence strengthens the claim that the radioreceptor assay would be a better technique to show correlation between plasma drug levels and clinical improvement.

However, this optimism may be premature, considering the complexities of receptor science, neuroleptic drugs, and psychiatric disease. To relate plasma "neuroleptic activity" to clinical response, several additional assumptions should be satisfied: (a) that the biochemical, physical, and physiological dopaminergic receptors of the bovine brain are identical to those in the human schizophrenic brain; (b) that the dopamine receptors of the striatal or caudate brain are identical to the mesolimbic ones; (c) that all schizophrenic abnormal behavior is explainable by altered dopamine receptor activity [this hypothesis is questionable, since some therapeutically effective antipsychotics are weak dopamine blockers, e.g. clozapine (36)]; and (d) that the parent compound and its metabolites are identical in their pharmacokinetics, transport through the blood-brain barrier, and regional distribution in the brain.

Neuroleptics in general possess anticholinergic, α-adrenergic-blocking, and antihistaminic activities in addition to their dopamine-blocking properties. The relative potencies of the different neuroleptics and their differential affinities to the cholinergic, α-adrenergic, histamine, and dopamine receptors have not been well studied. It is possible that the neuroleptic parent compound and the metabolites that bind to dopamine receptors in the in vitro assay and are measured and expressed as "neuroleptic activity," or that get into the brain, may preferentially bind to other receptors (cholinergic, α-adrenergic, and histamine), with consequent reduction in the amount of drug available for dopamine receptors. This will obviously affect the correlation of plasma "neuroleptic activity" and clinical improvement. To date, the published reports claiming a correlation between radioreceptor plasma concentration and clinical improvement are not convincing (37–41).

There are numerous metabolites of neuroleptics that may be pharmacologically active but have not been conclusively proven to be psychoactive. If these metabolites with less or no psychoactive activity possess moderate- or high-receptor binding affinity, plasma "neuroleptic activity" as measured by radioreceptor assay can obviously not relate precisely to clinical improvement. Serum levels by radioreceptor assay may be a poor way to monitor blood levels, because psychiatrists may elect not to push dosage in patients with high levels, even if there are logical reasons to suspect that the high levels may be due to less active metabolites, with inadequate levels of active compound.

It has been proposed that the radioreceptor assay would be a convenient and practical method for monitoring plasma levels of neuroleptics such as haloperidol and fluphenazine with few or insignificantly active metabolites, in contrast to chlorpromazine or thioridazine. This is discussed below.

Chronicity of Disease and Neuroleptic Treatment

If the plasma concentration of CPZ is a predictor of clinical response, then investigations on the wide variability of plasma concentration of CPZ after similar doses, and the failure of some patients to achieve adequate plasma concentrations of CPZ despite huge doses, become especially relevant. Abnormally low plasma levels of neuroleptic drugs have been reported in chronic schizophrenics by Smith et al (42). Prien et al (43) reported that chronic schizophrenic patients who had been hospitalized for ten years showed greater improvement on high CPZ doses (up to 2000 mg/day) than on low doses or placebo.

A number of studies (6, 44–48) using chronic psychiatric patients ill for over five years have shown abnormally low plasma levels of neuroleptic drugs (mostly CPZ) when compared to acute patients. It has been suggested that neuroleptic bioavailability is diminished and metabolism perhaps increased in such patients (3, 49, 50). Prolonged continuous treatment with neuroleptics has been implicated in the unusually low plasma levels of neuroleptics achieved in chronic institutionalized schizophrenics (44).

We reported that chronic schizophrenic patients achieved significantly lower plasma CPZ concentrations than did acute schizophrenics on similar doses (44). Data from 133 psychiatric patients in our study were submitted to multiple-regression analysis. With plasma CPZ as the dependent variable, the effects of independent variables (hospital, CPZ dose, presence or absence of anticholinergic medications, and years of neuroleptic treatment) were tested. The analysis showed that when all the independent variables are kept constant, the best predictor of plasma concentration is the dose of CPZ and that plasma concentration decreases with an increase in the duration of CPZ treatment. The analysis predicts that with prolonged CPZ treatment the plasma CPZ concentration will diminish 5–10% a year.

We attempted to determine whether chronic psychiatric patients would achieve higher plasma CPZ levels if the drug was given parenterally. After a one-month washout period (3), plasma CPZ pharmacokinetics after oral CPZ liquid concentration (400 mg) and intramuscular (i.m.) CPZ (100 mg) were compared in four chronic patients who had been under CPZ treatment for 15–30 years. The differences between the oral and parenteral values were analyzed by Student's paired-t test. There was no statistically significant difference in the total body clearance, plasma half-life, and volume of distribution between the oral and i.m. CPZ ($p > 0.05$). The plasma peak levels and total area under the curve after i.m. CPZ were significantly greater than after oral CPZ ($p < 0.01$).

The lack of statistically significant changes in plasma half-life, total clearance, and volume of distribution between oral and i.m. routes suggests that the low plasma concentrations of CPZ after oral administration in these chronically treated patients is entirely due to diminished oral bioavailability.

The calculated oral bioavailability in these chronic patients relative to the i.m. dose ranges from 6.2 to 13.6%, which is much lower than the 25% oral bioavailability reported by Hollister et al (51). Dahl (49) observed a decrease in CPZ plasma level after repeated dosing. His pharmacokinetic analysis suggested that the low plasma concentration could be due to induced metabolism of CPZ in the gut. Smith et al (42) also observed that there was no significant difference in the β-half-life between groups of patients with low and high plasma levels of butaperazine.

This diminished oral bioavailability could be due to an increased first-pass effect as a result of enzyme induction, to increased metabolism in the gut because of delayed gastric emptying, or to a biochemical or morphological action in the gastrointestinal mucosa, with consequent impairment of absorption.

Studies have indicated that biological changes in chronically treated schizophrenics significantly affect both the pharmacokinetics and pharmacodynamics of neuroleptics. It is commonly observed that chronic patients on very high doses of neuroleptics do better than those on low doses (52–57).

Lately, studies have indicated that striatal dopaminergic supersensitivity is a sequela of prolonged dopaminergic blockade with neuroleptics. This is the most popular theory for the development of tardive dyskinesis. Chouinard et al (58) have proposed that some dopaminergic supersensitivity develops in the mesolimbic dopaminergic receptors and expresses itself by a sudden return of psychotic symptoms upon withdrawal of medication or lowering of the neuroleptic dose. It was observed that in two patients extremely high plasma fluphenazine levels were required to reduce the psychopathology. Clearance of fluphenazine at the end of the postinjection interval induces a return of psychiatric manifestations, even if the blood levels are still high (>100 units haloperidol equivalent). Theoretically, this concentration should have been sufficient to control psychiatric symptoms in acute cases. This phenomenon suggests a significant increase in numbers of receptors, so that a much higher concentration of neuroleptics would be required to block all the receptors.

Hershey et al (48) studied the effect of a "drug holiday" (stopping neuroleptic medication for two weeks) on several parameters in six chronically treated schizophrenic patients using a placebo-controlled double-blind design. The parameters included peak-plasma CPZ, steady-state CPZ, psychiatric symptoms, withdrawal symptoms, extrapyramidal signs, and cognitive capacity. Drug holidays appeared to improve CPZ absorption, as shown by a more uniform onset of significantly higher CPZ plasma peaks after a post-holiday CPZ dose as compared to the pre-holiday dose. During the drug holiday, some mild withdrawal symptoms (restlessness, giddiness, agitation, autonomic symptoms) were noted in some patients. Others, who required diazepam for sedation, had shown high baseline BPRS scores. This is consistent with a report that the probability of relapse during drug holiday is related to the severity of illness (59).

Resumption of CPZ treatment after the holiday produced a worsening of extrapyramidal signs, greater sedation and hypotension, and alleviation of tardive dyskinesias. These observations indicate an increase in the bioavailability of CPZ to the tissues after the drug holiday. However, there was no appreciable change in the BPRS scores, possibly due to inadequate length of observation. Alternatively, this group of patients may be drug resistant, and have much higher plasma concentration requirements, comparable to the two patients reported by Chouinard et al (58).

This study suggests that drug holidays may improve both the pharmacokinetics and pharmacodynamics of neuroleptics; relapse seems not to be a major problem.

Neuroleptic and Anticholinergic Drug Interactions

Another controversial issue that has plagued CPZ plasma kinetic studies is the interaction between CPZ and trihexyphenidyl (THP; Artane), an anticholinergic drug used widely for treating Parkinson's disease since 1949. Since extrapyramidal adverse effects are often observed with neuroleptic treatment, anticholinergics are often routinely and prophylactically prescribed to prevent the occurrence of extrapyramidal symptoms.

In recent years, the prophylactic use of antiparkinsonian drugs with neuroleptics has been shown to be unnecessary in many patients (60–64). Several investigators have reported that only 10–25% of neuroleptic-treated patients withdrawn from antiparkinsonian medication exhibit a recurrence of side effects, and Singh and colleagues (65–67) showed a reversal of the therapeutic effects achieved with neuroleptics when anticholinergics were added to the therapeutic regimen. Klawans (68) has suggested that injudicious use of anticholinergics may contribute to the genesis of tardive dyskinesias in prolonged neuroleptic treatment.

Drugs with anticholinergic effects, such as imipramine, trihexyphenidyl, propantheline, orphenadrine, and desmethylimipramine, have been shown to lower the plasma concentration of concomitantly administered drugs (69–72). Animal and human evidence indicates that anticholinergic action slows gastric emptying and delays delivery of the drug to the site of absorption. If the drug is unmetabolized in the stomach and upper intestine, the absorption of the drug will be delayed but the area under the curve will not change. However, if drugs are degraded in an acid environment or metabolized by the gut, then the rate and magnitude of absorption will be diminished as a consequence of delayed gastric emptying. For this interaction to be demonstrated, the following criteria have to be met: (a) baseline gastric emptying should be normal before treatment; (b) the test drug has to be metabolized in the gastrointestinal tract; (c) there should be adequate plasma concentrations of the anticholinergic drug; (d) the test drug should be devoid of anticholinergic activity.

The chlorpromazine-trihexyphenidyl interaction was first suspected by Rivera-Calimlim et al (18) when five patients who were receiving trihexyphenidyl could not achieve CPZ plasma levels higher than 30 ng/ml despite high does of CPZ. In 1976 (19) this CPZ-THP interaction was shown in 12 out of 15 patients who were prescribed THP together with CPZ after two weeks of treatment with CPZ alone. The patients showed a mean drop of 44% in plasma

CPZ levels after two weeks on THP. The CPZ-THP interaction was then studied in experimental animals (70); the absorption and tissue distribution of orally administered [^{14}C]chlorpromazine (CPZ) in THP-treated rats and control rats were compared. Total radioactivity (CPZ) in the plasma and brain of rats treated with THP was significantly lower and total radioactivity in the stomach was significantly higher than in rats not previously treated with THP. Gastric emptying in rats treated with THP was significantly delayed as measured by gastric clearance of the marker [^{14}C]polyethene glycol. THP had no effect on transport of [^{14}C]CPZ in everted sacs of rats or on CPZ metabolism by liver homogenates. This study thus showed that THP lowers plasma tissue CPZ after oral administration by inhibiting gastric emptying, thus diminishing bioavailability of CPZ at the absorptive site.

The association of low plasma neuroleptic levels with concomitant anticholinergic therapy was subsequently shown by Loga (50), Chouinard et al (73), and Gautier et al (74). Loga suggested that orphenadrine lowers chlorpromazine concentration by increasing CPZ metabolism, since orphenadrine is known to increase significantly the plasma half-life of antipyrine. Morselli et al (75) observed in eight patients that plasma haloperidol is diminished by concomitant administration of trihexyphenidyl and that discontinuance of trihexyphenidyl caused a significant rise in plasma CPZ. Johnstone et al (76) showed in 20 patients that procyclidine, an anticholinergic, lowered plasma concentration of fluphenthixol.

However, several studies have failed to show an interaction between neuroleptics and anticholinergics (6, 77–79). Simpson et al (77) studied this interaction in a controlled double-blind split crossover design and did not find any lowering of plasma CPZ levels by trihexyphendiyl. These patients were chronic patients with a mean duration of hospitalization of 19.7 years. They showed very low plasma CPZ levels relative to dose and in all probability had been on chronic neuroleptic treatment.

Several studies have shown that chronically institutionalized patients achieve very low plasma CPZ levels despite high doses of CPZ, which could be due to the intrinsic anticholinergic effect of CPZ. Chlorpromazine, like other phenothiazines, has significant anticholinergic action and can slow gastric emptying per se and thus affect absorption. Thus, in patients who have been chronically treated with neuroleptics, baseline gastric emptying is already prolonged, so that the effect of the addition of antiparkinsonian drugs will not be dramatic enough to be appreciated. Furthermore, CPZ medication was shown to inhibit intestinal active transport of amino acids in vivo and in vitro in rats (80, 81). Considering the local anesthetic property, CPZ can possibly affect membrane permeability in the intestinal mucosa and inhibit passive absorption of other drugs.

Hence, in chronically treated CPZ patients, even the absorption of trihexyphenidyl or other anticholinergics may be diminished (82). This is another possible reason why CPZ-anticholinergic interaction may not be evident. It is noteworthy that studies that showed negative results for CPZ-anticholinergic interaction were all carried out in patients with initially low plasma concentrations of CPZ.

The conclusions of Simpson's study (77) were derived from statistical means of data generated from patients receiving variable doses and having undergone variable lengths of hospitalization. Inspection of individual data presented in this study shows that in over 50% of the patients plasma CPZ with trihexyphenidyl treatment was lower than without trihexyphenidyl in both steady-state and plasma-peak experiments.

Bolvig Hansen et al (78) studied plasma levels of perphenazine and its major metabolites during simultaneous treatment with anticholinergic drugs and reported no interaction. Plasma concentrations were measured at the seventh hour after the oral dose. If the CPZ-THP interaction is due to delayed gastric emptying after an oral dose of perphenazine, the peak time concentration will be more prompt in the group without concomitant anticholinergic than in the group with anticholinergic. Most likely by the seventh hour plasma concentrations in both groups would be comparable, since in the group with anticholinergic drug absorption is still going on because of delayed gastric emptying. This was shown by Morgan et al (69) in their study of the anticholinergic effect of imipramine on plasma kinetics of levodopa in rats and in man.

Again, one notices in this study unusually low baseline concentrations of perphenazine in all groups, but especially in the orphenedrine and biperidine group. Apparently these patients were chronically treated previous to the study with perphenazine, which in itself has intrinsic potent anticholinergic and antihistamine effects.

Kolakowska et al (6) likewise studied the interaction of benzhexol (trihexyphenidyl) in 13 chronic psychiatric patients with a history of 5–17 years of neuroleptic treatment. Plasma CPZ was measured before and after seven days' treatment with benzhexol. The study showed an increase in 12-hour and 23-hour plasma CPZ after benzhexol treatment. Seven patients had not received CPZ but were on other neuroleptic drugs and therefore were exposed to CPZ de novo during the study. The six patients who had been on CPZ for 8–17 years were given a placebo for 4–6 weeks before reinstating CPZ treatment in the study. In both groups, the increased plasma CPZ concentration seen after benzhexol could be the rise of plasma CPZ after simulated drug holidays reported in the study by Hershey et al (48).

In 1982, a statistical analysis of the effect of the anticholinergic THP on CPZ plasma levels in 38 acute psychiatric patients was reported (3). Each patient was prescribed an individual therapeutic dose of CPZ for four weeks. Eleven patients received THP (2 mg three times a day) in the first two weeks of the CPZ treatment; THP was then stopped for the next two weeks. Twenty-seven patients received the anticholinergic in the second two weeks. Plasma CPZ was assayed at the end of each week by the gas liquid chromatography with an electron-capture detector.

All patients had a decrease in plasma CPZ after THP treatment, and this decrease was significant at $p < 0.004$. There was an increase in plasma CPZ levels when the THP was withdrawn after two weeks' administration in 8 of the 11 patients. A one-way repeated analysis of covariance was used to test for anticholinergic effect.

The variables available for each patient were weekly plasma CPZ level, CPZ dosage for each week, anticholinergic for each week (yes/no), and years of CPZ treatment. The basic question considered by the analysis was the effect of anticholinergic drug on plasma CPZ level. The approach taken in analysis was to use a one-way repeated-measures (each patient is observed at two time points) analysis of covariance. Since the anticholinergic effect was not crossed with the trial (time) effect, no fixed effects were included in the analysis of variance. Only the random-effect "trial" (first two weeks/second two weeks) was included. The anticholinergic effect was a within-patient effect since each patient was observed both with and without anticholinergic. Histograms of the two plasma level variables indicated that a logarithmic transformation would reduce a certain amount of skewness in these variables, so that the assumption of normally distributed errors would not be violated. The dependent variables in the analysis were thus the logs of the two mean plasma levels for each patient. The analysis is summarized in Table 1.

As Table 1 indicates, the anticholinergic effect is highly significant. Furthermore, the sign of the regression coefficient for anticholinergic effect (recall that this variable was included as a covariate) indicated that patients not taking anticholinergic were predicted by the analysis of covariance model to have approximately 50% higher plasma levels (when all other independent variables are held constant). There was no trial (time) effect. Furthermore, dose did not account for a significant amount of variation within patients.

If it is true that anticholinergic-neuroleptic plasma kinetic interaction is only observed in acute patients who tend to achieve high concentrations of chlorpromazine and is absent in those who achieve very low plasma CPZ, then the clinical significance of this drug interaction in the two situations will be

Table 1   Effect of anticholinergic drugs on plasma CPZ level

Source	Sum of squares	DF	Mean square	F-ratio	P-value
Trial effect	.126	1	.126	2.83	.10
Anticholinergic	.448	1	.448	10.06	.004
Dose	.032	1	.032	.721	.40
Error	1.29	29	.045	—	—

different. The plasma CPZ lowering effect of anticholinergic drugs should be kept in mind when prescribing neuroleptics to acute cases so as to avoid inadequate concentrations of CPZ.

It had been a practice to prescribe anticholinergics routinely with neuroleptics to prevent extrapyramidal adverse effects. Because of this drug interaction, unnecessarily high doses of neuroleptics may be required to achieve clinical response in acute schizophrenic patients. On the other hand, in patients chronically treated with neuroleptics, dopaminergic hypersensitivity and cholinergic hyposensitivity may develop, so that prescribing anticholinergics may contribute to the induction of tardive dyskinesias and anticholinergic toxicity.

HALOPERIDOL

When Cooper reviewed the literature on antipsychotic plasma-level monitoring in 1978 (83), there were too few published studies on haloperidol (HDL) to recommend using drug-level measurements as a clinical tool. Since that time, however, a number of new analytic techniques have been introduced, and several groups have addressed the question of whether serum HDL levels correlate with dose and/or clinical response. Because haloperidol has no significant active metabolites, it is an ideal medication to use to study the relationship between clinical efficacy and neuroleptic levels. For adult schizophrenic patients, there is now evidence to suggest a therapeutic plasma range for HDL. While the exact limits for this range are still poorly defined, it appears that concentrations on either side of a "therapeutic window" may be associated with poor clinical response.

Assay Methods

Gas-liquid chromatographic (GLC) methods for measuring HDL have been described by Marcucci et al (84), Zingales (85), Forsman et al (86), Bianchetti et al (87), and Shvartsburd et al (88). The latter authors also demonstrated the usefulness of their GLC method (with nitrogen detection) in measuring red blood cell HDL levels in addition to plasma HDL levels.

Clark and others showed radioimmunoassay (RI) of HDL to be sensitive and specific (89), although they did not compare it to other analytic methods. Creese & Snyder developed the neuroleptic radioreceptor assay (NRRA) for antipsychotic drugs, including HDL (90). This assay is based on the ability of neuroleptic agents in serum to displace binding of tritiated ligand to brain dopamine receptors. Since HDL has no known active metabolite, the results of chemical (GLC) and biologic (NRRA) assays should be roughly comparable. Correlation coefficients of 0.75 or better have been reported when GLC and NRRA are compared (91, 92). Nevertheless, GLC has the advantage of greater sensitivity than the NRRA. GLC can reliably detect HDL concentrations of

0.5–1.0 ng/ml (92), while NRRA assays can rarely detect levels below 3 ng/ml–10 ng/ml (92). Rimon and others (93) showed the two biologic methods (NRRA and RI) to correlate poorly (r=0.51), although Creese & Snyder found the correlation to be good in the narrow range of 18–37 ng/ml (90). Rimon et al suggested that some patients have an immunoreactive metabolite of HDL that does not bind to receptors; conversely, other patients may have a receptor-active metabolite that is not immunoreactive (93).

More recently, high-pressure liquid chromatographic methods have been developed to measure HDL (94, 95), but the lower limit for useful quantitation with this method is similar to that of NRRA (2–3 ng/ml). A more sensitive (but more expensive) method is gas chromatography-mass spectrometry (GC-MS). It can accurately measure HDL levels in the range of 1 ng/ml, and it can perform the task in the presence of other drugs (96). Kurland et al found correlation coefficients of 0.73 and 0.97 when GC-MS and NRRA were compared in a group of schizophrenic patients (97).

Dose-Level Correlation

Using RI to measure HDL levels in pediatric patients, Morselli and his colleagues reported a poor correlation (r=0.56) between plasma levels and dose (mg/kg/day), but this could be explained by age-related differences in drug clearance in patients under the age of 20 (98). Using GLC to measure HDL levels in adults, Forsman et al also found a poor correlation (r=0.55) between plasma levels and dose (mg/kg/day), but their patient population was not defined in terms of age or clinical diagnosis (86). In adult schizophrenic patients, several authors have reported a good correlation between HDL levels and dose (mg/kg/day) over a wide range of doses using GLC (r=0.95), NRRA (r=0.83), or RI (r=0.90) (92, 99, 100). The next step will be to use these dose-level relationships to choose the starting dose for acutely psychotic patients. This method could potentially save time and prevent the persistent psychiatric distress associated with inadequate dosing.

Response-Level Correlation

The therapeutic range of HDL appears to vary as a function of the disease entity being treated. For example, Morselli and his co-workers (98) showed that children with motor tics or Gilles de la Tourette syndrome required lower levels of HDL to achieve a therapeutic response (1–3 ng/ml) than did children with psychoses (5–10 ng/ml). Similarly, Singer et al reported that older Gilles de la Tourette syndrome patients required about a tenth of the HDL dose (and level) that is required to treat young adults with schizophrenia (102).

The first authors to quote a therapeutic range for HDL in adults with psychiatric illnesses were Forsman & Ohman (103). They pointed out that the ranges vary according to the disease being treated. For example, the range for acutely psychotic patients was 0.8–32.9 ng/ml (mean=6.5), for chronically psychotic patients 0.6–12.1 ng/ml (mean=9.7), and for senile dementia 0.5–18.6 ng/ml (mean=3.4). The authors acknowledged the weaknesses of their study design (other antipsychotic drugs were permitted, and no baseline or followup psychiatric ratings were performed). Subsequent authors have taken care to control these factors.

Magliozzi et al (104), for example, had each patient examined at baseline by two raters using the brief psychiatric rating scale (BPRS) of Overall & Gorham (105). No other antipsychotic agents were permitted, and a final interview was performed 3–12 weeks later. Subjects were classified as responders if there was a 50% or greater decline in BPRS scores from baseline to the final determination. The authors reported a "therapeutic window" of 8–18 ng/ml because patients with lower or higher levels did not achieve therapeutic benefit by their criteria. Two criticisms can be leveled at this study: (a) the patients were diagnostically too heterogeneous (acute and chronic schizophrenia; subacute and chronic schizoaffective disorders); and (b) the timing of the followup examinations was too variable (3–12 weeks). Subsequent authors have been careful to control for these factors.

Extein et al (106) used only newly admitted acutely psychotic patients in their study (14 had schizophrenia and four had schizoaffective disorder). Each patient was examined at baseline and again at four weeks with the BPRS. Responders were defined as those showing a decline of 10 points or more on the BPRS. The authors reported a "therapeutic window" of 5–15 ng/ml even though two of their 12 responders had much higher levels and three of their six non-responders had levels within the "therapeutic window."

Smith et al (107) examined red blood cell levels of HDL in a fixed-dose study on inpatients with schizophrenia or schizoaffective disorder. Unfortunately, we do not know whether these patients had acute or chronic disease. The BPRS was done twice weekly and "estimated" BPRS scores for days 0 and 24 were used to compute the percentage improvement. Only three of their 26 patients had a 50% improvement or better. Nevertheless, the authors described a therapeutic "window" of 2.4–5.4 ng/ml for red blood cell levels of HDL at three weeks. They found a similar, though less significant, relationship between plasma HDL level and clinical response with a "window" of 5–14 ng/ml.

Some authors have suggested a broader "therapeutic window" than the 8–18 ng/ml range of Magliozzi et al (104) or the 5–15 ng/ml range of Extein et al (106). We examined psychotic patients who had deteriorated acutely with GLC and NRRA and found responders to have levels in the range of 10–40 ng/ml (92). We defined responders as those who had a 50% or greater decline in BPRS scores from the baseline to week two. Our patient population included those with acute and chronic schizophrenia, paranoid state, and schizoaffective disorder. Ericksen et al (108) compared low-dose to high-dose HDL treatment in a double-blind fashion. They found no difference in clinical improvement between those two groups as judged by total BPRS scores (reduction of about 30% was seen in both groups). Nevertheless, steady-state plasma levels in the low-dose group had a mean within the accepted "window" (9.9 mg/ml), while levels in the high-dose group were much higher (24.8 ng/ml). The latter patients thus improved with levels outside the currently accepted therapeutic range. Smith et al (107) showed that while an average improvement of 37% was seen in those with plasma HDL levels of 5–14 ng/ml, an average of 23% improvement was seen in those whose levels were above 14.1 ng/ml. There was a great deal of overlap between these two groups in the improvement seen in individual patients. It is also of interest to note that the six patients reported by Creese & Snyder had HDL levels by NRRA of 21–31 ng/ml (90).

With all this discussion of a "window," where is the evidence that high plasma HDL levels can be deleterious? Morselli et al (109) discussed the effects of high-dose HDL treatment in six patients with "resistant" paranoid schizophrenia. Oral doses were increased from 20 mg/day to 150 mg/day over seven weeks. Mean levels were initially within the "window" but quickly exceeded 40 ng/ml. None of the six patients improved clinically, and two patients developed increased psychomotor agitation and hallucinations with higher doses (and higher levels). These authors do not specify the exact levels obtained at the time of the clinical deterioration.

Bjorndal et al (100) also discussed the effects of high-dose HDL treatment in a group of chronic schizophrenics. Among 12 patients dosed with up to 120–240 mg/day of HDL for a twelve-week period, five deteriorated as judged by a rise in BPRS scores. Three of the high-dose patients exhibited attacks of violent aggression during which they struck fellow patients and staff. In all three of these patients, the aggression disappeared when their HDL doses were reduced by 50%. Unfortunately, the concomitant plasma levels achieved in these patients were not given. Extein et al (110) recently reported a schizophrenic patient in whom the initial antipsychotic effect of HDL was lost when the level reached 25.7 ng/ml. The antipsychotic effect was regained when the dose was adjusted so that the plasma levels came down to 10 ng/ml. All this suggests that high levels of HDL can indeed be deleterious.

FLUPHENAZINE

As early as 1961, Moore (111) used a naturalistic design to study the neuroleptic effect of oral fluphenazine in 174 patients aged 20–80 years. Doses ranged from 2.5 mg to 40 mg daily. Clinical improvement was observed as early as after one week of therapy in a few patients. Some improved after six weeks; some required continuous treatment up to eight months before improvement was observed.

One of the biggest problems in the maintenance treatment of chronic and remitting psychiatric patients is drug compliance. It is estimated that 30–70% of chronic patients fail to take their oral medication (112). This could explain the high incidence of relapse in outpatients. The introduction of parenteral depot fluphenazine is perhaps the most important advance in phenothiazine therapy since the introduction of chlorpromazine.

Fluphenazine decanoate and enanthate are long-acting versions of fluphenazine, a trifluoromethyl pipirazine derivative esterified with fatty acids for depot use. Fluphenazine is released to the blood stream after the hydrolysis of fluphenazine (FPZ) decanoate; it provides good control of symptoms in most chronic schizophrenic patients and reduces their rate of relapse (113–119). However, despite continuous treatment some 37% of chronic schizophrenics relapse within two years of starting treatment and 30–40% show extrapyramidal side effects. The plasma pharmacokinetics of fluphenazine in man has been studied using several methods of assay (120–123).

Using GLC-electron capture detector, fluphenazine was assayed in the plasma of six patients who were treated with parenteral fluphenazine decanoate (25–50 mg) every two weeks for an average of 2–4 weeks (121). Plasma concentrations ranging from 9–12 ng/ml were observed 7–14 days after injection. One patient achieved 15 ng/ml 24 hours after one injection of 50 mg FPZ decanoate.

Nasrallah et al (124) studied the relationship of plasma concentration of fluphenazine to clinical response and prolactin concentration in 10 chronic schizophrenic patients in a controlled study. There were wide intra- and interpatient variations in the plasma FPZ concentrations following an intramuscular dose of 50 mg. Concentrations from 6–28 ng/ml were observed within 1–6 hours after injection. Peak values occurred at different times in different patients. In most patients, daily oscillations of plasma concentrations from trace amounts to 22 ng/ml were observed. Two patients achieved 100 ng/ml, one at six days after injection and the other on the twenty-second day after injection. There was no relationship between fluphenazine concentration and prolactin plasma levels in these patients. Prolactin levels fluctuated but remained high for all patients throughout the period, including the days with undetectable plasma fluphenazine. There was no significant clinical change in any of the subjects in the study.

The kinetics of fluphenazine after fluphenazine dihydrochloride, enanthate, and decanoate administration to seven subjects were studied by Curry et al (120) using radioactive fluphenazine. Subjects who received fluphenazine hydrochloride orally achieved much lower concentrations than subjects who received the fluphenazine hydrochloride by intramuscular injection. The half-lives were shortest with the dihydrochloride (14–19 hours) and longest with the decanoate preparation (6–9 days). It appeared that the rate-limiting step in achieving plasma concentrations of depot fluphenazine is the clearance and release of the compound from the site of injection. There was no evidence of esters in plasma, urine, and feces. Jorgensen's group (125), using radioimmunoassay, studied two concentrations of fluphenthixol decanoate, 2% and 10%, in eight schizophrenic patients in a crossover design and showed no significant difference in the plasma concentration achieved by the two different concentrations. Maximum concentration was observed by 4–7 days. Tune et al (117), using the radioreceptor assay, monitored the serum levels of fluphenazine in nine chronic schizophrenic patients who received various doses of fluphenazine decanoate injected every two or three weeks. All these patients were in remission. Individual variations in plasma concentration were observed but intrapatient plasma concentrations tended to be stable. Concentrations were generally related to dose. Concentrations measured and expressed as chlorpromazine equivalents were amazingly low in this group of patients (<30 ng/ml) and yet maintained them in remission without significant adverse effects. Harris et al (126) reported plasma fluphenazine concentrations from oral and parenteral doses in 12 patients, measured by both high-pressure liquid chromatography (HPLC) and radioreceptor assay. NRRA was able to detect the drug in 94% of the samples. The sensitivity of the HPLC is 2 nanomolar fluphenazine and it detected no drug in all samples with less than 5 nM as measured by NRRA.

There was no correlation between doses (10 mg for oral and 25 mg depot injection every two weeks) and concentrations of fluphenazine. Plasma concentration of fluphenazine and metabolites appeared to correlate with clinical improvement, but the number of subjects was too small to be conclusive. Patients had florid symptoms of hallucinations and delusions and clinical improvement assessment was measured by the brief psychiatric rating scale.

Wiles & Gelder (122) claimed a correlation between the doses of fluphenazine decanoate (3 mg–75 mg weekly) and the mean plasma concentrations of fluphenazine measured by radioimmunoassay. In this complicated study, 33 patients were given different doses at different intervals. Examination of the raw data from three patients suggested that the plasma profile of patients receiving 25 mg/2 weeks was no different from that of patients receiving 12.5 mg/3 weeks, while one patient who received 25 mg/4 weeks achieved much higher concentrations. The raw data from the 33 patients showed a wide variation of plasma concentrations in patients within a dose level; some patients receiving 12.5 mg/week achieved much lower plasma concentrations than some who received 6.25 mg/week. These receiving 50 mg/week or higher had definitely higher plasma concentrations (3–6-fold) than those receiving 12.5 mg/week. It must be noted that the radioimmunoassay is not specific and can cross-react with both active and inactive metabolites.

A double-blind study to investigate the relationship of oral plasma fluphenazine and therapeutic response was conducted in 29 patients using GLC with nitrogen detector and acetylation procedure (127). There was no correlation between dose and plasma concentrations. Patients with less than 0.2 ng/ml and greater than 2.8 ng/ml deteriorated clinically, while patients in between these concentrations improved significantly. The study also showed no relationship between plasma concentration and extrapyramidal symptoms. The mean values of both the two-hour peak and the area under the curve of the six patients without dystonia were actually higher than for those with dystonia.

Megadoses and Neuroleptics

Certain chronic, drug-resistant schizophrenic patients respond to megadoses of neuroleptics. Whereas the majority of patients receive 25–50 mg FPZ i.m. every week or two weeks, a few patients may need doses up to 250–500 mg i.m. every two weeks. Itil (54) in 1970 reported the treatment of resistant schizophrenics with extremely high doses (up to 2000 mg daily) of fluphenazine hydrochloride.

Dencker et al (52) reported on the use of megadoses of fluphenazine enanthate in 30 chronic schizophrenics who also had been drug-refractory for 10 years. Fourteen patients responded so well that megadoses were continued as their treatment. The dose was 250–500 mg weekly, with withdrawal intervals, continued for 4–8 years. The total dosage received during the period ranged from 13.9–61.2 grams as ester. Plasma concentration was measured on four and five days after a megadose by ion-pair partition chromatography. Concentration ranged from < 0.4–55.1 ng/ml. Several parameters were monitored during the megadose treatment, such as skin and eye changes, EEG, ECG, chest X-rays, hematology, blood chemistry, and site of injections. The significant findings noted were leukopenia and low neutrophil percentage, EEG abnormalities, and ocular changes. Dyskinetic movements were usually slight. The authors concluded that the changes observed were not life-threatening and were not specific to megadose therapy.

Although megadoses have been tried and reported on (128, 129) from various parts of the world and have been shown to be beneficial for chronic drug-refractory non-responders compared to standard doses, careful evaluation of patient candidates for megadoses and judicious monitoring of side effects are indicated.

Effect of Age on Plasma Neuroleptic Concentration

Several reports (130–133) have shown that mentally ill children 7–15 years of age who were treated with neuroleptics achieved much lower plasma concentrations relative to dose than did adults. This observation is not unique for neuroleptics, however, since this is similarly observed with phenytoin, isoniazid, antibiotics, and tricyclic antidepressants. Studies have shown that children are rapid metabolizers of drugs. Recently (134), higher plasma-protein binding and a shorter plasma half-life of haloperidol (4–16 hours) were reported in children compared to adult values, which are 16–24 hours.

Our study (3) noted, however, that in six mentally ill children whose plasma concentrations were followed for 8–16 weeks, the optimum therapeutic CPZ plasma concentration (35–80 ng/ml) tended to be lower than values reported for adults (50–300 ng/ml).

Similarly, adverse effects were noted even in concentrations as low as 30 ng/ml. There was wide variations of plasma concentration on comparable doses, but plasma concentration increased with dose/kg body weight.

CONCLUSION

The dilemma of establishing a therapeutic range from neuroleptics in order to provide a guideline for psychiatric chemotherapy has not been resolved, despite experimental maneuvers to circumvent possible pitfalls in assay methodology, clinical design, and clinical diagnostic therapeutic assessment.

It is evident that there are significant individual variations in the pharmacokinetics and pharmacodynamics of the neuroleptics in psychiatric patients. Measurements of serum neuroleptic levels or "neuroleptic activity" are probably most useful in people who are not achieving optimum therapeutic benefit, those experiencing significant adverse effects, and those in whom poor compliance is suspected. Future studies are needed to define the limits of the therapeutic range for various sub-groups of psychiatric patients. High doses may be required in chronically treated patients and children because of bioavailability problems. However, clinical improvement and toxicity have been observed to occur at lower plasma concentrations in such patients than those required for patients showing acute deterioration in a chronic schizophrenic process. Maintenance treatment of chronic patients is conveniently and effectively achieved by long-acting parenteral fluphenazine. Bioavailability may improve with drug holidays in some patients and with megadoses in non-responding, treatment-resistant patients.

Early assessment of the treatment is needed (at 1–2 weeks) so that appropriate dosage adjustment can be made in non-responding patients. An important goal of monitoring neuroleptic levels in acutely psychotic patients is to shorten the duration of the patient's disability and hospital stay. Long-term studies will also be needed to see whether keeping patients at the low end of the therapeutic range can eventually reduce the incidence of tardive dyskinesia. To compulsively adhere to a rigid "therapeutic window" or therapeutic range without regard to clinical monitoring diminishes the usefulness of monitoring plasma concentrations of neuroleptics.

Literature Cited

1. Baldessarini, R. J. 1977. Anti-psychotic drugs. In *Chemotherapy in Psychiatry,* pp. 12–15. Cambridge, MA: Harvard Univ. Press
2. Usdin, E. 1971. The assay of chlorpromazine and metabolites in blood, urine, and other tissues. *Crit. Rev. Clin. Lab. Sci.* 2:347–91
3. Rivera-Calimlim, L. 1982. Problems in therapeutic blood monitoring of chlorpromazine. *Ther. Drug Mon.* 4:41–49
4. Curry, S. H., Marshall, J. H. L., Davis, J. M., Janovsky, D. S. 1970. Chlorpromazine plasma levels and effects. *Arch. Gen. Psychiatry* 22:289–96
5. Gelder, M., Kolakowska, T. 1979. Variability of response to neuroleptics in schizophrenia: Clinical, pharmacologic, and neuroendocrine correlates. *Compr. Psychiatry* 20:397–408
6. Kolakowska, T., Wiles, D. H., Gelder, M. G., McNeilly, A. S. 1976. Clinical significance of plasma chlorpromazine levels. II: Plasma levels of the drug, some of its metabolites and prolactin in patients receiving long-term phenothiazine treatment. *Psychopharmacology* 49:101–07
7. Sakurai, Y., Nakahara, T., Takahashi, R. 1975. Prediction of response to chlorpromazine treatment in schizophrenics. *Psychopharmacologia* 44:195–203
8. Mackay, A. V. P., Healey, A. F., Baker, J. 1974. The relationship of plasma chlorpromazine and its 7-hydroxy and sulphoxide metabolites in a large population of chronic schizophrenics. *Br. J. Clin. Pharmacol.* 1:425–30
9. Axelsson, S., Jonsson, S., Nordgren, L. 1975. Cerebrospinal fluid levels of chlorpromazine and its metabolites in schizophrenia. *Arch. Psychiatr. Nervenkr.* 221:167–70
10. Sakalis, G., Chan, T. L., Gershon, S., Park, S. 1973. The possible role of metabolites in the therapeutic response to chlorpromazine treatment. *Psychopharmacologia* 32:279–84
11. Sakalis, G., Curry, S. H., Mould, G. P., Lader, M. H. 1972. Physiologic and clinical effects of chlorpromazine and their relationship to plasma level. *Clin. Pharmacol. Ther.* 13:931–46
12. VanPutten, T., May, P. R. A., Jenden, D. J. 1981. Does a plasma level of chlorpromazine help? *Psychol. Med.* 11:729–34
13. Garver, D., Davis, J., Dekirmenjian, H., Jones, F., Casper, R., Haraszti, J. 1976. Pharmacokinetics of red blood cell phenothiazine and clinical effects. *Arch. Gen. Psychiatry* 33:862–66
14. Wode-Helgodt, B., Borg, S., Fyro, B., Sidvall, G. 1978. Clinical effects and drug concentrations in plasma and cerebrospinal fluid in psychotic patients treated with fixed doses of chlorpromazine. *Acta Psychiatr. Scand.* 58:149–73
15. Sved, S. 1969. The column chromatography of chlorpromazine and its metabolites in urine. *Clin. Biochem.* 2:369
16. May, P. R. A., VanPutten, T., Jenden, D. J., Yale, C., Dixon, W. J. 1981. Chlorpromazine blood and saliva levels and the outcome of treatment in schizophrenic patients. *Arch. Gen. Psychiatry* 38:202–07
17. Kaul, P. N., Clark, M. L. 1976. A novel approach to quantitative determination of submanomoles of psychoactive drugs in blood. In *Pharmacokinetics of Psychoactive Drugs,* ed. L. A. Gottschalk, S. Merlin, pp. 3–14. New York: Spectrum. 158 pp.
18. Rivera-Calimlim, L., Castaneda, L., Lasagna, L. 1973. Effect of mode of management on plasma chlorpromazine psychiatric patients. *Clin. Pharmacol. Ther.* 14:978–86
19. Rivera-Calimlim, L., Nasrallah, H., Strauss, J., et al. 1976. Clinical response and plasma levels: Effect of dose, dosage schedules and drug interactions on plasma chlorpromazine levels. *Am. J. Psychiatry* 133:646–52
20. Rivera-Calimlim, L., Gift, T., Nasrallah, H. A., Wyatt, R. J., Lasagna, L. 1978. Correlation between plasma levels of CPZ and clinical response of psychiatric patients. *Psychopharmacol. Commun.* 2:215–22
21. Wode-Helgodt, B., Borg, S., Fyro, B., Sidvall, G. 1978. Clinical effects and drug concentration in plasma and cerebrospinal fluid in psychotic patients treated with fluid doses of chlorpromazine. *Acta Psychiatr. Scand.* 58:149–73
22. Kane, J., Rifkin, A., Quitkin, F., Klein, D. 1976. Antipsychotic drug blood levels and clinical outcome. In *Progress in Psychiatric Drug Treatment,* ed. D. F. Klein, R. Gittelman-Klein, 2:399–408. New York: Brunner/Mazel. 653 pp.
23. Curry, S. H. 1981. Antipsychotic drugs I chlorpromazine: Pharmacokinetics, plasma levels and clinical response. In *Plasma Levels of Psychotropic Drugs and Clinical Response,* ed. G. D. Burrows, T. Norman, p. 95. New York: Marcel Dekker. 528 pp.
24. Cooper, T. B. 1978. Plasma level monitoring of antipsychotic drugs. *Clin. Pharmacokinetics* 3:14–38

25. May, P. R. A., VanPutten, T. 1978. Plasma levels of chlorpromazine in schizophrenia. *Arch. Gen. Psychiatry* 35:1081–87

26. Asberg, M., Montgomery, S. A., Perris, C., Schalling, D., Sedvall, G. 1978. A comprehensive psychopathological rating scale. *Acta Psychiatr. Scand.* Suppl. 271:5–27

27. Simpson, G. M., Angus, J. W. S. 1970. A rating scale for extrapyramidal side effects. *Acta Psychiatr. Scand.* Suppl. 212:11–19

28. Anavekar, S. N., Saunders, R. H., Wardell, W. M., Shoulson, I., Emmings, G. F., Cook, C. E., Gringeri, A. J. 1978. Parotid versus whole saliva in the prediction of serum total and free phenytoin concentration. *Clin. Pharmacol. Ther.* 24:629–37

29. Curry, S. H. 1980. Methodological pitfalls: The influence of experimental design on results. *Drug Concentrations in Neuropsychiatry. Ciba Found. Symp.* 74:35–49

30. Creese, I., Snyder, S. H. 1977. A simple and sensitive radioreceptor assay for antischizophrenic drugs in blood. *Nature* 270:180–82

31. Sakurai, Y., Nakahara, T., Takahashi, R. 1975. Prediction of response to chlorpromazine treatment in schizophrenics. *Psychopharmacology* 44:193–203

32. Sakurai, Y., Takahashi, R., Nakahara, T., Ikenaga, H. 1980. Prediction of response to and acute outcome of chlorpromazine treatment in schizophrenic patients. *Arch. Gen. Psychiatry* 37:1057–62

33. Sakalis, G., Chan, T. L., Sathananthan, G., Schooler, N., Goldberg, G., Gershon, S. 1977. Relationships among clinical response, extrapyramidal syndrome and plasma chlorpromazine and metabolite ratios. *Commun. Psychopharmacol.* 1:157–66

34. Phillipson, O. T., McKeown, J. M., Baker, J., Healey, A. F. 1977. Correlation between plasma chlorpromazine and its metabolites and clinical ratings in patients with acute relapse of schizophrenic and paranoid psychosis. *Br. J. Psychiatry* 131:172–84

35. Clark, M. L., Kaul, P. N. 1974. A preliminary report on clinical response and blood levels of chlorpromazine therapy in chronic schizophrenic patients. See Ref. 17.

36. Creese, I., Burt, D. R., Snyder, S. H. 1977. Dopamine receptors and average clinical doses. *Science* 194:546

37. Calil, V., Avery, D., Hollister, L., Creese, I., Snyder, S. 1979. Serum levels of neuroleptics measured by dopamine radioreceptor assay and some clinical observations. *Psychiatr. Res.* 1:39–44

38. Cohen, B., Lipinski, J., Harris, P., Pope, H., Friedman, M. 1980. Clinical use of the radioreceptor assay for neuroleptics. *Psychiatr. Res.* 1:173–78

39. Greenberg, J. S., Brown, W. A., Laughren, T. P., Krantz, J. 1983. Neuroleptic levels by radioreceptor assay and clinical response during treatment of acute exacerbation of schizophrenia: Some preliminary findings. *Psychopharmacol. Bull.* 19:74–76

40. Tune, L., Creese, I., Depaulo, J. R., Slavney, P., Coyle, J., Snyder, S. 1980. Clinical state and serum neuroleptic levels measured by radio-receptor assay in schizophrenia. *Am. J. Psychiatry* 137:187–90

41. Tune, L. E., McHugh, P. R., Coyle, J. T. 1982. Drug management in chronic schizophrenia. *Johns Hopkins Med. J.* 150:45–48

42. Smith, R. C., Crayton, J., Dekirmenjian, H., Klase, D., Davis, J. 1979. Blood levels of neuroleptic drugs in nonresponding chronic schizophrenic patients. *Arch. Gen. Psychiatry* 36:579–84

43. Prien, R. F., Cole, J. O. 1968. High dose chlorpromazine therapy in chronic schizophrenia. *Arch. Gen. Psychiatry* 18:482–95

44. Rivera-Calimlim, L., Gift, T., Nasrallah, H., Wyatt, R. J., Lasagna, L. 1978. Low plasma levels of CPZ in patients chronically treated with neuroleptics. *Common Psychopharmacol.* 2:113–21

45. Brown, W. A., Laughren, T., Chisholm, E., Williams, B. 1982. Low serum neuroleptic levels predict relapse in schizophrenic patients. *Arch. Gen. Psychiatry* 39:998–1000

46. VanPutten, T., May, P. R. A., Jenden, D. J. 1981. Plasma levels of chlorpromazine and clinical responses. *Psychopharmacol. Bull.* 17:113–15

47. VanPutten, T., May, T., Jenden, D. 1981. Does a plasma level of chlorpromazine help? *Psychol. Med.* 11:729–34

48. Hershey, L. H., Gift, T., Atkins, R. W., Rivera-Calimlim, L. 1981. Effect of drug holiday on plasma chlorpromazine levels in chronic schizophrenic patients. *Psychopharmacology* 73:355–58

49. Dahl, S. G. 1977. Pharmacokinetics after single and chronic dosage. *Clin. Pharmacol. Ther.* 21:437–48

50. Loga, S., Curry, S., Lader, M. 1975. Interactions of orphenadrine and pheno-

barbitone with chlorpromazine: Plasma concentrations and effects in man. *Br. J. Clin. Pharmacol.* 2:197–208

51. Hollister, L. E., Curry, S. H., Derr, J., Kanter, S. 1970. Plasma levels and urinary excretion of four different dosage forms of chlorpromazine. *Clin. Pharmacol. Ther.* 11:49–59

52. Dencker, S. J., Johansson, R., Lundin, L., Malm, U. 1978. High doses of fluphenazine enanthate in schizophrenia. A controlled study. *Acta Psychiatr. Scand.* 57:405–14

53. Dencker, S. J. 1976. High-dose treatment with neuroleptics in the acute phase of mental disease. *Proc. Roy. Soc. Med.* 69(Suppl. 1):32–34

54. Itil, T., Keskiner, A., Han, T., Gannon, P. 1970. Treatment of resistant schizophrenics with extreme high dosage fluphenazine hydrochloride. *Psychosomatics* 11:456–63

55. Kushner, T. 1966. Experience with greater than recommended doses of fluphenazine and triflupromazine. *Am. J. Psychiatry* 122:1061–62

56. McClelland, H. A., Farquharson, R. G., Leyburn, P., Schiff, A. A. 1976. Very high doses of fluphenazine decanoate: A controlled trial in chronic schizophrenia. *Arch. Gen. Psychiatry* 33:1435–39

57. Rifkin, A., Quitkin, F., Carillo, C., Klein, D. 1971. Very high dosage fluphenazine for nonchronic treatment-refractory patients. *Arch. Gen. Psychiatry* 25:398–403

58. Chouinard, G., Creese, I., Boisvert, D., Annable, L., Bradwejn, J., Jones, B. 1982. High neuroleptic plasma levels in patients manifesting supersensitivity psychosis. *Biol. Psychiatry* 17:849–52

59. Denber, H., Bird, E. G. 1955. Chlorpromazine in the treatment of mental illness. Side effects and relapse rates. *Am. J. Psychiatry* 112:465–68

60. Orlov, P., Kasparian, G., DiMascio, A., Cole, J. 1971. Withdrawal of antiparkinsonian drugs. *Arch. Gen. Psychiatry* 25:410–12

61. Klett, C. J., Caffey, F. 1972. Evaluating the long-term need for antiparkinson drugs by chronic schizophrenics. *Arch. Gen. Psychiatry* 26:372–79

62. McClelland, H. A., Blessed, G., Bhate, S., et al. 1974. The abrupt withdrawal of antiparkinson drugs in schizophrenic patients. *Br. J. Psychiatry* 124:151–59

63. Cahan, R. B., Parrish, D. D. 1960. Reversibility of drug-induced parkinsonism. *Am. J. Psychiatry* 116:1022–23

64. Mandel, W., Oliver, W. A. 1961. Withdrawal of maintenance antiparkinson drug in the phenothiazine-induced extrapyramidal reaction. *Am. J. Psychiatry* 118:350–51

65. Singh, M. M., Smith, J. 1973. Reversal of some therapeutic effects of an antipsychotic agent by an antiparkinson drug. *J. Nerv. Ment. Dis.* 157:50–52

66. Singh, M. M., Kay, S. R. 1974. Therapeutic antagonism between neuroleptics and anticholinergic antiparkinsonism agents in schizophrenia. *J. Bronx State Hosp.* 2:8–20

67. Singh, M. M., Kay, S. R. 1975. Therapeutic reversal with benztropine in schizoprenics: Practical and theoretical significance. *J. Nerv. Ment. Dis.* 60: 258–66

68. Klawans, H. L. 1973. The pharmacology of tardive dyskinesia. *Am. J. Psychiatry* 130:82–86.

69. Morgan, J. P., Rivera-Calimlim, L., Messiha, F., Sundaresan, P. R., Trabert, N. 1975. Imipramine mediated interference with levodopa aborption from the gastrointestinal tract in man. *Neurology* 25:1029–34

70. Rivera-Calimlim, L. Impaired absorption of chlorpromazine in rats given trihexyphenidyl. *Br. J. Pharmacol.* 56:301–05

71. Nimmo, J., Heading, R. C., Tothill, P., Prescott, L. F. 1973. Pharmacological modification of gastric emptying: Effects of propantheline and metaclopropamide on paracetamol absorption. *Br. Med. J.* 1:587–89

72. Consolo, S., Morselli, P. L., Zaccala, M., Garratini, S. 1970. Delayed absorption of phenylbutazone caused by desmethyl imipramine in humans. *Eur. J. Pharmacol.* 10:239–42

73. Chouinard, G., Annable, I., Casper, S. 1977. Anti-parkinsonian drug administration and plasma levels of penfluridol, a new acting neuroleptic. *Commun. Psychopharmacol.* 1:325–31

74. Gauwtier, J., Jus, A., Villanueve, A., Jus, K., Pures, P., Villanueve, R. 1977. Influence of antiparkinsonian drugs on plasma levels of neuroleptics. *Biol. Psychiatry* 12:389–99

75. Morselli, P. L., Bianchetti, G., Durand, G., LeHeuzey, M. F., Zarifian, E., Dugas, M. 1979. Haloperidol plasma level monitoring in pediatric patients. *Ther. Drug Monit.* 1:35–46

76. Johnstone, E. C., Bourne, R. C., Cotes, P. M., Crow, T. J., Ferrier, I. N., Owen, F., Robinson, J. D. 1980. Blood-levels of flupenthixol in patients with acute and chronic-schizophrenia. In *Drug Concentrations in Neuropsychiatry. Ciba Found. Symp.* 74:99–114

77. Simpson, G. M., Cooper, T. B., Bark, N., Sud, I., Lee, H. 1980. Effect of anti-parkinsonian medication on plasma levels of chlorpromazine. *Arch. Gen. Psychiatry* 37:205–08
78. Hansen, L. B., Elley, J., Christensen, T. R., Larsen, N. E., Naestoft, J., Hvidberg, E. F. 1979. Plasma levels of perphenazine and its major metabolites during simultaneous treatment with anticholinergic drugs. *Br. J. Clin. Pharmacol.* 7:75–80
79. El Yousef, M. K., Manier, D. H. 1974. The effect of benztropine mesylate on plasma levels of butaperazine maleate. *Am. J. Psychiatry* 131:471–72
80. Sundaresan, P. R., Rivera-Calimlim, L. 1977. Characterization of the effect of chlorpromazine on intestinal processes. I. Effect on L-methionine transport. *Biochem. Pharmacol.* 26:1411–15
81. Sundaresan, P. R., Rivera-Calimlim, L. 1978. Mechanism of chlorpromazine action on rat intestinal transport processes. *Biochem. Pharmacol.* 27:2781–86
82. Tune, L., Coyle, J. T. 1980. Serum levels of anticholinergic drugs in treatment of acute extrapyramidal side effects. *Arch. Gen. Psychiatry* 37:293–97
83. Cooper, F. B. 1978. Plasma level monitoring of antipsychotic drugs. *Clin. Pharmacokinetics* 3:14–38
84. Marcucci, F., Mussini, E., Airoldi, L., Fanelli, R., Frigerio, A., DeNadai, F., Bizzi, A., Rizzo, M., Morselli, P. L., Garattini, S. 1971. Analytical and pharmacokinetic studies on butyrophenones. *Clin. Chim. Acta* 34:321–32
85. Zingales, I. 1971. A gas chromatographic method for the determination of haloperidol in human plasma. *J. Chromatogr.* 54:15–24
86. Forsman, A., Martensson, E., Myberg, G., Ohman, R. 1974. A gas chromatographic method for determining haloperidol. *Arch. Pharmacol.* 286:113–24
87. Bianchetti, G., Morselli, P. L. 1978. Rapid and sensitive method for determination of haloperidol in human samples using nitrogen-phosphorus selective detection. *J. Chromatogr.* 153:203–09
88. Shvartsburd, A., Dekirmenjian, H., Smith, R. C. 1983. Blood levels of haloperidol in schizophrenic patients. *J. Clin. Psychopharmacol.* 3:7–12
89. Clark, B. R., Tower, B. B., Rubin, R. T. 1977. Radioimmunoassay of haloperidol in human serum. *Life Sci.* 20:319–26
90. Creese, I., Snyder, S. H. 1977. A simple and sensitive radioreceptor assay for anti-schizophrenic drugs in blood. *Nature* 270:180–82
91. Martin, D. M., Howard, E., Caswell, A. W., Bernot, D. C., Extein, I., Pottash, A. L. C., Gold, M. S. 1982. Dopamine radioreceptor assay and gas-liquid chromatographic analysis of haloperidol in human plasma. *Neurosci. Abstr.* 8:471
92. Miller, D. D., Hershey, L. A., Duffy, J. P. 1983. Serum haloperidol concentrations and clinical response in acute psychosis. *Drug Intell. Clin. Pharm.* 17:445
93. Rimon, R., Averbuch, I., Rozick, P., Fijman-Daniiovich, L., Kara, F., Desbert, H., Ebstein, R. P., Belmaker, R. H. 1981. Serum and CSF levels of haloperidol by radioimmunoassay and radioreceptor assay during high-dose therapy of resistant schizophrenic patients. *Psychopharmacology* 73:197–99
94. Miyazaki, K., Arita, T. 1981. High performance liquid chromatographic determination of haloperidol in plasma. *J. Chromatogr.* 223:449–53
95. Jatlow, P. I., Miller, R., Swigar, M. 1982. Measurement of haloperidol in human plasma using reversal-phase high-performance liquid chromatography. *J. Chromatogr.* 227:233–38
96. Maulin, M. A., Camsonne, R., Davy, J. P., Polipre, E., Marel, P., Debruyne, D., Bigot, M. C. 1979. Gas chromatography-electron-impact and chemicalionization mass spectrometry of haloperidol and its chlorinated homodogue. *J. Chromatogr.* 178:324–29
97. Kurland, A. A., Arramraju, W., Hanlon, T. E., Wildinson, E. H., Ng, K. 1981. A comparison of dopamine receptor blocking assay with plasma drug levels of haloperidol in schizophrenic patients. *J. Clin. Pharmacol.* 21:42–47
98. Morselli, P. L., Bianchetti, G., Durand, G., LeHeuzey, M. F., Zarifian, E., Dugas, M. 1979. Haloperidol plasma level monitoring in pediatric patients. *Ther. Drug Monit.* 1:35–46
99. Calil, H. M., Avery, D. H., Hollister, L. E., Creese, I., Snyder, S. H. 1979. Serum levels of neuroleptics measured by dopamine radioreceptor assay and some clinical observations. *Psychiatr. Res.* 1:39
100. Bjorndai, N., Bjerre, M., Gerlach, J., Kristjansen, R., Magelund, G., Oestrich, I. H., Wachrens, J. 1980. High dosage haloperidol therapy in chronic schizophrenic patients: a double-blind study of clinical response, side effects, serum haloperidol and serum prolactin. *Psychopharmacology* 67:17–23
101. Deleted in proof
102. Singer, H. S., Rabins, P., Tune, L. E., Coyle, J. F. 1981. Serum haloperidol

levels in Gilles de al Tourette syndrome. *Biol. Psychiatry* 16:79–84

103. Forsman, A., Öhman, R. 1977. Applied pharmacokinetics of haloperidol in man. *Curr. Ther. Res.* 21:396–411

104. Magliozzi, J. R., Hollister, L. E., Arnold, K. V., Earle, G. M. 1981. Relationship of serum haloperidol levels to clinical response in schizophrenic patients. *Am. J. Psychiatry* 138:365–67

105. Overall, J. E., Gorham, D. R. 1982. The brief psychiatry rating scale. *Psychol. Res.* 10:799–812

106. Extein, I., Augusthy, K. A., Gold, M. S., Pottash, A. L. C., Martin, D., Potter, W. Z. 1982. Plasma haloperidol levels and clinical responses in acute schizophrenia. *Psychopharmacol. Bull.* 18:156–58

107. Smith, R. C., Vroulis, G., Shvartsburd, A., Allen, R., Lewis, N., Schooler, J. C., Chojnacki, M., Johnson, R. 1982. RBC and plasma levels of haloperidol and clinical response in schizophrenia. *Am. J. Psychiatry* 139:1054–56

108. Ericksen, S. E., Hurt, S. W., Chang, S. 1978. Haloperidol dose, plasma levels, and clinical response: A double-blind study. *Psychopharmacol. Bull.* 14:15–16

109. Morselli, P. L., Zarifian, E., Cuche, H., Bianchetti, G., Cotterau, M. J., Deniker, P. 1980. Haloperidol plasma level monitoring in psychiatric patients. *Adv. Biochem. Psychopharmacol.* 24:529–36

110. Extein, I., Pottash, A. L. C., Gold, M. S. 1983. Therapeutic window for plasma haloperidol in acute schizophrenic psychosis. *Lancet* 1:1048–49

111. Moore, L. E. 1963. Fluphenazine in the treatment of hospitalized patients. *Am. J. Psychiatry* 119:987–88

112. Gittleman-Klein, R., Klein, D. C. 1968. In *Psychopharmacology: A Review of Progress*, ed. D. H. Efron. Washington DC: GPO

113. Ahlfors, U. G. 1973. Controlled clinical evaluation of depot neuroleptics. A double-blind trial with pipetiazine undecylenate and fluphenazine enanthate. *Acta Psychiatr. Scand.* (Suppl.) 241:95–99

114. Hirsh, S. R., Gaind, R., Rohde, P. D., Stevens, B. C., Wing, J. K. 1973. Outpatient maintenance of chronic schizophrenic patients with long-acting fluphenazine: Double-blind placebo trial. *Br. Med. J.* 1:633–736

115. Ayd, F. 1975. The depot fluphenazines: A reappraisal after 10 years' clinical experience. *Am. J. Psychiatry* 132:491–500

116. Westedt, B., Jorgensen, A., Wiles, D. 1982. A depot neuroleptic withdrawal study plasma concentration of fluphenazine and flupenthixol and relapse frequency. *Psychopharmacology* 78:301–04

117. Tune, L., Creese, I., Coyle, J., Pearlson, G., Snyder, S. 1980. Low neuroleptic serum levels in patients receiving fluphenazine decanoate. *Am. J. Psychiatry* 137:80–82

118. Wiles, D., Franklin, M., Dencker, S. J., Johansson, R., Lundin, L., Malm, U. 1980. Plasma fluphenazine and prolactin levels in schizophrenic patients during treatment with low and high doses of fluphenazine enanthate. *Psychopharmacology* 71:131–36

119. Johnson, D. A. W. 1977. Practical considerations in the use of depot neuroleptics. *Br. J. Hosp. Med.* 17:546–58

120. Curry, S.H., Whelpton, R., Schiffer, P. J., Vrancky, S., Schiff, A. A. 1979. Kinetics of fluphenazine after fluphenazine dihydrochloride enanthate and decanoate administration to man. *Br. J. Clin. Pharmacol.* 7:325–31

121. Rivera-Calimlim, L., Siracusa, A. 1977. Plasma assay of fluphenazine. *Psychopharmacol. Commun.* 2:233–42

122. Wiles, D. H., Gelder, M. G. 1980. Plasma fluphenazine levels by radioimmunoassay in schizophrenic patients treated with depot injections of fluphenazine decanoate. In *Advances Biochemical Psychopharmacology,* ed. F. Cattabeni, P. F. Spano, G. Racagni, E. Costa, 24:599–602. New York: Raven Press. 619 pp.

123. Javaid, J. I., Davis, J. M., Dysken, M. W., Janicak, P., Casper, R. 1983. Neuroleptic concentrations in schizophrenic patients: Measurement by radioreceptor assay and gas chromatography. *Psychopharmacol. Bull.* 19:72–74

124. Nasrallah, H. A., Rivera-Calimlim, L., Rogol, A. D., Gillen, J. C., Wyatt, R. J. 1978. Fluphenazine decanoate plasma concentrations and clinical response. *Psychopharmacol. Bull.* 14:46–47

125. Stauning, J. A., Jorgensen, A. 1979. Comparison of serum levels after intramuscular injection of 2% cis and 10% cis (2)-flupenthixol decanoate to patients. *Psychopharmacology* 65:69–72

126. Harris, P. A., Friedman, H. J., Cohen, B. M., Cooper, T. B. 1982. Fluphenazine blood levels and clinical response. *Biol. Psychiatry* 17:1123–30

127. Dysken, M. W., Javaid, J. T., Chang, S., Schaffer, C., Shabid, A., Davis, J. 1981. Fluphenazine pharmacokinetics

and therapeutic response. *Psychopharmacology* 73:205–10

128. Polvan, N., Yaqcioglu, V., Itil, M., Fink, M. 1969. High and very high doses of fluphenazine in the treatment of chronic psychosis. In *The Present Status of Psychotropic Drugs*, ed. A. Cerletti, pp. 495–97. Amsterdam: Excerpta Med. 572 pp.

129. Verhaegen, J. J. 1975. The long-term use of high doses of fluphenazine enanthate and fluphenazine decanoate. *Comp. Psychiatry* 16:357–62

130. Rivera-Calimlim, L., Griesbach, P. H., Perlmutter, R. 1979. Plasma chlorpromazine concentrations in children with behavioral disorders and mental illness. *J. Clin. Pharmacol.* 26:114–21

131. Morselli, P. L., Bianchetti, G., Durand, G., LeHeuzey, M. F., Zarifian, E., Dugas, M. 1979. Haloperidol plasma level monitoring in pediatric patients. *Ther. Drug Monit.* 1:35–46

132. Deleted in proof

133. Meyers, B., Tune, L., Coyle, J. 1980. Clinical response and serum neuroleptic levels in childhood schizophrenia. *Am. J. Psychiatry* 137:4

134. Morselli, P. L., ed. 1977. *Drug Disposition During Development*. New York: Spectrum. 490 pp.

Ann. Rev. Pharmacol. Toxicol. 1984. 24:387–423

ANTIARRHYTHMIC AGENTS: THE MODULATED RECEPTOR MECHANISM OF ACTION OF SODIUM AND CALCIUM CHANNEL-BLOCKING DRUGS

L. M. Hondeghem and B. G. Katzung

Department of Pharmacology, University of California, San Francisco, California 94143

INTRODUCTION

At the time of the last review of antiarrhythmic drugs in this series in 1975 (1), the important developments in the field centered around the "classical" agents: lidocaine, procainamide, quinidine, diphenylhydantoin (now phenytoin), and propranolol. That review properly emphasized the importance of new information regarding the effects of these agents on diseased tissue (e.g. obtained from infarcted hearts) or on normal tissue stressed in the muscle chamber (e.g. by depolarization with potassium). However, data and concepts available at that time were not sufficient to explain the important differences among the effects of these drugs on different types of cardiac tissue, or the difference in sensitivity of diseased and depolarized tissue as compared to normal tissue.

Since 1975, a modest revolution in antiarrhythmic drug development, research, and clinical application has occurred. The number of agents in active clinical use or investigation in the U.S. is now more than 18 (2, 3). In addition, a major new class of agents, the calcium channel blockers, has come into general use (4, 5). Furthermore, an attempt has been made to extend our understanding of the mechanism of action at the molecular level: the modulated receptor hypothesis (6, 7).

This review concentrates on the antiarrhythmic drug literature pertinent to an evaluation of the modulated receptor hypothesis. A number of general reviews

387

of the antiarrhythmic drug group have appeared in recent years (2, 8–14). In addition, numerous reviews and symposia have been published dealing with the calcium channel blocking agents (15–26).

MODULATED RECEPTOR HYPOTHESIS

The first crucial observation that led to the modulated receptor hypothesis for antiarrhythmic drug action was made by Weidmann in 1955 (Figure 1A). He observed that in the presence of cocaine, quinidine, procainamide, or diphenhydramine, cardiac sodium channels behave as if the voltage dependence of inactivation is shifted to more negative potentials (27).

A second milestone in the development of modulated receptor theory was the observation by Johnson & McKinnon in 1957 (Figure 1B) that the effect of quinidine upon $\dot{V}_{max}$ (maximum upstroke velocity) progressively increases with each successive action potential in a train (28), and the steady-state effect increases with increasing driving rate (Figure 1B). Furthermore, Heistracher showed that the reduction of $\dot{V}_{max}$ recovers exponentially between trains (29).

Thirdly, Chen et al (Figure 1C) showed that during diastole, use-dependent depression of $\dot{V}_{max}$ recovers slowly at depolarized potentials and more rapidly at more negative potentials (30).

These three observations have been confirmed for many of the sodium channel blocking antiarrhythmic drugs (see section on sodium channel blockers below) and for calcium channel blockers in cardiac tissue (see section on calcium channel blockade below) as well.

On the basis of these three key observations, and important studies in nerve (31, 32), it was concluded that the interactions of antiarrhythmic drugs with the cardiac sodium channel must be time and voltage dependent. One formulation of this notion is shown in Figure 1D. Specifically, the modulated receptor hypothesis (6, 7) postulates that (a) antiarrhythmic drugs bind to a receptor site on or very close to the transmembrane ionic channel; (b) the affinity of the receptor for the drug is modulated by the channel state and/or potential: rested (R), activated (A), and inactivated (I) channels (33) can have different kinetics of interaction with antiarrhythmic drugs; (c) drug-associated channels differ from drug-free channels in that they do not conduct and their voltage dependence is shifted to more negative potentials.

These modulated receptor postulates were expressed in a set of differential equations to obtain quantitatively testable predictions of drug action (7). Using a least square error search, we estimated the drug-receptor rate constants for quinidine and lidocaine (7). Although these rate constant estimates were based upon data from several laboratories, using various preparations and differing experimental conditions, they nevertheless were capable of satisfactorily predicting the effects of quinidine and lidocaine when used subsequently for data over a range of driving rates, recovery intervals, and holding potentials that had not previously been tested (34). At the time the literature search for the present review was completed, more than 100 studies had referred to the modulated receptor hypothesis to describe the action of ionic channel blockers. In the sections below we shall review the evidence for the hypothesis and call attention to some unanswered questions that require further research.

SODIUM CHANNEL BLOCKERS
Use-Dependent Block

Unless a sodium channel blocker has exactly the same affinity for rested, activated, and inactivated channels and does not alter the voltage and time dependence of gating when bound to the channel, its action on the sodium current will be use-dependent under appropriate conditions. Indeed, clinically useful antiarrhythmic drugs have a low affinity for rested channels and a high affinity for activated or inactivated channels. As a result, some block develops with each action potential, and recovery from block occurs during rest. Use-dependent block will occur whenever the rest interval is too short for complete recovery from block. It is thus not surprising that all sodium channel blockers studied so far have been found to cause use-dependent reduction of, and slowed rest-dependent recovery of, I_{Na}, $\dot{V}_{max}$, excitability, or conduction (Table 1). A few reports have appeared that suggest the absence of use-dependent block of sodium channel blocking drugs (91–94). However, in each of these, the apparent lack of use-dependent block can be explained by the experimental protocol used. Thus, a driving rate of 1 Hz at normal resting potential as used by Singh & Vaughan Williams (94) is too slow to observe marked use-dependent block in the presence of amiodarone, because at this membrane potential recovery from block proceeds so quickly that little block remains at the time of the next beat. As a result, Singh & Vaughan Williams observed only a small (but significant) reduction of $\dot{V}_{max}$. The use-dependent reduction of $\dot{V}_{max}$ by amiodarone becomes much more marked when the preparation is either depolarized (causing slower recovery from block) or driven at faster rates (providing more time for block to occur at depolarized potentials and less time for recovery between beats) (38). The latter observation is also supported by clinical findings: amiodarone usually has little effect upon ventricular conduction, but it may prolong pre-existing His-Purkinje delay (39) or induce tachycardia-dependent right bundle-branch block (95).

Lee et al (91) reported that therapeutic concentrations of lidocaine and quinidine substantially reduce the sodium current in a "tonic" fashion but cause very little use-dependent block. These authors used a holding membrane potential at which 70% of the channels in their preparation were inactivated.

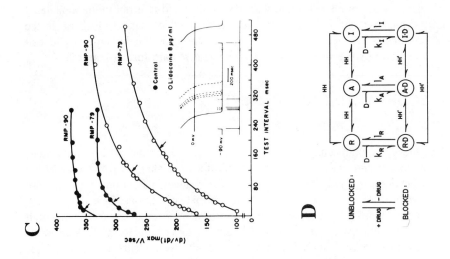

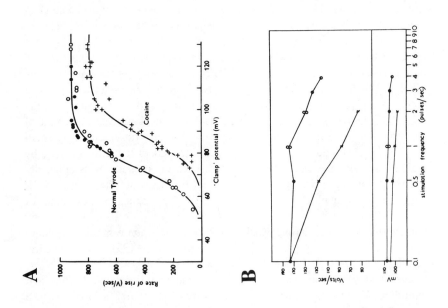

Table 1 Evidence for modulated receptor interaction with sodium channel blocking drugs

Drug	References
Alprenolol	35–37
Amiodarone	38,39
Aprindine	40–46
Disopyramide	47–51
Droperidol	52
Encainide	50,51,53
Ethmozin	54
Flecainide	51,55,56
Imipramine	35,57,58
Lidocaine and derivatives	30,35,49,51,59–69
Lorcainide	51
Mexiletine	50,51,69,71–76
Phenytoin	62,77,78
Prenylamine	36,79
Procainamide	35,49,51,62,80
Propafenone	81–83
Propranolol	37,60,62,84,85
Quinidine	30,34,37,49,51,62,86–88
Tocainide	35,37,49,51,61
Miscellaneous ß blockers	70,89,90

Since lidocaine and quinidine cause more block at depolarized potentials, and recovery from block occurs very slowly, block would remain close to the maximum possible under these conditions. Only limited use-dependent block can occur when "tonic" block is so great. Bean et al (96) used preparations clamped to more negative holding potentials and showed that marked use-dependent block develops in the presence of lidocaine. Similar findings were reported for quinidine by Colatsky (97).

Benzocaine has also been reported to lack use-dependence (92, 93). Benzo-caine has a very short recovery time constant from block: 105 msec at -95 mV, 27 msec at -120 mV (92). Consequently, unless the driving rate is rather fast, recovery from block will proceed to completion during diastole. In the studies by Sanchez-Chapula et al, the rest interval between clamp pulses was 500 msec, i.e. 4.7 times the time constant of recovery. Therefore, only about 1%

←

Figure 1 A: Antiarrhythmic drugs shift the $\dot{V}$max–mV curve to more negative potentials [to the right in this figure from (27)]. B: Antiarrhythmic drugs block in a use- or frequency-dependent fashion (28). C: Recovery from block is strongly voltage dependent (30). D: Modulated receptor schema: R = rested; A = activated or open; I = inactivated channels. R·D, A·D, and I·D represent the equivalent drug-associated channels. For more details see (6, 7).

use-dependent block would be predicted. In nerve, Schwarz et al (98) also failed to observe use-dependent block for benzocaine. It should be noted that, while they were driving the preparation at 5 Hz, the depolarizing pulse was only 1 msec in duration, leaving 199 msec available for recovery. In contrast, when stimulating at 10–100 Hz, use-dependent block was observed in the presence of benzocaine (99–102). In an unpublished study in cardiac tissue, we have found that the time constant of recovery from block by benzocaine can be lengthened by depolarization of myocardium. In guinea pig papillary muscle depolarized to −70 mV, benzocaine causes marked use-dependent block when stimulated at 5 Hz (Figure 2).

Thus, the evidence available so far is consistent with the claim that all sodium channel blockers exhibit use-dependent block under appropriate conditions, i.e. when "resting" block is maintained at a low level and diastolic interval is shorter than the recovery time.

Rested, Activated, and Inactivated Channel Blockade

Use-dependent block suggests different affinities for the individual channel states, i.e. state-dependent rate constants. (As noted below, an alternative or supplementary mechanism involves voltage-dependent rate constants of drug-receptor interaction. This mechanism is less well supported by the available evidence.) Although numerous investigators have discussed their results in terms of the modulated receptor hypothesis, only a few have estimated the affinities (or dissociation constants) for the individual states (see Table 2). In reviewing the literature we found two postulates that are consistently supported: (a) antiarrhythmic drugs have a low affinity for rested channels but a

Table 2 Dissociation constants for channel states and voltage shifts for several sodium channel blocking drugs

Drug	Kd_R (M)	Kd_A (μM)	Kd_I (μM)	V Shift (mV)	Method[a]	Reference
Amiodarone	0.1	1,000	20	50	G	38
Lidocaine	2.5	30	40	30	G	7
	2.5	92	37	25	G	61
	0.000 440	Large	10	19	NG	96
Mexiletine	∞		4		NG	71
Procainamide	1.85	37,000	370	50	G	80
Propafenone	0.3	1.0	0.5	55	G	103
Quinidine	∞	103	0	40	G	7
QX-314				30	NG	104

[a]G: global estimates of the four variables from experimental data; NG: non-global estimates from experimental data.

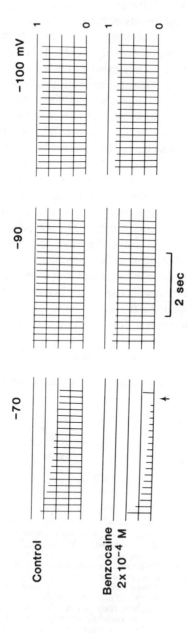

Figure 2   Use-dependent reduction of $\dot{V}$max by benzocaine (2×10^{-4}M) at 5 Hz. In each panel, normalized $\dot{V}$max for each action potential in a train of 20 are shown. Recovery from benzocaine block is so fast at -80 and -100 mV that little use-dependent block is observed. However, at -70 mV recovery is greatly slowed and use-dependent block becomes so marked that the preparation can no longer follow the stimulus train (see arrow). The resulting extra diastolic time provides for substantial recovery from block in the subsequent action potential.

relatively high affinity for the activated or inactivated channels or both; (b) unless the affinities for the three channel states are determined in a global fashion, the estimates for the affinity constant for any given state can be severely contaminated by the effects of the other states.

Open channel block may contaminate the estimates of the non-open state dissociation constants, because channel block can only be estimated by activating the channels. Therefore, block occurring during activation by the test pulse, but before the measured peak, will cause an overestimate of the actual block at the start of the test pulse. For example, a non-global estimate of rested block may underestimate the dissociation constant (overestimate rested affinity) by attributing open channel block to rested channel block. Quantitatively, approximately 10% of the total open channel time occurs before $\dot{V}_{max}$, and an even greater percentage before the peak of the sodium current. Any blockade of channels occurring during this time would be measured as apparent rested block. This effect can not be ignored, since studies in nerve have shown that open channels can have a high affinity for local anesthetics and that their blockade occurs with a time constant in the 100–1000 μsec range (105–111).

Inactivated state blockade may also contaminate non-global estimates of the affinity of rested or activated channels because many drugs have a very high affinity for the channel receptor in the inactivated state (i.e. a K_{d_I} in the μM range). To the extent that even a very small fraction of the drug-free channels are in the I state, a substantial fraction can nevertheless become trapped in the I·D (see Figure 1) state during rest (for the reason explained in Table 3). This

Table 3   Relation of inactivation voltage shift and rested state dissociation constant[a]

V-shift (mV)	K_{d_R} (M)
0	0.000 008 3
10	0.000 008 5
20	0.000 01
30	0.000 07
40	0.003 3
50	0.18
60	1.8

[a]The table shows the value of K_{d_R} (rested state dissociation constant) required if the first sodium current after an infinite rest period is to be reduced by 10%. Values were obtained using the modulated receptor equations (7) for a 1 μM drug concentration and resting potential of −90 mV. The affinities for activated and inactivated channels were set at zero. The voltage shift was varied from 0 to 60 mV. As the voltage shift is increased, the drug-associated channels behave as if they are more depolarized. This shifts the equilibrium between R.D. and I.D. (see Figure ID) toward the inactivated form, thus trapping progressively more channels in the I.D. pool. Consequently, to keep the total block less than 10%, the minimum rested state dissociation constant must progressively be increased, i.e. the affinity must be decreased.

also would appear as rested channel block. In cardiac tissue at room temperature, inactivation is substantially shifted to more negative potentials (92, 96, 112). Under these circumstances, rested block may be overestimated (91, 96) unless the holding potential is markedly hyperpolarized to remove all inactivation.

The voltage shift (discussed below) may also distort non-global estimates: it will translocate R·D channels to the I·D (see Figure 1) pool, again leading to an overestimate of the rested state affinity. A similar case can be made for distortion of the estimates for open or inactivated state affinities if non-global fitting is used. Because of these interactions, it is best to determine these affinities using a global least-square error search method (7).

RESTED BLOCK   The literature cited in the first section shows that at normal resting potentials therapeutic concentrations of clinically useful antiarrhythmic drugs reduce the sodium current very little, if at all, when the channels are not used, i.e. when they remain in the rested state. Using the modulated receptor equations (7), one can compute the effect of antiarrhythmic drugs under rest conditions (i.e. "tonic" block). Table 3 shows the minimum possible rested state dissociation constants that will result in a low (less than 10%) block of rested channels. As explained in Table 3, this estimate is strongly dependent on the magnitude of the voltage shift of inactivation. Thus, the model predicts that for a drug with a typical voltage shift of about 40 mV, the K_{d_R} must exceed 3 mM if little or no resting block is to occur. Experimentally, it has been observed that at normal resting potentials, concentrations of sodium channel-blocking drugs near the mM range are required to observe "tonic" block in heart. Similarly, when studying local anesthetics in nerve, tonic block is usually observed only when mM drug concentrations are applied [tonic block is usually the variable measured; for reviews see (113, 114)]. In contrast, when studying the effects of therapeutic concentrations of antiarrhythmic drugs (μM range), there is usually little tonic block at normal resting potential. It is thus not surprising that the estimates of rested state dissociation constants determined by global fitting for the drugs in Table 2 are rather large ($K_{d_R} > 0.1$M). Since all of these global fits were obtained in μM drug concentrations, estimates of these large dissociation constants cannot be accurate. Nevertheless, they can be interpreted as showing that the rested channel affinity for these antiarrhythmic drugs is too low to be measured accurately at therapeutic drug concentrations.

As noted above, unless all the state-dependent dissociation constants are determined simultaneously, i.e. by a global fitting procedure, serious overestimates of the rested state affinity are probable. When contributions from activation and inactivation block are excluded, rested channel block by therapeutic concentrations of antiarrhythmic drugs is found to be negligible. In Hodgkin-Huxley terminology, this can be interpreted as indicating that occupancy of the channel receptor by an antiarrhythmic drug is unlikely when the activation gate is closed and the inactivation gate is open. As a result, anti-arrhythmic agents that can exit from closed channels (e.g. neutral lipophilic drugs) will do so.

ACTIVATED CHANNEL BLOCK VERSUS INACTIVATED CHANNEL BLOCK   In nerve, open channel block was first convincingly demonstrated by Strichartz (31) for quaternary lidocaine derivatives. Lidocaine, quinidine, procainamide, and phenytoin have also been shown to block batrachotoxin-activated sodium .channels (115). Hille (6) proposed that the channel receptor is accessible through a hydrophilic pathway from the inside of the cell when the channel is open. Since sodium channels in heart behave very much like those of nerve (7) and since at body pH antiarrhythmic drugs exist in the neutral and charged forms, it is conceivable that the charged form could similarly block open cardiac sodium channels. However, because the free-running cardiac action potential lasts so long, direct measurement of "pure" open channel block, i.e. with minimal contamination by inactivation block, can only be done by using the voltage clamp technique to impose short pulses. Some evidence is available for specific agents.

Quinidine   Colatsky (97) showed that, in rabbit Purkinje fibers bathed in low sodium and at room temperature, the reduction in sodium current by quinidine (5 μg/ml) is mostly due to blockade of open channels. Moreover, lengthening of the pulses in the train from 50 to 5000 msec produced little additional block. This suggests that quinidine has a relatively low affinity for inactivated sodium channels. These observations are in agreement with earlier global estimates of the dissociation constants (7). In contrast, in ovine Purkinje fibers bathed in normal sodium and at body temperature, quinidine (10 μg/ml) caused a greater, but slowly developing (seconds), reduction of $\dot{V}_{max}$ as the pulse duration was increased (116). However, these authors also concluded that in therapeutic concentrations (< 2 μg/ml), inactivation block is less important and that the main mechanism of action of quinidine in reducing $\dot{V}_{max}$ must be block of open channels. We have also found that quinidine's block can increase with clamp duration in guinea pig papillary muscle (T. Matsubara et al, unpublished observation). However, the time constant of this slow phase of block (2–5 sec) is very similar to that of slow inactivation and has similar voltage dependence (117–118). This suggests that quinidine may promote slow inactivation. This voltage-dependent, slowly developing action of quinidine is different from all other drugs tested so far (see below): the block with other drugs develops much faster than with quinidine (hundreds of msecs instead of seconds; see below) and the extent and rate of inactivation block development is not strongly voltage dependent. To what extent "slow-inactivation block" by quinidine and other antiarrhythmic drugs may constitute an important mechanism of anti-arrhythmic drug action needs further investigation. Thus, for quinidine the order of affinity for the sodium channel states appears to be activated > inactivated >>> rested.

Lidocaine   A global fit based on $\dot{V}_{max}$ data (7) suggested that lidocaine has about equal affinities for activated ($K_{d_A} = 30$ μM) and inactivated ($K_{d_I} = 40$ μM) channels. Bean et al (96) have shown that lidocaine has indeed a very high affinity for inactivated sodium channels ($K_{d_I} = 10$ μM). The time constant of inactivation block at room temperature was a few hundred msec for 20 μM lidocaine, but shortened to only 10 msec for 200 μM drug. According to the modulated receptor model, when all the channels are in the I and I·D pools (Figure 1), the time constant for inactivation block is: $1/(k_I[D] + l_I)$, which shows that increasing the dose ([D]) may reduce the time constant. Sanchez-Chapula et al (92) also observed a high affinity and similar time constants for inactivated channel block by lidocaine.

In contrast to our initial estimates for lidocaine, neither Bean et al (96) nor Sanchez-Chapula et al (92) observed much activation block. This is not surprising, however, given their experimental protocol. A cationic drug in a hydrophilic transmembrane channel is expected to distribute according to the Boltzmann equation. As a consequence, concentration at the receptor site, and the blockade, will be more marked the more depolarizing the pulse (within limits) and vice versa (31, 32, 119, 120). Yeh & Narahashi (105) and Cahalan (121) directly demonstrated this effect experimentally in nerve and showed that it is mostly the rate constant l_A that is voltage dependent. For pancuronium and 9-aminoacridine the dissociation rate constant, l_A, becomes progressively smaller at more positive potentials. As a result, open channel block sharply declines as the clamp potential is made more negative, so that at -30 mV, the usual potential for clamp pulses in both of the above cardiac studies (92, 96), one might expect little activated channel block (120). In fact, in the one experiment in which Bean et al clamped to more positive levels ($+31$ mV) (see their Figure 9A), they too observed activation block for lidocaine. With free-running action potentials the membrane potential reaches positive levels while a substantial fraction of the sodium channels are still open, so a greater degree of activated channel block is expected to occur (122). Thus, lidocaine's affinities for the individual channel states appear to be: inactivated ≥ activated >>> rested. The exact relation between the first two may be influenced by pH (as discussed below).

Other drugs   Amiodarone (38) appears to cause little or no open channel block, since a fast train of 19 short pulses (5 msec at 3 Hz) results in no reduction of $\dot{V}_{max}$. In contrast, even a single long pulse (100–6000 msec) can markedly reduce $\dot{V}_{max}$ of a test pulse. Similarly, Sada (80), using a global search, has shown that procainamide elicits much less open channel block than lidocaine. Hence, for amiodarone and procainamide, the channel affinities appear to be best represented as: inactivated $>>$ activated $>>>$ rested.

Disopyramide, although in many respects similar to quinidine (123), is probably more of an inactivation blocker. Indeed, the percentage blocking effect of this drug increases with depolarization (124). In addition, hyperpolarization by reduced external potassium can increase disopyramide's effect (48). This anomalous effect can occur with inactivation blockers that have a long time constant of recovery from block. This may be due to the fact that reduced external postassium can lengthen the action potential duration and consequently promote inactivation block; this extra block can be observed on the subsequent beat.

According to Courtney's analysis (71), mexiletine also has a substantial affinity for the inactivated state ($K_{d_I} = 4$ μM). His analysis did not provide an estimate for open channel block.

Voltage Dependence

Rested sodium channels have a much lower affinity for antiarrhythmic drugs than depolarized (activated or inactivated) channels. In addition, the rate of recovery (re) from block is slower (the time constant, τ_{re}, is larger) the more depolarized the holding potential (Table 4). According to the modulated receptor hypothesis, the rate of recovery from block should be voltage dependent along two separate routes: (a) the I·D to I to R, and (b) the I·D. to R·D to R pathways (Figure 1D).

THE I·D TO I TO R PATHWAY   Since recovery from inactivation (I to R) is strongly voltage dependent (33, 127, 128), the recovery from block (I·D to I to

Table 4 Publications showing low drug-receptor affinity in rested channels and voltage dependence of recovery from block

Drug	References
Amiodarone	38
Benzocaine	92
Droperidol	52
Lidocaine	30,34,61,69,91,92,96,125,126
Mexiletine	73
Prenylamine	79
Procainamide	80
Quinidine	116
Tocainide	61

R) may, a priori, also be voltage dependent. However, the extent of the voltage dependence will appear very different for individual drugs. If the time constants of the I·D to I and I to R transitions are of the same order of magnitude, especially if $k_I > 0$ (e.g. lidocaine), the overall recovery process (I·D to I to R) will appear strongly voltage dependent. Indeed, from -85 to -70 mV, τ_{re} increased from about 200 to 500 msec (30, 61, 96). At more positive potentials, τ_{re} increases and, because of the high affinity of lidocaine for inactivated channels, most of the channels remain blocked. In contrast, when the time constant for the I·D to I process is much greater than that of the I to R transition, and especially if k_I is very small (e.g. quinidine), then after the initial fast recovery of the channels in the I pool the time constant of the global recovery process will approach $1/l_I$ (34, 116). Since the closed channel rate constants are not strongly voltage dependent (see below) the recovery will appear to be only slightly voltage dependent. In fact, over the -85 to -70 mV range, the τ_{re} for quinidine changes only from 5 to 7.5 sec (116).

THE I·D TO R·D TO R PATHWAY   As the membrane potential is made more negative and the voltage shift of drug-associated channels is overcome, an additional path for recovery becomes available: I·D to R·D to R (see Figure 1D). This pathway appears to be very fast: Hondeghem & Katzung (34) found that in the -120 to -140 mV range of resting potentials, recovery from quinidine block occurs so rapidly that it is not possible to induce use-dependent block with a 3 Hz pulse train, even if the concentration is increased to 16 μg/ml. Therefore, it appears that for quinidine, the recovery process shifts from a relatively slow process (on the order of 5 seconds) to a much faster recovery process (less than 50 msec) around -120 mV.

For lidocaine, the potential at which the recovery kinetics shift from slow to fast is less negative, and use-dependent block at 3 Hz disappears around -105 mV (34). Similar results were obtained for phenytoin (129) and benzocaine (see Figure 2).

For amiodarone (38) and aprindine (129), the hyperpolarization must be to at least -140 mV to attenuate use-dependent block. Thus, the latter two drugs appear to have a voltage shift larger than that for quinidine, while the voltage shifts for lidocaine, phenytoin, and benzocaine are smaller.

A shift in the voltage dependence of inactivation of drug-associated channels was proposed quite early in studies of cardiac tissue (27) and nerve (32). Recently, Weld et al (116) have questioned the existence of the voltage shift. However, the apparent voltage shift of inactivation, i.e. that, measured experimentally, ranges from zero (when no channels are blocked), to the actual shift that would be observed when all the channels are blocked. Unfortunately, since blocked channels do not conduct, the actual voltage shift cannot be measured directly. Since Weld et al combined μM concentrations of quinidine with slow driving rates, few channels would be blocked and, as expected, they observed only a small voltage shift (3 mV). Small concentrations of lidocaine also cause only a small apparent voltage shift [3.5 mV at 17 μM (30); 4.4 mV at 21 μM (69); 4.7 mV at 20 μM; and 5.8 mV at 40 μM (96)]. However, the shift increases as the dose is increased. Thus, at 1 mM lidocaine, Bean et al (96) observed a voltage shift of 22 mV in rabbit, and Payet et al (67), using 426 μM, measured a voltage shift of 40 $\pm$ 10 mV in rat. Although these direct experimental estimates may be somewhat contaminated by block occurring during the test pulse, the values are in fairly good argreement with estimates obtained from global fits: 25 mV (61) and 30 mV (7).

An important test of the voltage shift concept is the demonstration of open channel *unblocking*. The experiment requires that (*a*) a large fraction of channels be trapped in the drug-associated inactivated (I·D) pool; this is the normal consequence of rapid use-dependent blocking at normal or low resting potentials; and (*b*) a subsequent strong hyperpolarization be used to quickly translocate the blocked channels into the R·D pool. If an activation is then elicited so that the ratio of A·D channels to A channels exceeds the equilibrium ratio, one should observe activation unblocking. This was, in fact, demonstrated experimentally quite early by Strichartz (31) in nerve and by Gintant & Hoffman in cardiac fibers (130 and personal communication). In addition to demonstrating that a strong hyperpolarizing prepulse markedly enhances recovery from block, they showed that when the prepulse was within one millisecond of activation there was a substantial additional recovery from block. It is difficult to explain this result without invoking a voltage shift of inactivation and unblocking of the channel during the open state.

A second test of the voltage shift hypothesis is the prediction that the $\dot{V}_{max}$-V_m curve can exhibit a "bump," i.e. a double sigmoid contour (7) at certain rates in the presence of drugs. Such double-contoured $\dot{V}_{max}$-V_m curves have been reported (56, 131). This bump is most convincingly demonstrated with quaternary compounds. However, the presence of a bump is compatible with *either* a voltage shift *or* voltage-dependent drug rate constants (116). Both mechanisms are compatible with the modulated receptor hypothesis and predict a bump at appropriate driving rates. If the bump is such that at certain rates the $\dot{V}_{max}$-V_m curve shows a flat region (in the voltage range where all drug-free channels are fully recovered) between the two sigmoid regions, then this is easily explained by a *voltage shift*. The same characteristic would require an unusually complex *voltage dependence* of the rate constants.

It is quite possible that, in addition to a voltage shift, the drug binding and unbinding rate constants may also be voltage dependent. Thus, Starmer et al (132) have proposed a model that explicitly incorporates voltage-dependent rate constants. They assume that the drug is charged and consequently that its distribution in the sodium channel is governed by the Boltzmann equation, i.e.

is potential dependent. Such a proposal appears quite reasonable for the charged form of the drug interacting through the hydrophilic pathway (6) and has been demonstrated experimentally in nerve (105, 121). However, there is good evidence that the neutral form of the local anesthetics can also effectively block sodium channels (92, 93, also see Figure 2). As proposed by Hille (6), the uncharged molecule can move laterally through the lipid membrane to combine with the receptor in the inactivated channel. In this situation there is no reason to anticipate inactivated state block would be voltage (as opposed to state) dependent. In fact, it has been shown that block by amiodarone (38) and lidocaine (92, 96, 122) is mostly independent of voltage over a range of -40 to $+40$ mV, where channels are inactivated.

One experimental study noted above did report that the closed-state interactions (rested and inactivated) of quinidine are voltage dependent (116). However, the data analysis of that paper has been questioned (133). As noted above, the slow voltage-dependent block described (116) appears to have a voltage- and time-dependence similar to that of slow inactivation (117, 118).

In summary, the action of antiarrhythmic drugs is strongly voltage dependent for at least three reasons: (*a*) affinity of depolarized channels for antiarrhythmic drugs is much larger than that of rested channels; (*b*) recovery from block occurs much more slowly in inactivated than in rested channels; (*c*) inactivation of drug-associated channels is shifted to more negative potentials. Whether the association or dissociation rate constants of rested and inactivated states are also voltage-dependent will require further studies.

pH Effects

Most antiarrhythmic drugs are weak bases, with pKa ranging from 7.5 to 9.5. Thus, at physiological pH these drugs exist in both the cationic and the neutral form in the ratio determined by the Henderson-Hasselbalch equation. Many investigators have observed that the action of local anesthetics is pH dependent. Both the neutral (134) and the cationic forms of these drugs (135–137) have been proposed to be the active species. Hille (6) has made a very convincing case for the proposal that both the neutral and cationic species are active. The cationic drug can access the receptor only from the inside of the membrane and only when the channel is open. The neutral drug can interact with the receptor even if the channel is closed, gaining access to it through the lipophilic membrane phase. These observations have been confirmed in heart by Gliklich & Hoffman (138), who showed that in cardiac tissue, as in nerve, quaternary lidocaine derivatives are most effective when applied internally.

Small changes in pH can markedly alter the ratio of neutral-to-charged drug species. This in turn can alter the drug's effectiveness in several ways. First, external acidosis promotes the cationic drug form. Since this species partitions less readily into membranes (139), it is expected that the onset of drug action will be slowed (140). Furthermore, the equilibrium concentration in the membrane will be reduced under conditions of acidosis. Therefore, drugs that act primarily as blockers of the inactivated channel might have a reduced effect. On the other hand, acidosis may prolong the action potential, thereby providing a longer time for inactivation block to occur (141, 142). Since the concentration of neutral drug in the extracellular fluid is in equilibrium with the membrane concentration, external acidosis will, by translocation of drug from the sarcoplasmic pool to the extracellular pool, also reduce activation block (assuming the internal pH remains relatively unchanged) (143). Finally, external acidosis facilitates protonation of the receptor-bound drug (98, 144) and, since only neutral drug can dissociate from closed channels, recovery from block is expected to be slowed by acidosis. Indeed, Grant el al observed that when the extracellular pH was reduced from 7.4 to 6.9, the time constant of recovery from block was increased by 66% for quinidine (86) and over 100% for lidocaine (126). As a result, significant use-dependence occurs at slower heart rates. The net effect of acidosis will depend upon the relative importance of the reduction in block developed per action potential versus the increased persistence of block. Thus, Grant et al (86) observed little change in the potency of quinidine, whereas Nattel (144) found a small increase in potency. It therefore appears that for therapeutic concentrations of quinidine, the loss in activation block approximately balances the persistence of block at 1–2 Hz. In the case of lidocaine (which is also a potent inactivation blocker) block development may not be reduced much because of the lengthening of the action potential duration (141, 142). This together with the significant slowing of recovery can markedly potentiate the effect of lidocaine in acidosis (126, 144).

Usually, the intracellular pH is 0.2–0.3 units more acid than the external pH (145, 146). Since the neutral drug freely equilibrates across the cell membrane, one can calculate that the internal cationic concentration will be higher than the external. However, during cellular ischemia this pH gradient may be enhanced, resulting in a further relative increase of the cationic internal drug (147). Such an increase could markedly enhance activation block.

Finally, acidosis promotes the extrusion of intracellular potassium (148, 149). This may result in a marked increase of extracellular K^+, which in turn can produce substantial depolarization and enhance the voltage-dependent effect of antiarrhythmic drugs.

Conversely, alkalosis may tend to hyperpolarize the membrane potential and thereby reduce the effect of antiarrhythmic drugs. In addition, alkalosis promotes the neutral drug form, and recovery from block will occur more quickly (96). Alkalosis may also cause transient sequestration of drug from the aqueous phase into the lipid phase. For an activation blocker like quinidine, all these actions would be expected to reduce the effect. Alkalosis-inducing salts such as

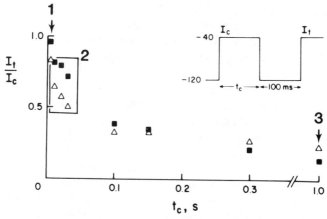

Figure 3   Effects of pH upon rate of development of block by lidocaine (200 μM) [Figure 10 from (96)]. Filled squares: pH = 7.0; open triangles:pH = 8.1. Alkalosis results in more activation block (1, arrow), faster development of inactivation block (2, box), and less steady-state block (3, arrow) (for explanation see text). Modified and reproduced from *The Journal of General Physiology* by copyright permission of The Rockefeller University Press and the authors.

sodium lactate have been traditionally used to combat toxicity caused by quinidine (150–151).

It should be noted, however, that under steady-state conditions external alkalosis will cause more neutral drug to dissolve in the membrane and thereby result in an increase in drug available for access to the inactivated channel receptor as well as an increase of internal drug concentration. As a result, activation block may actually become more marked and inactivation block may develop faster, but faster unblocking may result in less-steady–state block (see Figure 3).

Thus, the effects of pH can be quite complex. They will depend upon whether the change in pH is mostly intracellular or extracellular, whether the drug mostly blocks activated or inactivated channels, and the extent to which resting membrane potential and action potential duration are changed.

Structure-Activity Relationships

Traditional structure-activity analysis of local anesthetic (and antiarrhythmic) drugs have attempted to correlate physicochemical properties with a single "potency" figure. When block is measured in nerve by the usual techniques, the overall lipid solubility does correlate well with potency (113, 134, 135). However, the modulated receptor hypothesis predicts that a drug has three potencies, one for each of the channel states. Therefore, the reported single-value potencies must be intermediate between the lowest and the highest of the three state potencies. It is not surprising, therefore, that individual drugs can be reported as having very different potencies, depending upon the tissues used (71) or the experimental conditions. For example, chlorprocaine has been reported to be equal in potency to procaine (152) or four times as potent (114). This type of discrepancy would be greatly diminished if potencies were reported for well-defined standard experimental conditions or, better, if the potencies for the individual channel states were reported.

Recently, Courtney has shown that at 3 Hz antiarrhythmic drugs within a structural series, e.g. amides, may show a strong correlation between lipid solubility and potency (153). Non-amides appear generally more potent. Since the membrane potential of the cardiac cells was not voltage clamped in these studies, the potency of the inactivation blockers might have been altered by changes in action-potential duration.

The rate of block development can be roughly predicted on the basis of ionic charge on the local anesthetic molecule: quaternary compounds block rather slowly (93), while neutral compounds block much more quickly (92). For tertiary compounds the rate of block development appears intermediate and can be altered appropriately by pH (98).

For recovery from block, one would expect that lipophilic drugs, which can freely diffuse through the membrane, would exhibit the fastest recovery-time constant. However, Courtney has shown that the time constant of recovery correlates much better with molecular size than with lipid solubility (35). Sada & Ban (90) similarly showed that in a series of β-blockers the recovery time constant was more closely related to molecular weight than to lipid solubility. It appears that molecular weight and lipid solubility together can account for a significant part of the structure activity relations (over 20 drugs were analyzed in the above references). However, there must also be other important components. Firstly, several drugs deviate significantly from Courtney's molecular weight-lipid solubility rule (56, 89, 154). Secondly, it is possible to make small changes in compounds that only minimally alter their physicochemical properties, but nevertheless dramatically alter their electrophysiological blocking properties (155–157). Thirdly, stereoisomers that have identical physicochemical properties can nevertheless have markedly differing blocking properties (158). Clearly, in addition to the molecular weight-lipid solubility rule there must exist some stereoselective interactions between the receptor and the drugs (153). Unfortunately, no studies have yet correlated the modulated receptor affinities with various physicochemical properties of the drugs. We hope that by the time the next review in this series appears, it will be possible to give a more detailed account of quantitative structure analysis in relation to the channel receptor states.

CALCIUM CHANNEL BLOCKADE

There is now ample evidence (see reviews cited in introduction) showing that members of the verapamil, diltiazem, and nifedipine drug groups, as well as several inorganic polyvalent cations, reversibly diminish ion flux through membrane calcium channels as their primary effect. For several reasons, analysis of the mechanisms of this action is less complete than that of the sodium channel-blocking agents. Chief among these reasons is the still incomplete picture of physiological gating in the calcium channel (159–161). Second, there appear to be great differences between calcium channels in various species, between channels in different tissues of a given species, and even between channels in a given tissue at different stages of development (160, 161). Third, calcium influx through the membrane channels is modulated in many tissues by a variety of chemical agents (161, 163). Nevertheless, the kinetics and voltage-dependence of the cardiac calcium channel can be described *operationally* using conventional Hodgkin-Huxley variables and three states (rested, active, and inactivated) in analogy with the sodium channel (162, 164–166). Furthermore, considerable evidence is already available that suggests that the receptor for at least some of the organic calcium channel blockers is modulated by channel state or voltage. The modulated receptor hypothesis for the action of calcium channel blockers has recently been extended to smooth muscle (17, 167, 168). The most convincing evidence for the modulated receptor mechanism in the cardiac calcium channel comes from direct voltage clamp measurements of the calcium current (I_{si}), but the argument is also strongly supported by a marked frequency dependence of the negative inotropic action of verapamil and its congeners and of the effects of members of the verapamil and diltiazem groups on action potentials.

Use-Dependence

The earliest evidence suggestive of use-dependent blockade by calcium channel blockers can be found in studies of slow responses (169) and contractility (170–174). The first definitive evidence of use-dependent block of I_{si} was published by Ehara & Kaufmann (175) in a study of verapamil. This work was followed by a detailed study of D600 by McDonald et al (176) that fully confirmed the use-dependence as well as other modulated receptor characteristics of block by the verapamil congener. Subsequent voltage clamp studies have shown that diltiazem (177–179) as well as verapamil and its congeners (178, 180, 181) have strongly use-dependent effects on I_{si} in cardiac muscle. More recent studies of slow responses and force of contraction are fully consistent with this interpretation for papaverine (182, 183) and other calcium channel blockers (184, 185).

Voltage-Dependence of Recovery

Ehara & Kaufmann (175) in their voltage clamp study of verapamil showed that use-dependent block could be markedly reduced by a holding potential of -120 mV compared to the normal holding potential of -80 mV. The fact that this modulation of block represents the voltage dependence of the recovery from block produced by the activating-inactivating pulse was well demonstrated for D600 by McDonald et al (176). Trautwein and coworkers (180, 186) showed that blockade by AQA39 and by D600 was similarly removed by hyperpolarizing prepulses. A hyperpolarization of only 2 seconds to -90 mV was sufficient to reverse the AQA39 block, while 60 seconds at -90 mV was required for D600. At -140 mV, 2 seconds were sufficient to remove the D600 block. A similar voltage dependence has been reported for diltiazem (178). These results are consistent with a low affinity of these drugs for receptors in rested channels and a shift in the apparent inactivation curve to more negative levels. Similar results have been reported from the study of slow responses (187).

Is Drug-Receptor Affinity Higher in Activated or Inactivated Calcium Channels?

A recent study by Kanaya et al (178) showed that block by diltiazem and verapamil of I_{si} during a test pulse was markedly increased by increasing the duration of a depolarizing conditioning pulse from 100 msec to 2–3 seconds. This suggests that both drugs can block inactivated calcium channels. Moreover, for diltiazem this block could not be enhanced by increasing the voltage of a 30-msec conditioning pulse (one too short to result in much inactivation) from -30 to $+80$ mV. This was interpreted as evidence that the affinity of diltiazem for the inactivated channel is greater than the affinity for the channel in the open state. Lee & Tsien (177) similarly concluded that diltiazem mostly blocks inactivated calcium channels. Even at concentrations as high as 50 μM, they still could not demonstrate open channel block for this drug. In contrast, nitrendipine and D600 both caused a fast reduction of I_{si} upon opening of the channels. Lee & Tsien interpreted this as evidence for open channel block. It should be noted that under the conditions of their experiments (Ba^{2+} substituted for Ca^{2+}) inactivation is minimized, and consequently inactivation block would be minimized. Nevertheless, as in the case of the sodium channel blockers, it appears that some drugs (e.g. diltiazem) behave primarily as inactivated state blockers, while other drugs (e.g. verapamil, D600) also block open channels. It is not clear whether some drugs exclusively block open channels. Moreover, studies of single channel currents (188) have suggested that calcium channels flicker on and off for a period of time after sensing an activating voltage rather than opening only once, as is the case for sodium channels. If this is the case, then continuing development of block of calcium channels during a long depolarizing clamp might represent block of open flickering channels as well as inactivated ones. Patch clamp methods will probably be needed to resolve this problem.

Dihydropyridine Calcium Channel Blockers: A Special Case?

Several lines of evidence suggest that there may be important differences between the nifedipine family of drugs and other calcium channel blockers. For example, Schramm et al have reported (189) that a new dihydropyridine (BAY K 8644) has potent *positive* inotropic effects that are competitively inhibited by nifedipine. Second, receptor binding studies (190–194) suggest that nitrendipine and other members of the nifedipine family bind to a common receptor site that differs from but is allosterically linked to, the site or sites at which verapamil and diltiazem bind. Lee & Tsien (177) reported that the IC_{50} for I_{si} suppression was about 100-fold higher than the K_d reported for isotope binding studies. This is not totally unexpected, however, since binding studies determine dissociation constants in fully depolarized membrane fragments, i.e. the highest affinity state. In contrast, Lee & Tsien calculated binding in intact cells at -40 mV. Using computer fitting with our own data, we estimate binding to rested channels to have a dissociation constant in the mM to M range. Thus, as in the case of sodium channel blockers, apparent (measured) potencies can vary between the potencies of the lowest and highest affinity states. However, the possibility that the dihydropyridines produce a qualitatively different sort of blockade must be considered. Kohlhardt & Fleckenstein (195) and Bayer & Ehara (196) found that nifedipine produced a block of I_{si} that had the same apparent time constant of recovery as inactivated channels in the drug-free state. Unfortunately, these authors did not use very short or very long recovery intervals. Kass (197) reported that block of I_{si} in Purkinje fibers by nisoldipine was much less voltage-sensitive than block by D600. His protocol showed that, unlike D600 blockade, the nisoldipine-induced suppression of I_{si} was not removed by rests of up to 120 seconds at relatively negative holding potentials. Also in contrast to D600 results was the observation that use-dependence of the nisoldipine block was minimal or absent. Nitrendipine was similarly found to be almost devoid of use-dependent effect by Lee & Tsien (177) in their study of isolated ventricular cardiac cells when measured at a frequency of 0.05 Hz. In a report of slow responses in K^+-depolarized chick ventricle, Hachisu & Pappano (198) found that verapamil, but not nifedipine or nimodipine, caused a use-dependent block. However, the driving frequency in their experiments was only 0.1 Hz, which is too slow to detect use-dependent block if the recovery time constant of the dihydropyridines is less than 2–3 seconds. This point is clearly made by Lee & Tsien (177), who found a recovery time constant of only a few seconds at room temperature (20–22°C) for nitrendipine, thereby implying that use-dependence can occur with this drug. Molyvdas & Sperelakis (199) reported that mesudipine, another congener of nifedipine, manifested frequency-dependent block of slow responses for the first 20 minutes of exposure and frequency-independent block thereafter. In an earlier study of nifedipine, Kohlhardt & Haap (200) found that this agent caused a use-dependent depression of slow response action potential overshoot and upstroke velocity in rabbit AV node at a frequency of 0.2 Hz. Therefore, a firm conclusion should not be drawn regarding the state dependence of the block produced by the dihydropyridines until they have been studied over a broader range of driving rates. It is likely that most, if not all, of the calcium channel blockers will be found to have use dependence when they are studied at driving intervals shorter than the recovery time constant.

Site of Action of the Calcium Channel Blockers

The route traveled by a calcium channel blocker to its receptor site has certain parallels with that mapped out for the local anesthetics on the basis of their molecular structure and kinetics (6, 98). It is noteworthy that none of the useful calcium channel blockers are permanently charged and the amines all have pKa's of nine or less. All can be taken up by cells (201) and some structure-contractile activity analyses have been reported (174, 202, 203). These data suggest that the drugs must cross the cell membrane to gain access to their site of action. A study of D890 (the N-methyl quaternized derivative of D600) showed it to be without effect in a standard contractility assay (174). In an important extension of this approach, Hescheler et al (204) showed that extracellularly applied D890 had no effects on calcium-dependent electrical properties of guinea pig myocytes. In contrast, D600 at 50-fold lower concentrations markedly lowered and shortened the plateau of the action potential. However, when administered intracellularly by pressure injection, both drugs caused prompt suppressant effects. Furthermore, after a single pulse injection the block induced by D890 persisted, while that produced by D600 completely disappeared within nine minutes. These results suggest that, when in the charged form, drugs must access the verapamil receptor from the intracellular side of the membrane. No reports comparing intracellular and extracellular application of dihydropyridine drugs were found in our survey. However, Rosenberger & Triggle (205) reported that quaternary analogs of nifedipine were inactive in suppressing smooth muscle contraction, suggesting that these drugs also must cross a lipid barrier to gain access to their receptor.

As noted above, dissociation of uncharged local anesthetic drugs from the inactivated sodium channel probably takes place through the lipid phase of the membrane. Such studies require the availability of similar drugs with different lipid:water partition coefficients, or a single drug whose partition coefficient can be modified by pH manipulation. Whether size is a more important determinant of the recovery time constant than lipid solubility for calcium channel blockers, as it is for local anesthetics (35), will require further investigation. However, Pelzer et al (186) found that for the closely related drugs, D600 and AQA-39, the less lipophilic and slightly smaller molecule AQA-39 had the faster rate of dissociation.

APPLICATIONS OF THE MODULATED RECEPTOR HYPOTHESIS

Selective Depression of Depolarized Tissue

Arrhythmias are frequently associated with tissue depolarization caused by a variety of conditions, but especially ischemia (64, 206–213) and digitalis poisoning (214, 215). For several reasons, antiarrhythmic drugs are more depressant in depolarized tissue (Table 5). First, receptor binding of these drugs develops faster and dissociation occurs more slowly in depolarized myocardium. As a result, the clinician (under optimal circumstances) can choose a drug dose that will have relatively little effect on normally polarized tissue, which is necessary for normal conduction, while selectively depressing the depolarized tissue, which is responsible for the arrhythmia.

Second, although all antiarrhythmic drugs appear to shift inactivation and slow recovery, one would expect, other factors being equal, that an inactivation blocker would be more selective than an activation blocker when the major basis for the arrhythmia is depolarization.

Selective depression of depolarized tissue is now well accepted as a major mechanism of action of sodium channel-blocking antiarrhythmic drugs (2, 3, 63, 242, 255, 256).

Table 5 Evidence for selective depression as an effect of sodium channel blockers

Drug	References
Aprindine	41–43
Disopyramide	124,216,217
Encainide	218–220
Ethmozin	221
Flecainide	222–224
Imipramine	225
Lidocaine	30,34,61,62,69,93,96,226–246
Mexiletine	71,73,75,76,247,248
Phenytoin	62,227,249–251
Prenylamine	79
Procainamide	62,80
Propafenone	81,83
Propranolol	62,252
Quinidine	62,240
Tocainide	61,253,254

In the case of the calcium channel blockers, the situation is somewhat complicated by the very significant protective effect of these agents in metabolically compromised tissue (257–262). In several acute coronary occlusion and reperfusion models, diltiazem and verapamil are extremely effective in preventing arrhythmias (263–265). They are less effective in suppressing arrhythmias after they have started (266, 267). There are several possible explanations for this discrepancy; protection against depolarization caused by ischemia when given before occlusion or reperfusion is one (268).

Selective Depression of Tachycardias

During a rapid rhythm, i.e. one with short diastolic intervals, less recovery from drug-induced blockade can occur between beats than during a slower rhythm. Also, more activation and inactivation block develops. Hence, the shorter the cycle length, the greater the steady-state block of inward currents. Thus, given a drug with a long recovery time, e.g. quinidine, one can choose a dose that minimally reduces conduction at normal heart rates but suppresses conduction in a tachycardia. For some other drugs, e.g. lidocaine, the diastolic recovery from block at normal resting potential is so fast that they are not very effective in "filtering" tachycardias. Thus, it has been reported by numerous investigators that lidocaine is not a very effective agent in ventricular tachycardia in the absence of resting depolarization (269–271). However, lidocaine is still effective in preventing very fast arrhythmias, e.g. ventricular fibrillation (272). Nifedipine, which manifests little or no use dependence of blockade at slow and moderate driving rates, also turns out to be ineffective in reversing supraventricular tachycardias (273), the arrhythmia in which other calcium channel blockers are most effective.

Selective Depression of Early Extrasystoles

An early extrasystole can be viewed as a very rapid single beat tachyarrhythmia. Because the tachycardia is not sustained, a drug that produces a slowly increasing use-dependent block will not block such extrasystoles very effectively. The primary example of a drug that has such a pattern of slow in-slow out (SISO) blockade is quinidine. That is, development of block is slow and recovery during rest is also slow. In contrast, a drug like lidocaine can be described as fast in-fast out (FIFO), since it associates avidly with the receptor during the entire duration of the action potential and dissociates rapidly during diastole. Hence, a sufficiently early extrasystole will find a significant fraction of channels blocked—and will be suppressed—at doses of lidocaine that have little depressant effect on impulses in the normal rhythm. Therefore, for a given tolerable (minor) depression of the normal rhythm, a FIFO drug will provide much more depression during diastole than a SISO agent.

Instances often occur in which FIFOs are not quite effective, and the maximum tolerated level of a SISO also does not achieve the required suppression of the extrasystoles. It can be computed (34) that the combination of a FIFO agent (lidocaine or equivalent) with a SISO drug (quinidine) can provide a therapeutic efficacy not obtainable with maximum tolerated doses of either drug alone. This prediction has been confirmed by experimental (274) and by clinical studies (275, 276).

The other permutations of the rate in-rate out description are easily predicted. A slow in-fast out agent would be ineffective and would probably be dropped from study in early screening tests. In contrast, a fast in-slow out agent (rapid association, slow dissociation) might be expected to have a high degree of cumulation, i.e. would be a potent local anesthetic. If, however, such an agent was accidently administered systemically, it would be toxic to the myocardium at slow heart rates and relatively low plasma concentrations. Bupivicaine appears to be such a FISO drug (277).

Selective Depression on the Basis of Action Potential Duration

The experiments utilizing modulated receptor protocols described above show that certain drugs are nearly pure inactivation blockers, (e.g. amiodarone, benzocaine, diltiazem), others are nearly pure activation blockers (e.g. quaternary lidocaine derivatives, quinidine), while most of the drugs have significant affinity for the channel receptor in both states. Since the action potentials of all cardiac tissues have an upstroke of roughly comparable duration (1–2 msec), activation blockers are expected to be effective in all tissues. In contrast, the plateau of the action potential varies markedly in different cardiac cells (50–500 msec). The effect of an inactivation blocker will be more marked the longer the duration of the action potential plateau (13). Thus, inactivation blockers are expected to be more effective in Purkinje and ventricular myocardium than in atrial tissue. Moreover, if the inactivation blocker also has a fast diastolic recovery, the drug will produce an insignificant level of block in atrial tissue and will have little efficacy. Lidocaine in atrial tissue would therefore behave like a slow in-fast out drug; and it does have a low efficacy against atrial arrhythmias (234).

Antiarrhythmic Drug Interactions Caused by Receptor Modulation

Since many cardiac drugs can lengthen or shorten the cardiac action potential duration, it is predictable that these drugs might potentiate or antagonize the action of inactivation blockers. Thus, part of the positive interactions observed between quinidine and mexiletine (276) must result from the lengthening of the action potential duration caused by quinidine, which provides more time for inactivation block by mexiletine to occur. It will be important to see whether drugs that cause more marked lengthening will further amplify this synergistic action. Conversely, shortening of action potential duration would theoretically be of benefit in the treatment of toxicity caused by inactivation blockers.

In summary, modulated receptor concepts appear to be well supported by the available experimental evidence. However, the hypothesis cannot yet be considered to have been *proven* to be the sole or primary mechanism of the action of these drugs (278). Further tests over broader experimental conditions need to be carried out. One of the major advantages of the hypothesis is the wide range of testable predictions that can be generated. As noted above, many in vitro studies in the last five years have been designed on this basis. It is hoped that in the next five years, many more clinical as well as basic studies will test the hypothesis.

Acknowledgments

We thank James Moyer and Brian Katzung for computer help, Charles Cotner for graphics, and Deborah Noack and Virginia Hayes for word processing. Research has been funded in part by the USPHS and the American Heart Association. L. M. Hondeghem is an Established Investigator of the American Heart Association.

Literature Cited

1. Sasyniuk, B. I., Ogilvie, R. I. 1975. Antiarrhythmic drugs: Electrophysiological and pharmacokinetic considerations. *Ann. Rev. Pharmacol. Toxicol.* 15:131–55

2. Boyden, P. A., Wit, A. L. 1983. Pharmacology of the antiarrhythmic drugs. In *Cardiac Therapy*, ed. M. R. Rosen, B. F. Hoffman, pp. 171–234. Boston/Amsterdam: Martinus Nijhoff. 568 pp.

3. Hondeghem, L. M., Mason, J. W. 1982. Agents used in cardiac arrhythmias. In *Basic & Clinical Pharmacology*, ed. B. G. Katzung, pp. 138–54. Los Altos: Lange Medical Publ. 815 pp.

4. Fleckenstein, A. 1981. Fundamental actions of calcium antagonists on myocardial and cardiac pacemaker cell membranes. See Ref. 16, pp. 59–81

5. McAllister, R. G. Jr. 1982. Clinical pharmacology of slow channel blocking agents. *Prog. Cardiovasc. Dis.* 25:83–102

6. Hille, B. 1977. Local anesthetics: Hydrophilic and hydrophobic pathways for the drug-receptor reaction. *J. Gen. Physiol.* 69:497–515

7. Hondeghem, L. M., Katzung, B. G. 1977. Time- and voltage-dependent interactions of antiarrhythmic drugs with cardiac sodium channels. *Biochim. Biophys. Acta.* 472:373–98

8. Singh, B. N. 1977. Antiarrhythmic effects of local anesthetics and calcium antagonists. *Pharmac. Ther. C* 2:125–50

9. Hauswirth, O., Singh, B. N. 1979. Ionic mechanisms in heart muscle in relation to the genesis and the pharmacological control of cardiac arrhythmias. *Pharmacol. Rev.* 30:5–63

10. Zipes, D. P., Troup, P. J. 1978. New antiarrhythmic agents. Amiodarone, aprindine, disopyramide, ethmozin, mexiletine, tocainide, verapamil. *Am. J. Cardiol.* 41:1005–24

11. Scholz, H. 1981. Therapie der arrhythmien. Neue antiarrhythmika. *Verh. Dtsch. Ges. Kreislaufforsch.* 47:18–33

12. Surawicz, B. 1983. Pharmacologic treatment of cardiac arrhythmias: 25 years of progress. *J. Am. Coll. Cardiol.* 1:365–81

13. Hondeghem, L. M., Katzung, B. G. 1983. Mechanism of action of antiarrhythmic drugs. In *Function of the Heart in Normal and Pathological States,* ed. N. Sperelakis, Boston: Martinus Nijhoff. In press

14. Fleckenstein, A. 1977. Specific pharmacology of calcium in myocardium, cardiac pacemakers, and vascular smooth muscle. *Ann. Rev. Pharmacol. Toxicol.* 17:149–66

15. Henry, P. D. 1980. Comparative pharmacology of calcium antagonists: Nifedipine, verapamil and diltiazem. *Am. J. Cardiol.* 46:1047–58

16. Weiss, G. B. 1981. Sites of action of calcium antagonists in vascular smooth muscle. In *New Perspectives on Calcium Antagonists*, pp. 83–94. Bethesda: Am. Physiol. Soc. 241 pp.

17. Triggle, D. J. 1981. Calcium antagonists: Basic chemical and pharmacological aspects. See Ref. 16, pp. 1–18

18. Allen, J. C. 1982. The current status of the mechanism of the calcium channel antagonists. *Prog. Cardiovasc. Dis.* 25:133–40

19. Rahwan, R. G. 1983. Mechanisms of action of membrane calcium channel blockers and intracellular calcium antagonists. *Medicinal Res. Rev.* 3:21–42

20. Mitchell, L. B., Schroeder, J. S., Mason, J. W. 1982. Comparative clinical electrophysiologic effects of diltiazem, verapamil, and nifedipine: A review. *Am. J. Cardiol.* 49:629–35

21. Harris, P., Opie, L. 1971. *Calcium and the Heart*. London: Academic. 198 pp.

22. Braunwald, E. 1982. Mechanism of action of calcium-channel-blocking agents. *N. Engl. J. Med.* 307:1618–27

23. Reves, J. G., Kissin, I., Lell, W. A., Tosone, S. 1982. Calcium entry blockers: Uses and implications for anesthesiologists. *Anesthesiology* 57:504–18

24. Puech, P., Krebs, R. 1980. *New Therapy of Ischemic Heart Disease. 4th Int. Adalat Symp.* Amsterdam / Oxford / Princeton: Excerpta Med. 298 pp.

25. Flaim, S. F., Zelis, R. 1982. *Calcium Blockers. Mechanisms of Action and Clinical Applications*. Baltimore/Munich: Urban & Schrwarzenberg

26. Nayler, W. G., Horowitz, J. D. 1983. Calcium antagonists: A new class of drugs. *Pharmacol. Ther.* 20:203–62

27. Weidmann, S. 1955. Effects of calcium ions and local anesthetics on electrical properties of Purkinje fibers. *J. Physiol.* 129:568–82

28. Johnson, E. A., McKinnon, M. G. 1957. The differential effect of quinidine and pyrilamine on the myocardial action potential at various rates of stimulation. *J. Pharmacol. Exp. Ther.* 120:460–68

29. Heistracher, P. 1971. Mechanism of action of antifibrillatory drugs. *Naunyn-Schmiedebergs Arch. Pharmacol.* 269:199–212

30. Chen, C-M., Gettes, L. S., Katzung, B. G. 1975. Effect of lidocaine and quinidine on steady state characteristics and recovery kinetics of (dv/dt) max in guinea pig ventricular myocardium. *Circ. Res.* 37:20–29

31. Strichartz, G. R. 1973. The inhibition of sodium currents in myelinated nerve by quaternary derivatives of lidocaine. *J. Gen. Physiol.* 62:37–57

32. Courtney, K. R. 1975. Mechanism of frequency-dependent inhibition of sodium currents in frog myelinated nerve by the lidocaine derivative GEA 968. *J. Pharmacol. Exp. Ther.* 195:225–36

33. Hodgkin, A. L., Huxley, A. F. 1952. A quantitative description of membrane current and its application to conduction and excitation in nerve. *J. Physiol.* 117:500–44

34. Hondeghem, L. M., Katzung, B. G. 1980. Test of a model of antiarrhythmic drug action. Effect of quinidine and lidocaine on myocardial conduction. *Circulation* 61:1217–24

35. Courtney, K. R. 1980. Interval-dependent effects of small antiarrhythmic drugs on excitability of guinea-pig myocardium. *J. Mol. Cell. Cardiol.* 12:1273–86

36. Sada, H. 1978. Effect of phentolamine, alprenolol and prenylamine on maximum rate of rise of action potential in guinea-pig papillary muscles. *Naunyn-Schmiedebergs Arch. Pharmacol.* 304:191–201

37. Courtney, K. R. 1980. Antiarrhythmic drug design: Frequency-dependent block in myocardium. In *Molecular Mechanisms of Anesthesia*, ed. B. R. Fink, pp. 111–18. New York: Raven. 510 pp.

38. Mason, J. W., Hondeghem, L. M., Katzung, B. G. 1983. Amiodarone blocks inactivated cardiac sodium channels. *Pfluegers Arch.* 396:79–81

39. Rosenbaum, M. B., Chiale, P. A., Halpern, M. S., Nau, G. J., Przbylski, J. et al. 1976. Clinical efficacy of amiodarone as an antiarrhythmic agent. *Am. J. Cardiol.* 38:934–44

40. Moyer, J. W., Hondeghem, L. 1978. Rate rhythm and voltage dependent effects of aprindine: A test of a model of the mechanisms of action of antiarrhythmic drugs. *Proc. West. Pharmacol. Soc.* 21:57–61

41. Steinberg, M. I., Greenspan, K. 1976. Intracellular electrophysiological alterations in canine cardiac conducting tissue induced by aprindine and lignocaine. *Cardiovas. Res.* 10:236–44

42. Verdonck, F., Vereecke, J., Vlengels, A. 1974. Electrophysiological effects of aprindine on isolated heart preparations. *Eur. J. Pharmacol.* 26:338–47

43. Carmeliet, E. P., Verdonck, F. 1974. Effects of aprindine and lidocaine on transmembrane potentials and radioactive K efflux in different cardiac tissues. *Acta Cardiol. Suppl.* 18:73–90

44. Gilmour, R. F. Jr., Chikarev, V. N., Jurevichus, J. A., Zacharov, S. I., Zipes, D. P., Rosenshtraukh, L. V. 1981. Effect of aprindine on transmembrane currents and contractile force in frog atria. *J. Pharmacol. Exp. Ther.* 217:390–96

45. TenEick, R. E., Yeh, J. Z., Robertson, L. 1980. Cellular electrophysiological effects of aprindine on cat papillary muscle. *Fed. Proc.* 39:966

46. Yeh, J. Z., TenEick, R. E. 1980. Voltage dependent block of Na channels in cat papillary muscle and squid axon produced by aprindine. *Fed. Proc.* 39:966

47. Kojima, M. 1981 Effects of disopyramide on transmembrane action potentials in guinea-pig papillary muscles. *Eur. J. Pharmacol.* 69:11–24

48. Kojima, M., Ban, T., Sada, H. 1982. Effects of disopyramide on the maximum rate of rise of the potential (V_{max}) in guinea pig papillary muscles. *Jpn. J. Pharmacol.* 32:91–102

49. Man, R. Y. K., Dresel, P. E. 1979. A specific effect of lidocaine and tocainide on ventricular conduction of mid-range extrasystoles. *J. Cardiovasc. Pharmacol.* 1:329–42

50. Campbell, T. J. 1983. Resting and rate-dependent depression of maximum rate of depolarisation of (V_{max}) in guinea pig ventricular action potentials by mexiletine, disopyramide, and encainide. *J. Cardiovasc. Pharmacol.* 5:291–96

51. Campbell, T. J. 1983. Kinetics of onset of rate-dependent effects of Class I antiarrhythmic drugs are important in determining their effects on refractoriness in guinea pig ventricle, and provide a theoretical basis for their subclassification. *Cardiovasc. Res.* 17:344–52

52. Grant, A. O., Hondeghem, L. M., Katzung, B. G. 1978. Effects of droperidol on depolarization-induced automaticity, maximum upstroke velocity (V_{max}) and the kinetics of recovery of V_{max} in guinea-pig ventricular myocardium. *J. Pharmacol. Exp. Ther.* 205:193–203

53. Carmeliet, E. 1980. Electrophysiologic effects of encainide on isolated cardiac muscle and Purkinje fibers and on the Langendorff-perfused guinea-pig heart. *Eur. J. Pharmacol.* 61:247–62

54. Danilo, P. Jr., Langan, W. B., Rosen, M. R., Hoffman, B. F. 1977. Effects of the phenothiazine analog, EN-313, on ventricular arrhythmias in the dog. *Eur. J. Pharmacol.* 45:127–39

55. Kastor, J. A., Horowitz, L. N., Harken, A. H., Josephson, M. E. 1981. Clinical electrophysiology of ventricular tachycardia. *N. Engl. J. Med.* 304:1004–1020

56. Campbell, T. J., Vaughan Williams, E. M. 1983. Voltage- and time-dependent depression of maximum rate of depolarization of guinea-pig ventricular action potentials by two new antiarrhythmic drugs, flecainide and lorcainide. *Cardiovasc. Res.* 17:251–58

57. Weld, F. J., Bigger, J. T. Jr. 1980. Electrophysiological effects of imipramine on ovine cardiac Purkinje and ventricular muscle fibers. *Circ. Res.* 46:167–75

58. Rawling, D. A., Fozzard, H. A. 1979. Effects of imipramine on cellular electrophysiological properties of cardiac Purkinje fibers. *J. Pharmacol. Exp. Ther.* 209:371–75

59. Hondeghem, L. M., Lam, C. 1980. Selective depression of 2,4-dintrophenol depolarized canine Purkinje fibers by lidocaine. *Naunyn-Schmiedebergs Arch. Pharmacol.* 313:11–16

60. Courtney, K. R. 1979. Fast frequency-dependent block of action potential upstroke in rabbit atrium by small local anesthetics. *Life Sci.* 24:1581–88

61. Oshita, S., Sada, H., Kojima, M., Ban, T. 1980. Effects of tocainide and lidocaine on the transmembrane action potentials as related to external potassium and calcium concentrations in guinea pig papillary muscles. *Naunyn-Schmiedebergs Arch. Pharmacol.* 314:67–82

62. Wald, R. W., Waxman, M. B., Downar, E. 1980. The effect of antiarrhythmic drugs on depressed conduction and unidirectional block in sheep Purkinje fibers. *Circ. Res.* 46:612–19

63. Lazzara, R., Hope, R. R., El-Sherif, N., Scherlag, B. J. 1979. Effects of lidocaine on hypoxic and ischemic cardiac cells. *Am. J. Cardiol.* 41:872–78

64. El-Sherif, N., Scherlag, B. J., Lazzara, R., Hope, R. R. 1977. Re-entrant ventricular arrhythmias in the late myocardial infarction period. 1. Conduction characteristics in the infarction zone. *Circulation* 55:686–702

65. Ehring, G. R., Hondeghem, L. M. 1980. Structural similarities and cardiac electrophysiological differences between lidocaine and procainamide. *Proc. West. Pharmacol. Soc.* 23:163–66

66. Iven, H., Brasch, H. 1977. Effects of the local anesthetics Brufacain and Lidocaine on transmembrane action potentials, refractory period, and reactivation of the sodium system in guinea pig heart muscle. *Naunyn-Schmiedebergs Arch. Pharmacol.* 297:153–61

67. Payet, M. D. 1982. Effect of lidocaine on fast and slow inactivation of sodium cur-

rent in rat ventricular cells. *J. Pharmacol. Exp. Ther.* 223:235–40

68. Lamanna, V., Antzelevitch, C., Moe, G. K. 1982. Effects of lidocaine on conduction through depolarized canine false tendons and on a model of reflected reentry. *J. Pharmacol. Exp. Ther.* 221:353–61

69. Weld, F. M., Bigger, J. T. Jr. 1975. Effect of lidocaine on the early inward transient current in sheep cardiac Purkinje fibers. *Circ. Res.* 37:630–39

70. Sada, H., Ban, T. 1981. Frequency dependent block of nerve conduction by β-adrenergic blocking agents. *Arch. Int. Pharmacodyn. Ther.* 254:134–44

71. Courtney, K. R. 1981. Comparative actions of mexiletine on sodium channels in nerve, skeletal and cardiac muscle. *Eur. J. Pharmacol.* 74:9–18

72. Courtney, K. R. 1981. Significance of bicarbonate for antiarrhythmic drug action. *J. Mol. Cell. Cardiol.* 13:1031–1034

73. Hohnloser, S., Weirich, J., Antoni, H. 1982. Effects of mexiletine on steady-state characteristics and recovery kinetics of V_{max} and conduction velocity in guinea pig myocardium. *J. Cardiovasc. Pharmacol.* 4:232–39

74. Okuma, K., Sugiyama, S., Wada, M., Sugemoya, J., Nimi, N., et al. 1976. Experimental studies on the antiarrhythmic action of a lidocaine analog. *Cardiology* 61:283–97

75. Weld, F. M., Bigger, J. T. Jr., Swistel, D., Bordiuk, J., Lau, Y. H. 1979. Electrophysiological effects of mexiletine (Ko1173) on ovine cardiac Purkinje fibers. *J. Pharmacol. Exp. Ther.* 210:222–28

76. Sada, H., Ban, T., Oshita, S. 1980. Effects of mexiletine on transmembrane action potentials as affected by external potassium concentration and by rate of stimulation in guinea-pig papillary muscles. *Clin. Exper. Pharmacol. Physiol.* 7:583–93

77. Ehring, G. R., Hondeghem, L. M. 1978. Rate, rhythm and voltage dependent effects of phenytoin: A test of a model of the mechanisms of action of antiarrhythmic drugs. *Proc. West. Pharmacol. Soc.* 21:63–65

78. Courtney, K. R., Etter, E. F. 1983. Modulated anticonvulsant block of sodium channels in nerve and muscle. *Eur. J. Pharmacol.* 88:1–9

79. Ban, T., Kojima, M., Sada, H., Oshita, S. 1982. Effects of prenylamine on transmembrane action potentials as related to the changes in external porhtassium concentrations in guinea pig papillary mus-

cle. *J. Cardiovasc. Pharmacol.* 4:601–8

80. Sada, H., Kojima, M., Ban, T. 1979. Effect of procainamide on transmembrane action potentials in guinea-pig papillary muscles as affected by external potassium concentration. *Naunyn-Schmiedebergs Arch. Pharmacol.* 309: 179–90

81. Kohlhardt, M., Seifert, C. 1980. Inhibition of V_{max} of the action potential by propafenone and its voltage-, time- and pH-dependence in mammalian ventricular myocardium. *Naunyn-Schmiedebergs Arch. Pharmacol.* 315:55–62

82. Kohlhardt, M., Seifert, C. 1983. Tonic and phasic INa blockade by antiarrhythmics: Different properties of drug binding to fast sodium channels as judged from V_{max} studies with propafenone and derivatives in mammalian ventricular myocardium. *Pfleugers Arch.* 396:199–209

83. Ledda, F., Mantelli, L., Manzini, S., Amerini, S., Mugelli, A. 1981. Electrophysiological and antiarrhythmic properties of propafenon in isolated cardiac preparations. *J. Cardiovasc. Pharmacol.* 3:1162–73

84. Tarr, M., Luckstead, E. F., Jurewicz, P. A., Haas, H. G. 1973. Effect of propranolol on the fast inward sodium current in frog atrial muscle. *J. Pharmacol. Exp. Ther.* 184:599–610

85. Ban, T. 1977. A kinetic study of the effects of propranolol and N-propylajmaline on the rate of rise of action potential in guinea pig papillary muscles. *Jpn. J. Pharmacol.* 27:865–80

86. Grant, A. O., Trantham, J. L., Brown, K. K., Strauss, H. C. 1982. pH-dependent effects of quinidine on the kinetics of dV/dt-max in guinea pig ventricular myocardium. *Circ. Res.* 50:210–17

87. Ducouret, P. 1976. The effect of quinidine on membrane electrical activity in frog auricular fibres studied by current and voltage clamp. *Br. J. Pharmacol.* 57:163–84

88. Yeh, J. Z., Narahashi, T. 1976. Mechanism of action of quinidine on squid giant axon membranes. *J. Pharmacol. Exp. Ther.* 196:62–70

89. Sada, H., Ban, T. 1981. Effects of various structurally related β-adrenoceptor blocking agents on maximum upstroke velocity of action potential in guinea pig papillary muscles. *Naunyn-Schmiedebergs Arch. Pharmacol.* 317: 245–51

90. Sada, H., Ban, T. 1980. Effects of acebutolol and other structurally related β

adrenergic blockers on transmembrane action potential in guinea-pig papillary muscles. *J. Pharmacol. Exp. Ther.* 215:507–14

91. Lee, K. S., Hume, J. R., Giles, W., Brown, A. M. 1981. Sodium current depression by lidocaine and quinidine in isolated ventricular cells. *Nature* 291:325–27

92. Sanchez-Chapula, J., Tsuda, Y., Josephson, I. R. 1983. Voltage- and use-dependent effects of lidocaine on sodium current in rat single ventricular cells. *Circ. Res.* 52:557–65

93. Gintant, G. A., Hoffman, B. F., Naylor, R. E. 1983. The influence of molecular form of local anesthetic-type antiarrhythmic agents on reduction of maximum upstroke velocity of canine cardiac Purkinje fibers. *Circ. Res.* 52:735–46

94. Singh, B. N., Vaughan Williams, E. M. 1970. The effect of amiodarone, a new anti-anginal drug, on cardiac muscle. *Br. J. Pharmacol.* 39:657–67

95. Heger, J. J., Prystowsky, E. N., Jackman, W. M., Naccarelli, G. V., Warfel, K. A., et al. 1981. Amiodarone: Clinical efficacy and electrophysiology during long-term therapy for recurrent ventricular tachycardia or ventricular fibrillation. *N. Engl. J. Med.* 305:539–45

96. Bean, B. P., Cohen, C. J., Tsien, R. W. 1983. Lidocaine block of cardiac sodium channels. *J. Gen. Physiol.* 81:613–42

97. Colatsky, T. J. 1982. Quinidine block of cardiac sodium channels is rate- and voltage-dependent. *Biophys. J.* 37:343a

98. Schwarz, W., Palade, P. T., Hille, B. 1977. Local anesthetics. Effect of pH in use-dependent block of sodium channels in frog muscle. *Biophys. J.* 20:343–68

99. Strichartz, G. 1980. Use-dependent conduction block produced by volatile general anesthetic agents. *Acta Anaesthesiol. Scand.* 24:402–6

100. Courtney, K. R., Kendig, J. J., Cohen, E. N. 1978. Frequency-dependent conduction block: The role of nerve impulse pattern in local anesthetic potency. *Anesthesiology* 48:111–17

101. Rimmel, C., Walle, A., Kessler, H., Ulbricht W. 1978. Rates of block by procaine and benzocaine and the procaine-benzocaine interaction at the node of Ranvier. *Pfluegers Arch.* 376:105–118

102. Kendig, J. J., Courtney, K. R., Cohen, E. N. 1979. Anesthetics: Molecular correlates of voltage- and frequency-dependent sodium channel block in nerve. *J. Pharmacol. Exp. Ther.* 210:446–52

103. Hondeghem, L. M. 1983. See Ref. 82, appendix

104. Yeh, J. Z. 1978. Sodium inactivation mechanism modulates QX-314 block of sodium channels in squid axons. *Biophys. J.* 24:569–74

105. Yeh, J. Z. Narahashi, T. 1977. Kinetic analysis of pancuronium interaction with sodium channels in squid axon membranes. *J. Gen. Physiol.* 69:2293–323

106. Cahalan, M. D., Almers, W. 1979. Interactions between quaternary lidocaine, the sodium channel gates, and tetrodotoxin. *Biophys. J.* 27:39–56

107. Yeh, J. Z. 1982. A pharmacological approach to the structure of the sodium channel in squid axon. In *Proteins in the Nervous System: Structure and Function,* pp. 17–49. New York: Liss

108. Armstrong, C. M., Gilly, W. F. 1979. Fast and slow steps in the activation of sodium channels. *J. Gen. Physiol.* 74:691–711

109. Keynes, R. D., Rojas, E. 1974. Kinetics and steady-state properties of the charged system controlling sodium conductance in the squid giant axon. *J. Physiol.* 239:393–434

110. Lo, M-V. C., Shrager, P. 1981. Block and inactivation of sodium channels in nerve by amino acid derivatives. II. Dependence on temperature and drug concentration. *Biophys. J.* 35:1–16

111. Peganov, E. M., Khodorov, B. I. 1977. Vorootnyi tok v membrane perekhvata ranve v usloviiakh lineinoco izmeneniia membrannogo potentsiala *Biul. Eksp. Biol. Med.* 84:515–18

112. Brown, A. M., Lee, K. S., Powell, T. 1981. Sodium current in single rat heart muscles. *J. Physiol.* 318:479–500

113. Seeman, P. 1972. The membrane action of anesthetics and tranquilizers. *Pharmacol. Rev.* 24:583–655

114. Covino, B. G., Vassallo, H. G. 1976. *Local Anesthetics. Mechanisms of Action and Clinical Use.* New York: Grune & Stratton

115. Catterall, W. A. 1981. Inhibition of voltage-sensitive sodium channels in neuroblastoma cells by antiarrhythmic drugs. *Mol. Pharmacol.* 20:356–62

116. Weld, F. M., Coromilas, J., Rottman, J. N., Bigger, J. T. Jr. 1982. Mechanism of quinidine-induced depression of maximum upstroke velocity in ovine cardiac Purkinje fibers. *Cir. Res.* 50:369–76

117. Saikawa, T., Carmeliet, E. 1982. Slow recovery of the maximal rate of rise (V_{max}) of the action potential in sheep cardiac Purkinje fibers. *Pfluegers Arch.* 394:90–93

118. Clarkson, C. W., Mason, J. W., Matsubara, T., Moyer, J. W., Hondeghem, L.
M. 1983. Slow inactivation in guinea pig
ventricular myocardium. *Biophys. J.*
41:309a
119. Henderson, E. G., Reynolds, L. S. 1978.
Removal of slow sodium inactivation in
denervated and organ-cultured mouse
skeletal muscle: Modification by tetrodotoxin. *J. Pharmacol. Exp. Ther.*
207:1032–40
120. Lipicky, R. J., Gilbert, D. L., Ehren-
stein, G. 1978. Effects of yohimbine on
squid axons. *Biophys. J.* 24:405–22
121. Cahalan, M. D. 1978. Local anesthetic
block of sodium channels in normal and
pronase-treated squid giant axons. *Biophys. J.* 23:285–311
122. Hondeghem, L. M., Matsubara, T.
1984. Quinidine and lidocaine: Activation and inactivation block. *Proc. West.
Pharmacol. Soc.* 27 (In press)
123. Hashimoto, K., Satoh, H., Imai, S.
1980. Effects of etafenone and antiarrhythmic drugs on Na and Ca channels
of guinea pig atrial muscle. *J. Cardiovasc. Pharmacol.* 561–70
124. Kus, T., Sasynick, B. I. 1978. Disopyramide phosphate: Is it just another quinidine? *Can. J. Physiol. Pharmacol.*
56:326–31
125. Schmidtmayer, J., Ulbricht, W. 1980.
Interaction of lidocaine and benzocaine
in blocking sodium channels. *Pfluegers
Arch.* 387:47–54
126. Grant, A. O., Strauss, L. J., Wallace, A.
G., Strauss, H. C. 1980. The influence of
pH on the electrophysiological effects
of lidocaine in guinea pig ventricular myocardium. *Circ. Res.* 47:542–
50
127. Weidmann, S. 1955. The effect of the
cardiac membrane potential on the rapid
availability of the sodium-carrying system. *J. Physiol.* 127:213–24
128. Gettes, L. S., Reuter, H. 1974. Slow
recovery from inactivation of inward currents in mammalian myocardial fibres. *J.
Physiol.* 240:703–24
129. Hondeghem, L. M., Ehring, G. R.,
Moyer, J. W. 1978. Observations on the
nature of the voltage shift of antiarrhythmic drugs. *Proc. West. Pharmacol. Soc.*
21:67–69
130. Gintant, G. A., Hoffman, B. F. 1982.
Blockade of fast inward sodium current
by quaternary derivatives of lidocaine in
canine cardiac Purkinje fibers. *Biophys.
J.* 37:244a
131. Hondeghem, L. M., Katzung, B. G.
1977. A unifying model for the interaction of antiarrhythmic drugs with cardiac
sodium channels: Application to quini-

dine and lidocaine. *Proc. West. Pharmacol. Soc.* 20:253–56
132. Starmer, C. F., Grant, A. O., Strauss, H.
C. 1983. A model of the interaction of
local anesthetics with Na channels. *Biophys. J.* 41:145a
133. Courtney, K. R. 1983. Comments on
"Mechanisms of quinidine-induced depression of maximum upstroke velocity
in ovine cardiac Purkinje fibers" (Letters
to the Editor). *Circ. Res.* 52:232
134. Skou, J. C. 1954. Local anaesthetics. I.
The blocking potencies of some local
anaesthetics and of butyl alcohol determined on peripheral nerves. *Acta Pharmacol. Toxicol.* 10:281–91
135. Skou, J. C. 1954. Local anaesthetics.
Vol. II. Relation between blocking
potency and penetration of a mono-
molecular layer of lipoids from nerves.
Acta Pharmacol. Toxicol. 10:325–37
136. Narahashi, T., Frazier, D. T., Yamada,
M. 1970. The site of action and active
form of local anesthetics. I. Theory and
pH experiments with tertiary compounds. *J. Pharmacol. Exp. Ther.* 171:
32–44
137. Frazier, D. T., Narahashi, T., Yamada,
M. 1970. The site of action and active
form of local anesthetics. II. Experiments
with quaternary compounds. *J. Pharmacol. Exp. Ther.* 171:45–51
138. Glicklich, J. I., Hoffman, B. F. 1978.
Sites of action and active forms of lidocaine and some derivatives on cardiac
Purkinje fibers. *Circ. Res.* 43:638–51
139. Ritchie, J. M. 1975. Mechanism of action of local anaesthetic agents and
biotoxins. *Br. J. Anaesthesiol.* 47:191–
98
140. Nattel, S., Bailey, J. C. 1983. Time
course of the electrophysiological effects
of quinidine on canine cardiac Purkinje
fibers: Concentration dependence and
comparison with lidocaine and disopyramide. *J. Pharmacol. Exp. Ther.* 225:
176–80
141. Poole-Wilson, P. A., Langer, G. 1975.
Effect of pH on ionic exchange and function in rat and rabbit myocardium. *Am. J.
Physiol.* 229:570–81
142. Spitzer, K. W., Hogan, P. M. 1979. The
effects of acidosis and bicarbonate on action potential repolarization in canine
cardiac Purkinje fibers. *J. Gen. Physiol.*
73:199–218
143. Hille, B. 1977. The pH dependent rate
of action of local anesthetics on the node
of Ranvier. *J. Gen. Physiol.* 69:475–
96
144. Nattel, S., Elharrar, V., Zipes, D. P.,
Bailey, J. C. 1981. pH dependent electrophysiological effects of quinidine and

lidocaine on canine cardiac Purkinje fibers. *Circ. Res.* 48:55–61

145. Ellis, D., Thomas, R. C. 1976. Direct measurement of the intracellular pH of mammalian cardiac muscle. *J. Physiol.* 262:755–71

146. Bowman, W. C., Rand, M. J. 1980. *Textbook of Pharmacology*, Ch. 28, p. 17. Oxford: Blackwell. 2nd ed.

147. Bauman, J. L., Curtis, R. A., Covinsky, J. O. 1980. Effects of antiarrhythmics in ischemic models. *Am. Heart J.* 100:947–48

148. Skinner, R. B. Jr., Kunze, D. L. 1976. Changes in extracellular potassium activity in response to decreased pH in rabbit atrial muscle. *Circ. Res.* 39:678–83

149. Sperelakis, N., Lee, E. C. 1971. Characterization of (Na+,K+)ATPase isolated from embryonic chick hearts and cultured chick heart cells. *Biochim. Biophys. Acta* 233:562–79

150. Bellet, S., Harridan, G., Somylo, A., Lara, R. 1959. The reversal of cardiotoxic effects of quinidine by molar sodium lactate: An experimental study. *Am. J. Med. Sci.* 237:165–76

151. Bailey, D. J. Jr. 1960. Cardiotoxic effects of quinidine and their treatment. *Arch. Int. Med.* 105:13–22

152. Chernick, W. S. 1971. Local anesthetics. In *Drill's Pharmacology in Medicine*, ed. J. R. DiPalma, pp. 190–210. New York: Blakiston-McGraw Hill 4th ed.

153. Courtney, K. R. 1983. Quantifying antiarrhythmic drug blocking during action potentials in guinea-pig papillary muscle. *J. Mol. Cell Cardiol.* 15:749–57

154. Rudiger, H. J., Homburger, H., Antoni, H. 1981. Effects of a new antiarrhythmic compound [2-bensol-1-(2' disopropyl-amino-ethoxy-imino-cycloheptone hydrogen fumarate] on the electrophysiological properties of mammalian cardiac cells. *Naunyn-Schmidebergs Arch. Pharmacol.* 317:238

155. Ehring, G. R., Hondeghem, L. M. 1980. Structural similarities and cardiac electrophysiological differences between lidocaine and procainamide. *Proc. West. Pharmacol. Soc.* 23:163–66

156. Ehring, G. R., Hondeghem, L. M. 1981. Antiarrhythmic structure activity relationships in a series of lidocaine procainamide derivatives. *Proc. West. Pharmacol. Soc.* 24:221–24

157. Dangman, K. H., Hoffman, B. F. 1981. In vivo and in vitro antiarrhythmic and arrhythmogenic effects of N-acetyl procainamide. *J. Pharmacol. Exp. Ther.* 217:851–62

158. Yeh, J. Z. 1980. Blockage of sodium channels by stereoisomers of local anesthetics. In *Molecular Mechanisms of Anesthesia*, ed. R. Fink, pp. 35–44. New York: Raven

159. Reuter, H. 1979. Properties of two inward membrane currents in the heart. *Ann. Rev. Physiol.* 41:413–24

160. Hagiwara, S., Byerly, L. 1981. Calcium channel. *Ann. Rev. Neurosci.* 4:69–125

161. Reuter, H. 1983. Calcium channels modulation by neurotransmitters, enzymes and drugs. *Nature* 301:569–74

162. Tsien, R. W. 1983. Calcium channels in excitable cell membranes. *Ann. Rev. Physiol.* 45:341–58

163. Osterrieder, W., Brum, G., Hescheler, J., Trautwein, W., Flockerzi, V., Hofmann, F. 1982. Injection of subunits of cyclic AMP-dependent protein kinase into cardiac myocytes modulates Ca2+ current. *Nature* 298:576–78

164. Beeler, G. W. Jr., Reuter, H. 1970. Voltage clamp experiments on ventricular myocardial fibres. *J. Physiol.* 207:165–90

165. New, W., Trautwein, W. 1972. The ionic nature of slow inward current and its relation to contraction. *Pfluegers Arch.* 334:24–38

166. Trautwein, W., McDonald, T. F., Tripathi, O. 1975. Calcium conductance and tension in mammalian ventricular muscle. *Pfluegers Arch.* 354:55–74

167. Godfraind, T., Dieu, D. 1981. The inhibition by flunarizine of the norepinephrine—Evoked contraction and calcium influx in rat aorta and mesenteric arteries. *J. Pharmacol. Exp. Ther.* 217:510–15

168. Lowe, A., Matthews, E. K., Richardson, B. P. 1981. The calcium antagonistic effects of cyproheptadine on contraction, membrane electrical events and calcium influx in the guinea-pig taenia coli. *Br. J. Pharmacol.* 74:651–63

169. Wit, A. L., Cranefield, P. F. 1974. Effect of verapamil on the sinoatrial and atrioventricular nodes of the rabbit and the mechanism by which it arrests reentrant atrioventricular nodal tachycardia. *Circ. Res.* 35:413–25

170. Bayer, R., Hennekes, R., Kaufmann, R., Mannhold, R. 1975. Inotropic and electrophysiological actions of verapamil and D 600 in mammalian myocardium. I. Pattern of inotropic effects of the racemic compounds. *Naunyn-Schmiedebergs Arch. Pharmacol.* 290:49–68

171. Bayer, R., Kaufmann, R., Mannhold, R. 1975. Inotropic and electrophysiological actions of verapamil and D 600 in mammalian myocardium. II. Pattern of

inotropic effects of the optical isomers. *Naunyn-Schmiedebergs Arch. Pharmacol.* 290:69–80

172. Tritthart, H., Volkmann, R., Weiss, R., Fleckenstein, A. 1973. Calcium-mediated action potentials in mammalian myocardium. *Naunyn-Schmiedebergs Arch. Pharmacol.* 288:239–52

173. Ludwig, C., Nawrath, H. 1977. Effects of D-600 and its optical isomers on force of contraction in cat papillary muscles and guinea-pig auricles. *Br. J. Pharmacol.* 59:411–17

174. Mannhold, R., Steiner, R., Haas, W., Kaufmann, R. 1978. Investigations on the structure-activity relationships of verapamil. *Naunyn-Schmiedebergs Arch. Pharmacol.* 302:217–26

175. Ehara, T., Kaufmann, R. 1978. The voltage- and time-dependent effects of (–1)-verapamil on the slow inward current in isolated cat ventricular myocardium. *J. Pharmacol. Exp. Ther.* 207:49–55

176. McDonald, T., Pelzer, D., Trautwein, W. 1980. On the mechanism of slow calcium channel block in heart. *Pfluegers Arch.* 385:175–79

177. Lee, K. S., Tsien, R. W. 1983. Mechanism of calcium channel blockade by verapamil, D600, diltiazem and nitrendipine in single dialysed heart cells. *Nature* 302:790–94

178. Kanaya, S., Arlock, P., Katzung, B. G., Hondeghem, L. M. 1983. Diltiazem and verapamil preferentially block inactivated calcium channels. *J. Mol. Cell Cardiol.* 15:145–48

179. Tung, L., Morad, M. 1982. Frequency- and voltage-dependent block of tension and slow inward current in heart muscle by diltiazem. *Circulation* 66:II–293

180. Trautwein, W., Pelzer, D., McDonald, T. F., Osterrieder, W. 1981. AQA 39, a new bradycardic agent which blocks myocardial calcium (CA^{2+}) channels in a frequency- and voltage-dependent manner. *Naunyn-Schmiedebergs Arch. Pharmacol.* 317:228–32

181. Hume, J. R., Giles, W. 1981. Active and passive electrical properties of single bullfrog atrial cells. *J. Gen. Physiol.* 78:19–42

182. Sanguinetti, M. C., West, T. C. 1982. Comparison of papaverine and verapamil on frequence-dependent changes in V_{max} of K-depolarized ventricular tissue. *J. Cardiovasc. Pharmacol.* 4:791–802

183. Sanguinetti, M. C., West, T. C. 1982. Frequency-dependent depression of V_{max} of slow reponse action potentials by a high concentration of papaverine. *J. Cardiovasc. Pharmacol.* 5:125–30

184. Linden, J., Brooker, G. 1980. The influence of resting membrane potential on the effect of verapamil on atria. *J. Mol. Cell Cardiol.* 12:325–31

185. Borchard, U., Hafner, D. 1983. Difference in action of the calcium antagonists nifedipine and diltiazem on the slow response in ventricular myocardium. *Naunyn-Schmiedebergs Arch. Pharmacol.* 322:R28

186. Pelzer, D., Trautwein, W., McDonald, T. F. 1982. Calcium channel block and recovery from block in mammalian ventricular muscle treated with organic channel inhibitors. *Pfluegers Arch.* 394:97–105

187. Isenberg, G., Klockner, U. 1982. Isolated bovine ventricular myocytes. Characterization of the action potential. *Pfluegers Arch.* 395:19–29

188. Reuter, H., Stevens, C. F., Tsien, R. W., Yellen, G. 1982. Properties of single calcium channels in cardiac cell culture. *Nature* 297:501–04

189. Schramm, M., Thomas, G., Towart, R., Frankowiak, G. 1983. Novel dihydropyridines with positive inotropic action through activation of Ca2+ channels. *Nature* 303:535–37

190. Murphy, K. M. M., Gould, R. J., Largent, B. L., Snyder, S. H. 1983. A unitary mechanism of calcium antagonist drug action. *Proc. Natl. Acad. Sci. USA* 80:860–64

191. Holck, M., Thorens, S., Haeusler, G. 1983. Does [3H]-Nifedipine label the calcium channel in rabbit myocardium? *J. Receptor Res.* 3:191–98

192. DePover, A., Matlib, M. A., Lee, S. W., Dube, G. P., Grupp, I. L., et al. 1982. Specific binding of [3H]-nitrendipine to membranes from coronary arteries and heart in relation to pharmacological effects. Paradoxical stimulation by diltiazem. *Biochem. Biophys. Res. Commun.* 108:110–17

193. Ferry, D. R., Glossman, H. 1982. Identification of putative calcium channels in skeletal muscle microsomes. *FEBS Lett.* 148:331–37

194. Yamamura, H. I., Schoemaker, H., Boles, R. G., Roeske, W. R. 1982. Diltiazem enhancement of [3H]-nitrendipine binding to calcium channel associated drug receptor sites in rat brain synaptosomes. *Biochem. Biophys. Res. Comm.* 108:640–46

195. Kohlhardt, M., Fleckenstein, A. 1977. Inhibition of the slow inward current by nifedipine in mammalian ventricular myocardium. *Naunyn-Schmiedebergs Arch. Pharmacol.* 298:267–72

196. Bayer, R., Ehara, T. 1978. Comparative studies on calcium antagonists (VII). *Prog. Pharmacol.* 2:31–37
197. Kass, R. S. 1982. Nisoldipine: A new, more selective calcium current blocker in cardiac Purkinje fibers. *J. Pharmacol. Exp. Ther.* 223:446–56
198. Hachisu, M., Pappano, A. J. 1983. A comparative study of the blockade of calcium-dependent action potentials by verapamil, nifedipine, and nimodipine in ventricular muscle. *J. Pharmacol. Exp. Ther.* 225:112–20
199. Molyvdas, P-A., Sperelakis, N. 1983. Comparison of the effects of several calcium antagonistic drugs (slow-channel blockers) on the electrical and mechanical activities of guinea pig papillary muscle. *J. Cardiovasc. Pharmacol.* 5:162–69
200. Kohlhardt, M., Haap, K. 1981. The blockade of V_{max} of the atrioventricular action potential produced by the slow channel inhibitors verapamil and nifedipine. *Naunyn-Schmiedebergs Arch. Pharmacol.* 316:178–85
201. Pang, D. C., Sperelakis, N. 1983. Nifedipine, diltiazem, bepridil, and verapamil uptakes into cardiac and smooth muscles. *Eur. J. Pharmacol.* 87:199–207
202. Rodenkirchen, R., Bayer, R., Steiner, R., Bossert, F., Meyer, H., Moeller, E. 1979. Structure-activity studies on nifedipine in isolated cardiac muscle. *Naunyn-Schmiedebergs Arch. Pharmacol.* 310:69–78
203. Mannhold, R., Zierden, P., Bayer, R., Rodenkirchen, R., Steiner, R. 1981. The influence of aromatic substitution on the negative inotropic action of verapamil in the isolated cat papillary muscle. *Arzneim. Forsch.* 31:773–80
204. Hescheler, J., Pelzer, D., Trube, G., Trautwein, W. 1982. Does the organic calcium channel blocker D600 act from inside or outside on the cardiac cell membrane? *Pfluegers Arch.* 393:287–91
205. Rosenberger, L. B., Triggle, D. J. 1978. Calcium, calcium translocation and specific calcium antagonists. In *Calcium in Drug Action*, ed. G. B. Weiss, pp. 3–31. New York:Plenum. 366 pp.
206. Nguyen-Thi, A., Ruiz-Ceretti, E., Schanne, O. F. 1981. Electrophysiologic effects and electrolyte changes in total myocardial ischemia. *Can. J. Physiol. Pharmacol.* 59:876–83
207. Karagueuzian, H. S., Fenoglio, J. J. Jr., Weiss, M. B., Wit, A. L. 1980. Coronary occlusion and reperfusion: Effects on subendocardial cardiac fibers. *Am. J. Physiol.* 238:H581–93

208. Wit, A. L., Friedman, P. L. 1975. Basis for ventricular arrhythmias accompanying myocardial infarction. Alterations in electrical activity of ventricular muscle and Purkinje fibers after coronary artery occlusion. *Arch. Int. Med.* 135:459–72
209. Weiss, J., Shine, K. I. 1981. Extracellular potassium accumulation during myocardial ischemia: Implications for arrhythmogenesis. *J. Mol. Cell. Cardiol.* 113:699–704
210. Lazzara, R., El-Sherif, N., Scherlag, B. J. 1975. Disorders of cellular electrophysiology produced by ischemia of the canine His bundle. *Circ. Res.* 36:444–54
211. Carmeliet, E. 1978. Cardiac transmembrane potentials and metabolism. *Circ. Res.* 42:577–87
212. Janse, M. J., van Capelle, F. J. L., Morsink, H., Kleber, A. G., Wilms-Schopman, F., et al. 1980. Flow of "injury" current and patterns of excitation during early ventricular arrhythmias in acute regional myocardial ischemia in isolated porcine and canine hearts. Evidence for two different arrhythmogenic mechanisms. *Circ. Res.* 47:151–65
213. Janse, M. J., Cinca, J., Morena, H., Fiolet, J. W. T., Kleber, A. G., et al. 1979. The "border zone" in myocardial ischemia. An electrophysiologic, metabolic, and histochemical correlation in the pig heart. *Circ. Res.* 44:576–88
214. Ferrier, G. R. 1977. Digitalis arrhythmias: Role of oscillatory afterpotentials. *Prog. Cardiovasc. Dis.* 19:459–73
215. Rosen, M. R., Gelband, H., Hoffman, B. F. 1973. Correlation between effects of ouabain on the canine electrocardiogram and transmembrane potentials of isolated Purkinje fibers. *Circulation* 47:65–72
216. Danilo, P. Jr., Hordof, A. J., Rosen, M. R. 1977. Effects of disopyramide on electrophysiologic properties of canine cardiac Purkinje fibers. *J. Pharmacol. Exp. Ther.* 201:701–10
217. Yamada, S., Nishimura, M., Watanabe, Y. 1982. Electrophysiologic effects of disopyramide studied in a hypoxic canine Purkinje fiber model. *J. Electrocardiol.* 15:31–40
218. Gibson, J. K., Somani, P., Bassett, A. L. 1978. Electrophysiologic effects of encainide (MJ9067) on canine Purkinje fibres. *Eur. J. Pharmacol.* 52:161–69
219. Wong, S. S., Myerburg, R. J., Ezrin, A. M., Gelband, H., Bassett, A. L. 1982. Electrophysiologic effects of encainide on acutely ischemic rabbit myocardial cells. *Eur. J. Pharmacol.* 80:323–29
220. Elharrar, V., Zipes, D. P. 1982. Effects

of encainide and metabolities (MJ14030 and MJ9444) on canine cardiac Purkinje and ventricular fibers. *J. Pharmacol. Exp. Ther.* 220:440–47

221. Ruffy, R., Rozenshtraukh, L. V., Elharrar, V., Zipes, D. P. 1979. Electrophysiologic effects of ethmozin on canine myocardium. *Cardiovasc. Res.* 13:354–63

222. Cowan, J. C., Vaughan Williams, E. M. 1981. Characterization of a new oral antiarrhythmic drug, flecainide (R818). *Eur. J. Pharmacol.* 73:333–42

223. Hodges, M., Haugland, J. M., Granrud, G., Conrad, G. J., Asinger, R. W., et al. 1982. Suppression of ventricular ectopic depolarizations by flecainide acetate, a new antiarrhythmic agent. *Circulation* 65:879–85

224. Borchard, U., Boisten, M. 1982. Effect of flecainide on action potentials and alternating current-induced arrhythmias in mammalian myocardium. *J. Cardiovasc. Pharmacol.* 4:205–12

225. Brennan, F. J. 1980. Electrophysiologic effects of Imipramine and Doxepin on normal and depressed cardic Purkinje fibers. *Am. J. Cardiol.* 46:599–606

226. Allen, J. D., Brennan, F. J., Wit, A. L. 1978. Actions of lidocaine on transmembrane potentials of subendocardial Purkinje fibers surviving in infarcted canine hearts. *Circ. Res.* 43:470–81

227. Singh, B. N., Vaughan Williams, E. M. 1971. Effect of altering potassium concentration on the action of lidocaine and diphenylhydantoin on rabbit atrial and ventricular muscle. *Circ. Res.* 29:286–95

228. El-Sherif, N., Scherlag, B. J., Lazzara, R., Hope, R. R. 1977. Re-entrant ventricular arrhythmias in the late myocardial infarction period. 4. Mechanism of action of lidocaine. *Circulation* 56:395–402

229. Hondeghem, L. M., Cotner, C. L. 1978. Reproducible and uniform cardiac ischemia: Effects of antiarrhythmic drugs. *Am. J. Physiol.* 235:H574–80

230. El-Sherif, N., Lazzara, R. 1977. Reentrant ventricular arrhythmias in the late myocardial infarction period. 4. Mechanism of action of lidocaine. *Circulation* 56:395–402

231. Obayashi, K., Hayakawa, H., Mandel, W. J. 1975. Interrelationships between external potassium concentration and lidocaine effects on the canine Purkinje fibers. *Am. Heart J.* 89:221–26

232. Brennan, F. J., Cranefield, P. F., Wit, A. L. 1978. Effects of lidocaine on slow response and depressed fast response action potentials of canine cardiac Purkinje fibers. *J. Pharmacol. Exp. Ther.* 204:312–24

233. Rosen, M. R., Merker, C., Pippenger, C. E. 1976. The effects of lidocaine on the canine ECG and electrophysiologic properties of Purkinje fibers. *Am. Heart J.* 91:191–202

234. Rosen, M. R., Hoffman, B. F., Wit, A. L. 1975. Electrophysiology and pharmacology of cardiac arrhythmias. V. Cardiac antiarrhythmic effects of lidocaine. *Am. Heart J.* 89:526–36

235. Kimura, S., Nakaya, H., Kanno, M. 1982. Effects of verapamil and lidocaine on changes in action potential characteristics and conduction time induced by combined hypoxia, hyperkalemia and acidosis in canine ventricular myocardium. *J. Cardiovasc. Pharmacol.* 4:658–67

236. Lazzara, R., Hope, R. R., El-Sherif, N., Scherlag, B. J. 1978. Effects of lidocaine on hypoxia and ischemic cardiac cells. *Am. J. Cardiol.* 41:872–79

237. Nakaya, H., Hattori, Y., Kanno, H. 1980. Effects of calcium antagonists and lidocaine on conduction delay induced by acute myocardial ischemia in dogs. *Jpn. J. Pharmacol.* 30:587–97

238. Wang, C. M., James, C. A., Maxwell, R. A. 1979. Effects of lidocaine on the electrophysiological properties of subendocardial Purkinje fibers surviving acute myocardial infarction. *J. Mol. Cell. Cardiol.* 11:669–81

239. Kupersmith, J., Antman, F. L. Y., Hoffman, B. F. 1975. In vivo electrophysiologic effects of lidocaine in canine acute myocardial infarction. *Circ. Res.* 36:84–91

240. Chen, C-M., Gettes, L. S. 1976. Combined effects of rate, membrane potential, and drugs on maximum rate of rise (V_{max}) of action potential upstroke of guinea pig papillary muscle. *Circ. Res.* 38:464–69

241. Kupersmith, J. 1979. Electrophysiological and antiarrhythmic effects of lidocaine in canine acute myocardial ischemia. *Am. Heart J.* 97:360–66

242. Hondeghem, L. M., Grant, A. D., Jensen, R. A. 1974. Antiarrhythmic drug action: Selective depression of hypoxic cardiac cells. *Am. Heart J.* 87:602–5

243. Cardinal, R., Janse, M. J., VanEaden, I., Werner, G., Naumann, D. C., Durrer, D. 1981. The effects of lidocaine on intracellular and extracellular potentials, activation, and ventricular arrhythmias during acute regional ischemia in the isolated porcine heart. *Circ. Res.* 49:792–806

244. Gerstenblith, G., Scherlag, B. J., Hope, R. R., Lazzara, R. 1978. Effect of lidocaine on conduction in the ischemic His-Purkinje system of dogs. *Am. J. Cardiol.* 442:587–91

245. Avitall, B. 1979. Strength-interval curves of isolated rat papillary muscle during hypoxia and reoxygenation: Effect of lidocaine. *J. Electrocard.* 12: 353–60

246. Carson, D. L., Dresel, P. E. 1983. Effect of lidocaine on ventricular conduction in acutely ischemic dog hearts. *J. Cardiovasc. Pharmacol.* 5:357–63

247. Singh, B. N., Vaughan Williams, E. M. 1972. Investigations of the mode of action of a new antidysrhythmic agent (Ko1173). *Br. J. Pharmacol.* 44:1–9

248. Yamaguchi, I., Singh, B. N., Mandel, W. 1979. Electrophysiological actions of mexiletine on isolated rabbit atria and canine ventricular muscle and Purkinje fiber. *Cardiovasc. Res.* 13:288–96

249. Jensen, R. A., Katzung, B. G. 1970. Electrophysiological action of diphenylhydantoin on rabbit atria. Dependence on stimulation frequency, potassium, and sodium. *Circ. Res.* 26:17–27

250. Rosen, M. R., Danilo, P. Jr., Alonso, M. B., Pippenger, C. E. 1974. Effects of therapeutic concentrations of diphenylhydantoin on transmembrane potentials of normal and depressed Purkinje fibers. *J. Pharmacol. Exp. Ther.* 197:594–604

251. El-Sherif, N., Lazzara, R. 1978. Reentrant ventricular arrhythmias in the late myocardial infarction period. 5. Mechanism of action of diphenylhydantoin. *Circulation* 57:465–72

252. Pappano, A. J. 1970. Calcium-dependent action potentials produced by catecholamines in guinea pig atrial muscle fibers depolarized by potassium. *Circ. Res.* 27:379–90

253. Moore, E. M., Spear, J. F., Horowitz, L. N., Feldman, H. S., Moller, R. A. 1978. Electrophysiologic properties of a new antiarrhythmic drug—tocainide. *Am. J. Cardiol.* 41:703–9

254. Coltart, D. J., Berndt, T. B., Kernoff, R., Harrison, D. C. 1974. Antiarrhythmic and circulatory effects of Astra W36075, a new lidocaine like agent. *Am. J. Cardiol.* 34:35–41

255. Bigger, J. T. Jr., Hoffman, B. F. 1980. Antiarrhythmic drugs. In *Goodman and Gilmans's The Pharmacological Basis of Therapeutics,* ed. A. G. Gilman, L. S. Goodman, A. Gilman, pp. 761–92. New York: Macmillan. 6th ed.

256. Gettes, L. S. 1979. On the classification of antiarrhythmic drugs. *Mod. Concepts Cardiovasc. Dis.* 48:13–18

257. Bush, L. R., Romson, J. L., Ash, J. L., Lucchesi, B. R. 1982. Effects of diltiazem on extent of ultimate myocardial injury resulting from temporary coronary artery occlusion in dogs. *J. Cardiovasc. Pharmacol.* 4:285–96

258. Clarke, R. E., Christlieb, I. Y., Henry, P. D., Fischer, A. E., Nora, J. D., et al. 1979. Nifedipine: A myocardial protective agent. *Am. J. Cardiol.* 44:825–31

259. Fleckenstein, A. 1971. Specific inhibitors and promotors of calcium action in the excitation-contraction coupling of heart muscle and their role in the prevention or production of myocardial lesions. See Ref. 21, pp. 135–88

260. Henry, P. D., Schuchlieb, R., Borda, L. J., Roberts, R., Williamson, J. R., Sobel, B. E. 1978. Effects of nifedipine on myocardial perfusion and ischemic injury in dogs. *Circ. Res.* 43:372–80

261. Nayler, W. G., Grau, A., Slade, A. 1976. A protective effect of verapamil on hypoxic heart muscle. *Cardiovasc. Res.* 10:650–60

262. Saini, R. K., Antonaccio, M. J. 1982. Antiarrhythmic, antifibrillatory activities and reduction of infarct size after the calcium antagonist Ro 11–1781 (Tiapamil) in anesthetized dogs. *J. Pharmacol. Exp. Ther.* 221:29–36

263. Ribeiro, L. G. T., Brandon, T. A., Debauche, T. L., Maroko, P. R., Miller, R. R. 1981. Antiarrhythmic and hemodynamic effects of calcium channel blocking agents during coronary arterial reperfusion. Comparative effects of verapamil and nifedipine. *Am. J. Cardiol.* 48:69–74

264. Clusin, W. T., Bristow, M. R., Baim, D. S., Schroeder, J. S., Jaillon, P., et al. 1982. The effects of diltiazem and reduced serum ionized calcium on ischemic ventricular fibrillation in the dog. *Circ. Res.* 50:518–26

265. Weishaar, R. E., Bing, R. J. 1980. The beneficial effect of a calcium channel blocker, diltiazem, on the ischemic-reperfused heart. *J. Mol. Cell Cardiol.* 12:993–1009

266. Yamaguchi, I., Obayashi, K., Mandel, W. J. 1978. Electrophysiological effects of verapamil. *Cardiovasc. Res.* 12:597–608

267. Sheehan, F. H., Epstein, S. E. 1982. Effects of calcium channel blocking agents on reperfusion arrhythmias. *Am. Heart J.* 103:973–77

268. El-Sherif, N., Lazzara, R. 1979. Reentrant ventricular arrhythmias in the late myocardial infarction period. 7. Effect of

verapamil and D-600 and the role of the "slow channel". *Circulation* 60:605–15

269. Sverdlow, C. D., Echt, D. S., Winkle, R. A., Griffin, J. C., Ross, D. L., Mason, J. W. 1981. Incidence of acute antiarrhythmic drug efficacy at electrophysiologic study. *Circulation* 64:IV–137

270. Sverdlow, C. D., Blum, J., Winkle, R. A., Griffin, J. C., Ross, D. L., Mason, J. W. 1982. Decreased incidence of antiarrhythmic drug efficacy at electrophysiologic study associated with the use of third extrastimulus. *Am. Heart J.* 104:1004–11

271. Mason, J. W., Sverdlow, C. D., Winkle, R. A., Ross, D. L., Echt, D. S., et al. 1983. Ventricular tachyarrhythmia induction for drug selection; experience with 311 patients. *NIH Symposium on Antiarrhythmic Drug Therapy.* New York: Raven

272. Lie, K. I., Wellens, H. J., vanCapelle, F. J., Durrer, D. 1974. Lidocaine in the prevention of primary ventricular fibrillation. A double blind, randomized study of 212 consecutive patients. *N. Engl. J. Med.* 291:1324–26

273. Kawai, C., Konishi, T., Matsuyama, E., Okazaki, H. 1981. Comparative effects of three calcium antagonists, diltiazem, verapamil, and nifedipine, on the sino-atrial and atrioventricular nodes. Experimental and clinical studies. *Circulation* 63:1035–42

274. Moyer, J. W., Hondeghem, L. M. 1980. Effects of the combination of quinidine and lidocaine on the upstroke velocity of the cardiac action potential. *Proc. West. Pharmacol. Soc.* 23:159–61

275. Breithardt, G., Seipel, L., Abendroth, R. R. 1981. Comparison of antiarrhythmic efficacy of disopyramide and mexiletine against stimulus-induced ventricular tachycardia. *J. Cardiovasc. Pharmacol.* 3:1026–37

276. Duff, H. J., Roden, D., Primm, R. K., Oates, J. A., Woosley, R. L. 1983. Mexiletine in the treatment of resistant ventricular arrhythmias: Enhancement of efficacy and reduction of dose-related side effects by combination with quinidine. *Circulation* 67:1124–28

277. Albright, G. A. 1979. Cardiac arrest following regional anesthesia with etidocaine or bupivacaine. *J. Anesthesiol.* 51:285–87

278. Gettes, L. S. 1980. Editorial: Thoughts of a computerphobe. *Circulation* 61:1225–26

Ann. Rev. Pharmacol. Toxicol. 1984. 24:425–50

NEUROBEHAVIORAL TECHNIQUES TO ASSESS THE EFFECTS OF CHEMICALS ON THE NERVOUS SYSTEM[1]

Hugh A. Tilson and Clifford L. Mitchell

Laboratory of Behavioral and Neurological Toxicology, National Institute of Environmental Health Sciences, P. O. Box 12233, Research Triangle Park, North Carolina 27709

INTRODUCTION

Rationale for the Study of Behavior

Of the many organ systems potentially affected by hazardous agents, the nervous system is one of the most complex and probably the least understood. All bodily functions depend on processing sensory input and generating control output via the nervous system. The complexity of the interaction of the nervous system with other organ systems suggests that nervous system function should be among the first and most thoroughly assessed in cases of exposure to hazardous agents. However, the intricacy of the nervous system makes assessment difficult in at least two ways. First, there are many different functions that could be assessed, ranging from sensory alterations to motor deficits to associative dysfunction. Second, there are no or few guidelines for correlating most neurobehavioral functional deficits with specific neuropathological or neurochemical changes. The purpose of this review is to develop a rationale for the use and selection of behavioral tests to assess agents for potential neurotoxicity.

A cursory review of the current literature indicates that functional measures of central nervous system (CNS) integrity, in particular behavioral techniques,

---

[1]The US Government has the right to retain a nonexclusive, royalty-free license in and to any copyright covering this paper.

are being used with increasing frequency to determine the potential neurotoxicity of environmental agents. Mello (1) was among the first to argue that the behavior of the organism represents a functional integration of the nervous system and that nervous system capacity cannot be determined in histological or even physiological studies independent of behavioral analyses. Many researchers have subsequently pointed out the potential sensitivity of neurofunctional measures to study the deleterious effects of environmental agents (2–5).

In the past, the United States, Canada, and Western Europe placed heavy emphasis in chemical toxicity studies on defining pathological changes following exposure. However, in 1961, Elkins (6) published a paper comparing the maximum acceptable concentrations (MACs) of certain substances in the US with those in the Soviet Union. The higher values adopted by the US were believed to be due to the use of morphometric measures by that country (lethality, body weight loss), while the Soviets relied on functional measures (conditioned reflexes). Subsequent publications by Ruffin (7) and Brimblecombe (8) urged the use of behavioral measures in Western countries to establish MACs.

It is also interesting to note that Citovic (9), a student of Pavlov, reported in 1930 the use of conditioned reflexes to study the neurotoxic effects of gasoline and acetone. In the US, it was 1969 before Weiss & Laties (10) included a section on behavioral toxicology in their chapter on behavioral pharmacology in the *Annual Review of Pharmacology*. Since that time, behavioral toxicology has been the subject of numerous books, symposia, reviews, and book chapters in Western countries (1, 3–5, 11–20).

Scope of the Problem

In the US, the Chemical Abstracts Service Computer Registry contained over four million distinct entities as of 1977, and as many as 100,000 chemicals may be in everyday use by American industry. According to the National Institute for Occupational Safety and Health (NIOSH), more than 20 million people work with one or more chemicals known to be neurotoxic.

Although many of the chemicals that already exist in the environment and the approximately 1000 new chemicals introduced each year are probably not neurotoxic, we will inevitably be exposed to some that are. Many industrial chemicals will enter the environment as waste products discharged into the air, rivers, and lakes, while some will eventually appear as contaminants in food, water, and air. A few will also find their way into the food chain through carelessness or ignorance.

Obviously, an extensive assessment of all the possible chemical entities for potential behavioral and neurological toxicology is not a viable economic option. There is a need for a well-conceived screening program that would provide an initial indication of a chemical's potential to produce neurotoxicity.

The results of the screen could be used to prevent an agent from being employed inappropriately in the marketplace or to suggest additional studies that might provide a more detailed examination of the agent's effects.

Examples of Neurotoxicants

Before discussing specific criteria for the development of a screen for neurobehavioral toxicity, several general factors that may affect test results should be considered. Among these are choices of sex, age, species, and dosing parameters; they have been discussed in detail elsewhere (21–23). Another general consideration concerns the range of possible effects likely to be encountered when attempting to assess neurotoxic chemicals. The following sections illustrate this point by briefly providing examples of signs and symptoms reported in humans exposed to representative neurotoxicants and comparing these effects to those reported in animals exposed chronically to the same neurotoxicants. In the examples below, the rat is used as the animal model, since this or some other rodent species is likely to be used for screening.

INORGANIC LEAD   The neurotoxicity of inorganic lead has been known for many years. Encephalopathy has been reported following lead intoxication, as have tremors, disorientation, neuropathy, aphasia, blindness, convulsions, and coma (24). The neuropathy is primarily motor and histologically shows primary changes in the Schwann cells, with segmental disintegration beginning at the nodes of Ranvier (25, 26).

In spite of the well-documented effects of inorganic lead in adult humans, there have been relatively few studies on the effects of low-level exposure to lead in adult animals. High doses of systemically administered lead have been reported to produce motor impairment in a water maze (27) and alterations in the performance of schedule-controlled behavior (28). Lanthorn & Isaacson (29) reported reduced rates of spontaneous alteration in a maze as well as altered reactivity to handling. Pryor et al (30) used a battery of neurobehavioral tests with rats chronically exposed to lead acetate and found significant decreases in spontaneous motor activity (SMA) associated with decreases in body weight. Changes in responsiveness to noxious or nonnoxious stimuli were not detected by the battery of tests used by Pryor et al (30).

SOLVENTS   The neurotoxicity of the organic solvents has also been well-documented in humans. Neurological symptoms that follow exposure to these agents include paresthesia, reflex attenuation, symmetrical distal ascending motor weakness, and unsteady gait (31–33).

In rodents, several studies have been reported on the neurotoxic effects of acrylamide (30), which in many cases seems to be prototypic for this class of neurotoxicants. Using relatively simple measures of neuromotor function, repeated exposure to acrylamide has been reported to decrease forelimb grip strength and depress the hindlimb extensor reflex (34). Pryor et al (30) also reported that acrylamide decreased fore- and hindlimb grip strength, with impairment of the latter preceding alterations in the former. With prolonged exposure to acrylamide, more severe motor debilitation is seen and is quantified as disruption of motor coordination (negative geotaxis) and decreased motor activity (30, 34). Changes in responsiveness to noxious and nonnoxious stimuli have been observed but could not be demonstrated in the absence of motor weakness. The observation that acrylamide primarily affects neuromotor function has also been made by several investigators who have found acrylamide-induced hindlimb splay (35), altered gait (36), and impaired rotorod performance (37).

ORGANOCHLORINE INSECTICIDES   Included in the class of organochlorine insecticides are compounds with such widely divergent structures as DDT, chlordane, dieldrin, and chlordecone. Generally, these agents produce tremor, hyperexcitability, and convulsions at higher doses. Chlordecone is a polycyclic ketone formerly used to control fire ants and other insects. Workers exposed to large quantities of chlordecone exhibited a well-defined tremor associated with an ocular flutter (opsoclonus). In addition, exposed workers reported irritability and mild impairment of short-term memory (38). Taylor (39) has subsequently reported that virtually all of the effects produced by chlordecone are reversible.

There have been several studies on the neurobehavioral effects of chlordecone in laboratory animals. Acute or repeated exposure to chlordecone produces observable tremor in mice (40) and rats (41) and has been quantified using a spectral analysis technique by Gerhart et al (42). Hyperexcitability or irritability has been quantified in rodents as an increased startle response (30, 43, 44). Data concerning the effects of chlordecone on learning and memory are generally lacking, but Tilson et al (44) have reported that repeated exposure to chlordecone impairs the retention of a one-way shock avoidance task in rats. Some production workers exposed to high concentrations of chlordecone were observed to be ataxic. Neuromotor deficits have also been noted in animals; mice exposed to chlordecone display motor incoordination as measured by inability to balance on a bar (45). Reiter et al (43) reported that exposure of rats to chlordecone via the diet significantly decreased activity in the open field but increased activity in a residential maze. Pryor et al (30), however, did not observe chlordecone-induced alterations in an open-field–like apparatus.

METHYLMERCURY   Exposure to methylmercury has been reported to result in severe, irreversible damage to the CNS. The initial symptoms of methylmercury neurotoxicity consist of paresthesia, astereognosis, hearing and visual disorders, cerebellar ataxia, myoclonus, irritability, and memory impairment (46–48). Some of these effects were reported to be reversible depending upon the degree of exposure. Sensory deficits reportedly occur first, with constriction of the visual field being the most common visual deficit. The motor disturbances range from impairment of fine motor control to cerebellar ataxia and dysarthria.

In rodents, the neurobehavioral effects of methylmercury consist primarily of motor effects. Several investigators have observed a progressive weakness of the hindlimbs, followed by decreases in forelimb function (49–53). Grip strength was reported to be decreased in rats chronically dosed with methylmercury (30). Horizontally directed motor activity does not appear to be markedly affected by repeated exposure to methylmercury (54, 55), although MacDonald & Harbison (56) reported decreased motor activity in mice exposed to methylmercury via drinking water. Responsiveness to noxious stimuli is reportedly intact in methylmercury-exposed animals, even in the presence of gross neuromotor deficits (50, 55). Although extensive descriptions of the neurologic effects of methylmercury have been published, changes in reactivity have not been reported (50, 57). Pryor et al (30) did not observe a significant alteration in startle responsiveness to an acoustic stimulus in methylmercury-exposed rats. Few studies have been reported on the effect of methylmercury on conditioned behaviors. Hughes et al (58) reported that prepubescent rats exposed to a single dose of methylmercury were impaired in their ability to learn an active avoidance response at 70 days of age. Beliles et al (59), using a buzzer as a conditioned stimulus, chronically exposed rats to elemental mercury vapor and found decreased pole-climb response.

ORGANOLEADS   Alkylleads such as triethyl lead have been reported to produce degenerative changes in the cerebral cortex, cerebellum, and hippocampus of experimental animals (60, 61). The neurotoxic sequelae following exposure to organoleads have been well documented and include psychomotor disturbances, alterations in attention, and deficits in memory (62).

Several investigators have described the general effects of acute and short-term repeated exposure to organoleads in laboratory animals (62). In a recent paper, the effects of short-term repeated exposure to triethyl lead were quantified using several neurobehavioral tests (30). Triethyl lead was found to produce a phase of hyperexcitability characterized by increased startle responsiveness and altered responsiveness to noxious thermal stimuli, followed by a phase of hypoexcitability (63). Subsequent experiments found that triethyl lead facilitated the acquisition of a two-way shuttle box response but did not alter sensitivity to electric footshock applied to the grids of the chamber. Pryor et al (30) chronically dosed rats with triethyl lead and observed alterations in thermal sensitivity and a trend toward impaired performance of a conditioned pole-climb response.

As a further illustration of the range of possible neurotoxic effects, Table 1 summarizes a literature survey conducted by Damstra (64) in which the reported signs and symptoms following exposure of humans to a variety of neurotoxicants are listed. It is apparent from this table that the actions of toxic agents on both the central and peripheral nervous system are numerous and complex. In addition, it is evident that chemicals having widely different structures and industrial uses can produce similar effects. Finally, it is also apparent that many of the neurotoxic effects in humans are subjective, minor, and/or nonspecific.

This brief survey of human neurotoxicology and experimental neurobehavioral toxicology is reinforcing in the sense that, for some chemicals, there seems to be a reasonable correspondence between what can be quantified in humans and what can be detected in laboratory animals. However, there are major points of disparity, particularly in regard to the description of sensory and associative or cognitive deficits in an animal model, particularly rodents. Thus, although it seems possible to develop appropriate animal models for some of the neurotoxic effects observed in humans, it is not clear that a precise one-to-one relationship is possible.

SELECTION OF TESTS FOR NEUROBEHAVIORAL TESTING

Behavior Defined

Behavior can be conceptualized as the end-product of a variety of sensory, motor, and integrative processes occurring in the nervous system (65). Operationally, behavior can be defined as the movement of an organism or its parts within a temporal and spatial context. Thus, behavior can be thought of as being comprised of units termed responses, which can be further defined as whatever covaries with effective controlling variables. By definition, an aspect of the environment that controls behavior in a functional or lawful manner is a stimulus. Behaviorists study the relationship between stimuli, behavior, and the consequences of this behavior in the environment. The behavior of an organism at any point in time is determined by the currently active environment, as well as its previous experience with these or similar environmental conditions. A change in the environment, such as the superimposition of a chemical, has the capability to change the functional relationships that control behavior.

Classification of Behavioral Tests

One way to classify behavioral procedures is to define them according to the desired level of analysis. Table 2 indicates that techniques designed to detect

Table 1 Neurotoxic effects of representative agents in humans

Representative agent	Neurotoxic effects
1. Solvents	
Hexane, acrylamide	Ataxia, tremor, paresthesia, hypersomnia, slurring of speech, delirium/hallucinations
Carbon disulfide	Anosmia, paresthesia, depression
	Anxiety, psychoses
2. Organochlorine insecticides (chlordecone, DDT)	Ataxia, tremor, slurring of speech, euphoria/excitement, nervousness/irritability, depression/anxiety, mental confusion, memory disorders
3. Organophosphate esters	Ataxia, paresthesia, insomnia, slurring of speech, tinnitus, amblyopia, nystagmus, abnormal pupil reactions, nervousness/irritability, depression/anxiety, psychoses, memory disorders
4. Heavy metals	
Inorganic leads	Ataxia, tremor, pathological reflexes, paresthesia, hearing loss, abnormal pupil reactions, depression/anxiety
Mercury	Facial tic, tremor, insomnia, amblyopia, depression/anxiety
Manganese	Parkinsonism, tremor, paresthesia hypersomnia, euphoria/excitement, delirium/hallucinations, memory disorders
Cadmium	Anosmia
Arsenic	Hyperesthesia
5. Organometals	
Methylmercury	Ataxia, myoclonus, paresthesia, insomnia, slurring of speech, hearing loss, abnormal pupil reactions, mental confusion

the presence or absence of toxicity are generally different from those used to determine the degree of toxicity or the lowest level of a chemical required to produce a toxic effect. Obviously, those procedures used to detect the presence or absence of an effect are usually the most frequently used to screen for potential effects. Screening procedures used routinely to assess large numbers of environmental agents are typically inexpensive to perform, do not require extensive training of either the experimental animal or laboratory personnel, and permit the assessment of large numbers of subjects. On the other hand, these procedures are usually labor intensive, frequently require subjective measurements, often yield data on less than an interval scale, and may not be as sensitive to subtle neurobehavioral deficits as more complex (i.e. secondary) techniques.

Secondary level tests are generally thought to be more sensitive to subtle changes in neurobehavioral functioning than those used for screening and may be useful in experiments concerning mechanism of action or in estimating environmentally acceptable limits. They are, however, not cost effective under most conditions.

Criteria for Test Selection

Several general considerations should be taken into account in the selection of a test for screening. Because of the large number of chemicals to be tested and the fact that relatively large numbers of animals may have to be evaluated, tests should be relatively simple to perform and require cost-effective or inexpensive equipment. Screening tests should also require a relatively short time to perform and repeat testing on an individual animal in order to assess chronic, cumulative deficits at various intervals.

Validity is another important criterion for selecting tests. Tests must be discriminant where separate functions are supposed to be under evaluation and show convergence where the same functions are being assessed. In addition, results from a test using one species should be able to be extrapolated to another species. For example, acrylamide is known to produce peripheral neuropathy in the lower limbs of exposed humans. A valid screening test should show evidence for peripheral dysfunction in the hindlimbs of animals exposed to acrylamide. Valid tests should also show as few false positives and false negatives as possible.

Another criterion is that tests should be reliable. The level of measurement associated with a particular procedure frequently determines the reliability of the technique. Nominal or categorical ratings are perhaps the most difficult to provide reliability, while procedures that yield continuous measurements are the most objective and allow for the most precise quantification of error and consequently reliability. Of course, shortcomings with some measurements can be overcome through precise standardization of test conditions and the use

Table 2 Classification of behavioral techniques

Type of test	Advantages	Disadvantages
Screening	Cost-effective, does not require extensive training of animals or personnel; permits testing of large number of animals	Requires intensive labor input; tends to be subjective and often yields less than interval scale data; may be relatively insensitive to subtle effects
Secondary	Typically automated and objective; usually provides graded data; amenable to repeated measures designs; relatively sensitive to subtle neurotoxic effects	May be costly to perform because of equipment and training of animals and personnel; may not be amenable to testing large numbers of animals

of trained raters and interrater reliability scales. Insofar as economic constraints can be satisfied, techniques producing continuous data are clearly preferred. Ordinal or ranking procedures are somewhere in between category ratings and continuous scales of measurement.

Finally, it is important that behavioral tests be reproducible. Test results should be repeatable across subjects, across samples of subjects, and across laboratories. Also contained in the concept of reproducibility is the notion of sensitivity, which concerns the ability of a test to detect effects over a range of doses and especially to detect effects at lower doses.

Strategies for Neurobehavioral Testing

Two basic approaches have been suggested for screening for neurobehavioral toxicity. Butcher (66) was among the first to describe the possible use of an apical test, a single test that requires the successful integration of intact subsystems. An example of an apical test is schedule-controlled behavior, which typically utilizes intermittent reinforcement and establishes a dependency between the occurrence of a specific response and the presentation of a specific stimulus (e.g. food). Armstrong et al (67) used a fixed interval-fixed ratio schedule to examine the effects of chronic exposure to mercury vapor in pigeons. Daily exposure to mercury resulted in an altered response rate, which occurred several weeks prior to the appearance of overt toxicity. It is interesting to note that when the pigeons were sacrificed for histopathological study, there were no microscopically detectable lesions.

Thus, an apical test such as an operant schedule of reinforcement has obvious utility in detecting the presence of toxicity and it may do so prior to the onset of structural damage. However, a major problem associated with apical tests is that performance of these tasks depends on multiple neurobehavioral processes being intact. Thus, deficits in performance may be due to alterations in any one or more neurobehavioral functions (i.e. sensory, motor, motivational, associative). Furthermore, whatever appeal the apical test has initially is immediately offset by the low probability that a single test would be generally accepted by a majority of behavioral toxicologists.

The most frequently posited strategy for assessing agents for neurobehavioral toxicity is some form of sequential assessment. The depth to which a compound is studied depends on its eventual use and the known effects. The sequential approach provides for an initial level of evaluation, the extent of which varies according to the laboratory. For example, Weiss (68) and Evans & Weiss (12) proposed a three-tier approach that consists first of observational indices of neurotoxicity. These assessments are ratings of locomotor impairment, the presence or absence of tremor, ptosis and convulsions, alterations in various reflexes, and disorders of regulatory processes. In the schema proposed by Weiss & Evans, the second phase focuses on the specific functions that appear to be affected in the initial phase. Secondary tests assess specific sensory and motor functions using relevant state-of-the-art behavioral technology to quantify the neurobehavioral toxicity. Weiss (68) has also proposed a third phase of assessment, which focuses on human health studies.

Other investigators, such as Gad (69), have recommended an approach similar to that of Weiss & Evans, at least at the initial level of assessment. Gad proposed that a series of tests utilizing simple semi-quantitative measurements be used. These tests are in effect rating scales concerning the presence or absence of and in some cases the relative degree to which some reflexes are present. The second phase proposed by Gad consists of isolated tissue-preparation assays to establish the ability to differentiate between reversible and irreversible sensory-neural alterations.

Pavlenko (70) has also proposed three phases of testing. First, very simple methods to assess orienting and defensive reflexes, and corneal, pain, and other unconditioned reflexes are used in a tentative evaluation of potential neurotoxicity. The second phase determines the threshold and subthreshold quantities of potentially noxious substances. To accomplish this, procedures that assess higher order nervous system activity, such as conditioned reflex methods, are used. Finally, functional stress tests are employed to determine minor or latent functional changes and to study the mechanism of action of the neurotoxicant.

Reiter et al (71) have developed a Behavioral Toxicity Index based on the acute LD_{50} and experimentally derived ED_{50} values for a variety of behavioral tests. In this schema, a large index value (ratio) reflects a relatively specific behavioral toxicity and suggests that a behavioral change occurs at an exposure level below that producing overt toxicity. For the four insecticides tested (i.e. Baygon, Carbaryl, Chlordimeform, and Decamethrin), none of the four behavioral measures (i.e. figure-eight maze activity, schedule-controlled operant behavior, conditioned taste aversion, and activity in a radial arm maze) was uniquely sensitive. Ranking of the various tests overall indicated that the figure-eight maze and the schedule-controlled behavior were approximately equal in sensitivity and were more sensitive than the radial arm maze and flavor aversion procedures. The approach of using selective behavioral measures to establish a behavioral toxicity index appears to be successful, at least as it pertains to the compounds that were tested. More data are needed to determine its utility as a general screen for a wide variety of agents.

Mitchell and his colleagues (3, 14, 15) have proposed a two-tier approach to the assessment of potential neurotoxicants. Instead of relying on observational techniques at the first level of testing and then studying effects in greater detail following the detection of a behavioral change, these investigators propose judicious selection of tests at the initial phase based on several criteria. First, they propose that tests be considered for their inherent sensitivity, reliability, reproducibility, and validity. Second, tests should provide for an overview of nervous system functioning, i.e. tests should be chosen to evaluate a wide range of functions, from "simple reflexes" to more complex functions (including sensory function, motor strength, and coordination), reactivity (excitability), and associative factors. Recently, Pryor et al (30) reported on the results of a three-year study comparing the effects of eight chronically administered neurotoxicants (acrylamide, arsenic, chlordecone, methylmercury, monosodium salicyalte, lead acetate, triethyl lead, and tetraethyl tin) using a battery of tests (i.e. motor activity, startle to an air puff and acoustic stimulus, fore- and hindlimb grip strength, negative geotaxis, performance on a multisensory conditioned poleclimb shock-avoidance task, and body weights). For the compounds tested, these investigators found a reasonably good association between signs of neurotoxicity reported in humans and those neurobehavioral effects predicted in rodents.

EXAMPLES OF METHODS TO BE USED IN TESTING

Tests of Motor Function

Spontaneous motor activity in rodents has been extensively used in behavioral toxicology (2, 72). Movement within the living space or environment is a high probability response in animals and can easily be manipulated by environmental changes, including exposure to neurotoxicants. Although seemingly simple, locomotor activity is a very complex behavior comprised of a variety of motor acts, such as horizontally and vertically directed movement, sniffing, and grooming. Rating scales have been developed to fractionate motor activity into its relative components (73). The measures used most often in behavioral toxicology are horizontally and vertically directed activity (72). A large variety of devices, automated and unautomated, have been invented to measure motor activity, and quantitatively and qualitatively different effects can be observed following exposure to a neurotoxicant depending upon the apparatus used. Although it is premature to conclude that one technique or procedure is better than another, the figure-eight maze as utilized by Reiter and colleagues (2, 72) has been used extensively and successfully to detect effects produced by a number of chemicals.

Although Reiter and colleagues (2) have used the figure-eight maze as a residential maze to measure chemical effects on diurnal activity patterns, their most recent research has almost exclusively employed assessment during shorter time intervals. Elsner et al (74) have also reported a method for continuous monitoring of spontaneous locomotor patterns of rats. Using computer-assisted techniques, these investigators found that methylmercury treatment lowered activity during the night portion of the diurnal cycle.

Before going on to discuss other measures of motor function, some comment should be made concerning the meaning of data generated by procedures utilizing motor activity measurements. In some respects, motor activity can be viewed as an apical test (see above). As pointed out by Reiter (2), activity is not a unitary measure and a change in the frequency of this behavior could reflect toxicant-induced changes in any one or more sensory or motor functions, alterations in reactivity (excitability) or motivational states, or perturbations of a variety of regulatory states (i.e. diurnal cycles, energy balance of the animal). Thus, if a change in motor activity is observed, then additional tests are needed to determine the cause (i.e. is there a decrease in activity because the animal is paralyzed or is it because there is so much liver damage that the animal suffers from "general malaise").

Many types of screening tests are currently used to assess the effects of neurotoxicants on motor function. The most simple of these include observational assessments of body posture, muscle tone, equilibrium and gait, and righting reflexes (53, 69, 75). These tests are quantal or categorical at best and are generally subjective in nature.

A variety of other techniques have been developed to evaluate motor function in a less subjective fashion, including performance on a rotating rod (76), inclined screen, or plane (77); swimming to exhaustion (78); or suspension from a horizontal rod (79). One technique used with increasing frequency is quantification of hindlimb splay; Edwards & Parker (35) placed ink on the feet of rats, dropped them from a specified height, and measured the distance between the marked digits. Schallert et al (80) used a similar technique of inking the paws to evaluate abnormal gait in rats treated centrally with 6-hydroxydopamine.

Neurotoxicant-induced alteration in motor coordination has been evaluated by Pryor et al (30) using a negative geotaxis procedure, while the hindlimb extensor reflex was quantified using a method described by Cabe & Tilson (81). Grip strength is a frequently reported neurological sign in humans and fore- and hindlimb grip strength in rats and mice has been quantified using commercially available strain gauges (82).

One common neurological effect observed in animals exposed to neurotoxicants is tremor. A number of rating scales and semiquantitative procedures have been reported to measure tremor (42). Recently, a simple but expensive spectral analysis technique was reported that permits the rapid evaluation of tremor in freely moving animals (42).

More complicated techniques have been devised to measure motor deficits in laboratory animals. For example, Falk (83) used operant conditioning procedures to train animals to press a lever within a designated range of force for a given period. Falk and others (84) have used this procedure to study the effects of agents on fine motor control.

Tests for Sensory Function

Alterations in sensory processes, such as paresthesias or visual or auditory impairments, are frequently among the first signs of toxicity produced in humans exposed to toxicants. The most sensitive methods used to detect sensory deficits in animals involve psychophysical measurements to arrive at some estimation of the ability of an organism to make a differential response in the presence of a stimulus varied across some physical dimension (85). However, the great majority of psychophysical studies have been done in nonhuman primates and avian species rather than rodents.

One of the least complex approaches to the study of sensory deficits is based on the localization or orientation response. Marshall and his colleagues (86–88) have described a battery of observational tests in which a stimulus (a square of paper brought in from behind the animal's head over either eye, clicks presented close to and behind the ear, presentation of a strong odor on each side of the head, or pressing hairs calibrated to bend at a given force along various portions of the body surface) is presented and the presence or absence of a localization or orientation response to the source of the stimulus is recorded. Such techniques have been used to demonstrate sensory inattention as well as hyperexcitability in rats having lesions in various regions of the brain. Pavlenko (70) has described a variety of stimulus-elicited orientation reflexes used in the Soviet Union.

In spite of the fact that observational tests are simple to perform, they are labor intensive, especially if interrater reliability scales are used. Moreover, the scoring of the tests is frequently subjective and necessitates testing under blind conditions. Finally, the data are usually of a quantal nature (i.e. the response is scored as being either present or absent) or categorical (rating scores); thus, interpretation of the results is difficult, particularly in repeated measures designs.

Several attempts have been made to develop simple yet objective tests for sensory dysfunction in rodents. For example, depth perception has been assessed using a visual cliff procedure, which determines whether or not an animal will choose to step onto a nearby platform or floor ("shallow" floor) compared to one that may be perceived as being further away ("deep" floor) (89). Another simple test of visual function is the optokinetic drum, which relies on the optokinetic nystagmus or optomotor response (i.e. tracking a moving object with the eyes and head for a certain distance until the head is repositioned back into the frontal plane). This measure is believed to assess visual acuity (90), although there are little data reported using this technique to study toxicants. One screening test used by some investigators to assess hearing is the acoustic startle reflex, which consists of measuring the presence (and magnitude) or absence of the response to the presentation of a novel sound or tone (91). Pain sensitivity can be assessed using standard psychopharmacological techniques such as the tail flick or hot plate (30), while taste reactivity has been assessed using taste-aversion procedures (92).

Several more complicated paradigms have been proposed to assess sensory dysfunction in rodents. For example, maze and similar types of apparatus are frequently used to test for alterations in the performance of tasks based upon discrimination of sensory cues (93). On the basis of work done using visual cues, as well as work done with other sense modalities such as somesthesis (94, 95), mazes and maze-like apparatus appear to have some utility in evaluating sensory deficits in rats. However, as pointed out by Evans (93), care must be taken to determine the relative contribution of motor and higher level functions when interpreting results from such experiments.

One of the more objective ways to evaluate sensory deficits involves the use of operant technology. In these experiments, an animal is motivated by food or electric shock to make a response, such as a lever press. Eventually the animal learns to make the response only under certain stimulus conditions and, by varying the parameters of the stimuli, a graded stimulus-intensity response function curve can be determined. Of course, neurotoxicants with specific sensory effects would be expected to alter this curve. Auditory loss has been reported following exposure to kanamycin using such techniques (96, 97). Besides the procedures mentioned for auditory deficits, operant techniques have been used to study the effects of chemicals on light flicker discrimination (98), olfactory cues (99), and reactivity to electric shock (100).

Recently, Pryor et al (30) reported on the use of a multisensory conditioned avoidance response (CAR) to assess three sensory modalities concurrently in the same animal. In this procedure, a rat learns to climb or pull a rope to escape and then to avoid a noxious (1 mA) electric footshock. Eventually, the response is brought under the control of three conditioned stimuli (a 4-kHz tone, a low-intensity nonaversive current on the floor, .125 mA, and a change in the intensity of the chamber house light). Three intensities of each stimulus are presented during each series of trials on each day of testing, thereby permitting a quasipsychophysical response function to be generated. Once the animals are trained to make a response, they are exposed to a variety of toxicants and the change in response measured. A specific sensory neurotoxicant should have a specific effect on avoidance behavior controlled by one of the respective stimuli. Experiments with positive control manipulations (i.e. constant light in the home cage to alter visual function or repeated administration of kanamycin to produce hearing loss) have successfully demonstrated the validity of the technique. In a recent paper, Pryor et al (101) reported functional hearing loss associated with hair cell damage in the inner ear in rats exposed repeatedly to toluene.

Tests for Reactivity or CNS Arousal

One of the frequently reported indicators of neurotoxicity is nervousness and irritability (or, on the other hand, hypersomnolence and lethargy). One procedure frequently used to test for general responsiveness to environmental stimulation is the startle reflex. According to Davis and colleagues (91, 102), the startle reflex is mediated by a five-synapse pathway beginning at the auditory nerve and ending in the lower motor neurons. By using a supramaximal novel stimulus, a response having a short, reproducible latency occurring in virtually every animal can be elicited. The startle response can be influenced by changing the parameters of the eliciting stimulus and therefore has utility in psychophysical studies (see above).

Changes in the magnitude of the startle response have been associated with toxicant-induced alterations in CNS excitability. Increases [for chlordecone, see (43, 103)] and decreases [for PBBs, see (104)] have been reported. The startle response appears to be a relatively good indicator of general responsiveness when used under the appropriate conditions. However, other measures of neurological function should be considered when studying the startle response, since it is a reflex that contains a neuromuscular component.

Another procedure commonly used to determine changes in the excitability of the nervous system is to study alterations in responsiveness to chemically or electrically induced seizures. For example, changes in the threshold to produce maximal electroshock seizure (MES) have been shown in rats exposed during development to lead (105). Dyer et al (106) have shown that rats exposed to trimethyl tin were more sensitive to the effects of pentylenetetrazol, suggesting a general increase in seizure susceptibility.

Learning and Memory

The ability to learn and remember has obvious adaptive value for an organism. The capacity to learn permits an organism to escape or avoid aversive situations or approach desirable objects and to store the memory of these contingencies for use at some future time. The specificity of a toxic effect on learning must be interpreted within the context of the experimental design and in conjunction with controls that assess toxicant-induced effects on sensory, motor, and motivational processes.

Behavioral toxicologists have used a variety of experimental paradigms to assess learning/memory in laboratory animals. Briefly, procedures have been designed to determine acquisition using positive as well as negative reinforcing contingencies and to assess intermediate and long-term memory. A few working procedures have been developed to measure the ability to adjust to a new contingency once an initial task has been learned.

PROCEDURES USING NEGATIVE REINFORCEMENT   Aversive conditioning utilizing electric footshock has been used frequently in behavioral pharmacology and toxicology. Passive avoidance procedures involve training an animal to withhold a response to avoid being shocked. For example, Mactutus et al (107) used a multiple measure step-through passive avoidance procedure to assess learning/retention deficits in rats exposed neonatally to chlordecone. What is unique about the protocol they employed is that several measures (i.e. initial step-through latencies, frequency of head pokes, half crosses and full crosses, as well as the traditional latency to reenter the chamber after being shocked) were taken. In addition, retention over several time points (immediately and 72 or 144 hours after training) was assessed. A similar procedure has been used to assess retention deficits after trimethyl tin administration to adult rats (108) and following intraventricular administration of the cholinergic cytotoxicant AF64-A (109). The passive avoidance procedure has the advantage of being rapid and easy to perform without requiring extensive resources; it has the disadvantage of producing highly variable results if performed under inadequate test conditions or if the appropriate retention intervals are not used. Finally, we highly recommend that measurement be made on the nonassociative variables mentioned above, as well as evaluation of alterations in motivational factors, such as changes in pain thresholds to footshock.

One-way shock avoidance tasks require the animal to move from one compartment to another in order to escape or avoid being shocked. Once the response is made, the animal is placed back in the original compartment and the process is repeated. In one-way avoidance, the animal does not have to learn to return to the physical space where it has just been shocked. Using this type of test, Tilson et al (44) reported that rats exposed chronically to chlordecone learned to avoid as rapidly as controls, but displayed a significant retention deficit when retested several days later.

Another variant of the shock-motivated learning tasks is the two-way shuttle box paradigm. In this procedure, rats learn to shuttle from one compartment to another in order to escape or avoid electric footshock; however, unlike one-way avoidance, the animals have to learn to return to a compartment where they have just been shocked. It is interesting to note that differences in effects can be made between the one- and two-way procedures. For example, Sobotka et al (110) reported that rats exposed neonatally to lead performed as well as controls on a one-way shock avoidance task, but displayed significant deficits when required to learn a two-way avoidance task. Moreover, rats exposed to chlordecone chronically did not show deficits in two-way avoidance (R. Squibb, T. Burne, H. Tilson, unpublished observations), in spite of previous reports that similar exposure to chlordecone affected one-way avoidance (44).

In general, one- and two-way avoidance tasks are conducted in one training session or over several discrete massed trials, while retention is assessed in one or more trials at some point following demonstration of learning. A somewhat more complex learning task than either the one- or two-way avoidance procedures is the symmetrical Y-maze. In this procedure, a light or tone is activated in one of two arms not occupied by the animal, which has a predetermined amount of time to run to the proper arm of the maze or it will receive an electric shock. Not only does the animal have to learn when to run, but it must also learn where to run (111). The Y-maze has been used successfully by Vorhees (112) to study learning ability of rats exposed in utero to vitamin A.

The preceding techniques have all employed electric footshock as a negative reinforcer to promote learning. One procedure that uses another approach is the water maze. Animals are placed into a maze full of water and are required to learn a series of correct turns in order to gain access to an exit ramp. Learning trials are preceded by straight channel swimming trials as an adaptive procedure and to determine if there are measurable neuromotor deficits. Vorhees et al (113) detected learning deficits in animals exposed during development to vitamin A using a Biel water maze, while Zenick and his colleagues (114, 115) have found learning deficits in animals exposed to lead or mercury during development.

PROCEDURES USING POSITIVE REINFORCEMENT   Another approach to assessing learning abilities in animals is to use positive reinforcement, such as a food reward for a previously food-deprived animal. Mazes and similar apparatus have been used to demonstrate that animals will learn to make a response (i.e. move to a specific location or press a lever) to receive reinforcement. One procedure using positive reinforcement that shows promise in behavioral toxicology is the radial-arm maze (RAM). The RAM is a complex spatial learning task in which animals must "remember" a list of previously entered and non-entered feeders during a free-choice test session (116, 117). The most commonly used RAM consists of a circular arena from which eight equidistant arms radiate like spokes from a wheel. Each of the eight arms is baited at the beginning of a test session; the trial ends following consumption of all available pellets or after a fixed period of time has elapsed. The most effective strategy for solving the maze is to enter and eat in each of the arms only once. Recently, Walsh et al (108) reported that trimethyl-tin–exposed rats display impaired performance in this task and that the behavioral deficit may be due to an alteration in the integrity of limbic forebrain structures such as the hippocampus.

Another positive reinforcement procedure developed recently is the two-choice visual discrimination task described by Tilson et al (118). In this task, animals are trained in a discrete trial task to make a nose-poke-operant response in the presence of a visual cue located on one side of a cue panel. After the animal learns the correct discrimination, which occurs over a period of days, the contingency is reversed, i.e. a response to the side in which the cue lamp remains unlit is reinforced. Tilson et al (118) found that rats exposed to chlordecone during development showed a trend toward improved acquisition and were markedly different from the control rats in the way that they responded during the reversal phase of the test.

Naturally Occurring Behaviors

A general principle in psychology and animal behavior is that the behavior of an organism is likely to be stable and predictable given stable environmental conditions. Behaviors such as those that occur naturally in the home cage, such as eating, drinking, and general locomotor activity, are related to the ecological and evolutionary history of the organism.

One approach to the use of naturally occurring behaviors is to measure the repertoire of animals in their laboratory environment, i.e. in the homecage. Locomotor activity, food intake, and water intake can be easily quantified (119) and, once a stable pattern of homecage activity is established, toxicants can be introduced and the resulting alterations in behavior measured (3).

One naturally occurring response that has been proposed to screen for toxicants is geophagia, which is the ingestion of nonnutritive substances following conditions known to produce illness (120). Closely associated with geophagia is the conditioned taste aversion procedure. When rodents are given access to a flavored solution followed by exposure to a drug or toxicant, they often display an aversion upon subsequent presentation of the solution. Flavor aversions have been reported to occur following a number of environmentally relevant chemicals, such as arsenic, cadmium, copper sulfate, lead, methylmercury, chlordimeform, 2,4,5-T, acrylamide, physostigmine, and alkyltins (121, 122).

Silverman and colleagues (18, 123) have been proponents for the study of social behaviors in animals exposed to chemicals. These investigators record species-specific behaviors (i.e. exploration, sex-related activities, aggression, submission, etc.) of rats in an observation cage and measure toxicant-induced changes in the frequency of the behaviors. Through laborious and time-consuming observations and recordings, Silverman et al (123) were able to see significant changes in behaviors of animals exposed to methyl mercury via the diet (social behavior was decreased after 16–17 days of exposure to 75 ppm).

Alternative Approaches

Behavioral procedures described thus far have focused primarily on methods employed by researchers in Western countries. There is an equally important and vast literature on approaches used by investigators influenced by Sechenov and Pavlov (124, 125). In general, the Soviet Union and other countries pose the problems of neurobehavioral assessment in terms of physiological aspects of nervous system function.

As discussed earlier, Pavlenko (70) proposed simple tests of unconditioned responses as the first tier in neurobehavioral screening; tests of conditioned reflexes were proposed for later study. These tests involve various conditioned reflexes, such as those requiring shock or food motivation and induction processes of learning and acquisition. Although much of the terminology of the

Pavlovian-oriented researchers differs from that of the more behaviorist framework of the West, there is considerable convergence in the two approaches (12). Where they may differ is in how a behaviorally toxic effect is interpreted and later translated into regulations for the environment.

PROBLEMS AND RESEARCH NEEDS

Summary of Purpose and Scope

Numerous methods are available for use in toxicity assessment, yet several problem areas need to be resolved before there can be any agreement on a screening program. One significant question concerns the perceived goal of a screening program. It seems imperative that the large number of new chemicals introduced each year and the thousands of agents already in the environment need to be assessed for their effects on the nervous system. Neurobehavioral effects are significant in that, in some cases, a functional deficit may be observed prior to the onset of a more obvious toxic effect or before there is morphological damage.

If it is accepted that behavioral techniques have a place in the screening of toxic agents (along with those of other disciplines, especially neurophysiology), the next question concerns the choice of tests to be included in the screen. The purpose of the neurobehavioral screen is to provide an initial evaluation of the effect of agents on behavior and the nervous system so that neurotoxic agents will not reach the marketplace without proper warning. Thus, it is important that the tests used in the screen be sensitive, reliable, and reproducible as well as cost effective. It is important to realize that if insensitive techniques are used or if toxic effects observed in one laboratory cannot be reproduced in another, then resources have been wasted. More importantly, an insensitive screen could allow potentially neurotoxic agents to enter the environment. It is logical to assume that tests that are objective to perform (automated as much as possible) and yield continuous level data for analysis will contribute to the sensitivity and reliability of a battery of tests. Standardization of the protocols and conditions under which tests are performed will greatly assist in meeting the objectives of reliability and reproducibility.

Another objective in establishing criteria for neurobehavioral screening is that they should have some relevance to human toxicosis. One obvious way to accomplish this is to include a variety of tests that attempt to assess the wide range of signs typically observed in humans exposed to neurotoxicants. One approach toward this objective is to choose animal tests whose results can be applied to human neurobehavioral functions. Validation of test methods in neurobehavioral screening should be an empirical matter. Mitchell and his colleagues (3, 15, 16) have argued that validation of sensitive and reliable methodologies in animals (rats) is possible by first comparing compounds known to have specific neurotoxic effects in several tests chosen to overlap in terms of signs evaluated. The profile generated by such a comparison could be used to evaluate the sensitivity and selection of those tests assumed to measure the same neurobehavioral functions. This strategy permits test validation by showing the similarities between procedures assumed or purported to evaluate the same function and by providing a distinction between procedures assumed to measure different processes.

Problems Inherent in Behavioral Tests

One problem with the use and therefore selection of behavioral tests for screening is that it is often difficult to isolate the relative contributions of the various sensory, motor, arousal, or associative factors that may contribute to a behavioral toxic effect. For example, if a toxicant produces a decrease in the probability of a simple reflex, such as the orientation response to an auditory stimulus, the conclusion that hearing is affected depends upon concurrent measurement of motor dysfunction or responsiveness of the animals to nonaural environmental stimuli. In effect, a profile of neurobehavioral effects may be required in order to demonstrate the specificity of the neurotoxic lesion.

Another problem is that, with repeated exposure to a chemical, animals can adapt to its effects. As Norton (61, 125) points out, the effects of repeated exposure to a chemical may go undetected because of homeostatic mechanisms triggered by the presence of the agent. Furthermore, many organs possess an excess capacity that can be damaged and go undetected by functional tests. The so-called functional reserve of the central nervous system should be considered in the selection of tests for screening, perhaps by incorporating in the test procedures one or more conditions in which the system(s) or organism(s) is placed under some sort of stress. The combination of the test substance plus stress may result in a greater or detectable deficit in neurobehavioral function. Examples of stressors that have been used are ethanol and other drugs, muscular or work stress, exposure to cold, and auditory and electrical stimuli (70, 126).

Another problem that should be considered is that seemingly similar methods might yield different results. For example, Reiter et al (127) used two measures of locomotor activity (open field and residential maze) to evaluate the toxicity of chlordecone and triethyl tin. Chlordecone produced a dose-related decrease in the open field, whereas a dose-related increase was observed in residential maze activity. With triethyl tin, there was a dose-related decrease in residential maze activity but no change in activity in the open field. Thus, there were qualitative and quantitative differences in the two measures of locomotor activity.

Research Needs

In addition to the need for standardization and validation of tests discussed above, more emphasis needs to be placed on determining subpopulations at greatest risk. Most of the data in behavioral toxicology have been generated with young adult male animals. More emphasis needs to be placed on comparative effects in animals that may be predisposed to toxic insult (i.e. the very young, the elderly, the malnourished, females versus males).

Another area that deserves attention concerns the potential interactions of two or more chemical agents. In the environment, the probability of exposure to several toxicants exceeds the probability of being exposed to a single agent (i.e. Love Canal in the US). Although it is preferable to know more about the potential effects of toxicants when they are administered singly before studying the problems of mixtures, the reality of the environmental situation suggests that a strategy for the evaluation of mixtures be considered.

ACKNOWLEDGEMENT

The authors express their thanks to Ms. Nell Godfrey for expert preparation of this manuscript. The authors are also grateful to Drs. Kent Anger, Lawrence Reiter, Deborah Rice, and Gerhard Winneke for constructive comments and criticism on an earlier draft of this manuscript.

Literature Cited

1. Mello, N. K. 1975. Behavioral toxicology: A developing discipline. *Fed. Proc.* 34:1832–34
2. Reiter, L. 1978. Use of activity measures in behavioral toxicology. *Environ. Health Perspect.* 26:9–20
3. Tilson, H. A., Cabe, P. A. 1978. Strategy for the assessment of neurobehavioral consequences of environmental factors. *Environ. Health Perspect.* 26:287–99
4. Weiss, B., Laties, V., eds. 1975. *Behavioral Toxicology.* New York: Plenum
5. Zenick, H., Reiter, L. W., eds. 1977. *Behavioral Toxicology: An Emerging Discipline.* Research Triangle Park, NC: US Environ. Protect. Agency
6. Elkins, H. B. 1961. Maximum acceptable concentrations, a comparison in Russia and the United States. *Arch. Environ. Health* 2:45–55
7. Ruffin, J. B. 1963. Functional testing for behavioral toxicity: A missing dimension in experimental environmental toxicology. *J. Occup. Med.* 5:117
8. Brimblecombe, R. W. 1976. Behavioral toxicology in the evaluation of food safety. *Clin. Toxicol.* 9:731–43
9. Citovic, I. S. 1930. The procedure of studying the effects of oil products on the organism of animals. *Inst. Work Safety* 1:92
10. Weiss, B., Laties, V. 1969. Behavioral pharmacology and toxicology. *Ann. Rev. Pharmacology* 9:297–326
11. Bigami, G. 1976. Behavioral pharmacology and toxicology. *Ann. Rev. Pharmacol. Toxicol.* 16:329–66
12. Evans, H. L., Weiss, B. 1978. Behavioral toxicology. In *Contemporary Research in Behavioral Pharmacology,* ed. D. E. Blackman, D. J. Sanger, pp. 449–87. New York: Plenum
13. Geller, I., Stebbins, W. C., Wayner, M. J., eds. 1979. Proc. workshop on test methods for definition of effects of toxic substances on behavior and neuromotor function, San Antonio, Texas, 1979. *Neurobeh. Toxicol.* 1:1–225 (Suppl.)
14. Mitchell, C. L. 1978. Target organ toxicity: Nervous system. *Environ. Health Perspect.* 26:3–4
15. Mitchell, C. L., Tilson, H. A. 1982. Behavioral toxicology in risk assessment: Problems and research needs. *CRC Crit. Rev. Toxicol.* 10:265–74
16. Mitchell, C. L., Tilson, H. A., Cabe, P. A. 1982. Screening for neurobehavioral toxicity: Factors to consider. In *Nervous System Toxicology,* ed. C. Mitchell, pp. 229–36. New York: Raven
17. Norton, S. 1978. Is behavior or morphology a more sensitive indicator of central nervous system toxicity? *Environ. Health Prospect.* 26:21–27

18. Silverman, P. 1974. Behavioral toxicology. *New Sci.* 67:255–58
19. Tilson, H. A., Mitchell, C. L. 1980. Models for neurotoxicity. In *Reviews in Biochemical Toxicology*, ed. E. Hodgen, J. Bend, R. Philpot, pp. 265–300. New York: Elsevier/North Holland
20. Xintaras, C., Johnson, B. L., DeGroot, I., eds. 1974. *Behavioral Toxicology: Early Detection of Occupational Hazards.* Washington, DC: USGPO
21. NAS/NRC. 1970. *Evaluating the Safety of Food Chemicals.* Washington, DC: National Research Council
22. NAS. 1975. *Principles for Evaluating Chemicals in the Environment. A Rep. Comm. Working Conf. Principles Protocols Evaluating Chem. Environment.* Washington DC: National Academy of Sciences
23. WHO. 1978. *Environmental Health Criteria Series, No. 6, Part I—Report of a WHO Expert Committee.* Geneva: World Health Organization
24. Hicks, R. M. 1972. Air-borne lead as an environmental toxin, a review. *Chem. Biol. Interact.* 5:361–90
25. Lambert, P. W., Schochet, S. S. 1968. Demyelination and remyelination in lead neuropathy. *J. Neuropath. Exp. Neurol.* 27:210–20
26. Schlaepfer, W. W. 1969. Experimental lead neuropathy, a disease of the supporting cells in the peripheral nervous system. *J. Neuropath. Exp. Neurol.* 28:401–18
27. Brown, S., Dragann, N., Vogel, W. 1971. Effects of lead acetate on learning and memory in rats. *Arch. Environ. Health* 22:370–72
28. Shapiro, M. M., Tritschler, J. M., Ulm, R. A. 1973. Lead contamination: Chronic and acute behavioral effects in the albino rat. *Bull. Psychon. Soc.* 2:94–96
29. Lanthorn, T., Isaacson, R. L. 1978. Effects of chronic lead exposure in adult rats. *Physiol. Psychol.* 6:93–95
30. Pryor, G. T., Uyeno, E. T., Tilson, H. A., Mitchell, C. L. 1983. Assessment of chemicals using a battery of neurobehavioral tests: A comparative study. *Neurobehav. Toxicol. Teratol.* 5:91–117
31. Spencer, P. S., Schaumburg, H. H. 1974. A review of acrylamide neurotoxicity. Part I. Properties, uses and human exposure. *Can. J. Neurol. Sci.* 1:143–50
32. Spencer, P. S., Schaumburg, H. H. 1974. A review of acrylamide neurotoxicity. Part II. Experimental animal neurotoxicity and pathologic mechanisms. *Can. J. Neurol. Sci.* 1:152–69
33. Yamamura, Y. 1969. n-Hexane, poly-neuropathy. *Folia Psychiatr. Neurol. Jpn.* 23:45–57
34. Tilson, H. A., Cabe, P. A., Spencer, P. S. 1979. Acrylamide neurotoxicity in rats: A correlated neurobehavioral and pathological study. *Neurotoxicology* 1:89–104
35. Edwards, D. M., Parker, V. H. 1977. A simple, sensitive and objective method for early assessment of acrylamide neuropathy in rats. *Toxicol. Appl. Pharmacol.* 40:589–91
36. Jolicoeur, F. B., Rondeau, D. B., Barbeau, A., Wayner, M. J. 1979. Comparison of neurobehavioral effects induced by various experimental models of ataxia in the rat. *Neurobehav. Toxicol.* 1:175–78 (Suppl.)
37. Kaplan, M. L., Murphy, S. D. 1972. Effects of acrylamide on rotarod performance and sciatic nerve β-glucuronidase activity of rats. *Toxicol. Appl. Pharmacol.* 22:259–68
38. Taylor, J. R., Selhorst, J. B., Calabrese, V. P. 1980. Chlordecone. In *Experimental and Clinical Neurotoxicology.* ed. P. S. Spencer, H. H. Schaumburg, pp. 404–21. Baltimore, MD: Williams & Wilkins
39. Taylor, J. R. 1982. Neurological manifestations in humans exposed to chlordecone and follow-up results. *Neurotoxicology* 3:9–16
40. Huang, T. P., Ho, I. K., Mehendale, H. M. 1981. Assessment of neurotoxicity induced by oral administration of chlordecone in the mouse. *Neurotoxicology* 2:113–24
41. Baggett, J. M., Thureson-Klein, A., Klein, R. L. 1980. Effects of chlordecone on the adrenal medulla of the rat. *Toxicol. Appl. Pharmacol.* 52:313–22
42. Gerhart, J. M., Hong, J. S., Uphouse, L. L., Tilson, H. A. 1982. Chlordecone-induced tremor: Quantification and pharmacological analysis. *Toxicol. Appl. Pharmacol.* 66:234–43
43. Reiter, L. W., Kidd, K., Ledbetter, G., Gray, L. E., Chernoff, N. 1977. Comparative behavioral toxicology of Mirex and Kepone in the rat. *Toxicol. Appl. Pharmacol.* 41:143 (Abstr.)
44. Tilson, H. A., Byrd, N., Riley, M. 1979. Neurobehavioral effects of exposing rats to Kepone via the diet. *Environ. Health Perspect.* 33:321 (Abstr.)
45. Wang, T-P.H., Ho, I. K., Menhendale, H. M. 1981. Correlation between neurotoxicity and chlordecone (Kepone) levels in brain and plasma in the mouse. *Neurotoxicology* 2:373–81
46. Kurland, L. T., Faro, S. N., Siedler, H.

1960. Minamata disease. *World Neurol.* 1:370–95

47. Rustam, H., Handi, T. 1974. Methylmercury poisoning in Iraq. A neurological study. *Brain* 97:499–510

48. Tsubaki, T., Shirakawa, K., Hirota, K. 1973. Epidemiological and clinical studies on Minamata disease in Niigata. *Jpn. J. Med.* 12:119–25

49. Diamond, S. S., Sleight, S. D. 1972. Acute and subchronic methylmercury toxicosis in the rat. *Toxicol. Appl. Pharmacol.* 23:197–207

50. Herman, S. P., Klein, R., Talley, F. A., Krigman, M. 1973. An ultrastructural study of methylmercury-induced primary sensory neuropathy in the rat. *Lab. Invest.* 28:104–18

51. Klein, R., Herman, S., Brubaker, P. E., Lucier, G. W. 1972. A model of acute methylmercury intoxication in rats. *Arch. Path.* 93:408–18

52. Ohi, G., Nishigaki, S., Seki, H., Tamura, Y., Mizoguchi, I., Yagyu, H., Nagashima, K. 1978. Tail rotation, an early neurological sign of methylmercury poisoning in the rat. *Environ. Res.* 16:353–59

53. Snyder, D. R., Braun, J. J. 1977. Dissociation between behavioral and physiological indices of organomercurial ingestion. *Toxicol. Appl. Pharmacol.* 41:277–84

54. Morganti, J. B., Lown, B. A., Salvaterra, P., Massaro, E. J. 1976. Effects on open-field behavior of mice exposed to multiple doses of methylmercury. *Gen. Pharmacol.* 7:41–44

55. Salvaterra, P., Lown, B., Morganti, J., Marssaro, E. J. 1973. Alterations in neurochemical and behavioral parameters in the mouse induced by low doses of methylmercury. *Acta Pharmacol. Toxicol.* 33:177–90

56. MacDonald, J. S., Harbison, R. D. 1977. Methylmercury-induced encephalopathy in mice. *Toxicol. Appl. Pharmacol.* 39:195–205

57. Suzuki, T., Miyama, T. 1971. Neurological symptoms and mercury concentrations in the brain of mice fed with methylmercury salt. *Ind. Health* 9:51–58

58. Hughes, R., Belser, R., Brett, C. W. 1975. Behavioral impairment produced by exposure to subclinical amounts of methylmercury chloride. *Environ. Res.* 10:54–58

59. Beliles, R. P., Clark, R. S., Yuile, C. L. 1968. The effects of exposure to mercury vapor on behavior of rats. *Toxicol. Appl. Pharmacol.* 12:15–21

60. Niklowitz, W. J. 1974. Ultrastructural effects of acute tetraethyllead poisoning on nerve cells of the rabbit brain. *Environ. Res.* 8:17–36

61. Niklowitz, W. J., Yeager, D. W. 1973. Interference of Pb with essential brain tissue Cu, Fe and Zn as main determinant in experimental tetraethyllead encephalopathy. *Life Sci.* 15:897–905

62. Grandjean, P., Nielsen, T. 1979. Organolead compounds: Environmental health aspects. *Residue Rev.* 72:97–148

63. Tilson, H. A., Mactutus, C. F., McLamb, R. L., Burne, T. A. 1982. Characterization of triethyl lead chloride neurotoxicity in adult rats. *Neurobehav. Toxicol. Teratol.* 4:671–82

64. Damstra, T. 1978. Environmental chemicals and nervous system dysfunction. *Yale J. Biol. Med.* 5:457–68

65. Tilson, H. A., Harry, G. J. 1982. Behavioral principles for use in behavioral toxicology and pharmacology. See Ref. 16, pp. 1–27

66. Butcher, R. E. 1976. Behavioral testing as a method for assessing risk. *Environ. Health Perspect.* 18:75–78

67. Armstrong, R. D., Leach, L. J., Belluscio, P. R., Maynard, E. A., Hodge, H. C., Scott, J. R. 1963. Behavioral changes in the pigeon following inhalation of mercury vapor. *Am. Ind. Hyg. Assoc. J.* 24:366–75

68. Weiss, B. 1975. Behavioral methods for investigating environmental health effects. *Proc. Intl. Symp. Recent Adv. Assessment Health Effects Environ. Pollution, Paris, 1974*, pp. 2415–33, Luxenbourg: Comm. Europ. Committees

69. Gad, S. C. 1981. A sensory/neuro screen for use in industrial toxicology. *Toxicologist* 1:150

70. Pavlenko, S. M. 1975. Methods for the study of the central nervous system in toxicological tests. In *Methods Used in the USSR for Establishing Biologically Safe Levels of Toxic Substances*, pp. 86–108. Geneva: World Health Organization

71. Reiter, L. W., MacPhail, R. C., Ruppert, P. H., Eckerman, D. A. 1981. Animal models of toxicity: Some comparative data on the sensitivity of behavioral tests. In *Behavioral Consequences of Exposure to Occupational Environments, Proc. 11th Conf. Environ. Toxicol.* 11:11–23

72. Reiter, L., MacPhail, R. 1979. Motor activity: A survey of methods with potential use in toxicity testing. *Neurobehav. Toxicol. Teratol.* 1:53–66 (Suppl.)

73. Draper, W. A. 1967. A behavioral study of the homecage activity of the white rat. *Behaviour* 28:280–93

74. Elsner, J., Looser, R., Zbinden, G. 1979. Quantitative analysis of rat behavior patterns in a residential maze. *Neurobehav. Toxicol.* 1:163–74 (Suppl.)
75. Irwin, S. 1968. Comprehensive observational assessment. Ia. A systematic quantitative procedure for assessing the behavioral and physiological state of the mouse. *Psychopharmacologia* 13:222–57
76. Bogo, V., Hill, T. A., Young, R. W. 1981. Comparison of accelerod and rotorod sensitivity in detecting ethanol- and acrylamide-induced performance decrement in rats: Review of experimental considerations of rotating systems. *Neurotoxicology* 2:765–87
77. Wechkin, S., Elder, R. F., Furchgott, E. 1961. Motor performance in the rat as a function of age and prenatal X-irradiation. *J. Comp. Physiol. Psychol.* 54:658–59
78. Bhagat, B., Wheeler, M. 1973. Effect of nicotine on the swimming endurance of rats. *Neuropharmacology* 12:1161–65
79. Molinergo, L., Orsetti, M. 1976. Drug action on the "grasping reflex" and on swimming endurance: An attempt to characterize experimentally anti-depressant drugs. *Neuropharmacology* 15:257–60
80. Schallert, T., Whishaw, I. A., Ramirez, V. D., Teitelbaum, P. 1978. Compulsive, abnormal walking caused by anticholinergics in akinetic, 6-hydroxydopamine-treated rats. *Science* 199:1461–63
81. Cabe, P. A., Tilson, H. A. 1978. The hindlimb extensor response: A method for assessing motor dysfunction in rats. *Pharmacol. Biochem. Behav.* 9:133–36
82. Meyer, O. A., Tilson, H. A., Byrd, W. C., Riley, M. T. 1979. A method for the routine assessment of fore- and hindlimb grip strength of rats and mice. *Neurobehav. Toxicol.* 1:233–236
83. Falk, J. L. 1970. The behavioral measurement of fine motor control: Effects of pharmacological agents. In *Readings in Behavioral Pharmacology*, ed. T. Thompson, R. Pickens, R. A. Meich, pp. 223–36. New York: Appleton-Century-Crofts
84. Fowler, S. C., Price, A. W. 1978. Some effects of chlordiazepoxide and *d*-amphetamine on response force during punished responding in rats. *Psychopharmacology* 56:211–15
85. Stebbins, W. C. 1970. *Animal Psychophysics: The Design and Conduct of Animal Experiments*. New York: Appleton-Century-Crofts
86. Marshall, J. F. 1975. Increased orientation to sensory stimuli following medial hypothalamic damage in rats. *Brain Res.* 86:373–87
87. Marshall, J. F., Teitelbaum, P. 1974. Further analysis of sensory inattention following lateral hypothalamic damage in rats. *J. Comp. Physiol. Psychol.* 86:375–95
88. Marshall, J. F., Richardson, J. S., Teitelbaum, P. 1974. Nigrostriatal bundle damage and the lateral hypothalamic syndrome. *J. Comp. Physiol. Psychol.* 87:808–30
89. Sloane, S. A., Shea, S. L., Procter, M. M., Dewsbury, D. A. 1978. Visual cliff performance in 10 species of muroid rodents. *Anim. Learn. Behav.* 6:244–48
90. Wallman, J. 1975. A simple technique using an optomotor response for visual psychophysical measurements in animals. *Vision Res.* 15:3–8
91. Davis, M. 1980. Neurochemical modulation of sensory motor reactivity: Acoustic and tactile startle reflexes. *Neurosci. Biobehav. Rev.* 4:241–63
92. Kodama, J., Fukushima, M., Sakata, T. 1978. Impaired taste discrimination against quinine following chronic administration of theophylline in rats. *Physiol. Behav.* 20:151–55
93. Evans, H. L. 1978. Behavioral assessment of visual toxicity. *Environ. Health Perspect.* 26:53–58
94. Overmann, S. R. 1977. Behavioral effects of asymptomatic lead exposure during neonatal development in rats. *Toxicol. Appl. Pharmacol.* 41:459–71
95. Post, E. M., Yang, M. G., King, J. A., Sanger, V. L. 1978. Behavioral changes of young rats force-fed methylmercury chloride. *Proc. Soc. Exp. Biol. Med.* 143:1113–16
96. Chiba, Ando, K. 1976. Effects of chronic administration of kanamycin on conditioned suppression to auditory stimulus in rats. *Jpn. J. Pharmacol.* 26:419–26
97. Harpur, E. S., D'Arcy, P. F. 1975. The quantification of kanamycin ototoxicity in the rat using conditioned tone discrimination. *J. Pharm. Pharmacol.* 27:907–13
98. Schechter, M. D., Winter, J. C. 1971. Effects of mescaline and lysergic acid diethylamide on flicker discrimination in the rat. *J. Pharmacol. Exp. Ther.* 177:461–67
99. Wood, R. W. 1978. Stimulus properties of inhaled substances. *Environ. Health Perspect.* 26:69–76
100. Weiss, B., Laties, V. 1961. Changes in pain tolerance and other behavior pro-

duced by salicylates. *J. Pharmacol. Exp. Ther.* 131:120–29

101. Pryor, G. T., Dickinson, J., Rebert, C. S. 1983. Toluene-induced hearing loss in rats first exposed as weanlings or as young adults. *Toxicologist* 3:12 (Abstr.)

102. Davis, M. 1980. Neurochemical modulation of sensory motor reactivity: Acoustic and tactile startle reflexes. *Neurosci. Biobehav. Rev.* 4:241–63

103. Squibb, R. E., Tilson, H. A. 1982. Neurobehavioral changes in adult Fischer 344 rats exposed to dietary levels of chlordecone (Kepone): A 90-day chronic dosing study. *Neurotoxicology* 3:59–66

104. Tilson, H. A., Cabe, P. A. 1979. Studies on the neurobehavioral effects of polybrominated biphenyls in rats. *Ann. NY Acad. Sci.* 320:325–36

105. Fox, D. A., Overmann, S. R., Woolley, D. E. 1979. Neurobehavioral ontogeny of neonatally lead-exposed rats. II. Maximal electroshock seizures in developing and adult rats. *Neurotoxicology* 1:149–70

106. Dyer, R. S., Wonderlin, W. F., Walsh, T. J. 1982. Increased seizure susceptibility following trimethyltin administration in rats. *Neurobehav. Toxicol. Teratol.* 4:203–08

107. Mactutus, C. F., Unger, K., Tilson, H. A. 1982. Neonatal chlordecone exposure impairs early learning and memory in the rat on a multiple measure passive avoidance task. *Neurotoxicology* 3:27–44

108. Walsh, T. J., Miller, D. B., Dyer, R. S. 1982. Trimethyl tin, a selective limbic system neurotoxicant, impairs radial-arm maze performance. *Neurobehav. Toxicol. Teratol.* 4:177–84

109. Walsh, T. J., Tilson, H. A., Fisher, A., Hanin, I. 1983. AF64-A, a selective cholinergic neurotoxin, produces long-term learning and memory impairments. *Fed. Proc.* 41:755 (Abstr.)

110. Sobotka, T. J., Brodie, R. E., Cook, M. P. 1975. Psychophysiologic effects of early lead exposure. *Toxicology* 5:175–91

111. Ray, O. S., Barrett, R. J. 1975. Behavioral, pharmacological, and biochemical analysis of genetic differences in rats. *Behav. Biol.* 15:391–417

112. Vorhees, C. V. 1974. Some behavioral effects of maternal hypervitaminosis A in rats. *Teratology* 10:269–74

113. Vorhees, C. V., Brunner, R. L., McDaniel, C. R., Butcher, R. E. 1978. The relationship of gestational age to Vitamin A induced postnatal dysfunction. *Teratology* 17:271–76

114. Brady, K., Herrera, Y., Zenick, H. 1976. Influence of parental lead exposure on subsequent learning ability of offspring. *Pharmacol. Biochem. Behav.* 3:561–65

115. Zenick, R., Padick, Tokarek, T., Aragon, P. 1978. Influence of prenatal and postnatal lead exposure on discrimination learning in rats. *Pharmacol. Biochem. Behav.* 8:347–50

116. Olton, D. S., Becker, J. T., Handelman, G. E. 1979. Hippocampus, space, and memory. *Behav. Brain Sci.* 2:313–65

117. Olton, D. S., Becker, J. T., Handelman, G. E. 1980. Hippocampal function: Working memory or cognitive mapping. *Physiol. Psychol.* 8:239–46

118. Tilson, H. A., Squibb, R. E., Burne, T. A. 1982. Neurobehavioral effects following a single dose of chlordecone (Kepone) administered neonatally to rats. *Neurotoxicology,* 3:45–58

119. Premack, D., Kintsch, W. 1970. A description of free responding in the rat. *Learn Motiv.* 1:321–36

120. Mitchell, D., Beatty, E. T., Cox, P. K. 1977. Behavioral differences between two populations of wild rats: Implications for domestication research. *Behav. Biol.* 19:206–16

121. MacPhail, R. C. 1982. Studies on the flavor aversion induced by trialkyltin compounds. *Neurobehav. Toxicol. Teratol.* 4:225–30

122. Parker, L. A., Hutchison, S., Riley, A. 1982. Conditioned flavor aversions: A toxicity test of the anticholinesterase agent, physostigmine. *Neurobehav. Toxicol. Teratol.* 4:93–98

123. Silverman, A. P., Banham, P. B., Extance, K., Williams, H. 1981. Early change and adaptation in the social behaviour of rats given methylmercury in the diet. *Neurotoxicology* 2:269–81

124. Battig, K. 1976. Neurobiological and behavioral toxicity in animals. *Act. Nerv. Sup.* 18:270–74

125. Norton, S. 1982. Methods in behavioral toxicology. In *Principles and Methods of Toxicology,* ed. A. Hayes, pp. 353–73. New York: Raven

126. Lehrer, G. M. 1974. Measurement of minimal brain dysfunction. In *Behavioral Toxicology,* ed. C. Xintaras, C. Johnson, B. DeGroot, pp. 450–54. Washington, DC:USGPO

127. Reiter, L., Kidd, K. F., Gray, L. E., Chernoff, N. 1978. *The Use of Locomotor Activity Measurements as an Index of Toxicity: The Effects of Subacute Exposure to Kepone or Triethyl Tin.* Presented at US Workshop on Behavioral Toxicology, Sudzal, USSR

Ann. Rev. Pharmacol. Toxicol. 24:451–81

CYANIDE INTOXICATION AND ITS MECHANISM OF ANTAGONISM

James L. Way

Department of Medical Pharmacology and Toxicology, Texas A & M University College of Medicine, Medical Sciences Building, College Station, Texas 77843

INTRODUCTION

The biological studies on cyanide are unique in that they preceded the chemical preparation of the substance (1). The last comprehensive review on the pharmacology and toxicology of cyanide was written by Dr. Reid Hunt at Johns Hopkins University in 1923 (2); however, this review was written in German. Recently, other books and monographs on cyanide have appeared (3, 4). The present review is restricted to selected aspects of cyanide and is primarily concerned with a descriptive and interpretive appraisal of the status of cyanide intoxication and its mechanism of antagonism.

Cyanide has created complex problems for modern society and these problems have evolved not only from industrial pollution but, paradoxically, from an inadvertent attempt to resolve pollution problems (5). Its use as a suicidal, homicidal, chemical warfare, and genocidal agent is well known. Toxic problems have been associated with ingesting cyanide-containing foods, and occupational hazards have arisen as the industrial use of cyanide has increased. In medicine, it has created problems because some drugs with nitrile moieties liberate cyanide.

Much of the toxicological interest in cyanide has focused on its rapid lethal action; however, its most widely distributed toxicologic problems are due to its chronic toxicity from dietary, industrial, and environmental factors. Cyanide is not wholly a toxin synthesized by civilization, as it existed in prebiotic times and was involved in biogenesis. In addition, cyanide is produced by various organisms and plants in our environment and has a role in normal metabolism.

451

0362-1642/84/415-0451$02.00

DEDICATION

This review is in tribute to Dr. James Blake, the first American toxicologist (6, 7). James Blake and Claude Bernard were former students of François Magendie and both followed in the footsteps of their mentor in their continuing interest in elucidating the mechanism of action of cyanide. Dr. Blake was the first to demonstrate that the onset of cyanide action varied according to the route of administration. He also reported that the respiratory cessation produced by cyanide can be reversed by artificial respiration. Studies by Dr. Blake on cyanide were conducted at the University College in London. Subsequently he emigrated to the United States and continued his illustrious career in the development of a rational basis for the mechanism of intoxication of chemicals. It seems fitting that this review be dedicated to this pioneer for his contributions to toxicology in the United States. The history of cyanide has been reviewed elsewhere (8, 9).

POTENTIAL SOURCES OF CYANIDE INTOXICATION

Natural Causes

The release of hydrogen cyanide into our environment cannot be wholly related to human activity. A variety of natural sources release cyanide into the environment, and the contribution from these natural sources to overall human toxicity is difficult to evaluate. Prior to human habitation of this planet, hydrogen cyanide existed in higher concentrations in our atmosphere than it does presently; the basis for this statement is the existence of cyanide in the atmospheres of the sun and stars. Cyanide was one of the earliest polyatomic organic molecules detected in interstellar space (10, 11). It is one of the important precursors of the abiotic synthesis of essential biologic constituents such as amino acids, purines, and pyrimidines (12). Chemical emission investigation suggests that the original heteropolypeptides on earth may have been synthesized spontaneously from hydrogen cyanide and water without the involvement of amino acids as an intermediate (13). Other natural sources of cyanide are the various biologic organisms, such as bacteria, algae, fungi, and plants, that can form and excrete cyanide.

Various plants contain a high content of cyanogenic glycosides. The cyanide content can be high; some foods contain 100–8000 mg/kg of material. If the lethal dose of sodium cyanide in man is considered to be approximately 1 mg/kg, such high concentrations give reason for concern, because cyanide can predispose to various clinical diseases (14). Probably the most widely distributed major human food crop with a high content of cyanogenic glycosides is cassava or manioc (15, 16), one of the most important food crops in tropical countries. This food provides over 70% of the caloric intake in some diets.

Other foods also contain a high content of cyanogenic glycosides, e.g. fruit pits, sweet potato, corn, bamboo shoot, linseed, lima beans, and millet. Acute cyanide poisoning has occurred in the United States from the ingestion of almond-flavored milkshakes prepared from apricot kernels. Even in foods that do not normally contain cyanide, when hydrogen cyanide fumigation is used cyanide residue can persist in fumigated products for an extensive time period. In the United States, tolerances are set for hydrogen cyanide residue in various foods subjected to fumigation (17). However, because these various sources of cyanide are not generally recognized, the effect of low levels of cyanide on a long-term basis warrants concern.

Human-Related Causes

Cyanide wastes have contaminated our waterways and our drinking water. These wastes are produced by electroplating, the steel, aluminum, and paint industries, and certain mining operations. A series of litigations have been introduced in an attempt to control environmental contamination with cyanide. Regulation of the discharge of cyanide wastes into our waterways is included in the Federal Water Pollution Act (BL 92–500). The Environmental Protection Agency filed a Refuse Acts suit against the Armco Steel Company for the discharge of cyanide into the shipping channel in Houston, Texas, and successfully prosecuted this company (CA 70-H-1335). Presently there are other litigations pending against an aluminum company for allegedly contaminating the aquifer. Unlike in surface water, cyanide in the underground water table is not easily dissipated.

One of the sources of hydrogen cyanide in the air is the petrochemical industry. Recently, automobiles equipped with malfunctioning catalytic platinum converters have been reported by Bell Laboratory to produce hydrogen cyanide (18). Another source of hydrogen cyanide in the air is from home fires because of the increase in plastic contents in homes. Combustion of various plastics, such as polyurethane, liberates hydrogen cyanide upon pyrolysis (19). And lastly, one of the major sources for the inhalation of hydrogen cyanide affecting man is tobacco smoke. The use of low-tar, low-nicotine, or filter cigarettes does not reduce the hydrogen cyanide concentration in cigarette smoke.

Various drugs liberate cyanide to produce toxic signs and symptoms. For example, sodium nitroprusside is employed as a potent hypotensive agent in the management of hypertensive patients (20). This compound liberates significant quantities of cyanide to result in cyanide poisoning and deaths have occurred (21). Cyanide formation from sodium nitroprusside in rat liver mitochondrial preparations seems to require a reducing agent, such as ascorbic acid, reduced glutathione, and to a lesser extent NADH and NADPH (22). The decomposition of nitroprusside to liberate cyanide also has been reported to occur in blood by the interaction of nitroprusside ion with hemoglobin to yield cyanmethemoglobin and HCN (23). The reaction of hemoglobin with nitroprusside may be more complex than reported, as these workers were unable to establish stoichometry on the nitroprusside-hemoglobin reaction in even simple solutions, and questions have been raised with regard to the relative importance of the hemoglobin-nitroprusside interaction under in vivo conditions (24).

A cyanogenic glycoside, amygdalin (laetrile), has been used as an antineoplastic agent (25, 26) on the basis that it will be selectively hydrolyzed by a glucosidase to liberate cyanide, benzaldehyde, and sugar at the tumor site. The reports on this usage have been very controversial and have been refuted by various laboratories (27, 28). It has been proposed that tumor tissue is deficient in rhodanese to detoxify cyanide; therefore, it will be selectively attacked by cyanide, whereas normal cells contain a high concentration of rhodanese to detoxify cyanide, thereby preventing cell toxicity. This theory is rather simplistic and, furthermore, it is not substantiated by the facts. It has been reported that many tumor tissues are not selectively rich in β-glucosidase, nor do they contain a low concentration of rhodanese (27, 28). In addition, numerous studies indicate a lack of amygdalin antitumor activity in various model tumor systems (29–31).

Other agents shown to form cyanide include succinonitrile, which has been used as an antidepressant agent, and thiocyanate, an antithyroid agent (32). Thiocyanate can be oxidized to cyanide by peroxidase systems, but there is some controversy over whether the formation of cyanide from thiocyanate is real or an artifact. This controversy is normally trivial, since the amount of cyanide formed from thiocyanate is usually low in in vivo systems, so that the biologic significance of this reaction is minimal (33).

METHODOLOGY

In the assay of cyanide in body fluids, a number of factors need to be considered:

Tissue Selection and Storage

Cyanide is a reactive volatile nucleophile with a pKa of 9.2. This creates a variety of problems, as it can diffuse from tissue samples as well as bind to various components in the tissues. Tissue sampling techniques, storage, and cyanide analysis must be done with care if the results are to be reliable. Moreover, the organ distribution of cyanide varies considerably with the route of administration and the animal species injected (34, 35).

Which tissues to select for a toxicologic analysis of cyanide is controversial. Usually, whole blood is employed to analyze for cyanide concentration. This is considered to be the fluid of choice (36) in some laboratories. Other groups feel that cyanide content in whole blood has no apparent toxicologic significance (37) and yields invalid data because the analysis of cyanide in whole blood includes a large fraction of cyanide bound to a "biologically inactive form," cyanmethemoglobin. These latter groups probably are not cognizant of various factors. Studies between plasma, serum, and whole blood cyanide have been studied and the correlations between concentrations of cyanide in whole blood, serum, and plasma are quite consistent (34). Second, the concept of a stable, inert, inactive pool of cyanide is conceptionally erroneous. Not only is cyanide's mechanism of binding to red blood cells not clearly elucidated, but pharmacokinetic studies with cyanide and thiocyanate indicate that the blood cyanide concentration rapidly declines monoexponentially and is almost completely removed from blood within five minutes after intravenous injection (33, 38). Because the apparent volume of distribution of the compartment in which cyanide is converted to thiocyanate is in the central compartment and the initial rate of cyanide disappearance is very rapid, it appears likely that blood or tissue areas close to blood are necessary to explain blood cyanide biotransformation. Third, the advocates for the use of plasma rather than whole blood cyanide for analysis appear to base their opinions on the erroneous assumption that cyanide in plasma is free rather than bound, when in fact it has been shown that 60% of the cyanide in the plasma of the dog can be bound to plasma proteins (39). Fourth, cyanide has been found to attach more readily to serum albumin than to hemoglobin at neutral pH (40). Fifth, in small animal studies practicalities dictate the measurement of cyanide in whole blood samples. Finally, cyanide rapidly leaves serum and plasma, especially in the first 20 minutes (35). Although there is usually a good correlation between cyanide concentration in serum, plasma, and whole blood, on some occasions it may be worthwhile to measure cyanide both in whole blood and plasma, e.g. when the thiocyanate concentration is very high.

The other factors that influence analysis of cyanide are conditions of storage, duration, and temperature (41–43). Depending on the tissue to be analyzed, the delay of analysis can have considerable effect. For example, when cyanide is added to serum there is a rapid decrease in measurable cyanide concentration, and one hour after the addition of cyanide to serum the recovery is only one-third of the amount added, with the most rapid loss occurring during the first 20 minutes (44).

Detection and Estimation of Cyanide Concentration

There are a variety of sensitive methods for measuring cyanide in biological fluids. Most of these procedures are relatively convenient and sensitive, but each has its limitations. In most procedures, diffusion is used to trap the cyanide in the alkaline media prior to analysis. Care must be taken to ascertain that the presence of cyanide antidotes does not interfere with the cyanide analysis.

Probably the most frequently used colorimetric procedure is the oxidation of cyanide to a cyanogen, which is then interacted with a pyridine-pyrazolone mixture (45). The detection limit is approximately 0.004 μmole/ml. Sodium thiosulfate can interfere with the analysis of cyanide even after microdiffusion (45–47). The interfering material can be attributed to the conversion of sodium thiosulfate to polythionic acids upon sample acidification. The polythionates decompose to form sulfur dioxide and ultimately are diffused and trapped as sulfite (47). By using a buffered solution at pH 5.2 as the acidifying agent rather than sulfuric acid, it is possible to measure cyanide in the presence of sodium thiosulfate.

The potentiometric determination of cyanide using ion selective electrodes has become very popular, primarily because it is a convenient, rapid, and sensitive method of analysis (48). The more sensitive electrodes are those that contain a membrane of silver sulfide. Prior microdiffusion of biological samples containing cyanide is advisable to avoid interfering materials. Sodium thiosulfate also has been shown to interfere with the potentiometric analysis of cyanide due to an enhanced biotransformation of thiosulfate, particularly in the presence of blood, as this causes an artificially elevated cyanide concentration (49). The contaminant is sulfide, which can be removed by oxidation with hydrogen peroxide, and the excess hydrogen peroxide subsequently can be removed by sodium sulfite (49). It is important that the hydrogen peroxide be carefully removed, otherwise it will inactivate the ion selective electrode. With this method it is possible to measure samples in the range of 10^{-3}–10^{-6} M concentration range.

Spectrophotofluorometry is also a convenient, sensitive method for measuring cyanide in biological fluids, provided that prior microdiffusion is employed to isolate and concentrate the cyanide. Two fluorometric methods have been adapted to measuring cyanide in biologic fluids. One involves the catalytic conversion of pyridoxal to 4-pyridoxylactone (50, 51). Sodium thiosulfate interferes with the chemical conversion of this fluorophore. It is possible to circumvent this interference by using acetate buffer pH 5.2 as the acidifying agent. The mechanism for sodium thiosulfate interference is the formation of polythionic acids, as previously discussed; the sulfite anion then interacts with the aldehydic moiety. There are distinct advantages to the fluorometric method over the colorimetric method. The fluorometric method is more sensitive and requires fewer and more stable reagents than the colorimetric method. It should be pointed out that, in long-term preliminary studies, the apparent blood cyanide concentrations gradually increase more with 15% sulfuric acid as the acidifying agent than they do with pH 5.2 buffered solution containing sodium dodecylbenzylsulfate. The mechanism for this discrepancy has still not been elucidated (50). The primary disadvantage of the fluorometric method is its interference by extraneous fluorescent materials. Another fluorescent method with an advantage over pyridoxal uses para-benzoquinone (52, 53). The formation of these highly fluorescent cyanohydroquinone derivatives is not inhibited either by sulfite or by thiosulfate ion (52, 53). Approximately 0.001 μmole/ml of cyanide can be analyzed by this procedure. This fluorescent reaction (52, 53) adaptation to biologic methods (54) is a very sensitive, specific method; however, like many fluorometric methods, various small amounts of extraneous material in the laboratory can interfere with this determination.

The measurement of hydrogen cyanide directly by gas chromatography has been reported (55), but this method lacks sensitivity with most detectors. However, the use of chloramine-T to oxidize cyanide to cyanogen chloride for subsequent extraction with hexane has led to a sensitive, convenient method. The sensitivity of this method, which employs an electron capture detector and as little as 0.25 μg/ml, can be measured. Gas chromatographic techniques are not widely used for determining cyanide primarily because other methods are more convenient. However, the inherent sensitivity and selectivity of this method insure its application to specialized samples, particularly those requiring the differentiation of various cyanide species.

Cyanide also can be measured by indirect atomic absorption spectrometry. There are two methods: one procedure involves the formation of an insoluble metal cyanide compound; then the metal in the precipitate or the excess metal in the supernate is measured by atomic absorption spectrometry (56–58). In the other method, a relatively stable metal-cyanide complex is formed that is then extracted into an organic solvent and the metal content of the extract is determined. The sensitivity range for this type of determination is approximately 0.3–3.0 ppm. Indirect atomic absorption spectrophotometric method analyses are quite sensitive for measuring cyanide in biological fluids after prior preparation by microdiffusion. These methods are not widely used, probably because the method is indirect and because of the general adequacy and convenience of other methods.

TOXIC MANIFESTATIONS AND MECHANISM OF INTOXICATION

The toxic effect of cyanide has been attributed to its production of a histotoxic anoxia by the inhibition of cytochrome oxidase, the terminal oxidase of the mitochondrial respiratory chain (59–61). This is a reasonable assumption, because this enzyme occupies a critical position in cellular metabolism. With regard to the mechanism of lethal effects, it should be emphasized that cyanide poisoning very frequently is a massive poisoning, where the amount of cyanide greatly exceeds the minimal concentration necessary to inhibit cytochrome oxidase. In such intoxication many other enzymes and biological systems besides cytochrome oxidase probably are inhibited. A number of enzymes are equally or more sensitive to cyanide than cytochrome oxidase (62). Therefore, cyanide toxicity may not be a single biochemical lesion, but a complex effect on various enzyme systems involving Schiff base intermediates as well as metalloenzymes.

The mechanism of inhibition of cytochrome oxidase by cyanide is complicated, as this enzyme complex contains two heme A and two copper ions (63). The mechanism of cyanide inhibition has been studied intensively by various laboratories (64–66), and the reaction of this multimeric iron enzyme complex with cyanide has been found to involve a two-step reaction. The first step is the penetration of cyanide into a protein crevice, with initial binding of cyanide to the protein. The second step is the binding of the cyanide to the heme iron (66). Cyanide binds both to the oxidized and to the reduced form of the cytochrome oxidase. This toxic anion has a higher affinity for the oxidized form of the enzyme; however, it reacts more slowly with the oxidized form when compared with the reduced form. The cyanide probably reacts with the reduced form of cytochrome oxidase, which is subsequently oxidized to form the oxidized cyanide cytochrome oxidase complex. This latter complex is quite stable, but in the presence of reducing equivalents cyanide can readily dissociate from the enzyme inhibitor complex so that the cytochrome oxidase is reactivated (62).

There are enzymes that are more sensitive to cyanide than cytochrome oxidase. Two of these enzymes are nitrate reductase (67) and myoglobin (68). Some enzymes are almost as sensitive to cyanide as cytochrome oxidase, including horseradish peroxidase (69), yeast cytochrome c peroxidase (70), catalase (71), nitrite reductase (72), and ribulose diphosphate carboxylase (73). The basis for the inhibiting properties of cyanide may be attributed to its ability to complex with metals. Many of the enzymes sensitive to cyanide either contain molybdenum or iron. Other metalloenzymes that may be inhibited by cyanide are those that contain zinc or copper (62). Other mechanisms for cyanide inhibition may be attributed to chemical involvement between cyanide and a Schiff base intermediate, e.g. ribulose diphosphate carboxylase (73) and 2-keto-4-hydroxy glutarate aldolase (74), involving formation of a cyanohydrin intermediate.

Although extensive reports have been made on the effect of cyanide on cytochrome oxidase in in vitro systems, there is a paucity of information on the effect of cyanide on cytochrome oxidase in vivo (75–79). In vivo studies indicate that inhibition of cytochrome oxidase in various organs can occur. Brain cytochrome oxidase usually is measured, as the brain is one of the major target organs for cyanide. When the cyanide antidotes sodium nitrite and sodium thiosulfate were administered, no apparent inhibition of liver cytochrome oxidase activity occurred, even with a lethal dosage (77,

79). This observation may be due to various factors. The disposition of cyanide to sites of liver cytochrome oxidase localizations may be limited because of the high content and turnover number in the liver of rhodanese (80). Second, the cyanide-cytochrome oxidase multimeric complex may rapidly reactivate in the presence of rhodanese and sulfur donors due to cyanide biotransformation. Third, the physiological disposition of thiosulfate and nitrite-generated methemoglobin has a more limited distribution to brain than liver; this would result, therefore, in a higher sensitivity of brain tissue to cyanide, particularly since there is very little rhodanese in brain (77). These studies emphasize the importance of in vivo studies, as the data obtained in this way do not necessarily correlate with those found in in vitro biochemical studies.

A number of metabolic processes are known to be altered by cyanide in the intact animal and man. When cyanide inhibits cytochrome oxidase, this results in an alteration of a complex series of oxidative-reductive reactions in the cell; e.g. radiorespirometric studies using radioactive glucose (78) indicate that cyanide alters glucose catabolism, resulting in a 100% increase in the conversion of glucose by the pentose phosphate pathway, with a concomitant decrease in the breakdown of glucose by the glycolytic pathway (78). This shift from aerobic to anaerobic metabolism results in an increase in blood glucose and lactic acid, with a decrease in ATP/ADP ratio (75). The increased breakdown of glucose by the pentose phosphate pathway causes an increase in NADPH. This may represent a compensatory mechanism to maintain a balanced redox state, since an enhanced conversion of pyruvate to lactate is at the expense of NADH generated. In addition, cyanide causes an increase in phosphorylase activity as well as an increase in glucose production in the isolated perfused rat liver (81). Therefore, cyanide can alter carbohydrate metabolism, resulting in an increase in glycogenolysis and a shunting of glucose to the pentose phosphate pathway, by decreasing the rate of glycolysis and inhibiting the tricarboxylic acid cycle.

Physiologically, in cyanide intoxication one usually observes an initial hyperpnea followed by dyspnea and subsequently followed by convulsive seizures. Although cyanide is usually classified as a chemical producing a histotoxic anoxia, it probably also has an anoxic anoxia component. When a minimal lethal dose of cyanide is employed, the lethal effect is principally directed toward the central nervous system. At higher cyanide doses, cardiovascular signs occur. However, the brain is more sensitive to cyanide than the heart; in cases where a lethal dose has been administered, it has been frequently noted that the electrical activity of the brain has stopped and the heart is still beating. A considerable amount of information was available as early as 50 years ago on the in vivo physiological effects of cyanide (82–84). With regard to its effect on the chemoreceptors in the carotid body, cyanide promotes a slowing of the heart rate (85). Respiratory stimulation also can be promoted by cyanide by stimulation of the peripheral chemoreceptors (86). Cyanide causes an enhanced afferent discharge from the carotid chemoreceptors and this can be abolished with oxygen (87). Some of the more sensitive physiological parameters altered by cyanide are electrical changes in the heart (88) and brain (89), which can be partially inhibited with oxygen (90). Earlier studies on the ability of oxygen to reverse the effect of cyanide on EKG (88) could not be confirmed in subsequent studies (90). Additional studies have been made on the effect of cyanide on the cardiovascular system; these studies focused their major investigative efforts on the effects of cyanide on chemoreceptor reflexes and the effect of cyanide on the central nervous system (91–94).

A few correlations between electrical activity and cyanide can be made, e.g. in EEG tracings, the electrical changes produced by cyanide correlate with alterations in cellular energy. The administration of sodium cyanide can bring about a sudden loss of electrical activity, which is followed by a prolonged period of depressed abnormal wave amplitude (90). The role of oxygen in antagonizing electrical activity can be correlated with this ability to antagonize the lethal effects of cyanide. Small doses of cyanide have been reported to exert a direct effect on the activity of the respiratory neurons in the intact animal (95).

The pathologic changes that occur in cyanide poisoning vary with the dose, route, and duration of cyanide exposure (96). No specific pathological changes can clearly delineate cyanide intoxication. The most consistent lesion observed from cyanide poisoning is on the central nervous system. Studies in monkeys indicate lesions predominantly in the white matter and necrosis occur more frequently than demyelination (97–100). It seems that the white matter is the more sensitive tissue to cyanide, as lesions in rats were more apt to appear in the white matter at lower doses of cyanide. The cyanide encephalopathy lesions were attributed to the direct effect of a histotoxic anoxia and not to secondary changes due to neuronal dysfunction and edema. Pathologic changes also were observed to occur in the heart (101). The pathology observed in the myocardium was consistent with earlier studies (102) in man. Other lesions also were produced, presumably from cyanide. In tropical neuropathies, the pathologic findings reported that, when cassava is ingested as the major staple food (103), toxicity is manifested by demyelination, a decrease in conduction velocities of peripheral nerves, and changes in the auditory nerve.

Probably the more widely distributed adverse effects of cyanide are due to chronic toxicity. Chronic low-level exposure to cyanide produces various signs and symptoms that can loosely be called a chronic cyanide syndrome, which can be manifested in a variety of different forms. Since most of the evidence is epidemiological or based on field studies without controlled experimental conditions, it is difficult to assess precisely the contribution of cyanide to the clinical disease. Nevertheless, evidence is accumulating that is consistent with the presumption that cyanide intoxication is a major cause of various human diseases, although to say so is an oversimplification of a complex problem as there are other contributing factors. These disease entities may be due to high cyanide exposure, a depressed cyanide detoxification mechanism, various nutritional factors, or some combination of all these factors. Also, such abnormalities of detoxification may be ascribed either to inborn errors of metabolism or to a lack of substrate that can detoxify cyanide, which is secondary to the nutritional status.

Because of the widespread distribution of cyanide-containing sources and their implication as the etiology of various human diseases, this area of research is attracting a greater research effort. The involvement of cyanide in human diseases has been reviewed (104). Probably the best evidence of a human disease ascribed to cyanide is tobacco amblyopia. Visual abnormalities can be associated with a history of heavy smoking and a depletion of vitamin B_{12} (105). When this condition is treated with hydroxocobalamin, a cyanide antagonist, a reversal of the visual disturbance is observed (106) and plasma cyanocobalamin concentrations become elevated (107). Another clinical entity ascribed in part to cyanide exposure and a hereditary inborn error of metabolism is Leber's hereditary optic atrophy (108). When these individuals are exposed to a cyanide environment such as smoking, their plasma and urinary thiocyanate concentrations become lower than in normal individuals despite the fact that the enzymatic activity of liver rhodanese in the Leber's patients appears to be normal (109).

Probably the most widespread pathologic condition attributable to cyanide is tropical ataxic neuropathy associated with chronic cassava consumption. This is a diffuse degenerative neurological disease with peripheral and central signs. The signs and symptoms of this disease have been linked to cassava consumption and have been correlated with plasma thiocyanate concentrations (15, 16, 110, 111). Cassava is the major staple food in various tropical areas, and the plant has a high content of cyanogenic glycoside (linamarin). With continued ingestion over a period of time, tropical neuropathy gradually develops and the syndrome is characterized by optic atrophy, nerve deafness, and ataxia due to sensory spinal nerve involvement (112, 113). Other signs include scrotal dermatitis, stomatitis, and glossitis. In addition to dietary etiology, the cause of cyanide toxicity can be occupational, occurring in some industries when exposure to hydrogen cyanide is high (114, 115).

Experimental attempts have been made to show that cyanide is the etiological agent in human neuropathies (116, 117). Although these studies produced nerve lesions in rats similar to those observed in human disorders, it should be pointed out that the dosage required to produce damage in the rat was in the lethal range. In addition, in the rat the corpus callosum is more sensitive to cyanide than the optic nerve. This is quite different from human neuropathies, where the central nervous system involvement may result solely in optic disturbances. Lastly, with chronic cyanide ingestion, the thyroid may be affected due to enhanced formation of thiocyanate. The antithyroid properties of thiocyanate become manifest, and myxedema, thyroid goiter, and cretinism may occur (118).

CYANIDE ANTAGONISM

The antagonism of cyanide intoxication is an area that presently is receiving intensive investigation. However, most of the present concepts and basic classes of compounds were developed 50 to 150 years ago. Blake reported in 1840 that the lethal effects of cyanide can be antagonized by artificial respiration (6, 7). In 1888 it was reported that amyl nitrite was effective in antagonizing the lethal effects of cyanide (119), and by 1933 the use of sodium thiosulfate as the sulfur donor for rhodanese was described (120). This led to the studies by K. K. Chen employing a combination of amyl nitrite, sodium nitrite, and sodium thiosulfate as the antidote (121). Also, in 1894 cobalt was known to form a stable metal complex with cyanide and was used to antagonize cyanide (122).

In the last two decades a series of new cyanide antagonists have been developed. The protection afforded by these new antidotes would be of greater clinical interest if they could protect against the lethal effects of chemicals other than cyanide. Since a highly effective antidotal combination for cyanide is already available, the advantage of these new antidotes is relatively trivial. Since cyanide can act extremely rapidly, it is important to differentiate between the protective effects of these agents as an antidote for acute overdosage and as a prophylactic in chronic overdosage.

The cyanide antagonists are arbitrarily classified into compounds that metabolize or complex with cyanide and oxygen.

Biotransformation of Cyanide

Rhodanese initially was assumed to have a high substrate specificity for thiosulfate and to function solely to detoxify cyanide (120). Subsequently, this enzyme was found to catalyze a series of other reactions and has other biologic functions (123–126). Studies by two laboratories (121, 127) incorporated sodium thiosulfate into an antidotal combination to antagonize cyanide. Rhodanese is ideal from a toxicologic viewpoint, since the enzyme is present in large amounts (128), has a high turnover number, and catalyzes a reaction, at least with cyanide, that is essentially irreversible (129, 130). There is one limitation to the use of sodium thiosulfate as an antagonist: the selective distribution of the agonist (HCN) does not parallel that of the antagonist. Rhodanese is localized in the mitochondria, and the penetration of sodium thiosulfate to these sites is limited. In an attempt to reconcile these adverse disposition factors, crystalline rhodanese has been injected intravenously in combination with the sulfur donor to antagonize cyanide (131). In addition, various other sulfur donors have been employed (130).

During the past two decades, Westley and his associates have contributed much to our knowledge about the enzymic mechanism of the sulfurtransferases and their role in cyanide detoxication and other biologic functions (124–126, 132). The two sulfurtransferases that may play a role in the detoxification of cyanide are rhodanese and mercaptopyruvate sulfurtransferase. Although both sulfurtransferases can detoxify cyanide, the enzymic mechanism of the two reactions, the organ distribution, and the subcellular distribution of the enzymes are quite different. The basic reaction with rhodanese involves a transfer of a sulfane sulfur from the donor, thiosulfate, to the enzyme, forming a persulfide intermediate. Then the persulfide sulfur is transferred from the enzyme to the nucleophilic acceptor, in this case cyanide, to yield thiocyanate. Rhodanese does not have a high substrate specificity; there are many sulfur donors and other acceptors that can interact with rhodanese. The uniqueness of cyanide as a substrate is that this reaction is essentially irreversible, whereas with other nucleophilic acceptors the reactions are fully reversible. Westley and his associates have proposed a hypothesis that adds an intriguing perspective to the mechanism of cyanide detoxication and partially clarifies some of the puzzling features of the in vivo detoxification of cyanide with sodium thiosulfate. This detoxification reaction requires a source of sulfane sulfur, an ionized sulfur bonded to another sulfur, which reacts with cyanide, and there are various biological compounds that contain sulfane sulfur (132), e.g. thiosulfate, polythionates, thiosulfonates, persulfides, and elemental sulfur in the form of staggered-8 member rings (133). These sulfane-containing compounds in the presence of rhodanese rapidly equilibrate in the intact animal to form a sulfane pool that can react with cyanide. Sulfane sulfur may be derived from cysteine by mercaptopyruvate, which can then react with its sulfurtransferase. It should be emphasized that rhodanese not only can catalyze sulfane transfer to cyanide, but it also can interconvert these various forms of sulfanes. The sulfane carrier was postulated to be albumin because radioactive studies with sodium thiosulfate (133, 134) indicate that serum albumin interacts with elemental sulfur as it does with so many other hydrophobic biological substances. Moreover, this serum albumin sulfane sulfur carrier complex is in a form that can react with cyanide.

In summary, the proposal by Westley and associates implicates a serum albumin-sulfane carrier complex as playing a major role in cyanide detoxication mechanism operating in vivo. This proposal does not alter the importance of rhodanese in cyanide sulfur metabolism, but it does place it in a different perspective. Based on substantial experimental evidence, it infers that the action of sodium thiosulfate in antagonizing cyanide intoxication may also occur by an additional and alternative mechanism. The proposal is as follows: the source of the sulfane sulfur is derived from mercaptopyruvate via the mercaptopyruvate sulfurtransferase. The various forms of sulfane are then interconverted by rhodanese. The sulfane carrier that transports the sulfur formed in the liver and possibly other organs is serum albumin; the sulfane sulfur albumin complex is then reacted with cyanide.

This intriguing proposal warrants serious consideration because of the strength of the in vitro data and its conceptual importance to toxicologic mechanisms. The quantity of serum albumin and the rate constant for cyanolysis are consistent with the sulfur albumin complex for cyanide detoxication from the sulfane pool. Some preliminary in vivo data (33, 135) may be consistent with this proposal. Pharmacokinetic studies with cyanide and thiosulfate indicate that the conversion of cyanide to thiocyanate is predominantly in the central compartment, with a volume of distribution approximating that of the blood volume. The reaction rate is extremely fast and is consistent with the in vitro data by interaction with some of the sulfur albumin complex. An argument against this hypothesis is the fact that the cytochemical localization of rhodanese is perivascular (136). This infers that cyanide in blood is in close proximity to rhodanese. Also, a mechanism that transports thiosulfate in the rat liver mitochondria has been described (137).

Chemical Binding of Cyanide

NITRITES   The efficacy of amyl nitrite in protecting against cyanide poisoning in dogs was first reported in 1888 (119). This research went unnoticed, as it was published in a relatively obscure journal. However, when it was observed that cyanide interacts with methemoglobin to form cyanmethemoglobin and that methemoglobin reactivates cyanide-inhibited cytochrome oxidase, nitrite was utilized as an antidote against cyanide poisoning (121, 127). The basis for the antagonism of cyanide with the nitrites was biochemically sound (138). Cyanide has a low affinity for hemoglobin but a high affinity for methemoglobin. Nitrite generates methemoglobin, which then combines with cyanide to form cyanmethemoglobin.

The first nitrite employed to antagonize cyanide intoxication was amyl nitrite (119, 139), and subsequently sodium nitrite was used (121), the rationale being that, since therapy must be rapid, amyl nitrite could be inhaled while sodium nitrite was being prepared for intravenous administration. The efficacy of amyl nitrite in antagonizing cyanide intoxication has been questioned (140). The development of the rapid methemoglobin formers was prompted by various laboratories (140–143), which reported the limitations of using the nitrites in cyanide intoxication mainly because of the relatively slow rate of methemoglobin formation (92, 141). Subsequently, a series of investigations (140–143) led to the development of 4-dimethylaminophenol, DMAP, as the agent of choice.

It should be pointed out that methemoglobin can reactivate cyanide-inhibited cytochrome oxidase (75, 144). Although DMAP has many proponents because of its rapid rate of methemoglobin formation, other laboratories still indicate the efficacy of sodium nitrite as a cyanide antagonist over other methemoglobin formers and relate its superior efficacy to the more prolonged methemoglobenemia after sodium nitrite (145, 146). The mechanism for the enhanced protection of $NaNO_2$ over other methemoglobin formers is that, in the more rapid methemoglobin formers, mice were able to survive the initial acute cyanide challenge; however, they subsequently succumbed to the cyanide released rapidly from the cyanmethemoglobin pool. Also, the mechanism for the prolonged methemoglobinemia after sodium nitrite in mice and the greater cyanide protection afforded was attributed to a possible inhibition of methemoglobin reductase (146).

A discussion of methemoglobin formers and cyanide antagonists would not be complete without some reference to methylene blue, because misinformation still persists that methylene blue is an effective methemoglobin former and therefore an efficacious cyanide antagonist (147). Methylene blue is not an effective antidote (120), as it is a poor methemoglobin former (148–151).

The early rationale for the use of methemoglobin formers in cyanide antagonism was reasonable (152), particularly since sodium nitrite did protect against cyanide intoxication and methemoglobin formation did occur. Consequently, this mechanism has gone unquestioned for the past half century. Conceptually, this factor prompted the development of more rapid methemoglobin formers. However, the role of methemoglobin formation by nitrite should have been questioned, because the antidotal effect of nitrite is very rapid, whereas nitrite-generated methemoglobin formation is relatively slow. In low methemoglobin concentrations, the efficacy of nitrite in antagonizing cyanide is minimal (153, 154).

Recent studies suggest that methemoglobin formation by sodium nitrite may play a minimal, if any, role in the *therapeutic* antagonism of cyanide poisoning (153, 154). Moreover, sodium nitrite and sodium thiosulfate either alone or in combination are equally effective whether administered prophylactically or antidotally (155, 156). These studies prompted the consideration of alternative mechanisms for cyanide antagonism other than nitrite generation of methemoglobin formation. When methemoglobinemia was prevented by methylene blue pretreatment, sodium nitrite still protected efficaciously against cyanide poisoning (153, 154). These investigations infer that prophylactic studies under laboratory conditions, where sodium nitrite is given *prior* to cyanide to attempt to show maximal protective effect at maximal methemoglobin formation, methemoglobin does play a role in antagonizing the lethal effects of cyanide. However, this would not occur in cyanide poisoning if sodium nitrite was given *after* cyanide poisoning, as would normally occur. Under the latter conditions, the mechanism of action of sodium nitrite is due to some mechanism other than methemoglobin formation. This has important conceptual and practical implications for, if sodium nitrite is exerting its effect by a mechanism other than methemoglobin formation, this provides an opportunity for the development of a new class of cyanide antagonists. This area presently is being intensely investigated by various laboratories. The first logical alternative is to study the other known pharmacological properties of nitrites. Because nitrites are potent vasodilators, attention has focused on the vasogenic properties of various drugs as potential cyanide antagonists.

Investigation of vasogenic compounds as cyanide antagonists actually was initiated with chlorpromazine. Chlorpromazine has been reported to antagonize cyanide intoxication (157, 158) and the mechanism of this antagonism was attributed to the hypothermic properties of chlorpromazine (158), as various drugs protect against anoxia by lowering body temperatures (159). The protective effect of chlorpromazine could not be confirmed, either alone or with sodium nitrite (160); however, when chlorpromazine was administered with sodium thiosulfate, there was a striking potentiation against the lethal effects of cyanide. The mechanism of chlorpromazine in the antagonism of cyanide intoxication was found to be unrelated to hypothermia. The ability of chlorpromazine to antagonize cyanide in the presence of sodium thiosulfate was reversed by an α agonist, methoxamine (161, 162). This prompted the investigation of α blockade as a mechanism of cyanide antagonism. The α adrenergic blocking agent phenoxybenzamine subsequently was found to have almost identical properties to chlorpromazine as a cyanide antagonist. Similar to chlorpromazine, phenoxybenzamine possesses no antidotal property either alone or in combination with sodium nitrite; however, a striking potentiation was noted with sodium thiosulfate and to a lesser extent when it was added to the nitrite-thiosulfate combination. In addition, the antidotal effect of phenoxybenzamine, like that of chlorpromazine, can be reversed with methoxamine (161, 162). Subsequently, a series of different classes of vasogenic agents were examined against the lethal effects of cyanide in combination with sodium thiosulfate and/or sodium nitrite. Of all the vasodilators, only the ganglionic blocking agents and other α adrenergic blockers were observed to exhibit an antidotal effect. This includes examination of almost all classes of autonomic drugs, vasodilators such as papaverine, organic nitrates, and antihistaminic compounds. The reason why sodium nitrite but not other vasodilators should protect against the lethal effect of cyanide has still not been clearly elucidated, as methoxamine can reverse the antidotal effect of phenoxybenzamine but not that of sodium nitrite (161, 162).

COBALT COMPOUNDS   Cobalt ion is known to form a stable metal complex with cyanide and has been used in the treatment of cyanide poisoning (122,

163); however, the use of cobalt as a cyanide antidote has not received general support mainly because of the toxicity of cobalt ion. About a half century after their first use, interest in cobalt compounds was renewed when hydroxocobalamin was reported to antagonize the lethal effects of cyanide (164). A variety of cobalt-containing compounds have been tested against the lethal effects of cyanide, including hydroxocobalamin (164–167), cobalt histidine (168–170), cobalt chloride (171–173), and dicobalt ethylenediaminetetraacetic acid (Co_2 EDTA) (174–176). The use of cobalt-EDTA has been successful in treating cyanide poisoning in experimental and in clinical situations (174–178). Its use is based on the fact that cobalt ions form a stable complex with cyanide (179). More importantly, it was reported that the presence of the cobalt ion can reactivate the cyanide-inhibited cytochrome oxidase (180). This is an important observation, because cobalt itself can inhibit heme biosynthesis. The selection of cobalt-EDTA as the preferred cobalt compound is reasonable, since it was hoped that many of the toxic effects of cobalt ion could be minimized by administering this compound as a chelate. Whether the EDTA complex appreciably reduces the toxicity of cobalt is an area of controversy that has not been resolved. Also, since cobalt reacts directly with cyanide, this reaction should be quite rapid. It was believed that cobalt EDTA would have a distinct advantage as a cyanide antagonist over sodium nitrite, because of the relatively slow rate of methemoglobin generation by the nitrites.

CYANOHYDRIN FORMATION   Cyanide is a nucleophile known to interact with various carbonyl groups to form cyanohydrin intermediates. Sodium pyruvate was found to rapidly reverse the cyanide-inhibited respiration of the Ehrlich ascites tumor cells (181) and to antagonize the lethal effects of cyanide in mice (182). These relatively limited protective effects of sodium pyruvate alone were subsequently confirmed (183) and extended to detailed drug antagonism of cyanide in mice. The rationale for investigating sodium pyruvate is that it has many apparent theoretical advantages over other cyanide antagonists, i.e. sodium nitrite. Cyanide reacts directly with pyruvate to form a cyanohydrin derivative. Also, pyruvate is more apt to distribute to sites of cyanide localization, as there is a specific carrier for the active transport of pyruvate (183). However, sodium pyruvate is not as efficacious as sodium nitrite and does not enhance the protective effect of nitrite against the lethal effects of cyanide, but it does potentiate the antidotal effect of sodium thiosulfate. The addition of sodium pyruvate to the nitrite-thiosulfate antidotal combination further enhances the protective effect against cyanide. The value of sodium pyruvate as a potential cyanide antagonist is that it provides a different approach to the development of cyanide antidotes, an approach which is now being intensively investigated. As a possible supplement to the nitrite-thiosulfate combination, it provides a reason for decreasing the dose of sodium nitrite, as this antagonist has caused fatalities in susceptible individuals. In addition, no convulsions from cyanide were observed when sodium pyruvate was present (183). Sodium pyruvate or its analogs also has potential advantage over cobalt-EDTA employed clinically, in that it is less toxic and therefore a greater dose can be tolerated. This is of considerable importance when one calculates the ratio of antagonist to agonist.

Oxygen

Cyanide inhibits cytochrome oxidase (59, 60, 61), but if this were the sole mechanism of cyanide lethality there would be no rational basis for employing oxygen to treat cyanide intoxication. Furthermore, the substrate requirement of cytochrome oxidase requires an oxygen tension of only 70 mm Hg for maximal enzymatic activity (184). Nevertheless, oxygen has been advocated for the treatment of cyanide poisoning for many years. Unfortunately, in many of those studies the experimental designs were incomplete; consequently, the results obtained were not very convincing. None of these studies with oxygen were evaluated in combination with other known cyanide antagonists, e.g. sodium nitrite and/or sodium thiosulfate. It is only under these conditions that the striking protective effect of oxygen is realized, as oxygen potentiates the action of the nitrite-thiosulfate combination. Various reports have indicated that oxygen alone under atmospheric (185–188) or hyperbaric (89, 189, 190) conditions is beneficial in treating cyanide poisoning. Also, it was reported that oxygen can reverse the abnormalities of EKG and/or EEG tracings produced by cyanide (89, 90, 188, 189) and that hyperbaric oxygen can protect against the lethal effects of cyanide in mice (89, 189). Most of the early recommendations for the use of oxygen were as an adjunct rather than as an integral part of the treatment of cyanide poisoning. Oxygen alone has only minimal effects and enhances the protective effect of sodium thiosulfate to only a minor degree and does not do so at all for sodium nitrite, but it strikingly potentiates the effectiveness of the combination of sodium nitrite and sodium thiosulfate (90, 155, 191, 192). These studies have been confirmed in sheep (193) and by another laboratory using rats (194). Increased protection was observed as the oxygen concentration was increased from 20% to 100% (156), and no further increase in protection was noted with hyperbaric oxygen (4 ATA) (195). This protective effect of oxygen was observed not only prophylactically (90, 155, 191, 192, 195) but also therapeutically, after the signs and symptoms of cyanide poisoning were fully manifested (156, 193, 196).

It is important to recognize that oxygen at 1 ATA and 4 ATA can affect tissue metabolism. For example, it has been reported that α-ketoglutarate utilization from brain homogenate is inhibited within 20 minutes after oxygen administration (197) and changes in the concentration of glycolytic intermediates occur (198). In addition, biochemical lesions can be produced with hyperbaric oxygen with little evidence of toxicity under macroscopic or microscopic examination (199). These metabolic inhibitory effects of oxygen may provide a basis for the apparent great efficacy of oxygen as a cyanide antagonist.

One report indicates that oxygen did not enhance the protective effect against cyanide poisoning when pretreated with sodium thiosulfate (200), but the studies on which it is based suffer from inadequate experimental design and their conceptual basis may be questioned. A single dose of cyanide and a single dose of sodium thiosulfate were employed and percents survival were measured. As was indicated earlier, if adequate studies are to be conducted, a dose-response relationship should be established, particularly with cyanide, as the slope of the dose-response curve is quite steep. Second, if the efficacy of oxygen as a cyanide antagonist is to be evaluated, it would be reasonable to employ oxygen with the nitrite-thiosulfate combination rather than thiosulfate alone in order to see the most striking potentiation. Third, just because sodium thiosulfate or the nitrite-thiosulfate combination is enhanced by oxygen, this does not necessarily infer that the effect of oxygen is acting directly on sodium thiosulfate or the rhodanese enzyme, as the enzymatic conversion of cyanide to thiocyanate in the presence of rhodanese can occur without oxygen. Oxygen may be exerting its effect on alternative metabolic events unrelated to the rhodanese reaction.

Various physiologic effects of cyanide can be reversed with oxygen, as has already been discussed. Also, cyanide-induced encephalopathy has been described and oxygen has been reported to minimize these brain lesions (201). Studies on the effect of oxygen in altering the physiological action of cyanide were conducted in an attempt to elicit the effect of oxygen in combination with the classical cyanide antidotes under these conditions (90). Of all the physiological parameters measured, only the EEG was consistently sensitive enough to elicit differences between air and oxygen in dogs. Oxygen shortened the electrical silence produced by cyanide either alone, in combination with thiosulfate, or with the nitrite-thiosulfate combination, but not with sodium nitrite alone (90). In contrast, the protective effect of oxygen in preventing or reversing the EKG effects (188) and the respiratory changes (188) of cyanide (90) were not confirmed. The inability to confirm these changes probably reflects the higher dose of sodium cyanide employed.

Differences in biochemical parameters between air and oxygen also could be observed in vivo (76, 79). Inhibition in cytochrome oxidase activity was restored more rapidly in liver than in brain (77). Also, reactivation of cytochrome oxidase occurs more rapidly in oxygen than in air (79). In animals pretreated with nitrite-thiosulfate, brain but not liver cytochrome oxidase was inhibited by a lethal dose of cyanide (77). The mechanism for this surprising observation has not been elucidated. A dose-dependent cyanide inhibition of both brain and liver cytochrome oxidase was established, and oxygen shifted the dose-response curve to the right (79). Oxygen and air-treated animals displayed the same degree of cytochrome oxidase inhibition during the initial response to cyanide; however, the animals receiving air but not oxygen exhibited signs of cyanide intoxication (79). This suggests that the signs of cyanide intoxication do not parallel cytochrome oxidase inhibition and the appearance and disappearance of these effects are not necessarily dose-dependent (79). However, these differences between oxygen and air may be dose-related in certain physiologic changes that are induced by low cyanide concentration or that are sensitive to oxygen (188, 202–204), whereas neither oxygen nor air alters the physiologic changes induced by higher cyanide doses (90). Exposure to sublethal doses of cyanide can divert changes in carbohydrate intermediary metabolism to pathways that are less sensitive to cyanide (78). Further substantiation of the effect of oxygen in potentiating the protective effect against cyanide intoxication can be elicited in radiorespirometric studies in mice using radioactive glucose. Oxygen, but not air, when administered in combination with the nitrite-thiosulfate antidotal combination (205a), can completely reactivate glucose metabolism inhibited by cyanide. The rationale for these findings is that anoxic tissues induced by cyanide inactivation of cytochrome oxidase results in a shift from aerobic to anaerobic metabolism accompanied by a concomitant decreased production of carbon dioxide. Therefore, monitoring the respiratory excretion of carbon dioxide after the administration of uniformly labeled glucose appears to give a rough indication of the degree of metabolic inhibition produced by cyanide. The mechanism for the action of oxygen in reversing cyanide-inhibited glucose oxidation has not been elucidated (205a). Last, the disposition of cyanide does not appear to be a factor in eliciting the differences observed between air and oxygen (205). Although small differences were observed in the respiratory excretion of cyanide, actually this plays only a minor role, as only 4% of cyanide is excreted by the respiratory route. No differences were noted with regard to the urinary excretion or total body retention of sodium cyanide between air and oxygen. In summary, although oxygen can be established as a cyanide antagonist, the mechanism of action for its antidotal effect has not been elucidated.

TREATMENT

There are numerous effective cyanide antagonists; therefore, there is no unanimity of opinion on which is the most effective regimen. This is not surprising, as different experimental conditions and species of animals have been employed in testing the efficacies of different antidotes. Moreover, cyanide poisoning occurs with such frequency that the "successful" treatment of cyanide intoxication by a variety of methods has been reported.

Supportive Treatment

Because there are numerous specific antidotes for the treatment of cyanide poisoning, the importance of general supportive treatment is frequently overlooked. Although numerous reports on the signs and symptoms of cyanide poisoning exist, the fact remains that, in the absence of a suitable history, the diagnosis of cyanide poisoning is difficult. Blake (6, 7) indicated that artificial respiration is effective in protecting against cyanide poisoning. The value of general supportive treatment is particularly emphasized in one case report of a single incidence of a man ingesting potassium cyanide (206). Since the diagnosis of cyanide poisoning was not established, the only treatment employed was supportive. This study represents a rare, well-documented clinical study on cyanide poisoning in man that was successfully treated symptomatically. The dose of cyanide was established at 600 mg, and the blood level cyanide was reported to be 2.0 μg/ml 12 hours after admission to the hospital. The main emphasis is that even though effective antidotes are available, the general supportive treatment of any poisoning should not be ignored. This may be life-saving, particularly when the diagnosis of cyanide poisoning has not been documented.

Methemoglobin-Sulfur Sulfanes-Oxygen

The nitrite-thiosulfate antidotal combination is still one of the most effective treatments of cyanide poisoning, even though the specific mechanism of action of sodium nitrite and sodium thiosulfate are now being questioned.

The present dosage regimen of sodium nitrite-sodium thiosulfate combination recommended for humans still should be used with caution, as nitrite toxicity can occur. The administration of this antidotal combination, especially to children, must be done with caution (207). Presently, it is recommended that children weighing under 25 kg should be given an adjusted dose of sodium nitrite, as the usual dose is potentially lethal (207).

In veterinary practice, the proprietary mixture of sodium thiosulfate and sodium nitrite used to counteract cyanide poisoning can be vastly improved. These proprietary mixtures can protect against 6 LD_{50} doses of sodium cyanide; however, with adjustment of the dosage, it has been possible to raise the protection to 18 LD_{50} doses of sodium cyanide. These studies were conducted in sheep, as they are the range animal most apt to be poisoned by cyanide (171, 193).

The experience with the use of sodium nitrite and sodium thiosulfate as an antidotal combination in the treatment of cyanide poisoning and in clinical cases of intoxication has been summarized for humans in medical practice (207, 208) and for animals in veterinary practice (171, 193, 209). Oxygen should be employed in combination with sodium nitrite and sodium thiosulfate, as there appears to be no hazard in the use of oxygen and the procedure could be lifesaving. Its use in cyanide poisoning as a routine measure appears to be reasonable.

Objections to the nitrite-thiosulfate antidotal combination relate to the "slow onset of action" of nitrite and the purported surprisingly slow detoxifying capacity of thiosulfate (210). Conclusions on the slow onset of action of nitrite were based primarily on the rate of methemoglobin formation (142, 143). The validity of these analyses already has been addressed. Some researchers have indicated that these measurements may not necessarily be the most reliable parameters in assessing the therapeutic efficacy of the antidotal potential against the lethal effects of cyanide (90, 153, 154). Others advocate the use of DMAP in place of sodium nitrite, since it is a more rapid methemoglobin former (142, 143). Whether or not DMAP and thiosulfate provide more protection against the lethal effects of cyanide than nitrite and thiosulfate remains to be established.

Cobalt

Cobalt did not receive widespread acceptance as a cyanide antagonist, primarily because of its cardiac toxicity, until hydroxocobalamin (164) and subsequently cobalt EDTA were introduced (166, 174, 175, 210). Whether the two latter compounds have appreciably lowered toxicity on a molar basis is still an open question. Cobalt has been implicated as a contributory etiological factor in producing cardiomyopathy among heavy beer drinkers (211–214) because cobalt formerly was used as a beer additive. This was manifested by cardiac arrhythmias of both auricular and ventricular origin. This is of considerable concern, for when cobalt EDTA was employed in the treatment of cyanide intoxication, severe cardiac toxicity was observed and the most serious signs were related to ventricular arrhythmias (178, 215, 216). This finding places rather severe reservations on the use of cobalt EDTA in the treatment of cyanide poisoning.

Other studies also raise the question of whether sodium thiosulfate should be employed with cobalt EDTA or hydroxocobalamin, as sodium thiosulfate sharply enhances the antidotal effect of cobalt (170, 173, 210). The proprietary solution of cobalt EDTA is usually employed alone and contains no sulfane sulfur. Various laboratories in France and Germany have suggested that cobalt EDTA be employed as one of the cyanide antagonists, with the implication that a cobalt chelate or an aminophenol derivative (DMAP) in combination with sodium thiosulfate might replace the classic antidotal nitrite-thiosulfate combination.

It is important to note a species specificity with regard to susceptibility to cobalt. Whereas cobalt-thiosulfate combinations were much more effective than the nitrite-thiosulfate in mice (173), tolerance to cobalt salts were much lower in sheep (171, 193). It should be emphasized that cobalt exerts its antidotal effect primarily by combining directly with the cyanide ion; therefore, its action is dependent on the molar ratio of cobalt to cyanide. When the dose of cobalt was adjusted to a level that could be tolerated in sheep and the cobalt-thiosulfate combination then was administered to mice, it was found that the cobalt-thiosulfate combination was not as efficacious as before and the nitrite-thiosulfate antidotal combination was far superior in both mice and sheep (171, 173, 193). It should be emphasized that, unlike the addition of oxygen to the nitrite-thiosulfate antidotal combination, the addition of cobalt compounds as a cyanide antagonist may involve a substantial hazard. Even though cobalt can be lifesaving, a careful study of the toxicity of cobalt is essential, as its use under clinical conditions in cyanide poisoning may lead to severe cardiac toxicity (178, 215, 216).

The general assessment of the treatment of cyanide poisoning is blessed with a variety of antidotes that are very effective against the lethal effects of cyanide. For this reason there have been considerable differences of opinion with regard to the treatment of cyanide poisoning. The classic nitrite-thiosulfate treatment of cyanide poisoning developed 50 years ago is still one of the antidotal combinations of choice, particularly if it is employed with oxygen. Questions have been raised about the slow onset of action of sodium nitrite and methemoglobin formation and whether a more rapid methemoglobin former should be employed, i.e. dimethylaminophenol (DMAP). Whether DMAP is more effective than sodium nitrite in combination with sodium thiosulfate is still open to question, even though DMAP forms methemoglobin much more rapidly than sodium nitrite. Proponents for the use of cobalt-containing compounds such as hydroxocobalamin or cobalt EDTA, which are widely used in the United Kingdom, the Scandinavian countries, and Europe, stress the rapidity of action, since cobalt reacts directly with cyanide to form a stable complex in contrast to antidotes that act in an indirect manner and are dependent on the generation of methemoglobin. Concerns have been expressed with regard to the cardiac toxicity of these cobalt compounds, and some reservations about the use of cobalt exist for this reason.

In conclusion, there are a series of very effective cyanide antagonists that have been incorporated into the treatment of cyanide poisoning. There are some reservations with some of the cyanide antagonists and it is anticipated that more effective, safer cyanide antidotal combinations will be forthcoming, particularly since there is now a better basis for the experimental design of these antagonists.

ACKNOWLEDGMENT

Support for writing this review was derived from the National Institutes of Environmental Health Sciences, the National Science Foundation, and the US Army Medical Research and Development Command.

Literature Cited

1. Scheele, C. W. 1782. Försök beträffande det fargande ämnet i Berlinerblå. *Kongl Vetenskaps-Acad Handl* 3:264–75
2. Hunt, R. 1923. Cyanwasserstoff, Nitrilglukoside, Nitrile, Rhodanwasserstoff, Isocyanide. *Handbook Exp. Pharm.* 1:702–832
3. Way, J. L. 1978. Environmental assessment of cyanide. In *Reviews of the Environmental Effects of Pollutants. V: Cyanide*, ed. L. E. Towill, J. S. Drury, E. B. Whitfield, E. L. Galyan, A. S. Hammons, EPA-600/1–78–027, pp. 177–90. Washington, DC: US Government Printing Office
4. Vennesland, B., Conn, E. E., Knowles, C. J., Westley, J., Wissing, F. 1982. *Cyanide in Biology*. London: Academic. 548 pp.
5. Voorhoeve, R. J. H., Patel, C. K. N., Trimble, L. E., Kerl, R. J. 1975. Hydrogen cyanide production during reduction of nitric oxide over platinum catalysts. *Science* 190:149–51
6. Blake, J. 1839. Observations on the physiological effects of various agents introduced into the circulation as indicated by the hemodynamometer. *Edin. Med. Surg. J.* 51:330–45
7. Blake, J. 1840. Observations and experiments on the mode in which various poisonous agents act on the animal body. *Edin. Med. Surg. J.* 53:35–49
8. Earles, M. P. 1967. The introduction of hydrocyanic acid into medicine. A study in the history of clinical pharmacology. *Med. Hist.* 11:305–13
9. Sykes, A. H. 1982. Early studies on the toxicology of cyanide. See Ref. 4, pp. 1–9
10. Oro', J. 1972. Extraterrestrial organic analysis. *Space Life Sci.* 3:507–50
11. Oro', J., Rewers, K., Odom, D. 1982. Criteria for the emergence and evolution of life in the solar system. *Orig. Life* 12:285–305
12. Wolman, Y. 1972. Nonprotein amino acids from spark discharges and their comparison with the Murchison meteorite amino acids. *Proc. Natl. Acad. Sci. USA* 69:809–11
13. Nooner, D. W., Sherwood, E., More, M. A., Oro', J. 1977. Cyanamide mediated syntheses under plausible primitive earth conditions. Synthesis of peptides. *J. Mol. Evol.* 10:211–20
14. Levine, S. 1967. Experimental cyanide encephalopathy: Gradients of susceptibility in the corpus callosum. *J. Neuropath. Exp. Neurol.* 26:214–22

15. Osuntokun, B. O. 1980. A degenerative neuropathy with blindness and chronic cyanide intoxication of dietary origin. The evidence in Nigerians. In *Toxicology in the Tropics*, ed. R. L. Smith, E. A. Bababunmi, pp. 16–79. London: Taylor & Francis
16. Osuntokun, B. O., Monekosso, G. L., Wilson, J. 1969. Relationship of a degenerative tropical neuropathy to diet, report of a field study. *Br. Med. J.* 1:547–50
17. US Environmental Protection Agency. 1969. *EPA Compendium of Registered Pesticides III*, pp. 1–211. Washington DC: EPA
18. Voorhoeve, R. J. H., Patel, C. K. N., Trimble, L. E., Kerl, R. J. 1978. Hydrogen cyanide production during reduction of nitric oxide over platinum catalysts. *J. Cataly.* 54:102–5
19. Jellinek, H. A. G., Takata, K. 1977. Toxic gas evolution from polymers: Evolution of hydrogen cyanide from polyurethanes. *J. Polymer Sci.* 15:2269–88
20. Page, I. H., Corcoran, A. C., Dustan, H. P., Koppanyi, T. 1955. Cardiovascular action of sodium nitroprusside in animals and hypertensive patients. *Circulation* 11:188–98
21. Davis, D. W., Griess, L., Kadar, D., Stewart, D. J. 1975. A sudden death associated with the use of sodium nitroprusside for induction of hypotension during anaesthesia. *Can. Anaesth. Soc. J.* 22:547–52
22. Nakamura, S., Shin, T., Hirokata, U., Shigematsu, A. 1977. Inhibition of mitochondrial respiration by sodium nitroprusside and the mechanism of cyanide. *Br. J. Anaesth.* 49:1239–44
23. Smith, R. P., Kruszyna, H. 1974. Nitroprusside produces cyanide poisoning via a reaction with hemoglobin. *J. Pharmacol. Exp. Ther.* 191:557–63
24. Vesey, C. J., Cole, P. V., Simpson, P. J. 1977. Nitroprusside and cyanide. *Br. J. Anaesth.* 49:395
25. Marrone, J. A. 1962. Chemotherapy of inoperable cancer. *Exp. Med. Surg.* 20:279–308
26. Krebs, E. T. 1970. The nitrilosides (vitamin B_{17}): Their nature, occurrence and metabolic significance antineoplastics vitamin B_{17}. *J. Appl. Nutr.* 22:75–86
27. Greenberg, D. M. 1975. The vitamin fraud in cancer quackery. *West. J. Med.* 122:345–48
28. Lewis, J. P. 1975. Laetrile (informal opinion). *West J. Med.* 127:55–62

29. Laster, W. R., Schnabel, F. M. 1975. Experimental studies of the antitumor activity of amygdalin MF (NSC-15780) alone and in combination with β-glucosidase (NSC-128056). Cancer Chemother. Rep. Part 1 59:951–65

30. Wodnisky, I., Swiniarski, J. K. 1975. Antitumor activity of amygdalin MF (NSC-15780) as a single agent and with β-glucosidase (NSC-128056) on a spectrum of transplantable rodent tumors. Cancer Chemother. Rep. Part 1 59:939–50

31. Hill, G. J., Shine, T. E., Hill, H. Z., Miller, C. 1976. Failure of amygdalin to arrest B16 melanoma and BW5147. AKR Leukemia Cancer Res. 36:2102–107

32. Contessa, H. R., Santi, R. 1973. Liberation of cyanide from succinonitrile. The effect of ethanol. Biochem. Pharmacol. 22:827–32

33. Sylvester, D. M., Hayton, W. L., Morgan, R. L., Way, J. L. 1982. Effect of thiosulfate on cyanide pharmacokinetics in dogs. Toxicol. Appl. Pharmacol. 69:265–71

34. Ballantyne, B. 1975. Blood, brain and cerebrospinal fluid cyanide concentrations in experimental acute cyanide poisoning. J. Forensic Sci. Soc. 15:51–56

35. Ballantyne, B. 1983. Artifacts in the definitions of toxicity by cyanides and cyanogens. Fund. Appl. Toxicol. 3:400–08

36. Goenechea, S. 1982. Cyanide losses in samples of stored blood. Z. Rechtsmed. 88:97–101

37. Smith, R. P., Gosselin, R. E. 1976. Current concepts about the treatment of selected poisonings—Nitrite, cyanide, sulfide, barium, and quinidine. Ann. Rev. Pharmacol. Toxicol. 16:189–99

38. Sylvester, D. M., Sander, C., Hayton, W. L., Way, J. L. 1981. Alteration of the pharmacokinetics of sodium cyanide by sodium thiosulfate. Proc. West. Pharmacol. 24:135

39. Christel, D., Eyer, P., Hegemann, M., Kiese, M., Lorcher, W., Weger, N. 1977. Pharmacokinetics of cyanide in poisoning of dogs, and the effect of 4-dimethylaminophenol or thiosulfate. Arch. Toxicol. 38:177–89

40. McMillan, D. E., Svoboda, A. C. 1982. The role of erythrocytes in cyanide detoxification. J. Pharmacol. Exp. Ther. 221:37–42

41. Ballantyne, B. 1976. Changes in blood cyanide as a function of storage time and temperature. J. Forensic Sci. Soc. 16:305–10

42. Ballantyne, B. 1977. In vitro production of cyanide in normal human blood and the influence of thiocyanate and storage temperature. Clin. Toxicol. 11:173–93

43. Egekeze, J. O., Oehme, F. W. 1979. Direct potentiometric method for the determination of cyanide in biological fluids. J. Anal. Toxicol. 3:119–24

44. Ballantyne, B., Bright, J. E., Williams, P. 1973. An experimental assessment of decreases in measurable cyanide levels in biological fluids. J. Forensic Sci. Soc. 13:111–17

45. Epstein, J. 1947. Estimation of microquantities of cyanide. Anal. Chem. 19:272–74

46. Feldstein, M., Klendshoj, N. C. 1954. The determination of cyanide in biological fluids by microdiffusion analysis. J. Lab. Clin. Med. 44:166–70

47. Morgan, R. L., Way, J. L. 1979. Resolution of thiosulfate interference in cyanide determination. Toxicol. Appl. Pharmacol. 50:323–28

48. Frant, M. S., Ross, J. W., Riseman, J. H. 1972. Electrode indicator technique for measuring low levels of cyanide. Anal. Chem. 44:2227–30

49. Sylvester, D. M., Holmes, R. K., Sander, C., Way, J. L. 1982. Interference by thiosulphate with potentiometric analysis of cyanide in blood and its elimination. Toxicol. Appl. Pharmacol. 65:116–21

50. Morgan, R. L., Way, J. L. 1980. Determination of cyanide in biological fluids with pyridoxal. J. Anal. Toxicol. 4:78–81

51. Takanashi, S., Tamura, Z. 1970. Fluorometric determination of cyanide by the reaction with pyridoxal. Chem. Pharm. Bull. 18:1633–35

52. Guilbault, G. G., ed. 1976. Fluorescence Theory, Instrumentation, and Practice. New York: Dekker. 341 pp.

53. Guilbault, G. G., Kramer, D. N. 1965. Specific detection and determination of cyanide using various quinone derivatives. Anal. Chem. 37:1395–99

54. Ganjeloo, A., Isom, G. E., Morgan, R. L., Way, J. L. 1980. Fluorometric method for determination of cyanide in biological fluids with benzoquinone. Toxicol. Appl. Pharmacol. 55:103–07

55. Valentour, J. C., Aggarwal, V., Sunshine, I. 1974. Sensitive gas chromatographic determination of cyanide. Anal. Chem. 46(7):924–25

56. Danchik, R. S., Boltz, D. F. 1970. Indirect atomic absorption spectrometric methods for the determination of cyanide. Anal. Chim. Acta 49:567–69

57. Jungreis, E. 1969. Microdetermination

of cyanides by atomic absorption spectroscopy. *Isr. J. Chem.* 7:583–84

58. Manahan, S. E., Kunkel, R. 1973. An atomic absorption analysis method for cyanide. *Anal. Lett.* 6:547–53

59. Keilin, D. 1929. Cytochrome and respiratory enzymes. *Proc. Roy. Soc. Ser. B* 104:206–52

60. Keilin, D. 1966. *The History of Cell Respiration and Cytochrome*, pp. 204–24. Cambridge: Cambridge Univ. Press. 416 pp.

61. Warburg, O. 1931. Über nicht-hemmung der zellatmung durch blausaure. *Biochem. Z.* 231:493–97

62. Solomonson, L. P. 1982. Cyanide as a metabolic inhibitor. See Ref. 4, pp. 11–28

63. Hartzell, C. R., Beinert, H., van Gelder, B. F., King, T. E. 1978. Preparation of cytochrome oxidase from beef heart. *Methods Enzymol.* 53:54–66

64. Antonini, E. A., Brunori, M., Greenwood, C., Malstrom, B. G., Rotilio, G. C. 1971. The interaction of cyanide with cytochrome oxidase. *Eur. J. Biochem.* 23:396–400

65. Nicholls, P., Van Buuren, K. J. H., Van Gelder, B. F. 1972. Biochemical and biophysical studies on cytochrome aa_3. Binding of cyanide to cytochrome aa_3. *Biochim. Biophys. Acta* 275:279–87

66. Van Buuren, K. J. H., Nicholls, P., Van Gelder, B. F. 1972. Biochemical and biophysical studies on cytochrome aa_3. Reaction of cyanide with oxidized and reduced enzyme. *Biochim. Biophys. Acta* 256:258–76

67. Lorimer, G. H., Gewitz, H. S., Volker, W., Solomonson, L. P., Vennesland, B. 1974. The presence of bound cyanide in the naturally inactivated form of nitrate reductase of chlorella vulgaris. *J. Biol. Chem.* 249:6074–79

68. Ver Ploeg, D. A., Cordes, E. H., Gurd, F. R. N. 1971. Comparison of myoglobins from harbor seal, porpoise, and sperm whale. Mechanism and catalysis for addition of cyanide to myoglobins. *J. Biol. Chem.* 246:2725–33

69. Ellis, W. D., Dunford, H. B. 1968. The kinetics of cyanide and fluoride binding by ferric horseradish peroxidase. *Biochemistry* 7:2054–62

70. Erman, J. E. 1974. Kinetic and equilibrium studies of cyanide binding by cytochrome c peroxidase. *Biochemistry* 13:39–44

71. Galston, A. W. 1955. Plant catalase. *Methods Enzymol.* 2:789–91

72. Lafferty, M. A., Garrett, R. H. 1974. Purification and properties of the neurospora crassa assimilatory nitrite reductase. *J. Biol. Chem.* 249:7555–67

73. Marsho, T. V., Kung, S. D. 1976. Oxygenase properties of crystallized fraction 1 protein from tobacco. *Arch. Biochem. Biophys.* 173:341–46

74. Hasen, B. A., Dekker, E. E. 1976. Inactivation of bovine liver 2-keto-4-hydrooxyglutarate aldolase by cyanide in the presence of aldehydes. *Biochemistry* 15:2912–17

75. Albaum, H. G., Tepperman, J., Bodansky, O. 1946. The in vivo inactivation by cyanide on brain cytochrome oxidase and its effect on glycolysis and on the high energy phosphorus compounds in the brain. *J. Biol. Chem.* 164:45–51

76. Schubert, J., Brill, W. A. 1968. Antagonism of experimental cyanide toxicity in relation to the *in vivo* activity of cytochrome oxidase. *J. Pharmacol. Exp. Ther.* 162:352–59

77. Isom, G. E., Way, J. L. 1976. Lethality of cyanide in the absence of inhibition of liver cytochrome oxidase. *Biochem. Pharmacol.* 25:605–8

78. Isom, G. E., Liu, D. H. W., Way, J. L. 1975. Effect of sublethal doses of cyanide on glucose catabolism. *Biochem. Pharmacol.* 24:871–75

79. Isom, G. E., Way, J. L. 1982. Effect of oxygen on the antagonism of cyanide intoxication. Cytochrome oxidase, *in vivo*. *Toxicol. Appl. Pharmacol.* 65:250–56

80. Sorbo, B. H. 1951. On the properties of rhodanese. Partial purification, inhibitors and intracellular distribution. *Acta Chem. Scand.* 5:724–34

81. Jakob, A., Diem, S. 1974. Activation of glycogenolysis in perfused rat livers by glucagon and metabolic inhibitors. *Biochim. Biophys. Acta* 362:469–79

82. Bernthal, T. B., Bronk, D. W., Cordero, N., Gesell, R. 1928. The regulation of respiration. XVIII. The effects of low and high alveolar oxygen pressure and of sodium cyanide on the carotid and femoral flow of blood as studied with the continuous electrometric method. *Am. J. Physiol.* 83:435–44

83. Barcroft, J. 1931. The toxicity of atmospheres containing hydrocyanic acid gas. *J. Hyg.* 31:1–34

84. Dixon, M., Elliott, K. A. C. 1929. XC The effect of cyanide on respiration of animal tissues. *Biochem. J.* 23:812–30

85. Jacobs, L., Sampson, S. R., Comroe, J. H. 1971. Carotid sinus versus carotid body origin of nicotinic and cyanide bradycardia in the dog. *Am. J. Phys.* 220:472–76

86. Levine, S. 1975. Nonperipheral che-

moreceptor stimulation of ventilation by cyanide. *J. Appl. Phys.* 39:199–204

87. Von Euler, U. S., Liljestrand, G., Zotterman, Y. 1939. The excitation mechanism of the chemoreceptors of the carotid body. *Scand. Arch. Physiol.* 83:132–52

88. Cope, C., Abramowitz, S. 1960. Respiratory responses to intravenous sodium cyanide, a function of the oxygen-cyanide relationship. *Am. Rev. Resp. Dis.* 81:321–28

89. Ivanov, J. P. 1959. The effect of elevated oxygen pressure on animals poisoned with potassium cyanide. *Pharmacol. Toxicol.* (USSR) 22:476–79

90. Burrows, G. E., Liu, D. H. W., Way, J. L. 1973. Effect of oxygen on cyanide intoxication V: Physiologic effects. *J. Pharmacol. Exp. Ther.* 184:739–48

91. Paulet, G. 1960. *L'Intoxication cyanhydrique et son treatment*, pp. 48–51. Paris: Masson. 111 pp.

92. Offterdinger, H. 1970. Wirkung verschiedener blausaure-antidote auf den hersmuskel. *Naunyn-Schmiedebergs Arch. Pharmakol.* 266:416

93. Krasney, J. A. 1971. Cardiovascular responses to cyanide in awake sinoaortic denervated dogs. *Am. J. Physiol.* 220:1361–66

94. Calvelo, M. G., Abboud, F. M., Ballard, D. R., Abdel-Sayed, W. 1970. Reflex vascular responses to stimulation of chemoreceptors with nicotine and cyanide. *Circ. Res.* 27:259–76

95. Brodie, D. A. 1959. The effect of thiopental and cyanide on the activity of inspiratory neurons. *J. Pharmacol. Exp. Ther.* 126:264–69

96. Ballantyne, B. 1970. *Medicine, Science and the Law*, pp. 171–78. London: Sweet & Maxwell. 310 pp.

97. Hurst, E. W. 1940. Experimental demyelination of the central nervous system. 1: The encephalopathy produced by potassium cyanide. *Aust. J. Exp. Biol. Med. Sci.* 18:201–23

98. Hirano, A., Levine, S., Zimmerman, H. M. 1967. Experimental cyanide encephalopathy: Electron microscopic observations of early lesions in white matter. *J. Neuropathol. Exp. Neurol.* 26:200–13

99. Levine, S., Stypulkowski, W. 1959. Effect of ischemia on cyanide encephalopathy. *Neurology* 9:407–11

100. Levine, S. 1967. Experimental cyanide encephalopathy. *J. Neuropath. Exp. Neurol.* 26:214–22

101. Suzuki, T. 1968. Ultra structural changes of heart muscle in cyanide poisoning. *Tohoku J. Exp. Med.* 95:271–87

102. Wexler, J., Whittenberger, J. L., Dumke, P. R. 1947. The effect of cyanide on the electrocardiogram of man. *Am. Heart J.* 34:163–73

103. Osuntokun, B. O. 1972. Chronic cyanide neurotoxicity and neuropathy in Nigerians. *Plant Foods Hum. Nutr.* 2:215–66

104. Wilson, J. 1983. Cyanide in human disease: A review of clinical and laboratory evidence. *Fund. Appl. Toxicol.* 3:397–99

105. Wokes, F., Moore, D. F. 1958. Tobacco amblyopia. *Lancet* 2:526–27

106. Chisholm, I. A., Bronte-Stewart, J., Foulds, W. S. 1967. Hydroxocobalamin versus cyanocobalamin in the treatment of tobacco amblyopia. *Lancet* 2:450–51

107. Wilson, J., Linnell, J. C., Matthews, D. M. 1971. Plasma-cobalamins in neuroophthalmological diseases. *Lancet* 1:259–61

108. Wilson, J. 1963. Leber's hereditary optic atrophy. Some clinical and aetiological considerations. *Brain* 86:347–62

109. Wilson, J. 1965. Leber's hereditary optic atrophy. A possible defect of cyanide metabolism. *Clin. Sci.* 29:505–15

110. Clark, A. 1935. On the aetiology of pellagra and allied nutritional diseases. *West African Med. J.* 8:7–9

111. Monekosso, G. L., Wilson, J. 1966. Plasma thiocyanate and vitamin B_{12} in Nigerian patients with degenerative neurological disease. *Lancet* 1:1062–64

112. Money, G. L. 1958. Endemic neuropathies in the Epe district of southern Nigeria. *West Afr. Med. J.* 7:58–62

113. Osuntokun, B. O., Durowoju, J. E., McFarlane, H., Wilson, J. 1968. Plasma amino-acids in the Nigerian nutritional ataxic neuropathy. *Br. Med. J.* 3:647–49

114. El Ghawabi, S. H., Gaafar, M. A., El-Saharti, A. A., Ahmed, S. H., Malash, K. K., Fanes, R. 1975. Chronic cyanide exposure: A clinical, radioisotope, and laboratory study. *Br. J. Ind. Med.* 32:215–19

115. Chandra, H., Gupta, B. N., Bhargava, S. K., Clerk, S. H., Mahendra, P. N. 1980. Chronic cyanide exposure: A biochemical and industrial hygiene study. *J. Anal. Toxicol.* 4:161–65

116. Lessell, S. 1971. Experimental cyanide optic neuropathy. *Arch. Ophthalmol.* 86:194–204

117. Lessell, S., Kuwabara, T. 1974. Fine structure of experimental cyanide optic neuropathy. *Invest. Ophthalmol.* 13:748–56

118. Ermans, A. M., Delange, F., Van Der Velden, M., Kinthaert, J. 1972. Possible role of cyanide and thiocyanate in the

etiology of endemic cretinism. *Adv. Exp. Med. Biol.* 30:455–86

119. Pedigo, L. G. 1888. Antagonism between amyl nitrite and prussic acid. *Trans. Med. Soc. Va.* 19:124–31

120. Lang, K. 1933. Die rhodanbildung im tierkorper. *Biochem. Z.* 259:243–56

121. Chen, K. K., Rose, C. L., Clowes, G. H. A. 1933. Methylene blue, nitrites and sodium thiosulfate against cyanide poisoning. *Proc. Soc. Exp. Biol. Med.* 31:250–52

122. Antal, J. 1894. Experimentelle Untersuchungen zer Therapie die Cyanvergiftungen. *Arch. Med.* 3:117–28

123. Sorbo, B. 1975. Thiosulfate sulfurtransferase and mercaptopyruvate sulfurtransferase. In *Metabolic Pathways,* ed. D. M. Greenberg, 7:433–56. New York: Academic

124. Westley, J. 1973. Rhodanese. *Adv. Enzymol.* 39:327–68

125. Westley, J. 1977. Sulfur-transfer catalysis by enzymes. In *Bioorganic Chemistry,* ed. E. E. van Tamelen, 1:371–90. New York: Academic

126. Westley, J., Adler, A., Westley, L., Nishida, C. 1983. The sulfur transferases. *Fund. Appl. Toxicol.* 3:377–82

127. Hug, E. 1933. Accion del nitrito de sodio y del hyposulfite de sodio en el tratomiento de la intoxicación provacado por el cianura de potassio en el conejo. *Revta. Soc. Argent. Biol.* 9:91–97

128. Himwich, W. A., Saunders, J. P. 1948. Enzymatic conversion of cyanide to thiocyanate. *Am. J. Physiol.* 153:348–54

129. Sorbo, B. H. 1953. Crystalline rhodanese. I. Purification and physicochemical examination. *Acta Chem. Scand.* 7:1129–36

130. Sorbo, B. H. 1953. On the substrate specificity of rhodanese. *Acta Chem. Scand.* 7:1137–45

131. Clemedson, C., Hultman, H. I., Sorbo, B. 1955. A combination of rhodanese and ethanethiosulfonate as an antidote in experimental cyanide poisoning. *Acta Phys. Scand.* 35:31–35

132. Westley, J. 1980. Rhodanese and the sulfane pool. In *Enzymatic Basis of Detoxication,* ed. W. B. Jakoby, 2: 245–62. New York: Academic

133. Schneider, J. F., Westley, J. 1969. Metabolic interrelations of sulfur in proteins, thiosulfate, and cystine. *J. Biol. Chem.* 244:5735–44

134. Westley, J. 1981. Cyanide and sulfane sulfur. In *Cyanide in Biology,* ed. B. Vennesland, E. E. Conn, C. J. Knowles, J. Westley, F. Wissing, pp. 61–76. London: Academic

135. Myer, M., Tarr, B., Way, J. L. 1984. Mechanisms of cyanide antagonism. *Pharmacologist* (In press)

136. Sylvester, D. M., Sander, C., Way, J. L. 1981. Histochemistry of a sulfurtransferase. *Pharmacologist* 23:115

137. Crompton, M., Palmieri, F., Capano, M., Quagliariello, E. 1974. The transport of thiosulphate in rat liver mitochondria. *FEBS Lett.* 46:247–50

138. Wendel, W. B. 1932. Oxidation by erythrocytes and the catalytic influence of methylene blue. Methemoglobin and the effect of cyanide. *J. Biol. Chem.* 102:385–401

139. Chen, K. K., Rose, C. L., Clowes, G. H. A. 1933. Amyl nitrite and cyanide poisoning. *J. Am. Med. Assoc.* 100: 1920–22

140. Jandorf, B. J., Bodansky, O. 1946. Therapeutic and prophylactic effect of methemoglobinemia in inhalation poisoning by hydrogen cyanide and cyanogen chloride. *J. Ind. Hyg. Toxicol.* 28:124–32

141. Weber, H. D., Friedberg, K. D., Lendle, L. 1962. Beurteilung therapeutischer massnahmen bei der blausaureurevergiftung unter constanter cyanidinfusion. *Arch. Exp. Pathol. Pharmakol.* 244:1–16

142. Kiese, M., Weger, N. 1969. Formation of ferrihaemoglobin with aminophenols in the human for the treatment of cyanide poisoning. *Eur. J. Pharmacol.* 7:97–105

143. Weger, N. 1968. Aminophenole als Blausaure—Antidote. *Arch. Toxicol.* 49:50

144. Albaum, H. G., Tepperman, J., Bodansky, O. 1946. A spectrophotometric study of the competition of methemoglobin and cytochrome oxidase for cyanide *in vitro. J. Biol. Chem.* 163:641–47

145. Smith, R. P. 1967. The nitrite methemoglobin complex—Its significance in methemoglobin analyses and its possible role in methemoglobinemia. *Biochem. Pharm.* 16:1655–64

146. Kruszyna, R., Kruszyna, H., Smith, R. P. 1982. Comparison of hydroxylamine, 4-dimethlyaminophenol and nitrite protection against cyanide poisoning in mice. *Arch. Toxicol.* 49:191–202

147. Wendel, W. B. 1933. Methylene blue and cyanide poisoning. *J. Am. Med. Assoc.* 100:1054–55

148. Bodansky, O. 1951. Methemoglobinemia and methemoglobin-producing compounds. *Pharmacol. Rev.* 3:144–96

149. Naidler, J. E., Green, H., Rosenbaum, A. 1945. Intravenous injection of methylene blue in man with reference to its toxic symptoms and effect on electro-

cardiogram. *Am. J. Med. Sci.* 188:15–21

150. Rentsch, G., Wittekind, D. 1967. Methylene blue and erythrocytes in the living animal. Contribution to the toxicology at methylene blue and formation of Heinz bodies. *Toxicol. Appl. Pharmacol.* 11:81–87

151. Stossel, T. P., Jennings, R. B. 1966. Failure of methylene blue to produce methemoglobinemia *in vivo*. *Am. J. Clin. Pathol.* 45:600–4

152. Chen, K. K., Rose, C. L., Clowes, G. H. A. 1934. Comparative values of several antidotes in cyanide poisoning. *Am. J. Med. Sci.* 188:767–81

153. Way, J. L. 1983. Cyanide antagonism. *Fund. Appl. Toxicol.* 3:383–86

154. Holmes, R. K., Way, J. L. 1982. Mechanism of cyanide antagonism by sodium nitrite. *Pharmacologist* 24:182

155. Way, J. L., Gibbons, S. L., Sheehy, M. 1966. Effect of oxygen on cyanide intoxication. 1: Prophylactic protection. *J. Pharmacol. Exp. Ther.* 153:351–55

156. Sheehy, M., Way, J. L. 1968. Effect of oxygen on cyanide intoxication. III: Mithridate. *J. Pharmacol. Exp. Ther.* 161:163–68

157. Guth, P. S., Spirtes, M. A. 1958. Antagonism of cyanide intoxication by chlorpromazine. *Fed. Am. Soc. Exp. Biol.* 17:374

158. Levine, S., Klein, M. 1959. Effect of chlorpromazine on cyanide intoxication. *Proc. Soc. Exp. Biol. Med.* 102:192–94

159. Flacke, W., Mulke, G., Schulz, R. 1953. Beitrag zur Wirkung von Pharmaka auf die Unterdrucktoleranz. *Arch. Exp. Pathol. Pharmakol.* 220:469–76

160. Way, J. L., Burrows, G. E. 1976. Cyanide intoxication: Protection with chlorpromazine. *Toxicol. Appl. Pharmacol.* 36:1–5

161. Burrows, G. E., Way, J. L. 1976. Antagonism of cyanide toxicity by phenoxybenzamine. *Fed. Proc.* 35:533

162. Burrows, G. E., King, L., Tarr, S., Way, J. L. 1976. The protective effect of vasoactive compounds as cyanide antagonist. *Proc. Int. Congr. Toxicol.* 1:48

163. Meurice, J. 1900. Intoxication et desintoxication de differents nitriles par l'hyposulfite de soude et les sels metalliques. *Arch. Intl. Pharmacodyn.* 7:12–53

164. Mushett, C. W., Kelley, K. L., Boxer, G. E., Rickards, J. C. 1952. Antidotal efficacy of vitamin B_{12} (hydroxocobalamin) in experimental cyanide poisoning. *Proc. Soc. Exp. Biol. Med.* 81:234–37

165. Rose, C. L., Worth, R. M., Chen, K. K. 1965. Hydroxo-cobalamine and acute cyanide poisoning in dogs. *Life Sci.* 4:1785–89

166. Evans, C. L. 1964. Cobalt compounds as antidotes for hydrocyanic acid. *Brit. J. Pharmacol. Chemother.* 23:455–75

167. Friedberg, K. D., Grutzmacher, J., Lendle, L. 1965. Aquocobalamin (vitamin B_{12a}) als spezifisches blausaure antidot. *Arch. Intl. Pharmacodyn. Ther.* 154:327–50

168. Friedberg, K. D., Shukla, U. R. 1975. The efficiency of aquocobalamine as an antidote in cyanide poisoning when given alone or combined with sodium thiosulfate. *Arch. Toxicol.* 33:103–13

169. Mercker, H., Bastian, G. 1959. Kobaltuerbindungen zur entgiftung von blausaure. *Arch. Exp. Pathol. Pharmakol.* 236:449–58

170. Schwarzkopf, H. A., Friedberg, K. D. 1971. Zur beutteilung der blausaureantidote. *Arch. Toxicol.* 27:111–23

171. Burrows, G. E., Way, J. L. 1979. Cyanide intoxication in sheep: Antagonism with sodium nitrite, cobalt chloride, and sodium thiosulfate. *Am. J. Vet. Res.* 40:613–17

172. Smith, R. P. 1969. Cobalt salts: Effects in cyanide and sulfite poisoning and on methemoglobinemia. *Toxicol. Appl. Pharmacol.* 15:505–16

173. Isom, G., Way, J. L. 1972. Cyanide intoxication: Protection with cobaltous chloride. *Toxicol. Appl. Pharmacol.* 24:449–56

174. Paulet, G. 1957. Sur une nouvelle mise au point du traitemente de l'intoxication cyanhydrique. *Presse Med.* 65:573–76

175. Paulet, G. 1958. Intoxication cyanhydrique et chelates de cobalt. *J. Physiol.* (Paris) 50:438–42

176. Frankenberg, L., Sorbo, B. 1975. Effect of cyanide antidotes on the metabolic conversion of cyanide to thiocyanate. *Arch. Toxicol.* 33:81–89

177. Bartelheimer, E. W., Friedberg, K. D., Lendle, L. 1962. The potentialities of cobalt compounds for chemical reactions in relation to their toxicity and antidotal activity against hydrocyanic acid. *Arch. Intl. Pharmacodyn. Ther.* 139:99–108

178. Nagler, J., Provoust, R. A., Parizel, G. 1978. Hydrogen cyanide poisoning: Treatment with cobalt EDTA. *J. Occup. Med.* 20:414–16

179. Halpern, J., Guastalla, G., Bercaw, J. 1972. Some aspects of the chemistry of cobalt (I) cyanide and related complexes. *Coord. Chem. Rev.* 8:167–84

180. Tarkowski, S. 1966. Effect of cobalt on the inhibition of the cytochrome oxidase

activity by potassium cyanide. *Med. Prac.* 17:116–19

181. Cittadini, A., Galeotti, T., Terranova, T. 1971. The effect of pyruvate on cyanide inhibited respiration in intact ascites tumor cells. *Experientia* 27:633–35

182. Cittadini, A., Caprino, L., Terranova, T. 1972. The effect of pyruvate on the acute cyanide poisoning in mice. *Experientia* 28:943–44

183. Schwartz, C., Morgan, R. L., Way, L. M., Way, J. L. 1979. Antagonism of cyanide intoxication with sodium pyruvate. *Toxicol. Appl. Pharmacol.* 50:437–41

184. Stotz, E., Altschul, A. M., Hogness, T. R. 1938. The cytochrome C-cytochrome oxidase complex. *J. Biol. Chem.* 224:745–54

185. Karsten, A. 1934. Effect of cyanide on Black Hills trout. *Black Hills Eng.* 22:145–74

186. Gordh, T., Norberg, B. 1947. Studies on oxygen treatment in connection with experimental hydrocyanic poisoning. *Acta Physiol. Scand.* 13:26–34

187. Paulet, G. 1955. Valeur et mecanisms d'action de l'oxygenotherapie dans le traitement de l'intoxication cyanhydrique. *Arch. Intl. Physiol.* 63:340–60

188. Cope, C. 1961. The importance of oxygen in the treatment of cyanide poisoning. *J. Am. Med. Assoc.* 175:1061–64

189. Yungmeister, B. O. 1972. Complex oxygenbaric therapy for potassium cyanide poisoning. *Farmakol. Amidinovykh Soedin.*, pp. 96–101

190. Carden, E. 1970. Hyperbaric oxygen in cyanide poisoning. *Anaesthesia* 25:442–43

191. Way, J. L., Gibbon, S. L., Sheehy, M. 1966. Cyanide intoxication: Protection with oxygen. *Science* 152:210–11

192. Way, J. L., Gibbon, S. L., Sheehy, M. 1966. Effect of oxygen on cyanide intoxication. I: Prophylactic protection. *J. Pharmacol Exp. Ther.* 153:381–85

193. Burrows, G. E., Way, J. L. 1977. Cyanide intoxication in sheep: Therapeutic value of oxygen or cobalt. *Am. J. Vet. Sci.* 38:223–27

194. Savateen, N. V., Tonkopy, V. D., Frolov, S. F. 1969. Effect of oxygen at normal and increased pressure on the course of cyanide poisoning. *Farmakol. Toksik.* (USSR) 32:328–30

195. Way, J. L., End, E., Sheehy, M. H., Miranda, M., Feitknecht, U. F., Burrows, G. E., Gibbon, S. L., Bachand, R. 1972. Effect of oxygen on cyanide intoxication. IV: Hyperbaric oxygen. *Toxicol. Appl. Pharmacol.* 22:415–21

196. Sheehy, M., Gibbon, S. L., Way, J. L. 1966. Antagonism of cyanide intoxication: With oxygen in mice. *Pharmacologist* 8:218

197. Haugaard, N. 1965. Poisoning of cellular reaction by oxygen. *Ann. NY Acad. Sci.* 117:736–44

198. Horn, R. S., Williams, C. D., Haugaard, E. S., Haugaard, N. 1967. Toxic effects of oxygen on carbohydrate metabolism *in vitro. Fed. Proc. Am. Soc. Exp. Biol.* 26:709

199. Jamieson, D., Van den Brenk, H. A. S. 1962. Pulmonary damage due to high pressure oxygen breathing in rats. II: Changes in dehydrogenase activity in rat lung. *Aust. J. Exp. Biol. Med. Sci.* 40:51–56

200. Doherty, P. A., Riper, O. V., Berndt, W. O., Smith, R. P. 1979. Failure of oxygen to influence the metabolism or distribution of cyanide or of thiosulfate in mice. *Toxicol. Lett.* 4:25–29

201. Levine, S. 1959. Oxygen in the therapy of cyanide poisoning. *J. Am. Med. Assoc.* 170:1585

202. Brodie, D. A. 1959. The effect of thiopental and cyanide on the activity of inspiratory neurons. *J. Pharmacol. Exp. Ther.* 126:264–69

203. Fernandez, A. F., Gonzalez-Quintata, J., Russek, M. 1963. Effect of low concentrations of cyanide on Q_{O_2} of tissues slices. *Am. J. Physiol.* 204:314–16

204. Skene, W. G., Norman, J. N., Smith, G. 1966. Effect of hyperbaric oxygen in cyanide poisoning. In *National Academy of Sciences*, ed. I. W. Brown, B. G. Cox, pp. 705–10. Washington DC: NAS Public.1404

205. Burrows, G. E., Liu, D. H. W., Isom, G. E., Way, J. L. 1982. Effect of antagonists on the physiological disposition of sodium cyanide. *J. Toxicol. Environ. Health* 10:181–89

205a. Isom, G. E., Way, J. L. 1974. Effect of oxygen on cyanide intoxication. VI: Reactivation of cyanide-inhibited glucose metabolism. *J. Pharmacol. Exp. Ther.* 189:235–43

206. Graham, D. L., Laman, D., Theodore, J., Robin, E. D. 1977. Acute cyanide poisoning complicated by lactic acidosis and pulmonary edema. *Arch. Int. Med.* 137:1051–1055

207. Berlin, C. M. 1970. The treatment of cyanide poisoning in children. *Pediatrics* 46:793–96

208. Chen, K. K., Rose, C. L. 1952. Nitrite and thiosulfate in cyanide poisoning. *J. Am. Med. Assoc.* 149:113–19

209. Clawson, A. B., Bunyea, H., Couch, J.

F. 1934. Remedies for cyanide poisoning in sheep and cattle. *J. Wash. Acad. Sci.* 24:369–85

210. Friedberg, K. D. 1968. Antidote bei blausaurevergiftungen. *Arch. Toxicol.* 24:41–48

211. McDermott, P. H., Delaney, R. I., Egan, J. D., Sullivan, J. F. 1966. Mycardosis and cardiac failure in men. *J. Am. Med. Assoc.* 198:253–56

212. Kesteloot, H., Roelandt, J., Willems, J., Claes, J. H., Joossens, J. V. 1968. An inquiry into the role of cobalt in the heart disease of chronic beer drinkers. *Circulation* 37:854–64

213. Wiberg, G. S., Munro, I. C., Meranger, J. C., Morrison, A. B., Grice, H. C., Heggtveit, H. A. 1969. Factors affecting the cardiotoxic potential of cobalt. *Clin. Toxicol.* 2:257–71

214. Rona, G. 1971. Experimental aspects of cobalt cardiomyopathy. *Br. Heart J.* 33:171–74 (Suppl.)

215. Hilmann, B., Bardham, K. D., Bain, J. T. B. 1974. The use of dicobalt edetate (kelocyanor) in cyanide poisoning. *Postgrad. Med. J.* 50:171–74

216. Naughton, M. 1974. Acute cyanide poisoning. *Anaesth. Intens. Care* 4:351–56

Ann. Rev. Pharmacol. Toxicol. 1984. 24:483–500

MECHANISMS OF TERATOGENESIS

D. A. Beckman and R. L. Brent

Department of Pediatrics, Jefferson Medical College of Thomas Jefferson University,
Philadelphia, Pennsylvania 19107

MECHANISMS

The mechanisms of teratogenesis fall into two broad categories based on the etiology of the congenital malformations: (*a*) errors in genetic programming based on deviations in the genotype of the embryo or the low probability for error of a normal genotype; and (*b*) environmental agents or factors that interact with an embryo during the period of development (drugs, chemicals, radiation, hyperthermia, infections, abnormal maternal metabolic states, or mechanical factors).

The etiology of human malformations includes both genetic and environmental factors, but it also includes a large category labelled *unknown* (Table 1). Many geneticists believe that a significant proportion of congenital malformations of unknown etiology are polygenic (1, 2). Thus, malformations with an increased recurrent risk, such as cleft palate, anencephaly, spina bifida, congenital heart disease, pyloric stenosis, talipes equinovarus, and congenital dislocation of the hip, fit the criteria for polygenic inherited disease. They also happen to fit the criteria for multifactorial disease (1, 3). Included in the unknown category are malformations that occur spontaneously at a very low frequency simply on the basis of the probability of spontaneous errors of development. Thus, particular genotypes have an inherent malformation rate based on the fact that embryonic development is a very complicated process and has a variable but low probability of going awry just as DNA duplication, for example, is not an error-free process. The explanation for the etiology and mechanisms of teratogenesis for this large group of malformations with unknown etiology will depend upon identifying the genes involved in polygenic or plurogenic processes, identifying the interacting genetic and environmental

483

0362-1642/84/415-0483$02.00

Table 1 Etiology of human malformations observed during the first year of life[a]

Suspected cause	Percent of total
Genetic	
Autosomal genetic disease	15–20%
Cytogenetic (chromosomal abnormalities)	5%
Unknown	65%
Polygenic	
Multifactorial (genetic-environmental interactions)	
Spontaneous errors of development	
Synergistic interactions of teratogens	
Environmental	
Maternal conditions: diabetes, endocrinopathies, nutritional deficiencies, drug and substance addictions	4%
Maternal infections: rubella, toxoplasmosis, syphilis, herpes, cytomegalic inclusion disease	3%
Mechanical (deformations): abnormal uterus, amniotic bands, umbilical cord constrictions, disparity in uterine size and uterine contents	1–2%
Chemicals, drugs, radiation, hyperthermia	<1%

[a]References 4, 5

determinants of multifactorial traits, and identifying the mathematical risks for error during important embryonic processes of normal development. Until this can be accomplished, we will continue to label a large proportion of human malformations as having hypothetical etiologies.

The other two etiological categories of teratogenic agents, environmental and genetic, have different pathologic processes that result in embryopathology. Congenital malformations due to genetic etiology have a spectrum of pathologic processes that are the result of a gene deficiency, a gene abnormality, chromosome rearrangement, chromosome deletion, or chromosome excess that results in abnormal development. The pathologic nature of this process is determined before conception or at least before differentiation because of the presence of inherited or newly acquired genetic abnormalities. Although environmental factors may modify the development of the genetically abnormal embryo, the genetic abnormality is the predominant contributor to the pathologic process. Many genetic diseases in animals and man have been studied and we are able to determine the mechanism of teratogenesis of some hereditary malformations (i.e. T locus and Ah locus in the mouse and diaphragm aplasia and jejunal atresia in man). However, this review will not discuss the mechanisms involved in hereditary malformations but rather will discuss the mechanisms involved in malformations that are primarily environmentally produced.

Basic tenets of environmentally produced malformations are that teratogens or teratogenic milieus have certain characteristics in common:

1. *Stage sensitivity* indicates that susceptibility to teratogenesis varies during gestation so that the three stages of development have the following associated characteristics of teratogenesis: from fertilization through early post-implantation, the embryo has relatively few cells and a great capacity for the replacement of omnipotent cells. Thus, the effect of a teratogenic insult is typically an all-or-none phenomenon, because either the agent affects enough cells to result in embryolethality or so few cells are affected that the embryo is able to effectively repair itself. The second stage, the period of organogenesis (from day 18 through about day 60 of gestation in the human), is the period of greatest sensitivity to teratogenic insults and the period when anatomical malformations can be induced. The third stage, the fetal period, is characterized by cell depletion and growth retardation resulting from exposure to teratogenic agents after the major tissue and organ types have differentiated, although fetal death can be produced.

2. *Dose-response relationships* refer to the phenomenon that, as the exposure or dosage increases, frequency and severity of the teratogenic effects also increase.

3. *Threshold effects* refer to the dosage or level of exposure below which the incidence of death, malformation, growth retardation, or functional deficit is not statistically greater than that of controls (this is usually one to three orders of magnitude below the teratogenic dose).

4. *Genetic variability* in mammals determines differences in placental transport, absorption, metabolism, and distribution of an agent and accounts for variation in teratogenic effects among species and individuals.

5. *Infections* are exceptions to the basic tenets of teratogenesis. Infectious agents may not conform because the course of an infection is difficult to define in terms of period of exposure to the fetus and dose of the infectious agent to which the fetus is exposed at any one time. Therefore, dose-response relationships, threshold effects, and genetic variability have been impossible to demonstrate in the human.

Based on his review of the literature, Wilson (6, 7) proposed possible mechanisms of teratogenesis, summarized in Table 2. This list illustrates the many levels at which embryonic development is vulnerable to errors or disruptive influences. Unfortunately, this approach may generate some confusion when one attempts to determine etiology for the following two reasons: (*a*) the pathologic processes could result from genetic or environmental factors; and (*b*) the fact that an environmental agent can induce one of these pathologic processes does not guarantee that exposure will result in teratogenesis. Thus, while the listing summarized in Table 2 provides us with a format of theoretical teratogenic mechanisms, it does not relate these to known teratogens nor does it enable us to predict teratogenesis in the human if an agent exhibits one of these characteristics in an experimental test system.

We will first briefly discuss some of Wilson's proposed mechanisms to

Table 2   Mechanisms of teratogenesis as suggested by J. G. Wilson[a]

1.	Mutation: changes in the nucleotide sequence in DNA.
2.	Chromosomal aberations: alterations in the amount of DNA.
3.	Mitotic interference: a disturbance in the cell cycle.
4.	Altered nucleic acid synthesis and function: a disturbance in translation, transcription or DNA synthesis.
5.	Lack of precursors, substrates and coenzymes for biosynthesis: a general or specific nutritional deficiency.
6.	Altered energy sources: interference with the citric acid cycle or the terminal electron transport system.
7.	Enzyme inhibition: limited or specific enzyme inhibition.
8.	Osmolar imbalance: alterations in fluid pressures, viscosities, and osmotic pressures.
9.	Altered membrane characteristics: a disruption in membrane transport and permeability.
10.	Other mechanisms: an extensive list of possible mechanisms for which there is little scientific support.

[a]References 6, 7

illustrate the difficulty in using them to determine etiology and then we will discuss our current understanding of the mechanisms of teratogenesis of selected agents known to be teratogenic in man.

MUTATIONS, CHROMOSOMAL ABERRATIONS   The mutagenic effects listed in Table 2 are unlikely to play a role in the production of malformations following in utero exposure. Mutagens are more likely teratogenic due to their cytotoxic effects, which are related to cell destruction, and not to genetic changes that persist and affect embryonic development for many cell cycles in the developing embryo. While gene changes or chromosome abnormalities produced in eggs or sperm could result in embryopathology, they play little or no role when induced in somatic cells of the developing embryo except as they may cause cell death, retardation of differentiation, or mitotic delay.

ALTERED NUCLEIC ACID SYNTHESIS OR FUNCTION   Although there are no examples of subtle changes in the expression of genetic information due to exposures to environmental agents, the disruption of protein synthesis that must ensue from any significant disturbance in RNA or DNA synthesis or function would be of such great magnitude as to be incompatible with life.

The other proposed mechanisms listed in Table 2 similarly describe effects that may be attributable to an agent under defined experimental conditions. However, it is improbable that a drug, chemical, or other agent will have only one effect on a biological system. It is also improbable, even assuming that the mechanisms of action of a particular agent may be known, that an in utero exposure to that agent will result in congenital malformations without taking into consideration developmental state or dose. Rather than picking possible mechanisms of action from a list to test which fit the agent, a more useful approach is to study the effects of the agents in question to determine their mechanisms of action.

The following section briefly discusses what is known concerning the mechanisms of action of agents that have been proven to cause congenital malformations in man, summarized in Table 3.

TERATOGENIC AGENTS OF MAN

Alcohol

Jones et al (8) described fetal alcohol syndrome (FAS) in children with intrauterine growth retardation, microcephaly, maxillary hypoplasia, and reduction in the width of palpebral fissures (cardiac abnormalities were also seen). Approximately one-third of the children of alcoholic mothers had FAS (9, 10) and all of the affected children evidenced developmental delay (11).

A period of greatest susceptibility and a dose-response relationship have not yet been established (12). While consumption of six ounces of alcohol per day constitutes a high risk, FAS is not likely when the mother drinks less than two drinks (equivalent to two ounces of alcohol) per day (13). The human syndrome is likely to involve the direct effects of alcohol and its metabolite, acetaldehyde (14), and the indirect effects of genetic predisposition and poor nutrition. Alcoholism is also associated with smoking and the use of other drugs.

Aminopterin and Methotrexate

Aminopterin-induced therapeutic abortions have been shown to result in malformations (hydrocephalus, cleft palate, meningomyelocele) in some of the abortuses (15, 16). Three case reports of children receiving in utero exposure to aminopterin included observations of growth retardation, abnormal cranial ossification, high-arched palate, and reduction in derivatives of the first branchial arch (17, 18, 19).

Methotrexate (methylaminopterin) ingestion during the first two months (20) or for 5 days between the 8th and 10th weeks (21) resulted in the absence of the frontal bones, craniosynostosis, rib defects, and the absence of digits.

Both compounds are folic acid antagonists that inhibit dihydrofolate reductase, resulting in cell death during the S phase of the cell cycle (22). The clinical literature has been reviewed by Warkany (23).

Androgens

Masculinization of the external genitalia of the female has been reported following in utero exposure to large doses of testosterone (24), methyltestosterone (25), and testosterone enanthate (26). The masculinization is characterized by clitoromegaly with or without fusion of the labia minora.

Table 3 Teratogenic agents of man

Agents	Reported effects and/or associations	Comments
Alcohol	Fetal alcohol syndrome: intrauterine growth retardation, microcephaly; maxillary hypoplasia, reduction in width of palpebral fissure, mental retardation.	Direct cytotoxic effects of alcohol and acetaldehyde and indirect effects of alcoholism (poor nutrition, smoking, use of other drugs). Consumption of six ounces of alcohol or more per day constitutes a high risk.
Aminopterin, methotrexate	Hydrocephalus, cleft palate, meningomyelocele, intrauterine growth retardation, abnormal cranial ossification, reduction in derivatives of first branchial arch.	Folic acid antagonists that inhibit dihydrofolate reductase, resulting in cell death.
Androgens	Masculinization of female embryo: clitoromegaly with or without fusion of labia minora.	Effects are dose dependent; stimulates growth and differentiation of receptor containing tissue.
Coumarin derivates	Nasal hypoplasia, stippling of secondary epiphysis; intrauterine growth retardation, anomalies of eyes, hands, neck, variable CNS effects in gestation.	Metabolic inhibitor; bleeding is an unlikely explanation for effects. 10–25% risk from exposure during 8th–14th week of pregnancy.
Diethylstilbesterol	Masculinization of female, vaginal adenocarcinoma, anomalies of cervix and uterus. Affected males show hypotrophic testes, epidymal cysts, abnormal spermatozoa. Effects are dose-dependent.	Stimulates estrogen receptor-containing tissue, may cause misplaced tissue. 75% risk for vaginal adenosis for exposures before 9th week of pregnancy; risk of vaginal adenocarcinoma is low (1 in 10,000). 25% risk for anomalies in males (including minor variations).
Diphenylhydantoin	Hydantoin syndrome: hypoplastic nails and distal phalanges, cleft lip/palate, microcephaly, mental retardation.	Direct effect on cell membranes, folate and vitamin K metabolism. Wide variation in reported risk. Associations documented only with chronic exposure.
Methylmercury	Minamata disease: cerebral palsy, microcephaly, mental retardation, blindness.	Cell death due to inhibition of enzymes, especially sulfhydryl enzymes.

Table 3 (*continued*)

Agents	Reported effects and/or associations	Comments
Oxazolidine-2,4-diones	Fetal trimethadione syndrome: V-shaped eyebrows, low-set ears with anteriorly folded helix, high-arched palate, irregular teeth, central nervous system anomalies, developmental delay.	Affects cell membrane permeability. Wide variation in reported risk. Associations documented only with chronic exposure.
Polychlorinated biphenyls	Cola-colored children: pigmentation of gums, nails, and groin, hypoplastic deformed nails, intrauterine growth retardation.	Polychlorinated biphenyls and commonly occurring contaminants are cytotoxic.
Progestins	Masculinization of female embryo exposed to high doses.	Stimulates growth and differentiation of receptor-containing tissue.
Radiation	Microcephaly, mental retardation, eye anomalies, intrauterine growth retardation, visceral malformations depend on dose and stage of exposure.	Cell death and mitotic delay. Little or no risk with exposures of 5 rads or less of x-rays.
Tetracycline	Hypoplastic tooth enamel, tooth and bone staining	Effects seen only if exposure is during second or third trimester.
Thalidomide	Bilateral limb reduction defects (preaxial preferential effects, phocomelia), facial hemangioma, esophageal or duodenal atresia, anomalies of external ears, kidneys, and heart	Increased programmed cell death in the early limb bud causing retarded growth in the apical ectodermal ridge, especially in the preaxial border. Primary mechanism unknown. Very high risk of major malformations during critical periods.
Thyroid: Iodides, radioiodine, antithyroid drugs (propylthiouracil)	Hypothyroidism, goiter	Fetopathic effect specific for the thyroid. Metabolic block resulting in decreased thyroid hormone synthesis and gland development. Maternal intake of 12 mg of iodide per day or more increases the risk of fetal goiter.

To illustrate that androgens can only affect tissues with androgen receptors, inherited male pseudohermaphroditism is a syndrome in which the testes secrete normal amounts of testosterone but receptor binding in the target tissues is defective. The result is that genotypic males undergo feminine development (27). This is the same result that a lack of androgens has on the development of sex structures in the male (28). Thus, it can be seen that either an excess or a deficiency in androgens can have an effect only on those tissues with androgen receptors.

Coumarin Derivatives

Nasal hypoplasia following exposure to several drugs, including warfarin, during pregnancy was reported by DiSaia (29). Kerber et al (30) were the first to suggest warfarin as the teratogenic agent. Coumarin anticoagulants have since been associated with nasal hypoplasia, calcific stippling of the secondary epiphysis, and central nervous system abnormalities (31–33). Barr & Burdi (34) have described warfarin embryopathy and Warkany (35, 36), besides summarizing the clinical data, provides an excellent overview of the difficulties in relating a congenital malformation to an environmental cause. There is an estimated 25% risk for affected infants following exposure during the period from the 8th through the 14th week of pregnancy.

Coumarin has been shown to inhibit the formation of γ-carboxyglutamyl residues from glutamyl residues, decreasing the ability of proteins to bind calcium (37). The inhibition of calcium binding by proteins during embryonic/ fetal development, especially during a critical period of ossification, could explain the nasal hypoplasia, stippled calcification, and skeletal abnormalities of warfarin embryopathy (33).

Diethylstilbestrol (DES)

The first abnormality reported following exposure to diethylstilbestrol during the first trimester was clitoromegaly in female newborns (38). Much later, Herbst et al (39, 40) and Greenwald et al (41) reported an increased incidence of vaginal adenocarcinoma in female offspring following first-trimester expo- sures. Further studies revealed that almost all of the cancers occurred after 14 years of age and only in those exposed before the 18th week of gestation (42, 43). There is a 75% risk for vaginal adenosis for exposures occurring before the 9th week of pregnancy; however, the risk of developing the adenocarcinoma is extremely low (44).

Twenty-five percent of males exposed to DES in utero exhibited genital lesions and abnormal spermatozoa, but no malignancies have been observed (45). A review of the syndrome has been presented by Ulfelder (46).

DES is a very potent nonsteroidal estrogen and, as in the case of steroidal estrogens, must interact with the receptor proteins present only in estrogen-responsive tissues before exerting its effects by stimulating RNA, protein, and DNA synthesis. The alleged carcinogenic effect of DES is most likely indirect: DES exposure results in the presence of columnar epithelium in the vagina and this "misplaced tissue" may have a greater susceptibility to developing the adenocarcinoma.

Diphenylhydantoin

Exposure to diphenylhydantoin may involve a 10% risk for full syndrome and a 30% risk for some anomalies (47–49). While cleft lip and palate, congenital heart disease, and microcephaly have been reported, hypoplasia of the nails and distal phalanges are possibly specific malformations in up to 18% of the exposed fetuses (50, 51). Hanson et al (52) noted that, although the hydantoin syndrome is observed in 11% in their study, three times as many exhibit mental deficits. The hydantoin syndrome has been reviewed by Hanson et al (52). It should be mentioned that prospective studies demonstrate a much lower frequency of effects and some do not demonstrate any effect.

Factors associated with epilepsy may contribute to the etiology of these malformations: based on the United States Collaborative Perinatal Project and a large Finnish registry, the incidence of malformations was 10.5% when the mother was epileptic, 8.3% when the father was epileptic, and 6.4 when neither parent was affected (53).

Diphenylhydantoin affects ion movements to exert a stabilizing effect on cell membranes. There may also be some effect on folate and vitamin K metabolism (54).

Methylmercury

Mercury inactivates sulfhydryl enzymes by forming covalent bonds with sulfur present in sulfhydryl groups or divalent mercury can replace the hydrogen atom to form mercaptides. Mercury can further interfere with metabolism and function by combining with phosphoryl, carboxyl, amide, and amine groups to inhibit enzymes and precipitate proteins.

There have been several incidences of human exposures to methylmercury as an environmental pollutant or as a fungicide present on seed grain consumed by humans. In Minamata, Japan, the local population was exposed by ingesting fish caught in a bay heavily polluted by methylmercury. Cerebral palsy and associated microcephaly were the common features, with few other congenital defects (55, 56). Snyder (57) described the severe damage to the central nervous system in the offspring following ingestion by the pregnant mother of meat from a pig fed seed grain containing a mercurial fungicide. Seed grain containing a methylmercury fungicide was responsible for fetal exposures in Iraq, when pregnant women consumed bread inadvertently prepared using the seed grain (58, 59). Cerebral palsy and motor and mental impairments were reported.

Harada (60) has reviewed the clinical aspects of congenital Minamata disease.

Oxazolidine-2, 4-Diones

Trimethadione and paramethadione are antiepileptic oxazolidine-2, 4-diones that distribute uniformly throughout body tissues and exert their effects via the actions of their metabolites. These drugs affect cell membrane permeability and vitamin K-dependent clotting factors, but their primary mode of action is not known.

Zackai et al (61) described the fetal trimethadione syndrome characterized by developmental delay, V-shaped eyebrows, low-set ears with anteriorly folded helix, high-arched palate, and irregular teeth. German et al (62) reported similar findings plus cardiac anomalies. Feldman et al (63) and Goldman & Yaffe (64) have reviewed the clinical findings in the literature and from their own observations. There are wide variations in reported risk, with estimates as high as 80% for major or minor defects.

Polychlorinated Biphenyls

First identified in Japan in 1968 (65), then in Taiwan in 1979 (66), polychlorinated biphenyls (PCBs) consumed in contaminated cooking oil by pregnant women resulted in pigmented children (cola-colored) with low birth weight, pigmentation of the gums, nails, and groin, hypoplastic deformed nails, and conjunctivitis with an enlargement of the sebaceous glands of the eyelid (66).

Several circumstances have inhibited a full evaluation of PCB teratogenicity in the human: there are technical difficulties in measuring PCB concentrations; there are no dose-response data for the human; and PCBs are present in mixtures containing highly toxic products of degradation.

Rogan (66) has recently reviewed the effects of PCBs on human development.

Progestins

A few patients have an inadequate luteal response (deficient progesterone secretion) and it has been suggested that women with repeated abortions might benefit from progestins during the first trimester. The effects of progesterone on the human fetus are not well documented: there are only two case reports of masculinized female infants (67) and a few reports suggesting that progesterone may be associated with a low risk of hypospadias (68, 69).

In contrast to progesterone, some of the synthetic progestins have been reported to cause virilizing effects in the human. Exposure during the first trimester to large doses of 17-α-ethinyl-testosterone has been associated with masculinization of the external genitalia of female fetuses (70, 71). Similar associations result from exposure to large doses of 17-α-ethinyl-19-nortestosterone (norethadrone) (72) and 17-α-enthinyl-17-OH-5(10)estren-3-one (Enovid-R) (73). The synthetic progestins, like progesterone, can influence only those tissues with the appropriate steroid-receptor proteins. The preparations with androgenic properties will cause abnormalities in the genital development of females only if present in sufficient amounts during critical periods of development (70, 72). In 1959, Grumbach et al (73) pointed out that labio-scrotal fusion could be produced with large doses if the fetuses were exposed before the 13th week of pregnancy, while clitoromegaly could be produced after this period, illustrating that a specific form of maldevelopment can be induced only when the susceptible embryonic tissues are in a limited range of development. In a recent review, Wilson & Brent (74) presented evidence against the involvement of female sex hormones in nongenital teratogenesis.

Radiation

The effects of radiation are due to direct damage to the cell chromatin; they result in cell death or damage that is partially or completely repaired by the cell. The classical triad of effects of radiation are gross malformations, intrauterine growth retardation, and embryonic death, with each of these effects having a dose-response relationship and a threshold exposure below which no difference between an exposed and an unexposed control population can be demonstrated (75). Offspring born to patients receiving radiation therapy for various conditions exhibited growth retardation, eye malformations, and central nervous system defects (76–78). Microcephaly is probably the most common manifestation observed following in utero exposure to high levels of radiation in the human (79). Fetal exposure to radiation at Hiroshima resulted in microcephaly, growth retardation, and mental retardation (80–82). In his recent review of radiation teratogenesis, Brent (75) pointed out that no malformation of the limb, viscera, or other tissue has been observed unless the child also exhibits intrauterine growth retardation, microcephaly, or eye malformations.

The risk of major malformations is not increased by in utero exposure of 5 rads or less (75).

Tetracycline

The antimicrobial tetracyclines inhibit bacterial protein synthesis by preventing access of aminoacyl tRNA to the mRNA-ribosome complex (83).

Tetracycline crosses the placenta but is not concentrated by the fetus. Although tetracycline has been shown to discolor teeth (84), very high doses may depress skeletal bone growth and result in hypoplasia of tooth enamel (85).

Tetracylines complex with calcium and the organic matrix of newly forming bone without altering the crystalline structure of hydroxyapatite (85).

Thalidomide

Lenz & Knapp (86) and McBride (87) were the first to describe thalidomide-induced phocomelia. Limb defects resulted from exposure limited to a two-week period from the 27th to the 40th day of gestation: exposures from the 27th–30th days most often affected only the arms, while exposures from the 30th–33rd days (lower limb buds appear on about the 30th day) resulted in both leg and arm abnormalities (88). Although there was no association of central nervous system defects, other abnormalities included facial hemangioma, esophageal or duodenal atresia, and anomalies of the kidneys, heart, and external ears (86, 88, 89). A high proportion of the fetuses exposed during the critical period were affected.

McCredie & McBride (90) suggested that the limb-reduction defects exhibited a segmental pattern. McCredie (91) proposed that the segmental pattern was determined by the periperal nerves derived from the neural crest. McBride (92, 93) and Stokes et al (94) presented experimental evidence supporting an alternative proposal that the quantity of nerves was important: damage to the peripheral sensory nerves results in pre-axial abnormalities and greater damage results in amelia.

Stephens & McNulty (95) have confirmed that limb development exhibits a segmental pattern. However, recent studies by Streker & Stephens (96) have refuted the proposed role of peripheral nerve damage in thalidomide-induced embryopathy. A foil barrier was placed lateral to the chick neural tube to block the innervation of the wing field by the brachial plexus. A reduced source of innervation from spinal nerves anterior or posterior to the brachial plexus resulted in muscular atrophy but not in reductions or malformations of the skeleton of the wing. Therefore, both the proposal that the segmental pattern of the limb is determined by level-specific nerves and the proposal that diminished levels of innervation will result in skeletal malformations are untenable.

Lash & Saxen have postulated that thalidomide indirectly exerts its effects on limb chondrogenesis by acting upon the kidney primordia (97). Based upon an association between nephric tissue and limb development (98–100), Lash & Saxen (97) have in vitro evidence suggesting that thalidomide inhibits an interaction between metanephric tissue and associated mesenchymal tissue necessary for normal limb chondrogenesis.

The mechanism of thalidomide embryopathy is still controversial.

Thyroid: Iodides, Radioiodine, Antithyroid Drugs

Several drugs used to treat maternal hyperthyroidism (^{131}I and antithyroid drugs) and nonthyroid conditions (especially iodide-containing compounds for bronchitis and asthma) affect thyroid function. In utero exposure to these drugs may result in congenitally hypothyroid infants who will not reach their potential for physical or mental development unless treated very early following birth with thyroid hormone.

There are several case reports of congenital goiter due to in utero exposures to iodide-containing drugs (101, 102). Maternal intake of as low as 12 mg/day may result in fetal goiter (102). Iodinated contrast agents used for amniofetography have been reported to adversely affect fetal thyroid function (103).

Propylthiouracil and methimazole, used to treat thyrotoxicosis, readily cross the placenta (104). Methimazole has been associated with aplasia cutis (105, 106). Propylthiouracil is safer since the incidence of fetal goiter is low (107, 108) and there have been no observed detrimental effects on mental development (109, 110).

Radioactive iodine, ^{131}I, is a potential risk to the fetal thyroid, especially once the fetal thyroid begins to concentrate iodide at 10–12 weeks of gestation. In a retrospective study of fetuses accidentally exposed to ^{131}I during the first or first and second trimesters, six neonates out of 178 live births had hypothyroidism, while other anomalies were not statistically increased above the general population (111). Although there are few case reports in the literature, there is a definite risk of neonatal thyroid dysfunction.

Other

Although they are beyond the scope of this article, several infectious agents and maternal conditions have been associated with congenital malformations.

Rubella (112, 113), cytomegalovirus (114), toxoplasmosis (115), and syphilis (116) have all been shown to cause maldevelopment in the human. Similarly, maternal conditions such as starvation (117–119) and diabetes mellitus (120, 121) have been associated with an increased incidence of abnormalities. However, it may be difficult to determine whether a condition or a treatment for that condition during pregnancy is responsible for the malformed infant.

CONCLUSION

An estimate of the congenital malformations in man resulting from exposures to environmental agents as a single cause is 5–8% (4, 5, 122) and in combination with genetic components (multifactorial causes) is about 20% (123). We must continue to increase our knowledge of both the etiology and the mechanisms of teratogenesis so that avoidable exposures to known and possibly unrecognized environmental teratogens can be prevented in the future.

ACKNOWLEDGEMENTS

We thank Mrs. Yvonne G. Edney for secretarial assistance in the preparation of this manuscript. This work was supported in part by funds from the Foerderer Foundation, Harry Bock Charities, and NIH CA 29628.

Literature Cited

1. Carter, C. O. 1976. Genetics of common single malformations. *Br. Med. Bull.* 32:21–26
2. McKusick, V. A. 1978. *Mendelian Inheritance in Man.* Baltimore: Johns Hopkins Press. 975 pp. 5th ed.
3. Fraser, F. C. 1976. The multifactorial/threshold concept-uses and misuses. *Teratology* 14:267–80
4. Brent, R. L. 1976. Environmental factors: Miscellaneous. In *Prevention of Embryonic, Fetal, and Perinatal Disease*, ed. R. L. Brent, M. I. Harris, pp. 211–18. Bethesda, MD: DHEW Publ. No. (NIH) 76–853. 411 pp.
5. Brent, R. L. 1982. Drugs and pregnancy: Are the insert warnings too dire? *Contemp. OB-Gyn.* 20:42–49
6. Wilson, J. G. 1973. *Environment and Birth Defects.* New York: Academic. 305 pp.
7. Wilson, J. G. 1973. Mechanisms of teratogenesis. *Am. J. Anat.* 136:129–32
8. Jones, K. L., Smith, D. W., Ulleland, C. N., Streissguth, A. P. 1973. Pattern of malformation in offspring of chronic alcoholic mothers. *Lancet* 1:1267–71
9. Jones, K. L., Smith, D. W. 1973. Recognition of the fetal alcohol syndrome in early infancy. *Lancet* 2:99–101
10. Jones, K. L., Smith, D. W. 1975. The fetal alcohol syndrome. *Teratology* 12:1–10
11. Jones, K. L., Smith, D. W., Streissguth, A. P., Myrianthopoulos, N. C. 1974. Outcome in offspring of chronic alcoholic women. *Lancet* 1:1076–78
12. Mulvihill, J. J., Yeager, A. M. 1976. Fetal alcohol syndrome. *Teratology* 13:345–48
13. Streissguth, A. P., Landesman-Dwyer, S., Martin, J. C., Smith, D. W. 1980. Teratogenic effects of alcohol in humans and laboratory animals. *Science* 209:353–61
14. Veghelyi, P. V. 1983. Fetal abnormality and maternal ethanol metabolism. *Lancet* 2:53–54
15. Thiersch, J. B. 1952. Therapeutic abortions with a folic acid antagonist, 4-aminopteroylglutamic acid (4-amino P.G.A.). *Am. J. Obstet. Gynecol.* 63:1298–304
16. Goetsch, C. 1962. An evaluation of aminopterin as an abortifacient. *Am. J. Obstet. Gynecol.* 83:1474–77
17. Meltzer, H. J. 1956. Congenital anomalies due to attempted abortion with 4-aminopteroglutamic acid. *J. Am. Med. Assoc.* 161:1253
18. Warkany, J., Beaudry, P. H., Hornstein, S. 1959. Attempted abortion with aminopterin (4-aminopteroylglutamic acid). *Am. J. Dis. Child.* 97:274–81
19. Shaw, E. B., Steinbach, H. L. 1968. Aminopterin-induced fetal malformation: Survival of infant after attempted abortion. *Am. J. Dis. Child.* 115:477–82
20. Powell, H. R., Ekert, H. 1971. Methotrexate-induced congenital malformations. *Med. J. Aust.* 2:1076–77
21. Milunsky, A., Graef, J. W., Gaynor, M. F. 1968. Methotrexate-induced congenital malformations with a review of the literature. *J. Pediat.* 72:790–95
22. Skipper, H. T., Schabel, F. M. Jr. 1973. Quantitative and cytokinetic studies in experimental tumor models. In *Cancer Medicine*, ed. J. F. Holland, E. Frei III, pp. 629–50. Philadelphia: Lea & Febiger. 2018 pp.
23. Warkany, J. 1978. Aminopterin and methotrexate: Folic acid deficiency. *Teratology* 17:353–58
24. Grumbach, M. M., Conte, F. A. 1981. Disorders of sex differentiation. In *Textbook of Endocrinology*, ed. R. H. Williams, pp. 422–514. Philadelphia: W. B. Saunder. 1270 pp.
25. Moncrieff, A. 1958. Non-adrenal female pseudohermaphroditism associated with hormone administration in pregnancy. *Lancet* 2:267–68
26. Hoffman, F., Overzier, C., Uhde, G. 1955. Zur frage der hormonalen erzengung fotaler zwittenbildungen beim menschen. *Geburtshilfe Frauenheilkd.* 15:1061–70
27. Mauvais-Jarvis, P., Crepy, O., Bercovici, J. P. 1971. Further studies on the pathophysiology of testicular feminization syndrome. *J. Clin. Endocrinol. Metab.* 32:568–71
28. Jost, A. 1971. Embryonic sexual differentiation. In *Hermaphroditism, Genital Anomalies and Related Endocrine Disorders*, ed. H. W. Jones, W. W.

Scott, pp. 16–64. Baltimore: Williams & Wilkins. 564 pp. 2nd ed.

29. DiSaia, P. J. 1966. Pregnancy and delivery of a patient with a Starr-Edwards mitral valve prosthesis: Report of a case. *Obstet. Gynecol.* 29:469–72

30. Kerber, I. J., Warr, O. S., Richardson, C. 1968. Pregnancy in a patient with prosthetic mitral valve. *J. Am. Med. Assoc.* 203:223–25

31. Becker, M. H., Genieser, N. B., Finegold, M., Miranda, D., Spackman, T. 1975. Chondrodysplasia punctata. Is maternal warfarin therapy a factor? *Am. J. Dis. Child.* 129:360–62

32. Pettiflor, J. M., Benson, R. 1975. Congenital malformations associated with the administration of oral anticoagulants during pregnancy. *J. Pediat.* 86:459–62

33. Hall, J. G., Pauli, R. M., Wilson, K. M. 1980. Maternal and fetal sequelae of anticoagulation during pregnancy. *Am. J. Med.* 68:122–40

34. Barr, M., Burdi, A. R. 1976. Warfarin-associated embryopathy in a 17 week abortus. *Teratology* 14:129–34

35. Warkany, J. 1975. A warfarin embryopathy? *Am. J. Dis. Child.* 129:287–88

36. Warkany, J. 1976. Warfarin embryopathy. *Teratology* 14:205–9

37. Stenflo, J., Suttie, J. W. 1977. Vitamin K-dependent formation of gamma-carboxyglutamic acid. *Ann. Rev. Biochem.* 46:157–72

38. Bongiovanni, A. M., DiGeorge, A. M., Grumbach, M. M. 1959. Masculinization of the female infant associated with estrogenic therapy alone during gestation. Four cases. *J. Clin. Endocrinol. Metab.* 19:1004–11

39. Herbst, A. L., Ulfelder, H., Poskanzer, D. C. 1971. Adenocarcinoma of the vagina. Association of maternal stilbestrol therapy with tumor appearance in young women. *N. Engl. J. Med.* 284:878–81

40. Herbst, A. L., Kurman, R. J., Scully, R. E., Poskanzer, D. C. 1972. Clear-cell adenocarcinoma of the genital tract in young females. *N. Engl. J. Med.* 287:1259–64

41. Greenwald, P., Barlow, J. J., Nasca, P. C., Burnett, W. S. 1971. Vaginal cancer after maternal treatment with synthetic estrogens. *N. Engl. J. Med.* 285:390–92

42. Herbst, A. L., Scully, R. E., Robboy, S. J. 1975. Effects of maternal DES ingestion on the female genital tract. *Hosp. Prac.* 10:51–57

43. Herbst, A. L., Poskanzer, D. C., Robboy, S. J., Friedlander, L., Scully, R E. 1975. Prenatal exposure to stilbestrol: A

prospective comparison of exposed female offspring with unexposed controls. *N. Engl. J. Med.* 292:334–39

44. O'Brien, P. C., Noller, K. L., Robboy, S. J., Barnes, A. B., Kaufman, R. H., Tilley, B. C., Townsend, D. E. 1979. Vaginal epithelial changes in young women enrolled in the National Cooperative Diethylstilbestrol Adenosis (DESAD) Project. *Obstet. Gynecol.* 53:300–8

45. Gill, W. B., Schumacher, G. F. B., Bibbo, M. 1976. Structural and functional abnormalities in the sex organs of male offspring of mothers treated with diethylstilbestrol (DES). *J. Reprod. Med.* 16:147–53

46. Ulfelder, H. 1976. DES—transplacental teratogen—and possibly also carcinogen. *Teratology* 13:101–4

47. Speidel, B. D., Meadow, S. R. 1972. Maternal epilepsy and abnormalities of the fetus and newborn. *Lancet* 2:839–43

48. Fedrick, J. 1973. Epilepsy and pregnancy: A report from Oxford record linkage study. *Br. Med. J.* 2:442–48

49. Monson, R. R., Rosenberg, L., Hartz, S. C., Shapiro, S., Heinonen, O. P., Slone, D. 1973. Diphenylhydantoin and selected malformations. *N. Engl. J. Med.* 289:1049–52

50. Barr, M., Pozanski, A. K., Schmickel, R. D. 1974. Digital hypoplasia and anticonvulsants during gestation, a teratogenic syndrome. *J. Pediatr.* 4:254–56

51. Hill, R. M., Verniaud, W. M., Horning, M. G., McCulley, L. B., Morgan, N. F. 1974. Infants exposed in utero to antiepileptic drugs. *Am. J. Dis. Child.* 127:645–53

52. Hanson, J. W., Myrianthopoulos, N. C., Harvey, M. A. S., Smith, D. W. 1976. Risks to the offspring of women treated with hydantoin anticonvulsants, with emphasis on the fetal hydantoin syndrome. *J. Pediat.* 89:662–68

53. Shapiro, S., Hartz, S. C., Siskind, V., Mitchell, A. A., Stone, D., et al. 1976. Anticonvulsants and parental epilepsy in the development of birth defects. *Lancet* 1:272–75

54. Woodbury, D. M., Penry, J. K., Schmidt, R. P., eds. 1972. *Antiepileptic Drugs.* New York: Raven. 536 pp.

55. Matsumoto, H., Koya, G., Takeuchi, T. 1965. Fetal Minamata disease: A neuropathological study of two cases of intrauterine intoxication by a methylmercury compound. *J. Neuropathol. Exp. Neurol.* 24:563–74

56. Murakami, U. 1972. Organic mercury problem affecting intrauterine life. In

Advances in Experimental Medicine and Biology, ed. M. A. Klingberg, A. A. Abramovici, J. Chemke, 27:301–36. New York: Plenum. 559 pp.

57. Snyder, R. D. 1971. Congenital mercury poisoning. *N. Engl. J. Med.* 284:1014–16

58. Amin-Zaki, L., Elhassani, S., Majeed, M. A., Clarkson, T. W., Doherty, R. A., Greenwood, M. R. 1974. Intra-uterine methylmercury poisoning in Iraq. *Pediatrics* 54:587–95

59. Amin-Zaki, L., Majeed, M. A., Elhassani, S. B., Clarkson, T. W., Greenwood, M. R., Doherty, R. A. 1979. Prenatal mercury poisoning: Clinical observations over five years. *Am. J. Dis. Child.* 133:172–77

60. Harada, M. 1978. Minamata disease: Intrauterine methylmercury poisoning. *Teratology* 18:285–88

61. Zackai, E. H., Melman, W. J., Neiderer, B., Hanson, J. W. 1975. The fetal trimethadione syndrome. *J. Pediatr.* 87:280–84

62. German, J., Kowal, A., Ehlers, K. H. 1970. Trimethadione and human teratogenesis. *Teratology* 3:349–62

63. Feldman, G. L., Weaver, D. D., Lovrien, E. W. 1977. The fetal trimethadione syndrome. *Am. J. Dis. Child.* 131:1389–92

64. Goldman, A. S., Yaffe, S. J. 1978. Fetal trimethadione syndrome. *Teratology* 17:103–6

65. Kuratsune, M., Yoshimura, T., Matsuzaka, J., Yamaguchi, A. 1972. Epidemiologic study on Yusho, a poisoning caused by ingestion of rice oil contaminated with a commercial brand of polychlorinated biphenyls. *Environ. Health Perspect.* 1:119–28

66. Rogan, W. J. 1982. PCBs and colacolored babies: Japan, 1968, and Taiwan, 1979. *Teratology* 26:259–61

67. Hayles, A. B., Nolan, R. B. 1957. Masculinization of the female fetus, possibly related to administration of progesterone during pregnancy. *Proc. Staff Meet., Mayo Clin.* 32:200–3

68. Sweet, R. A., Schrott, H. G., Kurland, R., Culp, A. S. 1974. Study of the incidence of hypospadias in Rochester, Minnesota, 1940–1970, and a case-control comparison of possible etiologic factors. *Mayo Clin. Proc.* 49:52–58

69. Aarskog, D. 1979. Maternal progestins as a possible cause of hypospadias. *N. Engl. J. Med.* 300:75–78

70. Wilkins, L., Jones, H. W., Holman, G. H., Stempfel, R. S. 1958. Masculinization of the female fetus associated with administration of oral and intramuscular progestins during gestation: Non-adrenal female pseudohermaphrodism. *J. Clin. Endocrinol. Metab.* 18:559–85

71. Wilkins, L. 1960. Masculinization due to orally given progestins. *J. Am. Med. Assoc.* 172:1028–32

72. Jacobson, B. D. 1962. Hazards of norethindrone therapy during pregnancy. *Am. J. Obstet. Gynecol.* 84:962–68

73. Grumbach, M. M., Ducharme, J. R., Moloshok, R. E. 1959. On the fetal masculinizing action of certain oral progestins. *J. Clin. Endocrinol. Metab.* 19:1369–80

74. Wilson, J. G., Brent, R. L. 1981. Are female sex hormones teratogenic? *Am. J. Obstet. Gynecol.* 141:567–80

75. Brent, R. L. 1980. Radiation teratogenesis. *Teratology* 21:281–98

76. Goldstein, L., Murphy, D. P. 1929. Microcephalic idiocy following radium therapy for uterine cancer during pregnancy. *Am. J. Obstet. Gynecol.* 18:189–95, 281–83

77. Murphy, D. P., Goldstein, L. 1930. Micromelia in a child irradiated in utero. *Surg. Gynecol. Obstet.* 50:79–80

78. Dekaban, A. S. 1968. Abnormalities in children exposed to x-radiation during various stages of gestation: Tentative timetable of radiation injury to the human fetus. *J. Nucl. Med.* 9:471–77

79. Miller, R. W., Mulvihill, J. J. 1976. Small head size after atomic irradiation. *Teratology* 14:355–58

80. Miller, R. W. 1969. Delayed radiation effects in atomic bomb survivors. *Science* 166:569–74

81. Wood, J. W., Johnson, K. G., Omori, Y., Kawamoto, S., Keehn, R. J. 1967. Mental retardation in children exposed in utero to the atomic bombs in Hiroshima and Nagasaki. *Am. J. Public Health* 57:1381–90

82. Wood, J. W., Johnson, K. G., Omori, Y. 1967. In utero exposure to the Hiroshima atomic bomb. An evaluation of head size and mental retardation: Twenty years later. *Pediatrics* 39:385–92

83. Weisblum, B., Davies, J. 1968. Antibiotic inhibitors of the bacterial ribosome. *Bacteriol. Rev.* 32:493–528

84. Baden, E. 1970. Environmental pathology of the teeth. In *Thomas' Oral Pathology*, ed. R. J. Gorlin, H. M. Goldman, pp. 189–91. St. Louis: C. V. Mosby. 1139 pp. 6th ed.

85. Cohlan, S. Q., Bevelander, G., Tiamsic, T. 1963. Growth inhibition of prematures receiving tetracycline: Clinical and

laboratory investigation. *Am. J. Dis. Child.* 105:453–61

86. Lenz, W., Knapp, K. 1962. Thalidomide embryopathy. *Arch. Environ. Health* 5:100–5

87. McBride, W. G. 1961. Thalidomide and congenital abnormalities. *Lancet* 2:1358

88. McBride, W. G. 1977. Thalidomide embryopathy. *Teratology* 16:79–82

89. Knapp, K., Lenz, W., Nowack, E. 1962. Multiple congenital abnormalities. *Lancet* 2:725

90. McCredie, J., McBride, W. G. 1973. Some congenital abnormalities: Possibly due to embryonic peripheral neuropathy. *Clin. Radiol.* 24:204–11

91. McCredie, J. 1977. Sclerotome subtraction: A radiologic interpretation of reduction deformities of the limbs. In *Birth Defects: Original Article Series,* ed. D. Bergsma, R. B. Lowry, 13(3D):65–77. New York: Alan R. Liss. 298 pp.

92. McBride, W. G. 1974. Fetal nerve cell degeneration produced by thalidomide in rabbits. *Teratology* 10:283–92

93. McBride, W. G. 1976. Studies of the etiology of thalidomide dysmorphogenesis. *Teratology* 14:71–87

94. Stokes, P., Lykke, A. W., McBride, W. G. 1976. Ultrastructural changes in the dorsal root ganglia evoked by thalidomide, preceding limb development. *Experientia* 32:597–98

95. Stephens, T. D., McNulty, T. R. 1981. Evidence for a metameric pattern in the development of the chick humerus. *J. Embryol. Exp. Morphol.* 61:191–205

96. Strecker, T. R., Stephens, T. D. 1983. Peripheral nerves do not play a trophic role in limb skeletal morphogenesis. *Teratology* 27:159–67

97. Lash, J. W., Saxen, L. 1972. Human teratogenesis: In vitro studies on thalidomide-inhibited chondrogenesis. *Develop. Biol.* 28:61–70

98. Muchmore, W. 1957. Differentiation of trunk mesoderm in *Amblystoma maculatum.* II. Relation of the size of presumptive somite explants to subsequent differentiation. *J. Exp. Zool.* 134:293–314

99. Lash, J. W. 1963. Studies on the ability of embryonic mesonephros explants to form cartilage. *Develop. Biol.* 6:219–32

100. Lash, J. W. 1964. Normal embryology and teratogenesis. *Am. J. Obstet. Gynecol.* 90:1193–207

101. Martin, M. M., Rento, R. D. 1962. Iodide goiter with hypothyroidism in 2 newborn infants. *J. Pediatr.* 61:94–99

102. Carswell, F., Kerr, M. M., Hutchison, J. H. 1970. Congenital goiter and hypothyroidism produced by maternal ingestion of iodides. *Lancet* 1:1241–43

103. Rodesch, F., Camus, M., Ermans, A. M., Dodion, J., Delange, F. 1976. Adverse effect of amniofetography on fetal thyroid function. *Am. J. Obstet. Gynecol.* 126:723–26

104. Marchant, B., Brownlie, B. E. W., Hart, D. M., Horton, P. W., Alexander, W. D. 1977. The placental transfer of propylthiouracil, methimazole and carbimazole. *J. Clin. Endocrinol. Metab.* 45:1187–93

105. Milham, S. Jr., Elledge, W. 1972. Maternal methimazole and congenital defects in children. *Teratology* 5:125

106. Mujtaba, Q., Burrow, G. M. 1975. Treatment of hyperthyroidism in pregnancy with propylthiouracil and methimazole. *Obstet. Gynecol.* 46:282–86

107. Burrow, G. N. 1965. Neonatal goiter after maternal propylthiouracil therapy. *J. Clin. Endocrinol.* 25:403–8

108. Cheron, R. G., Kaplan, M. M., Lasen, P. R., Selenkow, H. A., Crigler, J. F. Jr. 1981. Neonatal thyroid function after propylthiouracil therapy for maternal Graves' disease. *N. Engl. J. Med.* 304:525–28

109. Burrow, G. N., Klatskin, E. H., Genel, M. 1978. Intellectual development in children whose mothers received propylthiouracil during pregnancy. *Yale J. Biol. Med.* 51:151–56

110. McCarroll, A. M., Hutchinson, M., McAuley, R., Montgomery, D. A. D. 1976. Long-term assessment of children exposed in utero to carbimazole. *Arch. Dis. Child.* 51:532–36

111. Stoffer, S. S., Hamburger, J. I. 1976. Inadvertent ^{131}I therapy for hyperthyroidism in the first trimester of pregnancy. *J. Nucl. Med.* 17:146–49

112. Gregg, N. M. 1941. Congenital cataract following German measles in the mother. *Trans. Ophthalmol. Soc. Aust.* 3:35–46

113. Korones, S. B. 1978. Congenital rubella—an encapsulated review. *Teratology* 14:111–14

114. Reynolds, D. W., Stagno, S., Alford, C. A. 1978. Congenital cytomegalovirus infection. *Teratology* 17:179–82

115. Larsen, J. W. Jr. 1977. Congenital toxoplasmosis. *Teratology* 15:213–18

116. Grossman, J. III. 1977. Congenital syphilis. *Teratology* 16:217–24

117. Smith, C. 1947. The effect of wartime starvation in Holland upon pregnancy and its product. *Am. J. Obstet. Gynecol.* 53:599–606

118. Smith, C. 1947. Effects of maternal undernutrition upon the newborn infant

in Holland (1944–1945). *J. Pediat.* 30: 229–43

119. Stein, Z., Susser, M., Saeger, G., Marolla, F. 1975. *Famine and Human Development. The Dutch Hunger Winter of 1944/45.* New York: Oxford Univ. Press. 284 pp.

120. Mills, J. L. 1982. Malformations in infants of diabetic mothers. *Teratology* 25:385–94

121. Chung, C. S., Myrianthopoulos, N. C. 1975. Factors affecting risks of congenital malformations. II. Effect of maternal diabetes. In *Birth Defects: Original Article Series,* ed. D. Bergsma, 11(10):23–35. Miami: Symposia Specialists. 38 pp.

122. Kalter, H., Warkanay, J. 1983. Congenital malformations. Etiologic factors and their role in prevention. (Second of two parts). *N. Engl. J. Med.* 308:491–97

123. Fraser, F. C. 1977. Relation of animal studies to the problem in man. In *Handbook of Teratology,* ed. J. G. Wilson, F. C. Fraser, 1:75–96. New York: Plenum. 476 pp.

Ann. Rev. Pharmacol. Toxicol. 1984. 24:501–24

MECHANISMS OF ACTION OF VANADIUM

Bohdan R. Nechay

Department of Pharmacology and Toxicology, University of Texas Medical Branch, Galveston, Texas 77550

INTRODUCTION

Vanadium is widely distributed, the twenty-first most abundant element in the Earth's crust, with an average content of 135 ppm. In sea water, vanadium ranks thirty-fourth in abundance, with an average concentration of only 2 ppb. Because it evolved as an essential element for certain forms of life and also because of its wide industrial use, the biological actions of vanadium are of interest to scientists. Excellent accounts of the history and previous knowledge of vanadium are available. (1–7).

The chemistry of vanadium is complex because the metal can exist in oxidation states from -1 to $+5$ and forms polymers frequently (8). Recently Rubinson (9) reviewed the material concerning the form of biochemically active vanadium. The following generalizations appear justified. At low-normal concentrations in mammals and birds, any free vanadium will be in hydrated, monomeric form. In the body fluids at pH 4–8, the predominant species will be VO_3^- ($+5$ oxidation state), vanadate (metavanadate). VO_3^- may enter certain cells by an anion transport system and be reduced by glutathione to VO^{2+} ($+4$ oxidation state), vanadyl. By way of speculation, the oxidation-reduction reactions may be as follows: $H^+ + VO_3^- + 2GSH \rightleftarrows VO^{2+} + G_2S_2 + OH^- + e^- + H_2O$. Extensive binding to extra- and intracellular ligands may be expected. Since phosphate and Mg^{2+} are ubiquitous in biological processes, VO_3^- as the analogue of phosphate and VO^{2+}, which resembles the size of Mg^{2+} (respective ionic radii: 0.60 and 0.65 Å), potentially have many biochemical and cellular sites of action. For example, vanadium compounds inhibit ATP phosphohydrolases, ribonuclease, adenylate kinase, phosphofructokinase, squalene synthetase, glyceraldehyde-3-phosphate dehydrogenase (10),

501

glucose-6-phosphatase (11), and phosphotyrosyl-protein phosphatase (12). The recent finding that VO_3^- is one of the most potent known inhibitors of Na^+ + K^+ ATPase (13–15), and a suggestion that vanadium may be a physiologic regulator of the Na^+ pump (16), have stimulated much research activity, and several reviews and editorials on the long-elusive role of vanadium in biology (9, 10, 17–25) have appeared.

This review is confined to selected aspects of vanadium interaction with transport ATPases and its expression on cellular, organ, and whole animal levels. For a biological perspective, updates on biochemistry, distribution, nutrition, and as yet unexplained observations on the effects of vanadium will be included. The symbol VO_3^- (for vanadate) will be used instead of the names of various salts of metavanadate (VO_3^-) or orthovanadate (VO_4^{3-}) employed in the works referenced.

DISTRIBUTION OF NATURALLY OCCURRING VANADIUM IN BIOLOGIC MATERIALS

The knowledge of vanadium content in biologic materials is far from complete. In addition to natural variability, inappropriate sensitivity of analytical methods, interference by other elements, nonavailability of standard reference materials in the past, and easy contamination of samples have contributed to a wide spread of vanadium values reported in the literature (26, 27). The most sensitive of commonly used methods for measuring vanadium are the techniques of neutron activation analysis (NAA) (26) and flameless atomic absorption spectroscopy (AAS) (28–9); detection limits are well under 1 ng of vanadium. The values given below are in ng per ml or g wet weight (5.1 = 10^{-7} M).

Humans

Byrne & Kosta (26) and Cornelis et al (27, 30) scrutinized published information on vanadium concentration in the blood plasma or serum (ranging from 0.016–570) and whole blood (ranging from 0.5–1500) of healthy individuals and concluded that much of the disparity in these figures was methodological. The lowest ever reported vanadium serum concentration determined by NAA ranged from 0.016–0.139 in 37 women and from 0.024–0.939 in 37 men (30). No correlation was found between vanadium content and age or serum concentrations of cholesterol, triglycerides, or lipoproteins. The lowest mean vanadium concentration determined by NAA in whole blood was 0.5 (26). Values recently obtained by AAS were 3 for serum (29), 8 for plasma (31), and 6 for whole blood (32). According to only a few measurements, erythrocytes appear to have a vanadium content similar to that of plasma (30, 32). By a photometric method, <1 to 11 (<1 to 24 in chimney sweepers) was found in whole blood

(33). Byrne et al (26, 34–36) reported (and compared with published values) the following vanadium concentrations (by NAA) in tissues and body fluids: bone and teeth, <1–8; liver, 5–19; kidney, 3–7; heart, 1; skeletal muscle, <1–7; spleen and thyroid, 3–4; pancreas, 14; brain, fat, urine, <1; lung, 13–140; hair, 12–87; bile, <1–2; dry feces, 141–2210; dry milk and colostrum, <1–1. Other workers reported: liver, 3–13 (NAA) (37); kidney, 67–194 (AAS) (38); placenta, 3 (photometry) (39). The US Environmental Protection Agency (40) listed vanadium ranges of 4–140 for hair and 4–625 for nails. Mean vanadium content in neonates' hair was 50 (NAA) (41). Vanadium concentrations in hair appear to be sensitive to environmental exposure (42). US city dwellers showed increased lung concentrations in the fifth and particularly sixth decades of life (43).

A recent estimate of the total body pool of vanadium in the "reference man" was 100–200 μg (26), in contrast to Schroeder's earlier calculation of 22 mg (4). The daily dietary intake of vanadium was estimated as 10–60 μg (26, 34, 44, 45), with excretion mainly in the feces and urine (45). The mean urinary output per 24 hours was 10 μg (29). Intake via air and water may be significant (6, 26).

Other Mammals (26, 28, 32, 46, 47)

Researchers have shown the following values in other mammals: bone, 20–40 (pig, sheep); bone marrow, <1 (pig); liver, 2–10 (beef, pig, rat); kidney, 9–34 (rat, pig, dog, rabbit); heart, <1–9 (pig, rat, rabbit); skeletal muscle, <1–14 (beef, pig, rabbit, horse); brain, <1–3 (rat, cow); lung, 5–25 (rabbit, beef); fat, <1–2 (pork); butter, 1; milk, <1–3; plasma, 2–5 (rat); gelatin, 9–43; whole mouse, 66.

Chicken (26, 28, 48)

Researchers have shown the following values in chicken: dry bone, 370–760; (turkey bone, 86); liver, 38; kidney, 18 (107 on 3.5 μg vanadium/g diet); heart, 5–9; light muscle, 2–22; dark muscle, 12; egg white, <1–2; egg yolk, 2–21.

Aquatic Animals (26, 28, 47, 49, 50)

Researchers have shown the following values in aquatic animals: salt water fish, 3–28 (cod, mackerel, sardines, tuna); fish bone, 125–2000 (mackerel, tuna); fresh water trout, 0.4; lobster, 5–43; scallop, 22; dry blue crab, mussels, oysters, white shrimp, 455–1840. Vanadium content in shrimp and oysters was higher in specimens taken from industrialized areas compared to nonindustrialized sections around Galveston Island, Texas (49). An extensive list of vanadium concentrations in other biological systems has been published (1).

Plants (26, 28, 32, 47)

Researchers have shown the following values in plants: numerous fruits, vegetables, nuts, oils, <1–5; lettuce, radish, spinach, 21–52; dill, 140; dill seed, 431; parsley, 790; cereals, grains, beans, flour, bread, <1–93; dry wild mushrooms, 50–2000 (26 species); dry *Amanita muscaria,* 51,000 (as amavadin) (1); cocoa powder, 610; dry tea leaf, 150; dry black pepper, 204–987; wine, 4–32; beer, 8; tobacco, 1000–8000 (10 types); drinking water <1–2.

DISTRIBUTION OF EXPERIMENTALLY ADMINISTERED VANADIUM

The most complete picture of vanadium distribution emerges from autoradiographic studies of sagittal sections of whole mice prepared five minutes to seven days after an intravenous injection of $^{48}V_2O_5$. These studies included pregnant mice (51). Half-life of ^{48}V in blood was <1 hour. Bones and teeth had the highest persistent concentrations of vanadium, which reached a peak 1–2 days after the injection; ^{48}V accumulated to the greatest extent in zones of ossification. [In a similar study on 7–9 day-old rats, the greatest ^{48}V uptake was found in parts of the teeth and bones, where rapid mineralization was taking place (52)]. In soft tissues, ^{48}V rose rapidly after the injection and declined faster than in bone. The highest concentrations were found in the kidney cortex, the liver with a spotty distribution, and the lung parenchyma, with no radioactivity in the bronchi. Medium levels of radioactivity were found in the skin and salivary glands, with low concentrations in skeletal and heart muscles, cartilage, spleen, and brain. Intestinal and urinary bladder contents were high in vanadium. In the pregnant mice, high concentrations of vanadium were visible in the placenta, especially the visceral yolk sac epithelium, the fetal skeleton, and the mammary gland. Other investigators (53–61) found similar distribution in selected organs of mice or rats after giving various vanadium compounds by different routes. Some accumulation in testes was also noted. A similar organ and subcellular distribution of vanadium after intravenous injections in rats of labelled cationic and anionic compounds with different vanadium oxidation states suggests an in vivo conversion of dissimilar vanadium compounds to common vanadium species (62–63). In blood, less than 5% of radioactivity was associated with erthrocytes and over 95% was in plasma; some vanadium was bound to transferrin [liver and spleen ferritins also bind vanadium (64, 65)]. In fractions of liver and kidney homogenates, nuclei contained the highest quantity of vanadium, followed in descending order by mitochrondria, cytosol, lysomes, and microsomes.

VO^{2+} is used in electron microscopy; it stains cytoplasmic organelles, collagen fibrils, glycogen granules, secretion granules, and ribosomes (66).

An autoradiographic study on fish of ^{48}V uptake from water showed an accumulation in skin, fins, intestines, liver, and bones. Vanadium content was low in the brain, eye, and muscles (47).

NUTRITIONAL IMPORTANCE

Vanadium is an essential nutrient for the chick and the rat (7, 67–71). Deficiencies have been induced in chicks and rats raised in vanadium-free isolator systems on diets containing <30 or <100 ng/g respectively. The requirement for growth probably lies between 50 and 500 ng/g. These figures appear high in view of the much lower vanadium content of most feeds (see the section on naturally occurring vanadium distribution above). However, in poultry farming too much vanadium is of concern because some rock phosphorus feed additives may contain high concentrations of vanadium; acceptable commercial chicken diets contain 1400–5400 ng V/g (72). Wild birds may obtain sufficient vanadium from grit and soil if their requirements are as high as those of chickens.

Vanadium-deficient chicks showed reduced vanadium concentrations in kidney, liver, and heart, reduced weight gain and feather growth, retarded skeletal development, increased plasma triglyceride concentrations and variably altered plasma concentrations of cholesterol. Signs of vanadium deficiency in the rat included impaired fertility, with a marked reduction in fourth-generation females and reduced pup survival. Deficiency in chicks and rats resulted in increased hematocrits. Evidence suggests that vanadium does not protect against experimental dental carries, as was once proposed (7, 35, 53).

Human diploid fibroblasts require 0.25 ng/ml of vanadium for optimal clonal growth. However, considerable background growth occurs in the absence of added VO_3^- (73). VO_3^- appears to act synergistically with epidermal growth factor in stimulating fibroblast DNA synthesis (74).

The mechanism of vanadium deficiency is not understood. No naturally occurring vanadium-deficiency disease has been described. No natural, functional mammalian or avian vanadium-containing metalloprotein is known.

$Na^+ + K^+$ ATPase

Vanadium has been known since 1965 to inhibit $Na^+ + K^+$ ATPase (75). However, it was shown only recently by three independent laboratories that certain vanadium compounds are among the most potent known inhibitors of this enzyme system (13–15). Cantley et al (13) and Quist & Hokin (15) tested VO_3^- because they identified it as an inhibitory contaminant present in certain ATP preparations (76–80). During a survey of metallic inhibitors of $Na^+ + K^+$ ATPase, Nechay & Saunders (14) worked with V_2O_5 dissolved in NaOH, which yields VO_3^- in solution, and discovered, together with Cantley et al (16), the inhibitory properties of this ion. In view of the physicochemical properties of vanadium, its interaction with $Na^+ + K^+$ ATPase, its nutritional requirement, and its distribution in tissues, Cantley et al (16, 81) postulated that VO_3^- is a potential regulator of the Na^+ pump. Beaugé & Glynn (76) also considered a similar physiologic role for the inhibitor contained in samples of ATP before it was identified as vanadium because its effect could be altered by K^+.

VO_3^- binds to one high- and one low-affinity site of the enzyme molecule [under optimal conditions the dissociation constants are 4×10^{-9} M and 5×10^{-7} M respectively (16, 82)] and interferes with the activity by slowing $E_2 \rightarrow E_1$ conformational change (83, 84). The high-affinity VO_3^- site corresponds to the low-affinity ATP site and vice versa (16); ATP reduces VO_3^- binding (85, 86) and inhibition (14, 16). Mg^{2+} is required for the binding of VO_3^- to the enzyme (80, 85) and inhibition of the $E_2 \rightarrow E_1$ conformational change (84), and it facilitates inhibition of the enzyme's activity (14–16, 87, 88). Na^+ promotes $E_2 \rightarrow E_1$ conformational change, interferes with VO_3^- binding (85), and opposes inhibition of enzymatic activity (14, 87). Na^+ may also act by displacing K^+ (87). An effect of K^+ in facilitating inhibition (14, 16, 87) may be to displace Na^+ from sites at which it activates the enzyme (88). K^+ is not required for VO_3^- binding (85). Ca^{2+} or Mn^{2+} can substitute for Mg^{2+} in promoting VO_3^- binding, although Ca^{2+} is less effective and Mn^{2+} more effective than Mg^{2+} (85, 86, 89). Cations (Tl^+, Rb^+, Cs^+, NH^+, Li^+) that substitute for K^+ as activators of the enzyme also increase VO_3^- inhibition (87, 90, 91).

Overall, in a model in which VO_3^- can bind only to the E_2 conformational state, agents that favor the E_2 state, such as Mg^{2+}, K^+, ouabain, and dimethyl sulfoxide, increase VO_3^- binding, whereas those that favor the E_1 state, such as ATP, Na^+, and oligomycin, decrease VO_3^- binding (85, 92–95). VO_3^- is able to promote the binding of ouabain to $Na^+ + K^+$ ATPase in the absence of ATP (89, 92); based on this finding, a potentially clinically useful method was developed for measuring the number of ouabain binding sites in muscle biopsies (96). VO_3^- was reported to lower pH optimum for isolated renal $Na^+ + K^+$ ATPase activity from 7.8 to 7.0 (97).

Agents that interfere with VO_3^- inhibition include bovine serum albumin (14), which probably acts by chelation; anions such as citrate (14) and EDTA (14, 98), which may displace the anionic VO_3^- from the enzyme; reducing agents such as glutathione (90, 99), ascorbate (14, 90), NADH, methylene blue, imipramine, and chlorpromazine (100, 101), which convert the VO_3^- to less active VO^{2+}; and catecholamines, which may both bind and reduce VO_3^- (15, 98, 102, 103, 235).

Incorporation of $Na^+ + K^+$ ATPase in lipid bilayers confers high ion channel conductance when a cation gradient is present across the planar membrane, and removal of the gradient results in low conductance. The high but not the low conductance state is inhibited by ouabain and VO_3^- (104).

In human erythrocytes (105, 106) and squid axons (107), VO_3^- is an effective inhibitor of the $Na^+ + K^+$ pump only when it interacts with the cytoplasmic surface of the $Na^+ + K^+$ ATPase, since VO_3^- binds to the phosphate site on the enzyme, located inside the cell. External K^+ (and Rb^+, Cs^+, NH^+, Li^+) controls VO_3^- inhibition of $Na^+ + K^+$ ATPase activity by an allosteric mechanism: low concentrations activate Na^+ efflux, high concentrations inhibit it (84, 105, 107).

$^{48}VO_3^-$ rapidly enters the erythrocyte, possibly by the same anion transport system as phosphate; there is also a slow equilibration process (56, 99, 106, 108). Inside the cell, VO_3^- is reduced nonenzymatically by glutathione (99), and probably by NADH, ascorbate, and catechols, to VO_3^- (56), a less active inhibitor of the $Na^+ + K^+$ ATPase activity (81, 90, 102, 109, 110). Similarly, entry of VO_3^- into rat adipocytes and its reduction to VO^{2+} has been reported (111). Also, after systemic administration of VO_3^- to rats, +4 is the predominant oxidation state of vanadium in homogenate of kidney and liver and subcellular liver fractions (112, 113). Binding of VO^{2+} to ATP (114, 115) and other phosphate and carboxyl ligands protects it from oxidation to VO_3^- (236), which would otherwise tend to occur at the intracellular pH. It is conceivable that the oxidation-reduction reactions could supply an appropriate concentration of free VO_3^- to modify the $Na^+ + K^+$ pump activity. However, the quantitative aspects and the physiologic control of free intracellular VO_3^- concentrations have yet to be established.

VO_3^- inhibits transepithelial Na^+ transport when applied at a high concentration (10^{-3} M) to the mucosal (but not to the serosal) surface of frog skin and toad bladder preparations (116, 117). Equally high VO_3^- concentration is required to inhibit $Na^+ + K^+$ ATPase activity in toad bladder homogenates. In keeping with the known ability of K^+ to promote the binding of VO_3^- and inhibition of enzyme activity, K^+ potentiates the VO_3^- effect on Na^+ transport in the toad bladder. VO_3^- exhibits delayed effects on both the Na^+ transport and the enzyme activity (117). The action of VO_3^- is not limited to $Na^+ + K^+$ ATPase, since it also blocks cyclic AMP-induced stimulation of Na^+ and water transport in amphibian epithelia (116, 118) and the H^+ pump in the turtle urinary bladder (119).

Of the 5b group of elements, niobate and tantalate are less effective $Na^+ + K^+$ ATPase (fish gills) inhibitors than VO_3^- (120).

$Ca^{2+} + Mg^{2+}$ ATPase

Studies have been done mainly on enzymes from sarcoplasmic reticulum of mammalian skeletal muscle and heart and from human erythrocytes. The red cell $Ca^{2+} + Mg^{2+}$ ATPase is several times more resistant to VO_3^- than $Na^+ + K^+$ ATPase (121). The $Ca^{2+} + Mg^{2+}$ ATPase of sacroplasmic reticulum requires at least 10 times higher concentration of VO_3^- for 50% inhibition than that of erythrocytes (122–124). It is generally agreed that Ca^{2+} induces conformational transition of $E_2 \rightarrow E_1$ and stabilizes the E_1 state (125). VO_3^- stabilizes the E_2 state and inhibits the Ca^{2+}-induced conformational change. VO_3^- binds to the Ca^{2+}-free enzyme in a process that requires Mg^{2+} and is competitively antagonized by phosphate and ATP; the high concentration of ATP required indicates binding of VO_3^- to the low-affinity binding site. A similar number of sites for VO_3^- binding and phosphorylation suggests that the stabilization of the Ca^{2+}-free conformation is due to formation of a stable E-Mg-V complex at the site of phosphorylation (123, 126). The activators of the enzyme Mg^{2+}, K^+, Na^+ and calmodulin facilitate inhibition by VO_3^-, while ATP and Ca^{2+} at concentrations higher than 5×10^{-5} M protect (121, 124, 127, 128). Li^+ does not substitute for K^+ in this system (121).

In reconstituted erythrocyte ghosts, intracellular VO_3^- (5×10^{-5} M) inhibits active Ca^{2+} efflux; this inhibition is promoted by intracellular Mg^{2+} and K^+ and is antagonized by extracellular Ca^{2+} (129). The sensitivity of the Ca^{2+} pump to VO_3^- in vesicles made of purified red cell $Ca^{2+} + Mg^{2+}$ ATPase is similar to that observed in whole erythrocytes ghosts (130). In the intact red cell, external VO_3^- (5×10^{-5} M) does not inhibit the Ca^{2+} pump (131). When exposed to 5×10^{-4} M VO_3^-, fresh erythrocytes become highly labelled with externally added Ca^{2+}, which suggests some penetration of VO_3^- into the cells as well as inhibition of the outwardly directed Ca^{2+} pumping ATPase (132). The VO_3^--induced accumulation of Ca^{2+} by red cells causes a massive efflux of K^+, suggesting either an activation of the Ca^{2+}-sensitive K^+ channel in the erythrocyte membrane (132) or that the intracellular VO^{2+} metabolite, similarly to Ca^{2+}, Mg^{2+}, and Pb^{2+}, can open the K^+ channel (133).

The newly characterized $Ca^{2+} + Mg^{2+}$ ATPase of dog heart sarcolemma is about as sensitive to VO_3^- (Ki = 0.5 µM) as the $Na^+ + K^+$ ATPase. This high VO_3^- sensitivity has been used to distinguish the Ca^{2+} ATPase activity of sarcolemmal vesicles from that of the contaminating sarcoplasmic reticulum vesicles in heart microsomal fractions. The sarcolemmal enzyme could be responsible for ejecting Ca^{2+} during resting conditions when its intracellular concentration is very low (134). Also, in the intestinal smooth muscle, two Ca^{2+} transport activities resembling the sarcoplasmic reticulum and sarcolemmal Ca^{2+} pumps have been differentiated by sensitivity to VO_3^- (135).

VO_3^- inhibits uncoupled (probably Ca^{2+} ATPase-dependent) Ca^{2+} efflux from squid axon (136) and isolated rat neurohypophyses (137). The Na^+-Ca^{2+} exchange is not affected. ATP-dependent Ca^{2+} uptake by microsomal fractions of rat salivary glands is inhibited by VO_3^- (138). Isolated from rat livers,

Ca^{2+}-pumping ATPase of the endoplasmic reticulum (139), but not that of plasma membrane (140), is sensitive to VO_3^-.

$H^+ + K^+$ ATPase

VO_3^- inhibits microsomal gastric mucosa K^+ ATPase, which is an expression of a part of the gastric H^+ pump; proton transport by gastric microsomal vesicles and acid secretion by gastric glands are also reduced (128, 141, 142). VO_3^- also inhibits urinary acidification by the turtle bladder; the mechanism has not been determined (119). A bacterial membrane-bound proton-translocating ATPase was found to be sensitive to VO_3^- (143).

DYNEIN ATPases

Dynein is the collective name for either Ca^{2+}- or Mg^{2+}-requiring high molecular weight ATPases associated with microtubules. They function in the transduction of the chemical energy provided by ATP hydrolysis into mechanical work such as ciliary and flagellar motility and may have roles in chromosome movement, exoplasmic transport, and the intracellular movement of membrane-bound vesicles (144, 145). The sources of dyneins studied in detail have been the flagella and cilia of the *Tetrahymena* and the sea urchin.

VO_3^- at concentrations on the order of 10^{-6}–10^{-7} M reversibly inhibits both the isolated dynein ATPase activity and the motility of demembranated sea urchin or porcine sperm flagella and sea urchin embryo cilia (146, 147). Mg^{2+}-activated dynein is over 30 times more sensitive to VO_3^- than the Ca^{2+}-activated one (146, 148, 149). The inhibition of Mg^{2+}-stimulated enzyme activity is noncompetitive with ATP (146, 148, 150), as is the reduction of flagellar beat frequency by VO_3^- (146). The intact sea urchin spermatozoa are not inactivated by 10^{-2} M VO_3^-, and those of the pig require 10^{-3} M VO_3^- for complete paralysis (147). Other observations extend and amplify these findings (151–157).

Myosin and actomyosin ATPases are not inhibited by VO_3^- concentrations below 5×10^{-4} M (13, 146). Other studies, however, have demonstrated an irreversible, slow-onset inhibition of myosin and actomyosin ATPases by millimolar concentrations of VO_3^-; the mechanism is the formation of a stable myosin-ADP-vanadium complex (158–160). The difference in kinetics and sensitivity to VO_3^- offers an opportunity for distinguishing between the actions of dynein and myosin in different forms of cell motility (146, 161).

VO_3^- at ~10^{-5} M has been shown to inhibit mitotic spindle in lysed cells (162) and translocation of pigment granules in permeabilized erythrophores (163) or when injected into the cell (164).

ADENYL CYCLASE

Cyclic AMP is formed by the catalytic action of adenyl cyclase and is inactivated by phosphodiesterase. VO_3^- ($>10^{-5}$ M), along with fluoride, catecholamines, vasopressin, prostaglandin E_1, parathyroid hormone, and glucagon, stimulates isolated adenyl cyclase activity from a variety of sources (165–170). The action of VO_3^- is not shared by V^{4+} and V^{3+} compounds (171) and is independent of hormones and inhibition of phosphodiesterase by theophylline (170, 172); it differs from that of fluoride (172–174). The postulated mechanism involves formation of an enzyme complex with VO_3^- via guanine nucleotide regulatory protein (174). Since VO_3^- does not attenuate the ability of hormone receptors to direct inhibition of adenyl cyclase, a routine inclusion of VO_3^- in studies directed at further elucidation of the mechanisms of receptor-mediated inhibition of the enzyme was suggested (172). One would expect VO_3^- to have cyclic AMP-mediated hormone-like effects in vivo. However, in toad bladder and skin, VO_3^- blocks cyclic AMP-induced (by vasopressin, theophylline, and exogeneous cyclic AMP) transepilial osmotic water flow by an unknown mechanism (116); it may also stimulate water flow in such systems (118).

Concentrations of VO_3^- in excess of 5 mM inhibit adenyl cyclase (172).

SMOOTH MUSCLE

In view of the dependence of vascular muscle tone on the electrogenic Na^+ pump, the effects of $Na^+ + K^+$ ATPase inhibitors on blood pressure are of great interest (175, 176). Indeed, an intravenous administration of VO_3^- acutely raises arterial blood pressure in rats (177, 178). Prolonged dietary administration of VO_3^- (100–200 ppm) to uninephrectomized rats produces hypertension that correlates positively with plasma vanadium concentrations ranging from 40–270 ng/ml (179). Note, however, that these vanadium levels are much higher than those encountered in human populations. In the dog or cat, intravenous VO_3^- infusions cause arterial hypertension, increased peripheral resistance, and a marked reduction of coronary, visceral, and renal blood flow, whereas the large arteries (femoral and carotid) escape constriction (180–183). There also may be centrally mediated effects of VO_3^- on blood pressure (184).

As expected of a $Na^+ + K^+$ ATPase inhibitor, VO_3^- (10^{-4} M) causes a contraction of isolated vascular smooth muscle preparations but does not inhibit the Na^+ pump (185–188). The VO_3^--induced contraction is blocked by a stilbene, an inhibitor of the anion transport system, suggesting an intracellular action of VO_3^- (185–188). Aortas of Dahl salt hypertension–sensitive rats react more vigorously to VO_3^- than do those from control rats (188).

It has been suggested that VO_3^- may act by inhibiting Ca^{2+} ATPase that controls intracellular Ca^{2+} concentrations (185). However, VO_3^- at a concentration as high as 10^{-4} M has been reported to have only minimal inhibitory effect on plasma membrane Ca^{2+} ATPase derived from rat mesenteric arteries and veins (189). VO_3^- also augments ^3H-norepinephrine release from the isolated pulmonary artery (190) and there is a pharmacological similarity between the contraction induced by VO_3^- and norepinephrine (187). Another observation is that actomyosin preparations of the carotid arteries of cattle contain VO_3^--sensitive phosphatase activity (191).

Intestinal smooth muscle may be more sensitive to VO_3^- than vascular muscle (185) and the VO_3^--induced contraction is inhibited by removal of external Ca^{2+} (192). Several vanadium compounds evoke contractions of the isolated rat vas deferens (193).

HEART

Since inhibition of $Na^+ + K^+$ ATPase has been implicated in the positive inotropic action of digitalis, there is much interest in the cardiac effects of VO_3^-. The subject has been clearly reviewed, and the reviewers concluded that VO_3^- has more action on the heart than does digitalis (17, 20). In intact dogs and cats, VO_3^- decreases the force of ventricular contraction, presumably due to a marked coronary constriction occurring at concentrations too low to have a direct effect on myocardium. In isolated cardiac muscle preparations, VO_3^- produces positive or negative inotropic effects, depending upon species, type of muscle, and experimental conditions; these actions do not appear to involve $Na^+ + K^+$ ATPase inhibition. VO_3^- stimulates adenyl cyclase and so can increase the concentration of cyclic AMP in cardiac muscle; this effect also seems to be unrelated to its inotropic actions. VO_3^- increases force of contraction of isolated rat atrial muscle by increasing the Mn^{2+}-sensitive superficial Ca^{2+} pool, which is related to the beat-to-beat control of force of contraction; on the other hand, VO_3^- lowers the force of contraction in guinea-pig atrial muscle by inhibiting slow Ca^{2+} channels (194). Compounds of vanadium in +4 and +3 oxidation states do not share with VO_3^- the positive inotropic effect on isolated cat papillary muscles and stimulation of adenyl cyclase (171).

High concentrations of VO_3^- ($>10^{-4}M$) may inhibit (like ouabain) or stimulate (like insulin) the uptake of K^+ by heart muscle cells from various species; both types of effects may be associated with the positive inotropic effect (195). It was shown previously for other tissues that VO_3^- mimics the stimulating effect of insulin on glucose oxidation (111) and transport, which appears to be associated with or mediated by a rise in cytoplasmic Ca^{2+} concentration (196). Another suggestion is that the stimulation by VO_3^- of rat heart protein kinase, which promotes the phosphorylation of the membranes of the sarcoplasmic reticulum, may play a role in strengthening myocardial contraction by increasing sarcoplasmic reticulum stores of Ca^{2+} (197).

In chemically skinned right-ventricle hog preparations, inorganic phosphate and VO_3^- interfere with the chemomechanical energy transformation of myosin (198).

KIDNEY

The renal effects of vanadium have been reviewed previously (21, 23); they include a mixture of hemodynamic and parenchymal actions and, like cardiac effects, are characterized by unexplained and profound species differences. VO_3^- produces a large diuresis in the rat but not in the dog (181, 199, 200) and cat (182, 183); vasoconstriction, lowering of renal blood flow, and glomerular filtration rate (GFR) are prominent. In the rat, GFR may rise simultaneously with increased renal peripheral resistance, suggesting a postcapillary vasoconstrictor effect (201); in the dog and cat only a fall of GFR was seen.

Most authors have speculated that the diuresis induced by VO_3^- in the rat is due to inhibition of $Na^+ + K^+$ ATPase, since the ouabain-sensitive Na^+ pump accounts for up to 50% of renal Na^+Cl^- reabsorption, the urinary electrolyte excretion pattern is typical for ouabain, and renal $Na^+ + K^+$ ATPase is exquisitely sensitive to VO_3^-. Vanadium accumulates in the kidney, although this may be mainly in the form of VO^{2+}, with less activity with respect to $Na^+ + K^+$ ATPase. Rats on 15–day diets containing 5 and 25 ppm VO_3^- had renal vanadium concentrations in excess of 10^{-5} M but showed no changes in fractional Na^+ excretion or $Na^+ + K^+$ ATPase activity in kidney homogenates (46). On the other hand, chickens on diets containing subtoxic (25–50 ppm) and toxic (100 ppm) concentrations of VO_3^- for 15 months had reduced renal $Na^+ + K^+$ ATPase in proportion to renal concentrations of vanadium; the potency of vanadium for $Na^+ + K^+$ ATPase was similar in vivo and in vitro, showing I_{50} of 5×10^{-6} M. Unfortunately, diuretic studies were not performed in these birds (48). These enzyme observations are also of interest in determining the mechanism of vanadium-induced nephrotoxicity, since generalized proximal tubular transport defects (Fanconi syndrome) may be associated with interference with the active Na^+ pump (202).

VO_3^- reduces renal renin secretion in rat kidney slices (203) and in volume-expanded dogs (199). It produces a striking phosphaturia in acutely parathyroidectomized rats (204). $Ca^{2+} + Mg^{2+}$ ATPase of the rabbit kidney is resistant to VO_3^- (205).

Beside the fact that urine is the major excretory route for vanadium (45), nothing is known about the renal handling of vanadium compounds.

EYE AND EAR

Topical application of VO_3^- lowers intraocular pressure in the rabbit and monkey, presumably by inhibition of $Na^+ + K^+$ ATPase in the ciliary body and consequent reduction of intraocular fluid formation (18, 206). It proved only marginally effective in human ocular hypertension (207). VO_3^- ($>10^{-4}$ M) also inhibits active Na^+ and Cl^- transport in the isolated frog cornea (208). An ATPase from toad retinal rod outer segments that may have a dynein function involved in light-controlled structural changes (photoreceptor ?) is sensitive to VO_3^- (209).

Ototoxicity of locally applied VO_3^- was studied in guinea pigs. Both the endocochlear and microphonic potentials are inhibited by ouabain. Although VO_3^- inhibits $Na^+ + K^+$ ATPase of stria vascularis in vitro, it causes an increase in the cochlear potential followed by a gradual decrease and a depression of the microphonic potential when applied perilymphatically. These results were interpreted to suggest that VO_3^- acts by depolarizing the hair cells of the organ of Corti (210, 211).

BRAIN

Whole brain mirosomal $Na^+ + K^+$ ATPase is several times less sensitive to VO_3^- than is the kidney or heart enzyme in four mammalian species (14); it is not known whether this is related to the presence of two types of $Na^+ + K^+$ ATPase in the brain (212) or to other factors. Consistent with inhibition of $Na^+ + K^+$ ATPase, VO_3^- interferes with the uptake of ^{3}H-norepinephrine by rat cerebral cortex slices; the high concentrations ($>10^{-4}$ M) required suggest poor intracellular penetration of VO_3^-. Vanadium intoxication in rats causes changes in brain catecholamine levels (213). VO_3^- (10^{-3} M) also diminishes muscarinic binding sites in homogenates of rat corpus striatum (214).

The signs of vanadium toxicity in man include tremor and central nervous system depression (215). A group of Scottish investigators suggest that manic-depressive disorders may be associated with increased vanadium levels and a genetically defective Na^+ pump (examined in lymphocytes and erythrocytes) hypersensitive to inhibitors (216–218). An editorial on the subject appeared in *Lancet* (19). Plasma vanadium concentrations in manic-depressed subjects were about twice that of normal controls and declined after recovery (31). Encouraging results were obtained in the therapy of manic-depressive psychosis with a low vanadium diet and therapy with EDTA or reducing agents, ascorbic acid, and methylene blue (219). Antidepressants such as imipramine and indalprine may also reduce VO_3^- to VO^{2+}. Other investigators extended these observations to several ATPases in erythrocytes of patients with affective disorders and found the best correlation between mood and Ca^{2+} ATPase activity (91).

MISCELLANEOUS

The common signs and symptoms of occupational industrial exposure to excess airborne vanadium are associated with the irritation of airways and conjunctiva and a green discoloration of the tongue. Recent measurements indicate that this may be accompanied by pronounced reversible reductions in forced vital capacity, forced expiratory volume, and forced mid-expiratory flow, together with increased urinary vanadium excretion (220). A few observations suggest that V_2O_5 particles may produce asthma, as judged by bronchiolar hyperreactivity to histamine (221). Alveolar macrophages isolated from rabbit lungs are inactivated only by very high concentrations ($>10^{-4}$ M) of V_2O_5 (222) and hence appear to offer a poor model for pulmonary toxicity testing of vanadium compounds. Green tongue may be due to deposition of hexaquo ion $[V(H_2O)_6]^{3+}$ (23).

In perfused rat livers, VO_3^- increases vascular resistance (at 3×10^{-5} M in the perfusate), decreases O_2 consumption, and reduces bile flow (at 6×10^{-5} M in the perfusate) (223). Some vanadium is excreted in the bile (224).

The effect of vanadium on drug biotransformation has been examined. Several hepatic microsomal mixed-function oxidase reactions are inhibited in vitro by VO_3^- with varying, generally low, effectiveness (225). Upon administration to mice, VO_3^-, and to a much lesser extent VO^{2+}, transiently inhibits oxidative demethylation of substrates of the cytochrome P-450-dependent monooxygenase system (226). Sulfite-induced lipid peroxidation is accelerated by VO_3^- (10^{-4} M) in several tissues (227).

Parathyroid hormone, prostaglandin E_2, 1,25-dihydroxycholecalciferol, and Na^+-stimulated Ca^{2+} release (resorption) from mouse bone is inhibited by ouabain and $\sim 10^{-5}$ M VO_3^- (228).

VO_3^- hyperpolarizes several types of cultured cells. This unique hyperpolarization is independent of Na^+, K^+, or the Na^+ pump, and requires $>10^{-5}$M VO_3^- for 50% effect (229).

The highest known accumulation of vanadium in any living system occurs in tunicate blood cells termed vanadocytes, reaching a concentration on the order of 1 M, or $\sim 10^8$ times higher than in sea water. The mechanism may involve entry of VO_3^- into acidic vacuoles where it is reduced by tunichrome and trapped as V^{4+}, and biologically unique V^{3+} states. The function of vanadocytes is unknown (10, 230, 231). Although crude petroleums contain vanadyl porphyrins of unknown origin, there is no convincing evidence that they have had, or currently have, functions as O_2 carriers or participate in photosynthetic reactions (232). Recently it was found that VO^{2+}, but not VO_3^-, enhances O_2

binding to bovine hemoglobin and myoglobin (233); the high vanadium concentration required ($>10^{-4}$ M) suggests that the effect is of no physiological significance.

Vanadocene dichloride, one of the numerous metallocene dihyalides, has an antiproliferative action in experimental mice leukemias (234).

CONCLUSIONS

Naturally occurring vanadium is among the lowest of trace elements in mammals (27, 30). Although nutritional essentiality has been established for the chicken and the rat, the physiologic role of vanadium remains unknown. It appears that vanadium exists in body fluids in $+5$ oxidation state as VO_3^- and intracellularly in $+4$ state as VO^{2+}. VO_3^- or VO^{2+} interferes with numerous enzymes involving phosphate at concentrations ranging from nM to mM. Of the enzymes studied, the most sensitive to VO_3^- is $Na^+ + K^+$ ATPase; this enzyme is more resistant to VO^{2+} than to VO_3^-. The proposal that vanadium may be a regulator of the Na^+ pump by means of a redox mechanism is yet to be proven. On the other hand, the differential sensitivity of various enzymes to vanadium has been exploited as an investigative tool. In general, it requires a large concentration ($>10^{-4}$ M) of VO_3^- outside the cell to influence even the sensitive intracellular enzymes. In the intact animal vasoconstriction is the most consistently observed pharmacologic-toxic effect of VO_3^-. There are obscure species differences in its renal, cardiac, and ocular actions: administration of VO_3^- may cause diuresis or antidiuresis, may have a positive or a negative inotropic effect on the heart, and may have variable effectiveness in reducing intraocular pressure. In spite of the recent advances, the understanding of vanadium effects remains incomplete because multiple mechanisms may be involved.

Literature Cited

1. Biggs, W. R., Swinehart, J. H. 1976. Vanadium in selected biological systems. In *Metals Ions in Biological Systems; Biological Actions of Metal Ions*, ed. H. Sigel, 6:141–96. New York: Dekker, 453 pp.
2. National Institute of Occupational Safety and Health. 1977. *Vanadium*. Washington DC: USDHEW, PHS, CDC. 142 pp.
3. National Research Council Committee on Biologic Effects of Atmospheric Pollutants. 1974. *Vanadium*. Washington DC: Natl. Acad. Sci. 117 pp.
4. Schroeder, H. A. 1974. *The Poisons Around Us*. Bloomington: Indiana Univ. Press. 144 pp.
5. Schroeder, H. A., Balassa, J. J., Tipton, I. H. 1963. Abnormal trace metals in man-vanadium. *J. Chron. Dis.* 16:1047–71
6. Waters, M. D. 1977. Toxicology of vanadium. *Adv. Mod. Toxicol.* 2:147–89
7. Underwood, E. J. 1977. *Trace Elements in Human and Animal Nutrition*, pp. 388–97. New York: Academic. 4th ed. 454 pp.
8. Clark, R. J. H. 1973. Vanadium. In *Comprehensive Inorganic Chemistry*, ed. C. Bailar Jr., et al, 3:491–551. New York: Pergamon. 1387pp.
9. Rubinson, K. A. 1981. Concerning the form of biochemically active vanadium. *Proc. R. Soc. London Ser. B* 212:65–84
10. Macara, I. G. 1980. Vanadium—An element in search of a role. *Trends Biochem. Sci.* 5:92–94

11. Singh, J., Nordlie, R. C., Jorgenson, R. A. 1981. Vanadate: A potent inhibitor of multifunctional glucose-6-phosphatase. *Biochim. Biophys. Acta* 678:477–82
12. Swarup, G., Cohen, S., Garbers, D. L. 1982. Inhibition of membrane phosphotyrosyl-protein phosphatase activity by vanadate. *Biochem. Biophys. Res. Commun.* 107:1104–9
13. Cantley, L. C. Jr., Josephson, L., Warner, R., Yanagisawa, M., Lechene, C., Guidotti, G. 1977. Vanadate is a potent (Na,K)-ATPase inhibitor found in ATP derived from muscle. *J. Biol. Chem.* 252:7421–23
14. Nechay, B. R., Saunders, J. P. 1978. Inhibition by vanadium of sodium and potassium dependent adenosinetriphosphatase derived from animal and human tissues. *J. Environ. Pathol. Toxicol.* 2:247–62
15. Quist, E. E., Hokin, L. E. 1978. The presence of two (Na⁺ + K⁺)-ATPase inhibitors in equine muscle ATP: Vanadate and a dithioerythritol-dependent inhibitor. *Biochim. Biophys. Acta* 511:202–12
16. Cantley, L. C. Jr., Cantley, L. G., Josephson, L. 1978. A characterization of vandate interactions with the (Na,K)-ATPase. Mechanistic and regulatory implications. *J. Biol. Chem.* 253:7361–68
17. Akera, T., Temma, K., Takeda, K. 1983. Cardiac actions of vanadium. *Fed. Proc.* 42:2984–88
18. Becker, B. 1980. Vanadate and aqueous humor dynamics. *Invest. Ophthalmol. Vis. Sci.* 19:1156–65
19. Editorial. 1981. Vanadium in manic-depressive illness. *Lancet* 2:511–12
20. Erdmann, E. 1980. Cardiac effects of vanadate. *Basic Res. Cardiol.* 75:411–12
21. Grantham, J. J. 1980. The renal sodium pump and vanadate. *Am. J. Physiol.* 239:F97–106
22. Hansen, O. 1983. Vanadate and phosphotransferases with special emphasis on ouabain/Na,K-ATPase interaction. *Acta Pharmacol. Toxicol.* 52:1–19
23. Phillips, T. D., Nechay, B. R., Heidelbaugh, N. D. 1983. Vanadium: Chemistry and the kidney. *Fed. Proc.* 42:2969–73
24. Sachs, G. 1980. Vanadate as a transport probe. *J. Lab. Clin. Med.* 96:379–81
25. Simons, T. J. B. 1979. Vanadate—A new tool for biologists. *Nature* 281:337–38
26. Byrne, A. R., Kosta, L. 1978. Vanadium in foods and in human body fluids and tissues. *Sci. Total Environ.* 10:17–30
27. Versieck, J., Cornelis, R. 1980. Normal levels of trace elements in human blood plasma or serum. *Anal. Chim. Acta* 116:217–54
28. Myron, D. R., Givand, S. H., Nielsen, F. H. 1977. Vanadium content of selected foods as determined by flameless atomic absorption spectroscopy. *J. Agric. Food Chem.* 25:297–300
29. Stroop, S. D., Helinek, G., Greene, H. L. 1982. More sensitive flameless atomic absorption analysis of vanadium in tissue and serum. *Clin. Chem.* 28:79–82
30. Cornelis, R., Versieck, J., Mees, L., Hoste, J., Barbier, F. 1981. The ultratrace element vanadium in human serum. *Biol. Trace Element Res.* 3:257–63
31. Dick, D. A. T., Naylor, G. J., Dick, E. G. 1982. Plasma vanadium concentration in manic-depressive illness. *Psychol. Med.* 12:533–37
32. Post, R. L., Hunt, D. P., Walderhaug, M. O., Perkins, R. C., Park, J. H., et al. 1979. Vanadium compounds in relation to inhibition of sodium and potassium adenosine triphosphatase. In *Na, K-ATPase Structure and Kinetics*, ed. J. C. Skou, J. G. Nørby, pp. 389–401. New York: Academic. 549 pp.
33. Kelm, W., Schaller, K. H. 1978. The quantitative determination of vanadium in blood samples of ecologically and occupationally exposed persons with a specific and sensitive method. *Wiss. Umwelt* 1:34–42
34. Byrne, A. R., Kosta, L. 1979. On the vanadium and tin contents of diet and human blood. *Sci. Total Environ.* 13:87–90
35. Byrne, A. R., Vrbič, V. 1979. The vanadium content of human dental enamel and its relationship to caries. *J. Radioanal. Chem.* 54:77–85
36. Byrne, A. R., Kosta, L., Dermelj, M., Tušek-Žnidarič, M. 1983. Aspects of some trace elements in human milk. In *Trace Elements: Analytical Chemistry in Medicine and Biology*, Vol. 2. Berlin: de Gruyter. In press
37. Cornelis, R., Mees, L., Hoste, M. J., Ryckebusch, J., Versieck, J., Barbier, F. 1979. Neutron activation analysis of vanadium in human liver and serum. In *Nuclear Activation Techniques in the Life Sciences 1978*, pp. 165–77 Vienna: Intl. Atomic Energy Agency
38. Corder, C. N. 1983. Vanadium levels in human kidney at autopsy. *Fed. Proc.* 42:627 (Abstr.)
39. Thürauf, J., Schaller, K. H., Syga, G., Weltle, D. 1978. The vanadium-concentration of the human placenta. *Wiss. Umwelt* 2:84–88

40. United States Environmental Protection Agency. 1979. *Toxic Trace Metals in Mammalian Hair and Nails*, pp. 130–32. Las Vegas, Nevada: Environ. Monitoring Sys. Lab. EPA-600/4–79–049. 185 pp.

41. Gibson, R. S., DeWolfe, M. S. 1979. The zinc, copper, manganese, vanadium, and iodine content of hair from 38 Canadian neonates. *Pediatr. Res.* 13:959–62

42. Creason, J. P., Hinners, T. A., Bumgarner, J. E., Pinkerton, C. 1975. Trace elements in hair, as related to exposure in metropolitan New York. *Clin. Chem.* 21:603–12

43. Tipton, I. H., Shafer, J. J. 1964. Statistical analysis of lung trace element levels. *Arch. Environ. Health* 8:58–67

44. Myron, D. R., Zimmermann, T. J., Shuler, T. R., Klevay, L. M., Lee, D. E., et al. 1978. Intake of nickel and vanadium by humans A survey of selected diets. *Am. J. Clin. Nutr.* 31:527–31

45. Tipton, I. H., Stewart, P. L., Dickson, J. 1969. Patterns of elemental excretion in long term balance studies. *Health Phys.* 16:455–62

46. Higashino, H., Bogden, J. D., Lavenhar, M. A., Bauman, J. W. Jr., Hirotsu, T., et al. 1983. Na-K-ATPase, and potassium adaptation in the rat. *Am. J. Physiol.* 244:F105–11

47. Söremark, R. 1967. Vanadium in some biological specimens. *J. Nutr.* 92:183–90

48. Phillips, T. D., Nechay, B. R., Neldon, S. L., Kubena, L. F., Heidelbaugh, N. D., et al. 1982. Vanadium-induced inhibition of renal Na^+, K^+-adenosinetriphosphatase in the chicken after chronic dietary exposure. *J. Toxicol. Environ. Health* 9:651–61

49. Blotcky, A. J., Falcone, C., Medina, V. A., Rack, E. P., Hobson, D. W. 1979. Determination of trace-level vanadium in marine biological samples by chemical neutron activation analysis. *Anal. Chem.* 51:178–82

50. LaTouche, Y. D., Bennett, C. W., Mix, M. C. 1981. Determination of vanadium in a marine mollusc using a chelating ion exchange resin and neutron activation. *Bull. Environ. Contam. Toxicol.* 26:224–27

51. Söremark, R., Ullberg, S. 1962. Distribution and kinetics of $^{48}V_2O_5$ in mice. In *The Use of Radioisotopes in Animal Biology and the Medical Sciences*, ed. N. Friend, pp. 103–14. New York: Academic. 563 pp.

52. Söremark, R., Ullberg, S., Appelgren, L.-E. 1962. Autoradiographic localization of vanadium pentoxide (V_2O_5) in developing teeth and bones of rats. *Acta Odontol. Scand.* 20:225–29

53. Bawden, J. W., Deaton, T. G., Chavis, M. 1980. In vivo and in vitro study of ^{48}V uptake in developing rat molar enamel. *J. Dent. Res.* 59:1643–48

54. Bogden, J. D., Higashino, H., Lavenhar, M. A., Bauman, J. W. Jr., Kemp, F. W., Aviv, A. 1982. Balance and tissue distribution of vanadium after short-term ingestion of vanadate. *J. Nutr.* 112:2279–85

55. Conklin, A. W., Skinner, S. C., Felten, T. L., Sanders, C. L. 1982. Clearance and distribution of intratracheally instilled vanadium compounds in the rat. *Toxicol. Lett.* 11:199–203

56. Hansen, T. V., Aaseth, J., Alexander, J. 1982. The effect of chelating agents on vanadium distribution in the rat body and on uptake by human erythrocytes. *Arch. Toxicol.* 50:195–202

57. Oberg, S. G., Parker, R. D. R., Sharma, R. P. 1978. Distribution and elimination of an intratracheally administered vanadium compound in the rat. *Toxicology* 11:315–23

58. Parker, R. D. R., Sharma, R. P. 1978. Accumulation and depletion of vanadium in selected tissues of rats treated with vanadyl sulfate and sodium orthovanadate. *J. Environ. Pathol. Toxicol.* 2:235–45

59. Parker, R. D. R., Sharma, R. P., Oberg, S. G. 1980. Distribution and accumulation of vanadium in mice tissues. *Arch. Environ. Contam. Toxicol.* 9:393–403

60. Peabody, R. A., Wallach, S., Verch, R. L., Lifschitz, M. 1980. Effect of LH and FSH on vanadium distribution in hypophysectomized rats. *Proc. Soc. Exp. Biol. Med.* 165:349–53

61. Wiegmann, T. B., Day, H. D., Patak, R. V. 1982. Intestinal absorption and secretion of radioactive vanadium ($^{48}VO_3^-$) in rats and effect of $Al(OH)_3$. *J. Toxicol. Environ. Health* 10:233–45

62. Sabbioni, E., Marafante, E. 1978. Metabolic patterns of vanadium in the rat. *Bioinor. Chem.* 9:389–407

63. Sabbioni, E., Marafante, E., Amantini, L., Ubertalli, L., Birattari, C. 1978. Similarity in metabolic patterns of different chemical species of vanadium in the rat. *Bioinorg. Chem.* 8:503–15

64. Chasteen, N. D., Theil, E. C. 1982. Iron binding by horse spleen apoferritin. A vanadyl (IV) EPR spin probe study. *J. Biol. Chem.* 257:7672–77

65. Sabbioni, E., Marafante, E. 1981. Relations between iron and vanadium metab-

olism: In vivo incorporation of vanadium into iron proteins of the rat. *J. Toxicol. Environ. Health* 8:419–29

66. Hayat, M. A. 1975. *Positive Staining for Electron Microscopy*, p. 221. New York: Van Nostrand Reinhold. 361 pp.

67. Davies, N. T. 1981. An appraisal of the newer trace elements. *Phil. Trans. R. Soc. London Ser. B* 294:171–84

68. Golden, M. H. N., Golden, B. E. 1981. Trace elements. *Br. Med. Bull.* 37:31–36

69. Hopkins, L. L. Jr., Mohr, H. E. 1971. The biological essentiality of vanadium. In *Newer Trace Elements in Nutrition*, ed. W. Mertz, W. E. Cornatzer, pp. 195–213. New York: Dekker. 438 pp.

70. Hopkins, L. L. Jr. 1974. Essentiality and function of vanadium. In *Trace Element Metabolism in Animals Vol. 2*, ed. W. G. Hoekstra, J. W. Suttie, H. E. Ganther, W. Mertz, pp. 397–406. Baltimore: University Park. 775 pp.

71. Mertz, W. 1974. The newer essential trace elements, chromium, tin, vanadium, nickel and silicon. *Proc. Nutr. Soc.* 33:307–13

72. Kubena, L. F., Phillips, T. D. 1983. Toxicity of vanadium in female leghorn chickens. *Poult. Sci.* 62:47–50

73. McKeehan, W. L., McKeehan, K. A., Hammond, S. L., Ham, R. G. 1977. Improved medium for clonal growth of human diploid fibroblasts at low concentrations of serum protein. *In Vitro* 13:399–416

74. Carpenter, G. 1981. Vanadate, epidermal growth factor and the stimulation of DNA synthesis. *Biochem. Biophys. Res. Commun.* 102:1115–21

75. Rifkin, R. J. 1965. In vitro inhibition of $Na^+ -K^+$ and Mg^{2+} ATPases by mono, di and trivalent cations. *Proc. Soc. Exp. Biol. Med.* 120:802–4

76. Beaugé, L. A., Glynn, I. M. 1977. A modifier of $(Na^+ + K^+)$ATPase in commercial ATP. *Nature* 268:355–56

77. Beaugé, L. A., Glynn, I. M. 1978. Commercial ATP containing traces of vanadate alters the response of $(Na^+ + K^+)$ ATPase to external potassium. *Nature* 272:551–52

78. Charney, A. N., Silva, P., Epstein, F. H. 1975. An in vitro inhibitor of Na-K-ATPase present in an adenosine triphosphate preparation. *J. Appl. Physiol.* 39:156–58

79. Hudgins, P. M., Bond, G. H. 1977. $(Mg^{2+} + K^+)$-dependent inhibition of NaK-ATPase due to a contaminant in equine muscle ATP. *Biochem. Biophys. Res. Commun.* 77:1024–29

80. Josephson, L., Cantley, L. C. Jr. 1977.

Isolation of a potent (Na-K)ATPase inhibitor from striated muscle. *Biochemistry* 16:4572–78

81. Cantley, L. C. Jr., Aisen, P. 1979. The fate of cytoplasmic vanadium. Implications on (Na,K)-ATPase inhibition. *J. Biol. Chem.* 254:1781–84

82. Cantley, L. C. Jr., Josephson, L., Gelles, J., Cantley, L. G. 1979. The active site structure of the Na, K-ATPase. See Ref. 32, pp. 181–91. New York: Academic

83. Glynn, I. M., Richards, D. E. 1982. Occlusion of rubidium ions by the sodium-potassium pump: Its implications for the mechanism of potassium transport. *J. Physiol.* 330:17–43

84. Karlish, S. J. D., Beaugé, L. A., Glynn, I. M. 1979. Vanadate inhibits $(Na^+ + K^+)$ATPase by blocking a conformational change of the unphosphorylated form. *Nature* 282:333–35

85. Robinson, J. D., Mercer, R. W. 1981. Vanadate binding to the (Na + K)-ATPase. *J. Bioenerg. Biomembr.* 13:205–18

86. Smith, R. L., Zinn, K., Cantley, L. C. Jr. 1980. A study of the vanadate-trapped state of the (Na,K)-ATPase. Evidence against interacting nucleotide site models. *J. Biol. Chem.* 255:9852–59

87. Bond, G. H., Hudgins, P. M. 1979. Kinetics of inhibition of NaK-ATPase by Mg^{2+}, K^+, and vanadate. *Biochemistry* 18:325–31

88. Bond, G. H., Hudgins, P. M. 1982. Low-affinity $(Na^+ + K^+)$-ATPase modulate inhibition of Na-ATPase by vanadate. *Biochim. Biophys. Acta* 687:310–14

89. Hansen, O. 1982. Studies on ouabain-complexed $(Na^+ + K^+)$-ATPase carried out with vanadate. *Biochim. Biophys. Acta* 692:187–95

90. Grantham, J. J., Glynn, I. M. 1979. Renal Na, K-ATPase: Determinants of inhibition by vanadium. *Am. J. Physiol.* 236:F530–35

91. MacDonald, E., LeRoy, A., Linnoila, M. 1982. Failure of lithium to counteract vanadate-induced inhibition of red blood cell membrane Na^+, K^+-ATPase. *Lancet* 2:774

92. Hansen, O. 1979. Facilitation of ouabain binding to $(Na^+ + K^+)$-ATPase by vanadate at in vivo concentrations. *Biochim. Biophys. Acta* 568:265–69

93. Hansen, O. 1979. Reactive states of the Na, K-ATPase demonstrated by the stability of the enzyme-ouabain complex. See Ref. 32, pp. 169–80

94. Hansen, O. 1980. Vanadate interaction

with Na, K-ATPase. An assay of serum vanadium based on the displacement of (^{48}V) vanadate from Na, K-ATPase. *Basic Res. Cardiol.* 75:455–59

95. Wallick, E. T., Lane, L. K., Schwartz, A. 1979. Regulation by vanadate of ouabain binding to (Na$^+$, K$^+$)-ATPase. *J. Biol. Chem.* 254:8107–09

96. Norgaard, A., Kjeldsen, K., Hansen, O., Clausen, T. 1983. A simple and rapid method for the determination of the number of ^{3}H-ouabain binding sites in biopsies of skeletal muscle. *Biochem. Biophys. Res. Commun.* 111:319–25

97. Michell, A. R., Taylor, E. A. 1982. The optimum pH of renal adenosine triphosphatase in rats: Influence of vanadate, noradrenaline and potassium. *Enzymes* 28:309–16

98. Wu, P. H., Phillis, J. W. 1979. Effects of vanadate on brain (Na$^+$ – K$^+$) ATPase and p - nitrophenylphosphatase - interactions with mono- and di-valent ions and with noradrenaline. *Int. J. Biochem.* 10:629–35

99. Macara, I. G., Kustin, K., Cantley, L. C. Jr. 1980. Glutathione reduces cytoplasmic vanadate. Mechanism and physiological implications. *Biochim. Biophys. Acta* 629:95–106

100. Vykočil, F., Teisinger, J., Dlouhá, H. 1980. A specific enzyme is not necessary for vanadate-induced oxidation of NADH. *Nature* 286:516–17

101. Vyskočil, F., Pilař, J., Zemková, H., Teisinger, J. 1982. Reduction of vanadate to vanadyl by methylene-blue, imipramine, and chlorpromazine in absence of NADH. *Lancet* 1:1078–79

102. Cantley, L. C. Jr., Ferguson, J. H., Kustin, K. 1978. Norepinephrine complexes and reduces vanadium (V) to reverse vanadate inhibition of the (Na,K)-ATPase. *J. Am. Chem. Soc.* 100:5210–12

103. Hudgins, P. M., Bond, G. H. 1979. Reversal of vanadate inhibition of NaK-ATPase by catecholamines. *Res. Commun. Chem. Pathol. Pharmacol.* 23:313–26

104. Last, T. A., Gantzer, M. L., Tyler, C. D. 1983. Ion-gated channel induced in planar bilayers by incorporation of (Na ,K)-ATPase. *J. Biol. Chem.* 258:2399–404

105. Beaugé, L. 1979. Vanadate-potassium interactions in the inhibition of Na, K-ATPase. See Ref. 32, pp. 373–87

106. Cantley, L. C. Jr., Resh, M. D., Guidotti, G. 1978. Vanadate inhibits the red cell (Na$^+$,K$^+$) ATPase from the cytoplasmic side. *Nature* 272:252–54

107. Beaugé, L., Dipolo, R. 1979. Vanadate

108. Heinz, A., Rubinson, K. A., Grantham, J. J. 1982. The transport and accumulation of oxyvanadium compounds in human erythrocytes in vitro. *J. Lab Clin. Med.* 100:593–612

selectively inhibits the K$_0^+$-activated Na$^+$ efflux in squid axons. *Biochim. Biophys. Acta* 551:220–23

109. North, P. E., Post, R. L. 1983. Two patterns of inhibition of (Na,K) ATPase by vanadyl ion. *Fed. Proc.* 42:1926

110. Vyskočil, F., Teisinger, J., Dlouhá, H. 1981. The disparity between effects of vanadate (V) and vanadyl (IV) ions on (Na$^+$ – K$^+$)-ATPase and K$^+$-phosphatase in skeletal muscle. *Biochem. Biophys. Res. Commun.* 100:982–87

111. Degani, H., Gochin, M., Karlish, S. J. D., Shechter, Y. 1981. Electron paramagnetic resonance studies and insulin-like effects of vanadium in rat adipocytes. *Biochemistry* 20:5795–99

112. Johnson, J. L., Cohen, H. J., Rajagopalan, K. V. 1974. Studies of vanadium toxicity in the rat. Lack of correlation with molybdenum utilization. *Biochem. Biophys. Res. Commun.* 56:940–46

113. Sakurai, H., Shimomura, S., Fukuzawa, K., Ishizu, K. 1980. Detection of oxovanadium (IV) and characterization of its ligand environment in subcellular fractions of the liver of rats treated with pentavalent vanadium (V). *Biochem. Biophys. Res. Commun.* 96:293–98

114. Sakurai, H., Goda, T., Shimomura, S. 1982. ^{31}P- and ^{13}C-NMR study of the ATP (adenosine triphosphatase)-vanadyl complex. *Biochem. Biophys. Res. Commun.* 108:474–78

115. Sakurai, H., Goda, T., Shimomura, S., Yoshimura, T. 1982. ATP (adenosine triphosphate)-vanadyl complex. *Biochem. Biophys. Res. Commun.* 104:1421–26

116. De Sousa, R. C., Grosso, A. 1979. Vanadate blocks cyclic AMP-induced stimulation of sodium and water transport in amphibian epithelia. *Nature* 279:803–4

117. Walker, M. D., Phillips, T. D. 1983. Effects of vanadate and vanadyl on sodium transport in toad urinary bladder. *Toxicologist* 3:75 (Abstr.)

118. Arruda, J. A. L., Westenfelder, C. 1983. Effect of vanadate water transport by the toad bladder. *Life Sci.* 32:1879–84

119. Arruda, J. A. L., Sabatini, S., Westenfelder, C. 1981. Vanadate inhibits urinary acidificion by the turtle bladder. *Kidney Int.* 20:772–79

120. Bell, M. V., Sargent, J. R. 1979. The

partial purification of sodium-plus-potassium ion-dependent adenosine triphosphatase from the gills of *Anguilla anguilla* and its inhibition by orthovanadate. *Biochem. J.* 179:431–38

121. Bond, G. H., Hudgins, P. M. 1980. Inhibition of red cell Ca^{2+}-ATPase by vanadate. *Biochim. Biophys. Acta* 600:781–90

122. Hagenmeyer, A., Wierichs, R., Bader, H. 1980. Vanadate inhibition of the Ca^{++}-ATPase of sarcoplasmic reticulum from pig heart. *Basic Res. Cardiol.* 75:452–54

123. Pick, U. 1982. The interaction of vanadate ions with the Ca-ATPase from sarcoplasmic reticulum. *J. Biol. Chem.* 257:6111–19

124. Wang, T., Tsai, L. I., Solaro, R. J., Grassi de Gende, A. O., Schwartz, A. 1979. Effects of potassium on vanadate inhibition of sarcoplasmic reticulum Ca^{2+}-ATPase from dog cardiac and rabbit skeletal muscle. *Biochem. Biophys. Res. Commun.* 91:356–61

125. Pick, U., Karlish, S. J. D. 1982. Regulation of the conformational transition in the Ca-ATPase from sarcoplasmic reticulum by pH, temperature, and calcium ions. *J. Biol. Chem.* 257:6120–26

126. Dupont, Y., Bennett, N. 1982. Vanadate inhibition of the Ca^{2+}-dependent conformational change of the sarcoplasmic reticulum Ca^{2+}-ATPase. *FEBS Lett.* 139:237–40

127. Barrabin, H., Garrahan, P. J., Rega, A. F. 1980. Vanadate inhibition of the Ca^{2+}-ATPase from human red cell membranes. *Biochim. Biophys. Acta* 600:796–804

128. O'Neal, S. G., Rhoads, D. B., Racker, E. 1979. Vanadate inhibition of sarcoplasmic reticulum Ca^{2+}-ATPase and other ATPases. *Biochem. Biophys. Res. Commun.* 89:845–50

129. Rossi, J. P. F. C., Garrahan, P. J., Rega, A. F. 1981. Vanadate inhibition of active Ca^{2+} transport across human red cell membranes. *Biochim. Biophys. Acta* 648:145–50

130. Niggli, V., Adunyah, E. S., Penniston, J. T., Carafoli, E. 1981. Purified (Ca^{2+}−Mg^{2+})-ATPase of the erythrocyte membrane reconstitution and effect of calmodulin and phospholipids. *J. Biol. Chem.* 256:395–401

131. Szasz, I., Sarkadi, B., Enyedi, A., Gárdos, G. 1981. Ca-transport and CaMg-ATPase activity in human red cell preparations. *Acta Biol. Med. Ger.* 40:429–36

132. Varecka, L., Carafoli, E. 1982. Vanadate-induced movements of Ca^{2+} and K$^+$

in human red blood cells. *J. Biol. Chem.* 257:7414–21

133. Siemon, H., Schneider, H., Fuhrmann, G. F. 1982. Vanadium increases selective K$^+$-permeability in human erythrocytes. *Toxicology* 22:271–78

134. Caroni, P., Carafoli, E. 1981. The Ca^{2+}-pumping ATPase of heart sarcolemma. Characterization, calmodulin dependence, and partial purification. *J. Biol. Chem.* 256:3263–70

135. Wibo, M., Morel, N., Godfraind, T. 1981. Differentiation of Ca^{2+} pumps linked to plasma membrane and endoplasmic reticulum in the microsomal fraction from intestinal smooth muscle. *Biochim. Biophys. Acta* 649:651–60

136. DiPolo, R., Rojas, H. R., Beaugé, L. 1979. Vanadate inhibits uncoupled Ca efflux but not Na-Ca exchange in squid axons. *Nature* 281:228–29

137. Nordmann, J. J., Zyzek, E. 1982. Calcium efflux from the rat neurohypophysis. *J. Physiol.* 325:281–99

138. Kanagasuntheram, P., Theo, T. S. 1982. Parotid microsomal Ca^{2+} transport subcellular localization and characterization. *Biochem. J.* 208:789–94

139. Famulski, K., Carafoli, E. 1982. Ca^{2+} transporting activity of membrane fractions isolated from the postmitochondrial supernatant of rat liver. *Cell Calcium* 3:263–81

140. Iwasa, Y., Iwasa, T., Higashi, K., Matsui, K., Miyamoto, E. 1982. Demonstration of a high affinity Ca^{2+}-ATPase in rat liver plasma membranes. *Biochem. Biophys. Res. Commun.* 105:488–94

141. Faller, L. D., Malinowska, D. H., Rabon, E., Smolka, A., Sachs, G. 1981. Mechanistic studies of the gastric (H$^+$ + K$^+$)-ATPase. *Prog. Clin. Biol. Res.* 73:153–74

142. Faller, L., Jackson, R., Malinowska, D., Mukidjam, E., Rabon, E., Saccomani, G., Sachs, G., Smolka, A. 1982. Mechanistic aspects of gastric [H$^+$ + K$^+$]-ATPase. *Ann. NY Acad. Sci.* 402:146–63

143. Yoshimura, F., Brodie, A. F. 1981. Interaction of vanadate with membrane-bound ATPase from mycobacterium phlei. *J. Biol. Chem.* 256:12239–42

144. Gibbons, I. R. 1982. Dynein ATPases. *Prog. Clin. Biol. Res.* 80:87–93

145. Johnson, K. A., Porter, M. E. 1982. Transient state kinetic analysis of the dynein ATPase. *Prog. Clin. Biol. Res.* 80:101–06

146. Gibbons, I. R., Cosson, M. P., Evans, J. A., Gibbons, B. H., Houck, B., et al. 1978. Potent inhibition of dynein adenosinetriphosphatase and of the motility of

cilia and sperm flagella by vanadate. *Proc. Natl. Acad. Sci. USA* 75:2220–24

147. Kobayashi, T., Martensen, T., Nath, J., Flavin, M. 1978. Inhibition of dynein ATPase by vanadate, and its possible use as a probe for the role of dynein in cytoplasmic motility. *Biochem. Biophys. Res. Commun.* 81:1313–18

148. Shimizu, T. 1981. Steady-state kinetic study of vanadate-induced inhibition of ciliary dynein adenosinetriphosphatase activity from Tetrahymena. *Biochemistry* 20:4347–54

149. Shimizu, T. 1982. Further investigations on the vanadate-induced inhibition kinetics of enzyme activity of ciliary dynein from tetrahymena. *Prog. Clin. Biol. Res.* 80:107–12

150. Anderson, S. A., Purich, D. L. 1982. A reinvestigation of dynein ATPase kinetics and the inhibitory action of vanadate. *J. Biol. Chem.* 257:6656–58

151. Goodenough, U. W., Heuser, J. E. 1982. Substructure of the outer dynein arm. *J. Cell Biol.* 95:798–815

152. Majumder, G. C. 1981. Enzymic characteristics of ecto-adenosine triphosphatase in rat epididymal intact spermatozoa. *Biochem. J.* 195:103–10

153. Penningroth, S. M. 1982. Dependence of flagellar relaxation on the hydrolysis of ATP. *Prog. Clin. Biol. Res.* 80:121–26

154. Penningroth, S. M., Cheung, A., Olehnik, K., Koslosky, R. 1982. Mechanochemical coupling in the relaxation of rigor-wave sea urchin sperm flagella. *J. Cell Biol.* 92:733–41

155. Rikmenspoel, R., Orris, S. E., Isles, C. A. 1981. Effects of vanadate, Mg^{2+} and electric current injection on the stiffness of impaled bull spermatozoa. *J. Cell. Sci.* 51:53–61

156. Satir, P., Wais-Steider, J., Lebduska, S., Nasr, A., Avolio, J. 1981. The mechanochemical cycle of the dynein arm. *Cell Motil.* 1:303–27

157. Warner, F. D., McIlvain, J. H. 1982. Binding stoichiometry of 21S dynein to A and B subfiber microtubules. *Cell Motil.* 2:429–43

158. Goodno, C. C. 1979. Inhibition of myosin ATPase by vanadate ion. *Proc. Natl. Acad. Sci. USA* 76:2620–24

159. Goodno, C. C., Taylor, E. W. 1982. Inhibition of actomyosin ATPase by vanadate. *Proc. Natl. Acad. Sci. USA* 79:21–25

160. Kawamura, T., Tawada, K. 1982. Dissociation of actomyosin by vanadate plus ADP, and decomposition of the myosin-ADP-vanadate complex by action. *J. Biochem.* 91:1293–98

161. Yamin, M. A., Tamm, S. L. 1982. ATP reactivation of the rotary axostyle in termite flagellates: Effects of dynein ATPase inhibitors. *J. Cell Biol.* 95:589–97

162. Cande, W. Z., Wolniak, S. M. 1978. Chromosome movement in lysed mitotic cells is inhibited by vanadate. *J. Cell. Biol.* 79:573–80

163. Stearns, M. E., Ochs, R. L. 1982. A functional in vitro model for studies of intracellular motility in digitonin-permeabilized erythrophores. *J. Cell Biol.* 94:727–39

164. Beckerle, M. C., Porter, K. R. 1982. Inhibitors of dynein activity block intracellular transport in erythrophores. *Nature* 295:701–03

165. Grupp, G., Grupp, I., Johnson, C. L., Wallick, E. T., Schwartz, A. 1979. Effects of vanadate on cardiac contraction and adenylate cyclase. *Biochem. Biophys. Res. Commun.* 88:440–47

166. Hackbarth, I., Schmitz, W., Scholz, H., Wetzel, E., Erdmann, E., et al. 1980. Stimulatory effect of vanadate on cyclic AMP levels in cat papillary muscle. *Biochem. Pharmacol.* 29:1429–32

167. Krawietz, W., Werdan, K., Erdmann, E. 1980. Stimulation of human cardiac adenylate cyclase by vanadate. *Basic Res. Cardiol.* 75:433–37

168. Pertseva, M. N., Kuznetsova, L. A., Mazina, T. I., Plesneva, S. A. 1982. Study of functional properties of the catecholamine-sensitive adenylate cyclase system in embryonic skeletal muscle. *Biokhimiia* 47:1678–86

169. Schmitz, W., Hackbarth, I., Scholz, H., Wetzel, E. 1980. Effects of vanadate on the c-AMP system of the heart. *Basic Res. Cardiol.* 75:438–43

170. Schwabe, U., Puchstein, C., Hannemann, H., Sochtig, E. 1980. Activation of adenylate cyclase by vanadate. *Nature* 277:143–45

171. Schmitz, W., Scholz, H., Erdmann, E., Krawietz, W., Werdan, K. 1982. Effect of vanadium in the +5, +4 and +3 oxidation states on cardiac force of contraction, adenylate cyclase and $(Na^+ + K^+)$-ATPase activity. *Biochem. Pharmacol.* 31:3853–60

172. Lichtstein, D., Mullikin-Kilpatrick, D., Blume, A. J. 1982. Modification of neuroblastoma X glioma hybrid NG108–15 adenylate cyclase by vanadium ions. *Biochem. Biophys. Res. Commun.* 105:1157–65

173. Johnson, R. A. 1982. Changes in pH sensitivity of adenylate cyclase specifi-

cally induced by fluoride and vanadate. *Arch. Biochem. Biophys.* 218:68–76

174. Krawietz, W., Downs, R. W. Jr., Spiegel, A. M., Aurbach, G. D. 1982. Vanadate stimulates adenylate cyclase via the guanine nucleotide regulatory protein by a mechanism differing from that of fluoride. *Biochem. Pharmacol.* 31:843–48

175. Fleming, W. W. 1980. The electrogenic Na$^+$, K$^+$-pump in smooth muscle: Physiologic and pharmacologic significance. *Ann. Rev. Pharmacol. Toxicol.* 20:129–49

176. Hamlyn, J. M., Ringel, R., Schaeffer, J., Levinson, P. D., Hamilton, B. P., et al. 1982. A circulating inhibitor of (Na$^+$ + K$^+$) ATPase associated with essential hypertension. *Nature* 300:650–52

177. Day, H., Middendorf, D., Lukert, B., Heinz, A., Grantham, J. 1980. The renal response to intravenous vanadate in rats. *J. Lab. Clin. Med.* 96:382–95

178. Hatfield, M., Churchill, P. 1981. Renal vascular and tubular effects of vanadate in the anesthetized rat. *J. Pharmacol. Exp. Ther.* 217:406–10

179. Steffen, R. P., Pamnani, M. B., Clough, D. L., Huot, S. J. Muldoon, S. M., et al. 1981. Effect of prolonged dietary administration of vanadate on blood pressure in the rat. *Hypertension* 3 (Suppl. 1):173–78

180. Borchard, U., Greeff, K., Hafner, D., Noack, E., Rojsathaporn, K. 1981. Effects of vanadate on heart and circulation. *J. Cardiovasc. Pharmacol.* 3:510–21

181. Inciarte, D. J., Steffen, R. P., Dobbins, D. E., Swindall, B. T., Johnston, J., et al. 1980. Cardiovascular effects of vanadate in the dog. *Am. J. Physiol.* 239:H47–56

182. Larsen, J. A., Thomsen, O. Ø. 1980. Vascular effects of vanadate. *Basic Res. Cardiol.* 75:428–32

183. Larsen, J. A., Thomsen, O. Ø. 1980. Vanadate-induced oliguria and vasoconstriction in the cat. *Acta Physiol. Scand.* 110:367–74

184. Hom, G. J., Chelly, J. E., Jandhyala, B. S. 1982. Evidence for centrally mediated effects of vanadate on the blood pressure and heart rate in anesthetized dogs. *Proc. Soc. Exp. Biol. Med.* 169:401–05

185. Hudgins, P. M., Bond, G. H. 1981. Alteration by vanadate of contractility in vascular and intestinal smooth muscle preparations. *Pharmacology* 23:156–64

186. Ozaki, H., Ueda, F., Urakawa, N. 1982. Inhibitory effects of vanadate on the con-

tractile responses in vascular smooth muscle. *Eur. J. Pharmacol.* 80:317–22

187. Ozaki, H., Urakawa, N. 1980. Effects of vanadate on mechanical responses and Na-K pump in vascular smooth muscle. *Eur. J. Pharmacol.* 68:339–47

188. Rapp, J. P. 1980. Aortic responses to vanadate: Independence from (Na,K)-ATPase and comparison of Dahl salt-sensitive and salt-resistant rats. *Hypertension* 3 (Suppl. 1):168–72

189. Kwan, C. Y. 1982. Mg^{2+}- or Ca^{2+}-activated ATPase activities of plasma membranes isolated from vascular smooth muscle. *Enzymes* 28:317–27

190. Török, T. L., Rubányi, G., Vizi, E. S., Magyar, K. 1982. Stimulation by vanadate of [^{3}H] noradrenaline release from rabbit pulmonary artery and its inhibition by noradrenaline. *Eur. J. Pharmacol.* 84:93–97

191. Ehlers, D. 1981. Isolation and characterization of phosphatases from vascular smooth muscle. *Acta Biol. Med. Ger.* 40:1087–93

192. Ueda, F., Kishimoto, T., Ozaki, H., Urakawa, N. 1982. Dual actions of vanadate on high K-induced contraction in guinea-pig taenia coli. *Jpn. J. Pharmacol.* 32:149–57

193. Garcia, A. G., Jurkiewicz, A., Jurkiewicz, N. H. 1981. Contractile effect of vanadate and other vanadium compounds on the rat vas deferens. *Eur. J. Pharmacol.* 70:17–23

194. Stemmer, P., Akera, T., Brody, T. M. 1983. Vanadate effects Mn^{2+}-sensitive but not ryanodine-sensitive, calcium pools in isolated rat and guinea pig heart muscle. *Fed. Proc.* 42:633 (Abstr.)

195. Werdan, K., Bauriedel, G., Fischer, B., Krawietz, W., Erdmann, E., et al. 1982. Stimulatory (insulin-mimetic) and inhibitory (ouabain-like) action of vanadate on potassium uptake and cellular sodium and potassium in heart cells in culture. *Biochim. Biophys. Acta* 597:79–93

196. Clausen, T., Andersen, T. L., Stürup-Johansen, M., Petkova, O. 1981. The relationship between the transport of glucose and cations across cell membranes in isolated tissues. XI. The effect of vanadate on ^{45}Ca-efflux and sugar transport in adipose tissue and skeletal muscle. *Biochim. Biophys. Acta* 646:261–67

197. Catalan, R. E., Martinez, A. M., Aragones, M. D., Godoy, J. E., Robles, A., et al. 1982. Effects of vanadate on heart protein kinase. *Biochem. Med.* 28:353–57

198. Herzig, J. W., Peterson, J. W., Solaro, R. J., Ruegg, J. C. 1981. Phosphate and

vanadate reduce the efficiency of the chemomechanical energy transformation in cardiac muscle. *Adv. Exp. Med. Biol.* 151:267–81

199. Lopez Novoa, J. M., Garcia, J. C., Cruz-Soto, M. A., Benabe, J. E., Martinez-Maldonado, M. 1982. Effect of sodium orthovanadate on renal renin secretion in vivo. *J. Pharmacol. Exp. Ther.* 222:447–51

200. Lopez-Novoa, J. M., Mayol, V., Martinez-Maldonado, M. 1982. Renal actions of orthovanadate in the dog. *Proc. Soc. Exp. Biol. Med.* 170:418–26

201. Kumar, A., Corder, C. N. 1980. Diuretic and vasoconstrictor effects of sodium orthovanadate on the isolated perfused rat kidney. *J. Pharmacol. Exp. Ther.* 213:85–90

202. Gonick, H. C. 1982. Pathophysiology of human proximal tubular transport defects. *Klin. Wochenschr.* 60:1201–11

203. Churchill, P. C., Churchill, M. C. 1980. Vanadate inhibits renin secretion from rat kidney slices. *J. Pharmacol. Exp. Ther.* 213:144–49

204. Westenfelder, C., Hamburger, R. K., Garcia, M. E. 1981. Effect of vanadate on renal tubular function in rats. *Am. J. Physiol.* 240:F522–29

205. Doucet, A., Katz, A. I. 1982. High-affinity Ca-Mg-ATPase along the rabbit nephron. *Am. J. Physiol.* 242:F346–52

206. Krupin, T., Becker, B., Podos, S. M. 1980. Topical vanadate lowers intraocular pressure in rabbits. *Invest. Ophthalmol. Vis. Sci.* 19:1360–63

207. Krupin, T., Podos, S. M., Becker, B. 1983. Ocular effects of vanadate. In *Glaucoma Update,* ed. G. K. Krieglstein, W. Leydhecker, 2:25–29. Berlin: Springer-Verlag

208. Candia, O. A., Podos, S. M. 1981. Inhibition of active transport of chloride and sodium by vanadate in the cornea. *Invest. Ophthalmol. Vis. Sci.* 20:733–37

209. Thacher, S. M. 1981. Transient phosphorylation by ATP of a 160,000 dalton protein in rod outer segment of Bufo Marinus. *Biochim. Biophys. Acta* 648:199–205

210. Marcus, D. C., Demott, J. E., Kobayashi, T., Ge, X.-X., Thalmann, R. 1981. Specificity of action of vanadate to the organ of Corti. *Hearing Res.* 5:231–43

211. Marcus, D. C., Ge, X.-X., Thalmann, R. 1982. Comparison of the non-adrenergic action of phentolamine with that of vanadate on cochlear function. *Hearing Res.* 7:233–46

212. Sweadner, K. J. 1979. Two molecular forms of (Na$^+$ + K$^+$)-stimulated ATPase in brain. Separation and difference in affinity for strophanthidin. *J. Biol. Chem.* 254:6060–7

213. Witkowska, D., Brzeziński, J. 1979. Alteration of brain noradrenaline, dopamine and 5-hydroxytryptamine during vanadium poisoning. *Pol. J. Pharmacol. Pharm.* 31:393–98

214. Danielsson, E., Unden, A., Bartfai, T. 1983. Ortho–vanadate induces loss of muscarinic cholinergic binding sites. *Biochem. Biophys. Res. Commun.* 110:567–72

215. Done, A. K. 1979. Of metals and chelation. *Emerg. Med.* 11:186–218

216. Naylor, G. J. 1983. Vanadium and affective disorders. *Biol. Psychiatr.* 18:103–12

217. Naylor, G. J., Smith, A. H. W. 1981. Vanadium: A possible aetiological factor in manic depressive illness. *Psychol. Med.* 11:249–56

218. Naylor, G. J., Smith, A. H. W. 1981. Defective genetic control of sodium-pump density in manic depressive psychosis. *Psychol. Med.* 11:257–63

219. Narsapur, S. L., Naylor, G. J. 1983. Methylene blue. A possible treatment for manic depressive psychosis. *J. Affect. Disorders* 5:155–61

220. Lees, R. E. M. 1980. Changes in lung function after exposure to vanadium compounds in fuel oil ash. *Br. J. Industr. Med.* 37:253–56

221. Musk, A. W., Tees, J. G. 1982. Asthma caused by occupational exposure to vanadium compounds. *Med. J. Austr.* 20:183–84

222. Medinsky, M. A., Cuddihv, R. G., Hill, J. O., McClellan, R. O. 1981. Toxicity of selenium compounds to alveolar macrophages. *Toxicol. Lett.* 8:289–93

223. Thomsem, O. Ø., Larsen, J. A. 1982. Comparison of vanadate and ouabain effects on liver hemodynamics and bile production in the perfused rat liver. *J. Pharmacol. Exp. Ther.* 221:197–205

224. Sabbioni, E., Marafante, E., Rada, J., Gregotti, C., Dinucci, A., et al. 1981. Biliary excretion of vanadium in rats. *Toxicol. Eur. Res.* 3:93–98

225. Beyhl, F. E. 1982. Action of ammonium *meta* vanadate on the activities of hepatic drug-metabolizing enzymes *in vitro*. *Biochem. Pharmacol.* 31:1458–61

226. Heide, M., Legrum, W., Netter, K. J., Fuhrmann, G. F. 1983. Vanadium inhibits oxidative drug demethylation in vivo in mice. *Toxicology* 26:63–71

227. Inouye, B., Morita, K., Ishida, T., Ogata, M. 1980. Cooperative effect of sulfite

and vanadium compounds on lipid perox-idation. *Toxicol. Appl. Pharmacol.* 53: 101–07

228. Krieger, N. S., Tashjian, A. H. Jr. 1983. Inhibition of stimulated bone resorption by vanadate. *Endocrinology* 113:324–28

229. Lichtstein, D., Mullikin-Kilpatrick, D., Blume, A. J. 1982. Hyperpolarization of neuroblastoma-glioma hybrid NG108–15 by vanadium ions. *Proc. Natl. Acad. Sci. USA* 79:4202–6

230. Macara, I. G., McLeod, K., Kustin, K. 1979. Isolation, properties and structural studies on a compound from Tunicate blood cells that may be involved in vana-dium accumulation. *Biochem. J.* 181: 457–65

231. Macara, I. G., McLeod, G. C., Kustin, K. 1979. Vanadium in tunicates: Oxy-gen-binding studies. *Comp. Biochem. Physiol. A* 62:821–26

232. Caughey, W. S. 1973. Iron porphyrins-hemes and hemins. In *Inorganic Bio-chemistry,* ed. G. L. Eichhorn, 2:797–831. Amsterdam: Elsevier. 1263 pp.

233. Sakurai, H., Goda, T., Shimomura, S. 1982. Vanadyl (IV) ion dependent en-hancement of oxygen binding to hemo-globin and myoglobin. *Biochem. Bio-phys. Res. Commun.* 107:1349–54

234. Köpf-Maier, P., Wagner, W., Hesse, B., Köpf, H. 1981. Tumor inhibition by metallocenes: Activity against leukemias and detection of the systemic effect. *Eur. J. Cancer* 17:665–69

235. Nieder, G. L., Corder, C. N., Culp, P. A. 1979. The effect of vanadate on hu-man kidney potassium dependent phos-phatase. *Naunyn-Schmiedebergs Arch. Pharmacol.* 307:191–97

236. Nechay, P. S. E., Nanninga, L. B., Nechay, B. R. 1984. Binding of vanadyl to intracellular ligands. *Fed. Proc.* (Abstr.). In press

Ann. Rev. Pharmacol. Toxicol. 1984. 24:525–33

REVIEW OF REVIEWS

E. Leong Way

Department of Pharmacology, University of California,
San Francisco, California 94143

NEW JOURNALS AND INFORMATION RETRIEVAL

There seems to be no end to the announcements of new journals, particularly volumes related to drugs. These additions place an increasing burden on libraries already hampered in recent years by severe budgetary restrictions. Publishers, confident of a captive audience, have not hesitated to support the spawning of new journals. This proliferation, plus current administrative economic policies, have forced libraries to be more selective in their purchases. The library of my own institution, the University of California at San Francisco, has one of the largest holdings in health sciences periodicals in the country, subscribing to nearly 4000 journals. Although numerous new journals on drugs have existed for at least two years, if not longer, many are not on our subscription list; fifteen years ago, acquisition of a new primary source journal was nearly automatic. Small wonder that the libraries at private institutions, with limited budgets, are beset with major problems in maintaining a viable collection.

Some relatively new pharmacologic journals include: *Pharmacotherapy, Pharmacological and Biochemical Properties of Drug Substances, Research Communications in Substance Abuse, Developmental Pharmacology and Therapeutics*, the *International Journal of Clinical and Pharmacological Research, Acta Pharmacologica Sinica*, the *International Journal of Crude Drug Research, Clinical Neuropharmacology*, the *Journal of Medical Therapeutics, Drug Development Research*, the *Journal of Clinical Psychopharmacology, Theory in Psychopharmacology, Pediatric Pharmacology, Methods and Findings in Experimental and Clinical Pharmacy*, the *Annual Drug Data Report, Investigational New Drugs*, the *Journal of Anticancer Agents, Drug Development Research, Reviews in Pure and Applied Pharmacological Sciences, Biopharmaceutics and Drug Disposition, Drug Nutrient Interactions, Drugs of*

525

0362-1642/84/415-0525$02.00

the Future, Clinical Pharmacy of Clinical Therapeutics, Immunopharmacology, the *International Journal of Immunopharmacology,* the *Journal of Immunopharmacology,* the *Journal of Autonomic Pharmacology,* the *Journal of Cardiovascular Pharmacology,* and the *Journal of Clinical Psychopharmacology and Therapeutic Drug Monitoring.* Some recent journals in the area of toxicology include the *Journal of Applied Toxicology, Fundamental and Applied Toxicology, Veterinary and Human Toxicology, Drug and Chemical Toxicology, Aquatic Toxicology, Human Toxicology,* the *Journal of the American College of Toxicology, Neurotoxicology, Drug Chemical Toxicology,* and *Regulatory Toxicology and Pharmacology.*

As information is generated more and more rapidly, the burden of keeping up with the literature becomes greater each year. This has led to increased efforts to develop new services that not only can publish information faster but also will provide easier access to information already published. Terrant describes the electronic technology that has had a striking impact on reducing the cost of publishing (1). This technology includes hardware (especially computers), software, storage devices, word processors, communications media, micrographics, audio and video devices, and input/output devices. He predicts that in the future data-oriented information will proliferate and that this information will be submitted by authors in computer-readable form. Increased technology will lead to improvements in data processing and wider application of the data-base approach. Dissemination of information will be enhanced by more customized packaging and by increased computer-based publishing of materials that can be delivered on-line or on computer-readable media.

ALLELOPATHIC AGENTS

Putnam has authored a fascinating account of allelopathic chemicals (2). The term alludes to agents used for chemical warfare between plants whereby one plant releases chemicals that have an adverse effect on neighboring plants. For example, sorghum is grown to produce allelopathic chemicals that control the growth of certain types of weeds. In addition, the succession of various plant species in old fields and in cut-over forests has long intrigued ecologists; the appearance and disappearance of species and the changes in dominance by species has been shown to be related in part to allelopathy. A wide variety of allelopathic compounds exist; Putnam mentions thirteen types with varying herbicidal effects. These natural products can be useful for either suppressing weeds or imparting weed resistance and can thereby affect crop growth and nitrogen fixation. Not only do allelopathogens have important argicultural applications, but I believe these highly potent substances might find utility as pharmacologic tools and therapeutics agents.

ANTIBIOTICS

Combined antibiotic therapy in the treatment of certain serious bacterial and polymicrobic infections is a well-accepted treatment modality. Establishing the proper combination to use and the condition to treat is difficult, however. Isenberg and associates (3) review the problems in correlating in vitro with clinical studies to demonstrate synergetic effects between combinations of antibiotics and present the results of a comprehensive cooperative study attempting to resolve some of these problems. They conclude that the efficacy of a single antibiotic for a specific infection cannot be used to predict its behavior in combination. A combination may be effective not only against organisms usually susceptible but also against some resistant bacterial species that are resistant to the individual components of the combination.

RATIONAL BASIS FOR ANTIHYPERTENSIVES

Beyer & Peuler (4) provide a perspective on the current understanding of the factors that relate to hypertension in people and laboratory animals. The interactions of several physiologic systems relating to the modulation of blood pressure and to the prevention and treatment of essential hypertension are emphasized. Dietary control of weight and salt intake are vitally important with or without drugs. When arterial pressure cannot be controlled by weight and salt regulation, combined therapy modulating vasoconstriction and volume reduction should be instituted.

In a concise review, Freis (5) gives a critical, balanced analysis of the pros and cons for treating mild hypertension. There is a growing body of opinion that all patients with hypertension—no matter how mild or uncomplicated—should be treated. Freis provides some staggering statistics on the results of putting this policy into practice. He estimates that at least 40 million people have a diastolic pressure between 90–99 mm Hg and most are asymptomatic. He anticipates poor drug compliance from such persons; those who do comply are subject to the risks of drug toxicity. The addition of 40 million patients to lifelong treatment programs would cost about $20 billion a year based on a conservative estimate of $500 per patient per year for drugs, professional services, and laboratory tests. Consequently, Freis proposes a compromise approach. Since myocardial infarction is the most frequent complication in mild hypertension, only subjects having additional multiple risk factors (cigarette smoking, left ventricular hypertrophy, hypercholesteremia, and glucose intolerance) should have drug therapy. He recommends beginning the treatment with a diuretic alone but, should complications develop, the regimen can be intensified with additional drugs and adjunct measures.

OPIOPEPTINS

Endorphin is the generic term originally proposed for endogenous peptides having opioid-like activity, but the appellation has not gained universal acceptance and has often been associated with the peptide series related to β-endorphin. In view of the fact that three distinct families of opioid peptides with separate biochemical and neuronal pathways are now recognized, we propose using *opiopeptins* as a generic term to cover the three types classified as enkephalinergic, dynorphinergic, and endorphinergic.

A concise and informative review of the three opiopeptin types is provided by Höllt, who describes the current state of knowledge on their processing, distribution, and receptor selectivity (6). All native opioids isolated from mammals thus far belong to one of three families with distinct precursors. Pro-opiomelanocortin (POMC) is the common precursor for β-endorphin and ACTH; pro-enkephalin A is the common precursor for met-enkephalin and leu-enkephalin as well as for several larger residues having potent opioid-like activity and containing either leu-enkephalin or met-enkephalin as fragments; prodynorphin (or pro-enkephalin B) is the precursor of leu-enkephalin and a number of larger fragments containing leu-enkephalin, such as dynorphin A, dynorphin B, α-neo-endorphin, and β-neo-endorphin.

The peptides belonging to POMC are localized mainly in the pituitary gland, from where they are released into the circulation in response to hypothalamic activation. POMC-derived peptides are also localized in the arcuate nucleus of the hypothalamus. Axons of these cells project to the amygdala nuclei and the midbrain periaqueductal gray area. In contrast, peptides derived from pro-enkephalin A and B have a much more ubiquitous distribution in the central nervous system, and their sites correspond fairly well to opioid recognition or binding sites in the thalamus, hypothalamus, striatum, brainstem, and spinal cord. Although enkephalin A and enkephalin B appear to have pathways in close proximity and might even co-exist in some neurons, the hypothalamic-posterior pituitary pathways contain essentially pro-enkephalin B. A single precursor peptide can generate peptides with different receptor selectivities; furthermore, the selectivity changes as the processing continues. This suggests that the processing enzymes play a key role in determining the relative receptor specificity of the processed peptide.

Shah & Donald have edited a volume entitled *Endorphins and Opiate Antagonists in Psychiatric Research* (7). They attempt to gain wider appeal by adding *Clinical Implications* to the title. Progress in the latter area has been agonizingly slow, however, and in order to give substance to the book, the authors have had to cover basic considerations in detail. In contrast, the rate of progress in this facet of the subject has been so phenomenal that much of the information is dated. In a major oversight, no mention is made of the highly significant and potent peptide dynorphin, identified in 1979. However, my criticism about obsolescence is attenuated in part by the editors' attempt to place emphasis on the clinical aspects of the peptides. The shelf life of this volume will be short but it can be recommended. Its main value rests in its summary of the field to 1980, its comprehensive biobibliography, and its provocative, if not always solidly based, concepts.

Essays by some 93 authors are included. So many contributors usually require a heavy editorial hand to insure a standard of quality in the presentations. However, a perusal of this work makes it obvious that the editors have given the writers free rein because there is much redundancy and some inconsistency among the chapters.

Most of the clinical topics in the volume deal with either the use of narcotic antagonists for reducing a postulated hyperactive state in the endogenous opioid peptides or the application of β-endorphin for a putative hypofunctional state. The bulk of the clinical investigations concern the role of opioid peptides in the treatment of schizophrenia and depression. The results are paradoxical in the sense that both narcotic antagonists and β-endorphin have been reported to alleviate certain, albeit different, signs and symptoms of schizophrenia. It appears that either agent might be palliative in some aspects of the disorder, but the benefits are minimal and the effects probably do not influence the primary pathologic processes. A better case can be made for the use of β-endorphin in the panic states, since the locus ceruleus is concerned mainly with central noradrenergic activity and opiates have been established to have inhibitory effects at the site. A plausible case can be argued for hypoendorphinergism in chronic pain states, although the supporting data are rather thin. In sum, the data are suggestive but not definitive and more controlled studies are in order.

The basic contributions to the volume in general have more substance than the clinical studies and are informative. There is substantial data indicating that some opioid peptides can modulate the analgetic effect of opiates even though they may not be active per se. The evidence now points overwhelmingly to the fact that a family of opioid receptors exists with varying sensitivities to different agonists. Despite being peptides, a good body of evidence supports the fact that central sites can be affected and responses to most opiopeptins can be obtained after peripheral administration.

A hypothesis that might decrease the number of subsets of opioid receptors is contained in the model proposed by Lee and her associates for the β-endorphin receptor (8). Based on both pharmacologic and binding data, β-endorphin is suggested to combine at a locus having both a μ and an δ recognition site. The authors argue that since β-endorphin is as potent as morphine in the guinea-pig ileum and as potent as the enkephalins in the mouse vas deferens, and since β-endorphin displaces either type of ligand equally well and is in turn displaced to about the same degree by opiate alkaloids and the enkephalins, β-endorphin must combine simultaneously with at least two sites. Structure-activity relationship studies are cited to indicate that an intact β-endorphin molecule is required for expressing full biological as well as binding activity. Thus, shortening the β-endorphin chain by removing the middle peptide sequences reduces biologic activity and binding. Also, modifications of the five N-terminal amino acids with the methionine-enkephalin sequence reduces both binding to brain tissue and biological potency and, although less critical, sequential removal of C-terminal amino acids also results in a gradual decrease in binding and pharmacologic activity. As a consequence, Lee and her colleagues suggest that the site of β-endorphin resides at its N-terminus and at another site 14–24 carbons removed, the first site being the δ-site where the enkephalins bind and the second being the μ-site where alkaloidal agonists can interact. Although each of these two types of ligands can exhibit activity by binding to its respective receptor, β-endorphin must bind simultaneously at both sites. Thus, the β-endorphin receptor is viewed as a complex containing both μ- and δ-binding loci. Based on other evidence, the authors further propose that the enkephalin site may be associated with a protein and the morphine site with a lipid. This concept has the advantage of unifying a great deal of information hitherto explained in terms of multiple opiate receptors, but like all other operational postulates, good and bad, it needs to be verified by the isolation of the receptor.

ANALGETICS

Lednicer has edited a monograph, entitled *Central Analgetics;* it is the inaugural volume in the series *Chemistry and Pharmacology of Drugs* (9). Topics for subsequent volumes include diuretics, cardiovascular agents, and antineoplastic agents. The series is aimed toward research chemists, pharmacologists, and graduate students. In the Lednicer volume the coverage of the field is incomplete. Four areas related to opiate-like analgetics and opioid peptides are discussed; the treatment of these subject matters falls somewhere between that of a chapter in a comprehensive textbook and an in-depth review. In general, the chapters are readable and informative and the errors noted are generally remarks made in passing on details not related to the main thrust of the chapter.

The first chapter, authored by Mohrland and concerned with neuronal sites and pathways involved in analgetic action, is readable and fairly comprehensive. It emphasizes primarily the aspects of pain concerned with its perception. Such an approach can hardly be faulted, because the knowledge on this facet of the topic is the most extensive. However, the uninitiated might gain a distorted perspective of the field, since it is well recognized that opiates also act by altering reactivity to pain and, even though the information is sparse in this area, this component might well be more important for pain relief than altering the perception of noxious stimuli.

In the second chapter, Vonvoigtland extends the discussion of the possible sites where analgetics might act and implicates substance P as the excitatory substance in sensory neurons. He suggests that potentially useful analgetics might be developed by looking for agents that selectively inhibit substance P release or block its receptor. He also describes animal techniques for testing analgetic activity and recommends that binding assays be utilized for screening compounds. However, insofar as in vitro procedures for purposes of screening are concerned, none approaches the usefulness of the isolated guinea-pig ileum assay. Indeed, the latter preparation can be applied to prediction of the tolerance and physical dependence properties of opioid agonists as well as to differentiate the type of opioid receptor that may be involved in the effect.

The final two chapters by Lednicer include a discussion of the potential of centrally acting regulatory peptides as analgetics. He describes the structure-activity relationships of the enkephalins as analgetics, enkephalinase inhibitors, releasers, and precursors. He speculates on the design of antagonists based on hypothetical conformations of agonist receptors and on the manners in which the compounds may interact with the models. He gives undue credit to the usefulness of receptor binding assays for establishing multiple opioid receptors, whereas in fact the evidence in quantity and quality is derived from the intact animal and isolated organ preparations. The final chapter provides a historic and chemical perspective on the structure, synthesis, and development of analgetic agents.

DRUG DEPENDENCE

The February issue of *Drug and Alcohol Dependence* commemorates its tenth birthday (10). Instead of publishing original papers, the editor, Hans Halbach, invited leading researchers in the field from five continents to write about the major problems in chemical dependencies that have been solved or need resolving. Some twenty-five essays from investigators in both basic and clinical disciplines were the result; their topics range from receptors to behavior to epidemiology.

Craig & Baker have edited a volume dealing with the treatment of and research on drug-dependent patients (11). With the present administration's desire to emphasize medical and social problem-solving at the local level and the imposition of severe budgetary cutbacks on prevention and treatment programs for the drug-dependent patient, the appearance of the book is timely and should be especially welcomed by workers in the field. The contents range from fairly comprehensive critical reviews of certain facets of drug dependence to highly speculative essays. Treatment of heroin addicts is the main topic of interest; the alcoholic and other drug misusers are dealt with only cursorily.

Most of the pharmacologic information in this volume appears to be relevant and accurate and the psychosocial discussions are provocative and challenging. Dorus reviews opiate withdrawal techniques and their outcomes. His minimization of the abstinent state reflects unfamiliarity with handling the severely abstinent subject. While opiate abstinence is usually not life-threatening, the heavily dependent subject is a picture of abject misery after discontinuing the drug. Hyperthermia, hyperpnea, diarrhea, and vomiting are hardly innocuous and contribute to marked fluid loss that must be corrected. Fortunately, such cases are rarely seen in this country.

Lahmeyer's brief encapsulation of methadone maintenance is interesting and informative. Since its introduction by Dole & Nyswander in 1964, the importance of methadone for maintenance of the heroin recidivist has become widely recognized. Methadone gets the largest number of addicts off the street and into rehabilitative therapy more quickly, more successfully, and more cheaply than any other approach except perhaps the punitive methods used in totalitarian regimes. Non-drug intervention modalities, however successful they may be, are costly in man hours and in monies. Methadone alone, of course, cannot do the job of long-term treatment and adjunct measures can be crucial for achieving success. Such approaches, which may or may not include drugs, are covered in the chapters on residential treatment (Zarcone), behavioral treatment (Ross & Callner), group therapy (Craig), family therapy (Stanton), therapeutic communities (Bale), and defining goals (Lorei). These accounts overlap to a considerable degree and most include a description of trade techniques. Other treatment topics include a chapter on the management of addictions to psychoactive medication (Heilman, Hermos, & Bachrach) and urine analysis (Wang). The aim of most of these approaches is to promote total abstinence from drugs, but prolonging intervals between relapses is a more realistic goal.

The misuse of drugs is a characteristic peculiar to the human species and occurs in certain persons who find themselves unable to cope with stresses imposed by societal and economic pressures. Several contributors attempt to identify and define the personality variable of these individuals. Such assessments are likely to evoke controversies because they cannot be completely objective. Attitudes about drug taking vary with place and time and as a result the prevailing mores of a societal generation become a paramount factor in why and how many individuals take drugs. Much of the interpretation of these studies cannot be applied to global generalizations. Examples include the neuropsychologic assessments of drug use (Mider & Lewis) and the conclusions resulting from a comparison of the personalities of heroin and polydrug users (Penk & Robinowitz). The most tenuous presentation is the attempt to link the personality of the gambler with that of the drug taker (Custer).

Literature Cited

1. Terrant, S. W. 1983. Publishing scientific information: Today and tomorrow. *Chem. Eng. News* 61:51–58
2. Putnam, A. R. 1983. Allelopathic chemicals. *Chem. Eng. News* 61:34–45
3. Isenberg, H. D., Sampson-Scherer, J., Leeland, R., Titsworth, E., Beskid, G., et al. 1982. Correlation of the results of antibiotic synergy and susceptibility testing in vitro with results in experimental mouse infection. *Crit. Rev. Microbiol.* 10:1–76
4. Beyer, K. H., Peuler, J. D. 1982. Hypertension: Perspectives. *Pharmacol. Rev.* 34:287–314
5. Freis, E. D. 1982. Should mild hypertension be treated? *N. Engl. J. Med.* 307:306–9
6. Höllt, V. 1983. Multiple endogenous opioid peptides. *Trends Neurol. Sci.* 6:24–26
7. Shah, N. S., Donald, A. G., eds. 1982. *Endorphins and Opiate Antagonists in Psychiatric Research: Clinical Implications.* New York: Plenum. 488 pp.
8. Smith, A. P., Lee, N. M., Loh, H. H. 1983. The multiple site β-endorphin receptor. *Trends Pharmacol.* 4:163–64
9. Lednicer, D., ed. 1982. *Central Analgetics.* New York: Wiley. 219 pp.
10. Halbach, H., ed. 1983. Special issue heralding the second decade of this journal. *Drug Alcohol Depend.* 11(1):1
11. Craig, R. J., Baker, S. L., eds. 1982. *Drug Dependent Patients: Treatment and Research.* Springfield, Ill.: Thomas. 397 pp.

SUBJECT INDEX

535

CUMULATIVE INDEXES

CONTRIBUTING AUTHORS, VOLUMES 20–24

CHAPTER TITLES, VOLUMES 20–24